MW01295119

Surgeons as Educators

Tobias S. Köhler • Bradley Schwartz
Editors

Surgeons as Educators

A Guide for Academic Development and Teaching Excellence

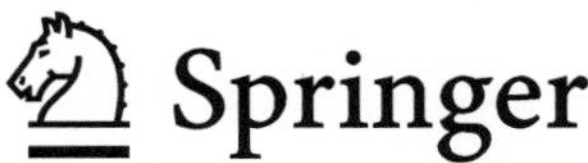

Springer

Editors
Tobias S. Köhler
Urology
Mayo Clinic
Rochester, MN
USA

Bradley Schwartz
Department of Surgery, Urology
Southern Illinois University School
of Medicine
Springfield, IL
USA

ISBN 978-3-319-64727-2 ISBN 978-3-319-64728-9 (eBook)
https://doi.org/10.1007/978-3-319-64728-9

Library of Congress Control Number: 2017959585

Printed on acid-free paper

This Springer imprint is published by Springer Nature
The registered company is Springer International Publishing AG
The registered company address is: Gewerbestrasse 11, 6330 Cham, Switzerland

"Upon the subject of education, not presuming to dictate any plan or system respecting it, I can only say that I view it as the most important subject which we as a people can be engaged in... For my part, I desire to see the time when education, and by its means, morality, sobriety, enterprise and industry, shall become much more general than at present, and should be gratified to have it in my power to contribute something to the advancement of any measure which might have a tendency to accelerate the happy period."

– Abraham Lincoln, March 9, 1832

Dr. Köhler would like to dedicate this book to his parents and to all of his former mentors and teachers that are too numerous to name. He would also like to thank all of the medical students, residents, and fellows with whom he had the opportunity to teach and indeed learn from in turn.

Dr. Schwartz would like to dedicate this book to his parents and his two sons for always emphasizing the value of both teaching and learning, thereby making him better at both. Also, to all of the students he has taught over the years, most notably his urology residents, for being given the opportunity to influence both physicians and patients for generations leaving an indelible carbon footprint.

Preface

"Let each become all that he or she is capable of being through education." – Anonymous

The average surgeon may operate on 5000–10000 patients if he or she is lucky enough to have a healthy and fruitful career. But a surgeon educator who teaches, trains, and mentors medical students, residents, and fellows easily influences an exponentially greater number of patients. Thus it is paramount that surgeons have the skills to teach the next generation of surgeons – not only on how to tie a knot, but also how to handle the unexpected, how to remain calm under pressure, how to be professional, and when and when not to operate.

Yet, many surgeons have had no formal training in how to teach. Further, current surgical educators are dealing with ever-increasing challenges to teach more in less time. A few of these challenges include the restriction on resident duty hours, educational core competencies, ever-changing science and technology, generational differences, electronic health records, patient safety, and pay for performance criteria.

This book is designed to help the reader (surgeons, program directors, or anyone involved in medical student, resident, or fellow education) understand the principles of contemporary surgical education and skills and is laid out into 3 main sections.

Section 1 "Foundations of Teaching" provides the reader with an introduction to teaching and lays a foundation for subsequent chapters on which the reader can build. From basic principles of how we learn to how we assess complex medical procedures, the reader gains insight on the basics of teaching. Section 2 "Program Optimization" describes how to assess and assure quality in both clinical practice and in teaching. Section 3 "Lessons and Insights of Surgical Education" details how to actually teach and provides examples of the art of teaching in the surgical field.

The ultimate goal of this book is to prepare the reader to excel in education and thus be able to positively influence patient care well beyond that of any one individual and hopefully perpetuate the teaching and learning culture in our field for generations.

Rochester, MN, USA — Tobias S. Köhler
Springfield, IL, USA — Bradley Schwartz

Contents

Contributors

Wesley Baas, MD Southern Illinois University, Carbondale, IL, USA

Jennifer Bartlett, ST J Roland Folse MD Surgical Skills Center at Southern Illinois University School of Medicine, Springfield, IL, USA

Sumeet Batra, MD, MPH Cook Children's Healthcare System, Fort Worth, TX, USA

Joseph Blessman, MSII Southern Illinois University School of Medicine, Springfield, IL, USA

Timothy C. Brand, MD, FACS Madigan Army Medical Center, Tacoma, WA, USA

Karen Broquet, MD, MHPE Southern Illinois University School of Medicine, Springfield, IL, USA

Jon A. Chilingerian, PhD Brandeis University, Heller School, Waltham, MA, USA

Public Health and Community Medicine at Tufts School of Medicine, Boston, MA, USA

Organizational Behavior and Health Care Management at INSEAD, Fontainebleau, France

Kristin L. Chrouser, MD, MPH Minneapolis VA Health Care Center, University of Minnesota, Department of Urology, Minneapolis, MN, USA

Anna T. Cianciolo, PhD Southern Illinois University School of Medicine, Department of Medical Education, Springfield, IL, USA

Jessica Dai University of Washington, Department of Urology, Seattle, WA, USA

Matthew Davis, MD Southern Illinois University, Carbondale, IL, USA

Karen M. Devon, MD, MSc, FRCSC Department of Surgery, Faculty of Medicine, University of Toronto, Toronto, ON, Canada

Joint Center for Bioethics, Dalla Lana School of Public Health, University of Toronto, Toronto, ON, Canada

Women's College Hospital, Toronto, ON, Canada

University Health Network, Toronto, ON, Canada

Laura M. Douglass Montefiore Medical Center, Bronx, NY, USA

Danuta I. Dynda, MD Division of Urology/Center for Clinical Research, Southern Illinois University School of Medicine, Springfield, IL, USA

James Feimster, MD General Surgery, Southern Illinois University School of Medicine, Springfield, IL, USA

Ethan L. Ferguson Department of Urology, Indiana University, Indianapolis, IN, USA

Sabha Ganai, MD, PhD, FACS Department of Surgery, Southern Illinois University School of Medicine, Springfield, IL, USA

Evalyn I. George, BS Henry M. Jackson Foundation/Madigan Army Medical Center, Tacoma, WA, USA

Nikhil K. Gupta, MD Rutgers-Robert Wood Johnson Medical School, Piscataway Township, NJ, USA

Susan Hallbeck, PhD, PE, CPE Department of Health Sciences Research, Division of Health Care Policy and Research, Mayo Clinic, Rochester, MN, USA

Robert D. and Patricia E. Kern Center for the Science of Health Care Delivery, Mayo Clinic, Rochester, MN, USA

Department of Surgery, Mayo Clinic, Rochester, MN, USA

Sevann Helo, MD Surgery, Division of Urology, Albany Medical College, Albany, NY, USA

Collin Hitt, PhD Department of Medical Education, Southern Illinois University School of Medicine, Springfield, IL, USA

Bradley Holland, MD Division of Urology/Center for Clinical Research, Southern Illinois University School of Medicine, Springfield, IL, USA

Tobias S. Köhler, MD, MPH, FACS Urology, Mayo Clinic, Rochester, MN, USA

Alison C. Keenan Department of Urology, University of Wisconsin-Madison, Madison, WI, USA

Janet Ketchum, CST J Roland Folse MD Surgical Skills Center at Southern Illinois University School of Medicine, Springfield, IL, USA

Jeanne L. Koehler, PhD Department of Medical Education, Southern Illinois University School of Medicine, Springfield, IL, USA

Joel F. Koenig, MD Children's Mercy Hospital, Kansas City, MO, USA

Thomas G. Leffler Department of Urology, University of Wisconsin-Madison, Madison, WI, USA

Bethany Lowndes, PhD, MPH Department of Health Sciences Research, Division of Health Care Policy and Research, Mayo Clinic, Rochester, MN, USA

Robert D. and Patricia E. Kern Center for the Science of Health Care Delivery, Mayo Clinic, Rochester, MN, USA

Carol F. McCammon, MD, MPH Department of Emergency Medicine, EVMS, Norfolk, VA, USA

Kurt McCammon, MD Department of Urology, EVMS, Norfolk, VA, USA

Elspeth M. McDougall, MD, FRCSC, MHPE University of British Columbia,Gordon & Leslie Diamond Health Care Centre, Vancouver, BC, Canada

Alexandria D. McDow, MD General Surgery, Southern Illinois University School of Medicine, Springfield, IL, USA

Patrick H. McKenna Department of Urology, University of Wisconsin-Madison, Madison, WI, USA

John D. Mellinger, MD Department of Surgery, Southern Illinois University School of Medicine, Springfield, IL, USA

Melanie Hammond Mobilio Wilson Centre, University Health Network, Toronto, ON, Canada

Carol-anne Moulton Wilson Centre, University Health Network, Toronto, ON, Canada

Department of Surgery, University of Toronto, Toronto, ON, Canada

Division of General Surgery, University Health Network, Toronto, ON, Canada

Toronto General Hospital, Toronto, ON, Canada

Amanda C. North Montefiore Medical Center, Bronx, NY, USA

Yasser A. Noureldin, MD, MSc, PhD WWAMI Institute for Simulation in Healthcare (WISH), University of Washington, Seattle, WA, USA

Urology Department, Benha University, Benha, Egypt

Jamie S. Padmore, DM, MSc Georgetown University School of Medicine and MedStar Health, Washington, DC, USA

Carla M. Pugh, MD, PhD, FACS Department of Surgery, University of Wisconsin School of Medicine and Public Health, Madison, WI, USA

David J. Rea, MD, FACS Division of General Surgery, Department of Surgery, Department of Surgery, Southern Illinois University School of Medicine, Springfield, IL, USA

Michael R. Romanelli, MA Southern Illinois University School of Medicine, J Roland Folse MD Surgical Skills Center, Springfield, IL, USA

Carrie Ronstrom, BS University of Minnesota Medical School, Minneapolis, MN, USA

Hilary Sanfey, MB, BCh, MHPE, FACS SIU School of Medicine, Department of Surgery, Springfield, IL, USA

Bradley Schwartz, DO, FACS Department of Urology at Southern Illinois University School of Medicine, Springfield, IL, USA

Bradley F. Schwartz, DO, FACS Department of Surgery, Urology, Southern Illinois University School of Medicine, Springfield, IL, USA

Anna Skinner, PhD Black Moon, LLC, Louisville, KY, USA

Matthew Smith, DO Division of General Surgery, Department of Surgery, Southern Illinois University School of Medicine, Springfield, IL, USA

Mathew Sorensen University of Washington, Department of Urology, Seattle, WA, USA

Emily Sturm, MD Department of Surgery, Southern Illinois University School of Medicine, Springfield, IL, USA

Chandru P. Sundaram, MD Department of Urology, Indiana University School of Medicine, Indianapolis, IN, USA

Robert M. Sweet, MD, FACS WWAMI Institute for Simulation in Healthcare (WISH), University of Washington, Seattle, WA, USA

UW Medicine, Department of Urology, University of Washington, Seattle, WA, USA

Charles Welliver, MD Surgery, Division of Urology, Community Care Physicians, The Urological Institute of Northeastern NY, Albany, NY, USA

Part I

Foundations of Teaching

"See One, Do One, Teach One?" A Story of How Surgeons Learn

1

Anna T. Cianciolo and Joseph Blessman

It is November. The skies have grown sullen and gray, and a bone-deep chill suffuses the air. A young surgical resident, seeking to impress his girlfriend, has decided to cook her a pot roast, a favored comfort food of his family for generations. As his roommate looks on, he carefully cuts a quarter inch off both ends of the roast and places it in the pan. "Why did you cut off the ends?" his roommate asks. The resident pauses, looks at the knife and strips of excess beef, and shrugs. "My mom always did it that way, and I learned from her."

The dinner date was a success, but his roommate's question nagged the resident's mind. The next time he spoke to his mother, he asked, "Mom, how do you cook a pot roast?" His mother proceeded to explain, adding, "You cut off both ends before placing it in the pan." "But why?" the resident asked. His mother replied, "That's how your grandmother did it, and I learned it from her." At Thanksgiving dinner a few weeks later, the resident, still curious and unable to find an answer online, asked his grandmother, "When you cook a pot roast, why do you cut both ends off the meat?" Before she could answer, the resident's grandfather piped up, "I never could get a pan big enough for your Nana's pot roasts, so she trimmed the meat to make them fit!"

Versions of this pot roast parable are shared to convey the importance of critical thinking to awareness, adaptability, innovation, and change. In surgical education, stepping back from the pursuit of simple, straightforward training prescriptions to ask "Why?" and grapple with "What's going on here?" leads to seeing learning in new, more insightful ways and opening up possibilities to take trainee development

A.T. Cianciolo, PhD (✉)
Southern Illinois University School of Medicine, Department of Medical Education, 913 N Rutledge St., PO Box 19681, Springfield, IL, USA, 62794-9681
e-mail: acianciolo@siumed.edu

J. Blessman, MSII
Southern Illinois University School of Medicine, Springfield, IL, USA

T.S. Köhler, B. Schwartz (eds.), *Surgeons as Educators*,
https://doi.org/10.1007/978-3-319-64728-9_1

to the next level [52]. One could ask, for example, why is "see one, do one, teach one" held up as a time-honored approach to training technical skill? Are today's training objectives and conditions the same as in 1890, when William Halsted founded the surgical residency on this model [36]? Considering the dizzying array of technology in the modern operating theater, is observing a procedure once enough for a trainee to go on and successfully perform the procedure and then teach it to others? If the answer to this question is no [54], how many repetitions are needed and how can they be provided in light of patient safety concerns and restricted duty hours? What kind of repetitions "count" as practice? The Accreditation Council for Graduate Medical Education's recently established Next Accreditation System [47] also has raised this question: How do we know if practice is actually making surgeons competent?

Theorists in medical education make it their business to ask questions. They explore learning in all its complexity so as to enable a thoughtful, purposeful approach to developing others [26, 42]—an approach in which understanding and practical solutions evolve as people share evidence and insight from grappling with educational problems in their local setting [52]. At the program level, learning theory may be used to inform decision making on training standards and policy, as well as the adoption of educational infrastructure and technology [34]. At the individual or team level, understanding how people learn may help surgical educators adapt instructional and assessment strategies to best suit the needs of their trainees, their patients, and their service. Learning theory has been used, for example, to explore how the old "see one, do one, teach one" adage may be updated to improve learning outcomes in the modern surgical training context [36].

Documenting all the questions that theorists have asked about learning, and the answers they have produced, far exceeds the scope of this chapter. Instead, this chapter tells a single story of how surgical trainees develop by weaving multiple theories together. It is a story that emerges out of stepping back from the immediate, practical tasks at hand, carefully examining all that is going on, and packaging that complex reality into a narrative about learning that can be readily understood and shared with others. It is a tale of how environmental conditions, supervisory methods, and trainee characteristics cooperate to produce surgical expertise. The purpose of telling this story is to present surgical educators inclined to ask questions with answers they can use to enrich their thinking and to approach educational improvement with an attitude of experimentation and innovation. Ideally, this story also will inspire educators to contribute to theory as an important way of developing the next generation of surgeons [8]. Much of this story likely will seem familiar, perhaps even obvious, like traveling down a neatly paved road, but hopefully it also is a bit unsettling, like the urge to follow that road around the bend to a destination not yet envisioned.

The Surgical Learning Context

Our story opens in the teaching hospital, a demanding place by any measure. Here, trainees commonly encounter an "unfiltered immersion experience" ([25], p. 105), where they are simultaneously learners and functional members of the surgical team. Learning occurs on the job, in full context, within a group of providers that is hierarchical, interprofessional, and frequently changing [9]. Focused technical skill development must fit within a mandated 80-h workweek along with clinical paperwork, quality improvement projects, scientific research, and teaching junior peers, which requires maximum efficiency in the face of numerous distractions and unexpected events [9, 25]. Technologies used to perform procedures are constantly evolving, changing the organization of surgical work and requiring the development of new skill [9, 49]. To accelerate skill acquisition, training supplements immersive learning with skills laboratories, simulation exercises, and didactics such as grand rounds and journal clubs [25]. Workload is high at all levels of the hierarchy; this is a setting where learning to work fatigued during training is believed necessary to meet the demands of future independent practice [16].

With learners on the care team, educators must balance the obligation to provide a high volume of safe, quality care with the mission to develop trainees at all levels, from medical student to fellow [32, 51]. Trainees' performance is assessed regularly [29] using methods that range from written tests to direct observation of real or simulated performance and assessors that range from supervisors and peers to non-physician providers, medical students, and patients [58]. Surgical educators are held accountable for high-risk, high-stakes outcomes, which depend not only on their technical skill but also successful team coordination and careful regulation of trainees' graded responsibility in patient care. The operating theater provides opportunities for educators and trainees to work closely together on technical skill in practice [6, 63], but even here the decision to entrust trainees with independent activities that will enhance their learning depends on many factors that differ with each procedure, trainee, and educator [8, 30, 32, 51].

In sum, the surgical learning context offers opportunities for and places constraints on trainee development that differ vastly from the classroom [8, 20, 40]. To support educational decision making, theory must be able to explain how performance improvement happens *here* [42]. General theories applicable to surgical education explore what expertise looks like and the kind of practice it requires [5, 19, 24]. They examine how social dynamics influence what is learned, how, when, and from whom [3, 12, 38, 59], how workplace characteristics shape learning processes [7, 21], how experience can be structured to promote optimal learning outcomes [11, 35], and how learners play an active role in their own development [13, 57, 64]. Theory specific to surgical learning illustrates how this more general understanding may be extended by asking questions about its fit to the surgical learning context.

The Quest for Surgical Expertise

The plot of our story centers on our protagonist, the trainee, who is challenged with a quest: to become a surgical expert. To accomplish this mission, the trainee must go beyond graduating from a series of training programs, beyond having spent years in scrubs and operating rooms, and beyond being told by his peers that his experience makes him an expert [22, 44]. Rather, his quest for expertise is accomplished when he consistently exhibits superior performance, as reflected indirectly by successful patient outcomes or, more directly, by the effective completion of directly observed surgical tasks in real or simulated settings [23].

In a complex world ruled by uncertainty, however, consistency is difficult to achieve; patients' anatomy differs, care teams turn over, technology changes, and procedures can dramatically and unexpectedly intensify in the blink of an eye. Expert surgeons distinguish themselves by confronting this uncertainty—proactively ordering and prioritizing tasks to mitigate risk and managing distractions, thereby creating the conditions for staying calm under pressure [37]. Like King Arthur brandishing the sword he drew from stone, surgical experts challenge uncertainty with a firm grasp on their capabilities and limitations, slowing down and intensifying their focus in response to prevailing conditions and knowing when to seek help, if necessary [44–46]. Their expert judgment comprises a cycle of information seeking, critical evaluation, and course correction, as needed, making them responsive to the inconsistency inherent in surgery and able to maintain superior performance and positive outcomes [17, 46]).

Surgical expertise, then, comprises not only a demonstrated level of performance but a way of thinking—a way of approaching a complex, high-stakes endeavor whose defining characteristic is uncertainty so as to continue growing and achieve positive results consistently. Beyond this, formal competency standards for surgical trainees cover a range of capability much broader than technical knowledge and skill [1], to include interpersonal skill and professional attitudes, values, and behaviors. These standards, reflecting evolving notions of medical competency [17, 31, 42, 56], reveal that surgical expertise is now viewed as much as a social achievement as it is a technical one (e.g., [9, 15, 32, 53]). That is, expert surgeons are recognized not only by what they can do and how they do it but also the kind of practitioner they are and how they fit within their professional community.

The Journey Inward

No quest can be completed without a journey, the series of trials the protagonist must endure to achieve his aims. The quest for surgical expertise is no different, requiring approximately 10 years of "intense involvement" in surgical skill acquisition, including thousands of operations ([22], p. 114). Intense involvement comprises long-term engagement in deliberate practice—continuous, motivated engagement in clearly defined tasks with performance feedback and opportunities to repeat, refine, and improve [24]. However, although the notion of "practice makes perfect" would seem to apply naturally to surgical learning, this is not the whole story. The protagonist's journey is never solitary; his path is shaped by his interactions with the story's other characters.

In the surgical learning context, interactions with other members of the care team are essential to determining trainees' access to practice opportunities, the degree of challenge they experience, and the support and feedback they receive [20, 25]. All of these things influence trainees' participation in work and the learning they derive from it [8, 21]. In addition, trainees' observations of their role models provide

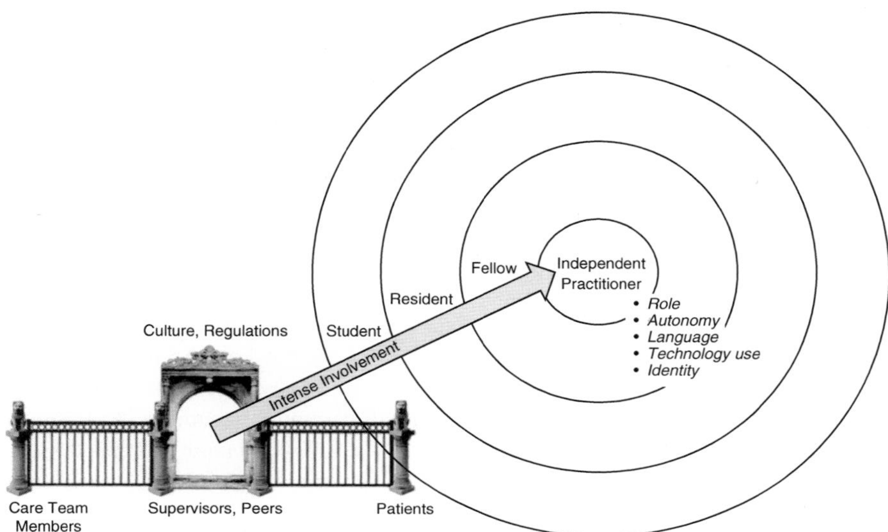

Fig. 1.1 Moving inward within a community of clinical practice

valuable information about surgical culture—the values, beliefs, and behaviors that must be adopted to become a recognized member of the professional community [8, 32, 40]. Importantly, technology also plays a role in how surgeons see their patients, their work, and their own capabilities; trainees must learn how to manipulate these tools and, in turn, are manipulated by them [9, 55]. Essential learning that does not resemble deliberate practice therefore emerges from social interactions [8, 32] and is shaped by the learning environment [9, 61]. Beyond being an approach to practicing technical skills, then, intense involvement reflects deepening learner participation in the personal, social, and technological context of surgical work.

Consider Fig. 1.1, which depicts the surgical learning context as a "community of clinical practice" in which a trainee's progress toward expertise is reflected in movement from the periphery of the community toward its center [15, 20, 32]. Shown at the center of the community is the independent practitioner, a person identifiable by her role, that is, the community's expectations for her knowledge, attitudes, values, and behavior as professional surgeon, her autonomy to manage uncertainty by exercising judgment and making decisions to mitigate risk, the language she uses to communicate with members of the community—which is distinct from the language she uses outside the community—her use of specialized tools and technology to perform her work, and her self-identification as a full community member.

Our independent practitioner arrived at the center of her community after starting out on the periphery as a medical student and gradually deepening her participation over the course of her training [32]. Throughout this process, characteristics of the surgical learning context served as a gateway to her progress. Professional culture and formal regulations dictated her level and type of direct involvement in surgical work. For example, her procedural practice with real patients as a medical student was limited to observing passively, gaining a feel for anatomy and pathology, holding retractors, and occasional suturing, with more intensive hands-on practice of procedures occurring in the skills lab [10, 40]. As she moved inward in the community, constraints on her practice with real patients lifted, with trips to the skills lab becoming less frequent and involvement in simulations increasing as the scope of her responsibility broadened to teams and more advanced technologies. Supervisors, care team members, peers, and patients offered formal and informal learning opportunities and feedback along the way, enhancing her ability to meet meaningful work challenges and increasing her confidence, motivation, and commitment to participation [21]. Importantly, she influenced these gatekeepers by proactively seeking learning opportunities, demonstrating her motivation and capability to improve, and gradually assuming of the mantle of community member [32, 41, 61].

The reader should be cautioned that in today's rapidly changing surgical workplace, a single-journey story is a convenient oversimplification [26]; sequels and spin-offs are needed to accurately characterize how surgeons progress to the center of multiple parallel communities of clinical practice, crossing the boundaries between them in order to maintain a coherent but flexible sense of themselves as a professional [9]. To take the science-fiction feel a step further, one could also consider how learning to use surgical technology grants trainees special access to the inner circle by enabling them to participate in the community's definitive work [55], much as gaining control of the "force" is necessary to being a member of the Jedi Order in the fictional *Star Wars* series. Using a more grounded example, it is interesting to contemplate how laparoscopic instruments and minimally invasive techniques mediate perceptions of the body—once directly seen and felt, anatomy is visualized through 2- and 3D displays—such that the surgeon controls what the rest of the team sees [49]. This unique perceptual capability signals her status as surgeon, further distinguishing her from other team members and the less experienced trainees who look on.

The Moral of Our Story: Implications for Surgical Education

At this point in our story, the practically minded reader is likely asking the question of greatest interest to busy educators: How is all this going to help me improve education *now*? [48] A key lesson we can take away from thoughtfully considering the surgical learning context, the quest for surgical expertise, and the journey into communities of clinical practice is that theory calls us to rethink what surgical learning *is*. Rather than taking it to be the acquisition of technical knowledge and skills by a lone physician in isolation, we can think of learning instead as participation in the surgical profession in all of its technical, personal, and social respects [38, 42, 59]. Another key lesson is that learning and practice happen simultaneously in the teaching hospital and, in so doing, require the workplace to be structured and organized

- All trainees have a functional and valued role on the surgical team, from Day 1, with meaningful work and an appropriate level of challenge.
- Educators serve as coaches, mentors, and role models, guiding trainees' deepened participation in surgical work.
- Roles and expectations for trainees are made clear from the outset and revisited periodically as conditions change.
- Educators and trainees continuously work collaboratively to set and monitor progress toward learning objectives.
- Trainees signal readiness to deepen participation through making themselves useful and internalizing the values, attitudes, and behaviors of the profession.
- Trainees learn in teams with attendings, peers, and other healthcare providers to promote implicit learning and enculturation.
- On-the-job training is supplemented with external learning opportunities designed to improve consequential work performance via lower-stakes practice.
- On-the-job and supplemental education are interleaved to maximize training efficiency and promote deepened participation in surgical work.
- Supplemental skills training employs a deliberate practice approach.
- Specific approaches to training are continuously examined to ensure that they are working as expected and adapted as needed.
- The workplace community of clinical practice espouses the same standards and ideals against which trainees are evaluated.
- Experiences with training are shared among educators within and across institutions to promote continuous educational quality improvement and learning about how surgeons learn.

Fig. 1.2 Educational implications of how surgeons learn

in a way that supports both endeavors [8, 21, 33]. Viewing trainee development in this way has clear implications for surgical education, as itemized in Fig. 1.2.

First, even the most junior learners, medical students on their surgical clerkship, should be viewed as having a legitimate role in the workplace [8, 21, 42]. Legitimacy occurs when community members—educators, peers, and other healthcare providers—recognize and facilitate all trainees' capacity to demonstrate "total dedication" to patients, learning, and the profession [62]. Specifically, trainees should be included in meaningful clinical work that is appropriately challenging and that involves interaction with—and implicit learning from—the whole of the clinical team and patients [8, 18, 21]. In addition, allocation of work and dedicated learning opportunities outside of the clinical context, such as skills lab and simulation exercises, should be sequenced and prioritized with learners' deeper participation in the workplace as the ultimate goal [25]. Lower-risk activities should precede more consequential ones to promote both safety and learning [8, 21]. To accelerate skill development, a deliberate practice approach—featuring performance goals, direct observation, feedback, and opportunities to improve—should be employed [10, 23].

In all these things—allocating work, structuring learning, fostering deliberate practice, and role modeling—surgical educators must act as a coach and mentor, ensuring trainee confidence and a smooth progression from the periphery inward [17, 21, 25]. Importantly, trainees also have an essential role that of figuring out how to “fit in” by seeking learning opportunities, improving their technical skill, making themselves useful, observing others, and internalizing the values, attitudes, and behaviors of the profession [8, 32, 40]. Educators may enhance trainees’ ability to self-develop by orienting them to their role and community expectations, fostering a positive learning climate, collaboratively setting clear learning objectives, and conducting goal-driven observation and feedback [21, 40].

Several chapters in this volume provide detailed guidance for designing, implementing, and evaluating educational approaches consistent with the general implications described above. However, an important but easily overlooked moral of our story is this: one cannot assume that specific prescriptions for surgical education will achieve the same performance outcomes across settings or even across time within the same setting [52]. The surgical learning context is always changing, and the implementation of workplace curricula in practice often is influenced by factors that educational designers did not anticipate or cannot control [8, 48]. For example, a training program’s assessment culture can shape trainees’ approach to learning in ways that do not conform to expectations or produce improved clinical performance [2, 43]. Moreover, the direct observation and feedback central to meaningful performance assessment and deliberate practice are practically nonexistent in the clinical workplace [14, 27, 50, 60], and major reforms in medical education cannot take place until they are [28]. Trainees, however, do observe closely [8, 32], and they may accept as normal the interpersonal conflict and professional silos they witness, despite official statements labeling such values, attitudes, and behaviors undesirable [39].

Epilogue

To conclude, the story of how surgical trainees develop does not have an ending; there will always be questions to ask and new understanding and implications that emerge from applying the answers to education. Consistently achieving desired performance outcomes requires periodically reconsidering what we are trying to accomplish and making refinements both to our interventions and to the setting in which they are situated [26, 52]. It is essential that people intrigued by surgical learning continue to ask “Why?” and “What’s going on here?” so as to continually deepen understanding about surgeons’ development and support efforts to design education that works. The reader may find it interesting to learn that surgical education has become a field of study in its own right, with its own specialized degree programs [34], which indicates the depth and breadth of knowledge about surgical learning that has been developed to date.

Ultimately, knowledge about surgical learning is given meaning by its impact on surgical performance [48], an endeavor greatly facilitated by educators themselves using theory to try something new, taking a close look at what happens, and sharing detailed stories about what they see [17]. Participatory action research is a mode of theory development that features educators at the very center of inquiry, using a cycle of data collection, reflection, and action to build knowledge about how people learn in a given setting [4]. Practically speaking, this knowledge helps educators understand whether or how to adapt an educational approach so that it is successful in a given time and place. Participatory action research demonstrates that theory development and practice improvement are tightly interwoven community activities in which educators have an important part.

At this point, learning about surgical learning through participation within a community should sound very familiar. Like expert surgeons constantly honing their skills, educators continually seeking to improve trainee development are, by the very nature of their pursuits, committed to working at the edge of uncertainty, a place where time is slowed [52] and the invisible—the state of affairs we take for granted—becomes visible and open to inspection [17, 34]. Pausing in the midst of ongoing activity to ask "Why?" and "What's going on here?" empowers the educator to adapt to changing circumstances, ask for help when needed, and consistently achieve success. Understanding and improving how surgeons learn is, one might say, as far away as a close look.

References

1. Accreditation Council for Graduate Medical Education & American Board of Surgery. The general surgery milestone project. Chicago: ACGME; 2015. Available at: http://www.acgme.org/portals/0/pdfs/milestones/surgerymilestones.pdf.
2. Al-Kadri HM, Al-Kadi MT, van der Vleuten CPM. Workplace-based assessment and students approaches to learning: a qualitative inquiry. Med Teach. 2013;35:S31–8.
3. Bandura A. Social learning theory. Englewood Cliffs: Prentice Hall; 1977.
4. Baum F, MacDougall C, Smith D. Participatory action research. J Epidemiol Community Health. 2006;60(10):854–7.
5. Bereiter C, Scardamalia M. Surpassing ourselves: an inquiry into the nature and implications of expertise. Chicago: La Salle: Open Court; 1993.
6. Bezemer J, Cope A, Kress G, Kneebone R. Holding the scalpel: achieving surgical care in a learning environment. J Contemp Ethnogr. 2014;43(1):38–63.
7. Billett S. Constituting the workplace curriculum. J Curric Stud. 2006;38(1):31–48.
8. Billett S. Learning through health care work: premises, contributions and practices. Med Educ. 2016;50:124–31.
9. Bleakley A. Learning and identity in the professional world of the surgeon. In: Fry H, Kneebone R, editors. Surgical education: theorising an emerging domain. New York: Springer; 2011. p. 183–97.
10. Boehler ML, Schwind CJ, Rogers DA, Ketchum J, et al. A theory-based curriculum for enhancing surgical skillfulness. J Am Coll Surg. 2007;205:492–7.
11. Boud D, Keogh R, Walker D. Reflection: turning experience into learning. London: Kogan Page; 1985.
12. Brown JS, Collins A, Duguid P. Cognition and the culture of learning. Educ Res. 1989;18(1): 32–42.
13. Butler DL, Winne PH. Feedback and self-regulated learning: a theoretical synthesis. Rev Educ Res. 1995;65(3):245–81.
14. Chisholm CD, Whenmouth LF, Daly EA, Cordell WH, Giles BK, Brizendine EJ. An evaluation of emergency medicine resident interaction time with faculty in different teaching venues. Acad Emerg Med. 2004;11(2):149–55.
15. Cope, A, Bezemer, J, Mavroveli, S, & Kneebone, R (2017). What attitudes and values are incorporated into self as part of professional identity construction when becoming a surgeon?. Academic Medicine, ePub ahead of print.

16. Coverdill JE, Bittner JG IV, Park MA, Pipkin WL, Mellinger JD. Fatigue as impairment or educational necessity? Insights into surgical culture. Acad Med. 2011;86(Suppl 10):S69–72.
17. Cristancho SM, Apramian T, Vanstone M, Lingard L, Ott M, Forbes T, Novick R. Thinking like an expert: surgical decision making as a cyclical process of being aware. The American Journal of Surgery. 2016;211(1):64–69.
18. de Cossart L, Fish D. Cultivating a thinking surgeon: new perspectives on clinical teaching, learning and assessment. Shrewsbury: TFM; 2005.
19. Dornan T, Scherpbier AJJA, Boshuizen HPA. Supporting medical students workplace learning: experience-based learning (ExBL). Clin Teach. 2009;6(3):167–71.
20. Dreyfus HL, Dreyfus SE. A five-stage model of the mental activities involved in directed skill acquisition (res. Rep. No. ORC-80-2). Washington, DC: Air Force Office of Scientific Research; 1980.
21. Egan T, Jaye C. Communities of clinical practice: the social organization of clinical learning health: an interdisciplinary. J Soc Study Health, Illn Med. 2009;13(1):107–25.
22. Eraut M. Learning from other people in the workplace. Oxf Rev Educ. 2007;33(4):403–22.
23. Ericsson KA. The surgeon's expertise. In: Fry H, Kneebone R, editors. Surgical education: theorising an emerging domain. New York: Springer; 2011. p. 107–21.
24. Ericsson KA. Acquisition and maintenance of medical expertise: a perspective from the expert-performance approach with deliberate practice. Acad Med. 2015;90:1471–86.
25. Ericsson KA, Krampe RT, Tesch-Römer C. The role of deliberate practice in the acquisition of expert performance. Psychol Rev. 1993;100(3):363–406.
26. Gofton W, Regehr G. Factors in optimizing the learning environment for surgical training. Clin Orthop Relat Res. 2006;449:100–7.
27. Goldszmidt M, Faden L. Is medical education ready to embrace the socio-material? Med Educ. 2016;50:162–4.
28. Holmboe ES. Faculty and the observation of trainees clinical skills: problems and opportunities. Acad Med. 2004;79(1):16–22.
29. Holmboe ES, Batalden P. Achieving the desired transformation: thoughts on next steps for outcomes-based medical education. Acad Med. 2015;90(9):1215–23.
30. Holmboe ES, Sherbino J, Long DM, Swing SR, Frank JR. The role of assessment in competency-based medical education. Med Teach. 2010;32(8):676–82.
31. Holzhausen Y, Maaz A, Cianciolo AT, ten Cate O, Peters H. A conceptual model of the entrustment decision making process. Perspect Med Educ. 2017;6(2):119–26.
32. Jarvis-Selinger S, Pratt DD, Regehr G. Competency is not enough: integrating identity formation into the medical education discourse. Acad Med. 2012;87(9):1185–90.
33. Jaye C, Egan T, Smith-Han K. Communities of clinical practice and normalising technologies of self: learning to fit in on the surgical ward. Anthropol Med. 2010;17(1):59–73.
34. Kennedy TJT, Regehr G, Baker GR, Lingard LA. Progressive independence in clinical training: a tradition worth defending? Acad Med. 2005;80(10 Suppl):S106–11.
35. Kneebone R, Fry H. The environment of surgical training and education. In: Fry H, Kneebone R, editors. Surgical education: theorising an emerging domain. New York: Springer; 2011. p. 3–17.
36. Kolb DA. Experiential learning: experience as the source of learning and development. Englewood Cliffs: Prentice-Hall; 1984.
37. Kotsis SV, Chung KC. Application of see one, do one, teach one concept to surgical training. Plast Reconstr Surg. 2013;131(5):1194–201.
38. Land R, Meyer JHF. The scalpel and the 'mask': threshold concepts in surgical education. In: Fry H, Kneebone R, editors. Surgical education: theorising an emerging domain. New York: Springer; 2011. p. 91–106.
39. Lave J, Wenger E. Situated learning: legitimate peripheral participation. Cambridge: Cambridge University Press; 1991.
40. Lingard L, Reznick R, DeVito SE. Forming professional identities in the health care team: discursive constructions of the 'other' in the operating room. Med Educ. 2002;36(8):728–34.

41. Lyon P. Making the most of learning in the operating theater: student strategies and curricular initiatives. Med Educ. 2003;37:680–8.
42. Lyon P. A model of teaching and learning in the operating theatre. Med Educ. 2004;38:1278–87.
43. Mann K. Theoretical perspectives in medical education: past experience and future possibilities. Med Educ. 2011;45:60–8.
44. Miller A, Archer J. Impact of workplace-based assessment on doctors' education and performance: a systematic review. British Med J (Online). 2010;341:c5064.
45. Moulton CE, Regehr G, Mylopoulos M, MacRae HM. Slowing down when you should: a new model of expert judgment. Acad Med. 2007;82:S109–16.
46. Moulton CE, Regehr G, Lingard L, Merritt C, MacRae H. Slowing down when you should: initiators and influences of the transition from the routine to the effortful. J Gastrointest Surg. 2010a;14:1019–26.
47. Moulton CE, Regehr G, Lingard L, Merritt C, MacRae H. Staying out of trouble in the operating room: remaining attentive in automaticity. Acad Med. 2010b;85:1571–7.
48. Nasca TJ, Philibert I, Brigham T, Flynn TC. The next GME accreditation system – rationale and benefits. N Engl J Med. 2012;366(11):1051–6.
49. Norcini J. Understanding learning in the workplace for those who practise: we can't wait another 50 years. Med Educ. 2016;50:18–20.
50. Nyssen A. Integrating cognitive and collective aspects of work in evaluating technology. IEEE Trans Syst, Man, and Cybern—Part A: Syst Hum. 2004;34(6):743–8.
51. Osman NY, Walling JL, Mitchell VG, Alexander EK. Length of attending-student and resident-student interactions in the inpatient medicine clerkship. Teach Learn Med. 2015;27(2):130–7.
52. Raja AJ, Levin AV. Challenges of teaching surgery: ethical framework. World J Surg. 2003;27:948–51.
53. Regehr G. A user's guide to reading the scholarship of anesthesia education. Can J Anesth. 2012;59:132–5.
54. Rogers DA, Lingard L, Boehler ML, Espin S, Klingensmith M, Mellinger JD, Schindler N. Teaching operating room conflict management to surgeons: clarifying the optimal approach. Med Educ. 2011;45:939–45.
55. Rohrich RJ. See one, do one, teach one: an old adage with a new twist. Plast Reconstr Surg. 2006;118(1):257–8.
56. Rowell D. The sociomateriality of expertise: an exploratory study of trauma surgeons. 2015. Dissertations available from ProQuest. Paper AAI3746344. http://repository.upenn.edu/dissertations/AAI3746344.
57. Saba GW, Villela TJ, Chen E, Hammer H, Bodenheimer T. The myth of the lone physician: toward a collaborative alternative. Ann Fam Med. 2012;10(2):169–73.
58. Schön DA. The reflective practitioner: how professionals think in action. New York: Basic Books; 1983.
59. Schuwirth LWT, van der Vleuten CPM. Conceptualising surgical education assessment. In: Fry H, Kneebone R, editors. Surgical education: theorising an emerging domain. New York: Springer; 2011. p. 75–90.
60. Wenger E. Communities of practice: learning, meaning, and identity. Cambridge, UK: Cambridge University Press; 1998.
61. Williams R, Dunnington G. Assessing the ACGME competencies with methods that improve the quality of evidence and adequacy of sampling. ACGME Bulletin. 2006;19(5 Pt 2):38–42.
62. Woods NN, Mylopoulos M, Brydges R. Informal self-regulated learning on a surgical rotation: uncovering student experiences in context. Adv Health Sci Educ. 2011;16:643–53.
63. Wyatt TR, Bowen J, Mann K, Regehr G, Cianciolo AT. Conversation starter: coming in from the cold: physician professional development as deepening participation in the healthcare community. Teach Learn Med. 2016;28(4):358–61.
64. Zemel A, Koschmann T. Put your fingers right in here: learnability and instructed experience. Discourse Studies. 2014;16(2):163–83.
65. Zimmerman BJ, Schunk DH, editors. Self-regulated learning and academic achievement: theory, research, and practice. New York: Springer; 1989.

2 Surgical Curriculum Development

Carol F. McCammon and Kurt McCammon

As the landscape of medical practice in the United States rapidly changes with the advent of patient safety and quality mandates in parallel with cost reduction efforts, medical education is at risk of harm and requires diligent attention to keep up with these demands to protect the needs of learners and support high-quality programs in the current fluctuating environment [1]. Great responsibility rests on the shoulders of medical educators to assess these shifting circumstances to enhance and protect the learning experience through curriculum development to ensure the best educational outcomes.

An educational curriculum is defined as a planned educational experience through a particular course of study and involvement. It is important to understand that medical educators have a professional and ethical obligation to meet the needs of their learners, the patients served, and the society as a whole. In order to develop the most appropriate curriculum for learners, a logical systematic approach to curriculum development will help achieve this outcome. A six-step process is recommended in the development of an educational curriculum. These steps include:

1. Conduct a needs assessment.
2. Set well-defined goals and objectives.
3. Determine instructional method(s).
4. Create instructional materials.
5. Teach the learners.
6. Evaluate student and resident performance and the effectiveness of teaching methods and the curriculum as a whole.

C.F. McCammon, MD MPH
Department of Emergency Medicine, EVMS, Norfolk, VA, USA

K. McCammon, MD (✉)
Department of Urology, EVMS, Norfolk, VA, USA
e-mail: mccammka@evms.edu

T.S. Köhler, B. Schwartz (eds.), *Surgeons as Educators*,
https://doi.org/10.1007/978-3-319-64728-9_2

In developing a curriculum for any program is it important to recognize that there are different "levels" of the curriculum that need to be addressed. Any curriculum must satisfy the requirements of the institution, the program, and the specific rotation within the program and must also be effective at the instructional level as well. Each aspect is important to the overall educational outcome, and each level should be reviewed regularly.

Developing or changing an educational curriculum is an arduous task and requires careful planning before any initial work to ensure the curriculum achieves the desired results and that efforts are focused and streamlined. The initial phase in the process is a thorough needs assessment, which is crucial in the development of a successful curriculum. The needs assessment will identify differences and gaps between the existing knowledge of the learner and the goal of the learning encounter. In essence, the needs assessment provides a blueprint that will give guidance during curriculum development.

To conduct a quality needs assessment, one must first determine the needs of the target population (the learners) and the current results of the existing situation. Then, articulate what the desired outcome looks like. The distance between the current results and the desired outcome is the actual need [2]. Determine what concepts and skills are required for the resident to learn during the training period based on the desired range of mastered knowledge and skills expected by each milestone and by the time of graduation from the program.

The advantages of performing a needs assessment include validation of the need for the curriculum itself or for a change in the curriculum [2]. A well-developed needs assessment will make every other phase of curriculum development much simpler as this is the most opportune time to anticipate problems and difficulties in the remaining phases of curriculum development and implementation. The needs assessment will improve educational efficiency and affords measurable outcomes to confirm curriculum effectiveness. It also allows for identification of curricular strategies and methods for testing knowledge and skills at educational intervals. A beneficial side product of the needs assessment is that it creates an opportunity for those interested to design and develop educational research.

There are a number of ways to conduct a needs assessment. These can include primary data acquisition through direct surveys, informal discussions, in-depth interviews, focus group discussions, self-assessments, and pre- and post-test assessments from cohorts of current residents, students, academic faculty, and community faculty. An often even more valuable resource to tap is the cohort of graduates from the program, as their experience and perceptions of the program provide a unique perspective and significance to curriculum improvement efforts. The advantage of using primary data lies in the direct relevance of the information obtained to the specific program and will answer the exact questions of the curriculum planners as focused on the needs of the learners. Additionally, secondary data can be helpful to the curriculum developers during the needs assessment. Secondary data is information that is readily available and has already been collected by another source. Sources of secondary data include expert reviews, graduate medical education guidelines and resources (e.g., ACGME and RRC), and medical and educational literature. Secondary data provides the advantage of immediate availability for use; most is readily accessible and inexpensive and reduces collection time. However, secondary data may fail to address the specific needs of the program and its target population and thus may not be generalizable to all academic situations.

Many academicians in graduate medical education (GME) fail to begin curriculum planning with a needs assessment for a number of reasons, with the most common a lack of confidence in what way to proceed. Although the reasons for a needs assessment are recognized, hesitation exists because of uncertainty in the process, limited resources, financial constraints, and lack of time to dedicate to the effort. Occasionally, a sense that the needs of the program and the individual learners are already clear to the planners may preclude the developers from taking the time to perform the needs assessment. This paternalistic misperception is a significant pitfall to be wary of, as effective educators cannot presume to understand the perspective and needs of the target population without their input. Additionally, changes to the curriculum that are implemented without the benefit of a needs assessment are subject to great scrutiny if there are problems identified after the changes are applied. It is difficult to defend actions taken without careful and thoughtful planning. Furthermore, it is difficult to define success or failure of curriculum changes if outcome measures have not been clearly defined through the process of conducting the needs assessment.

Specific to a urologic surgical residency, some areas of needs assessment content targeted to the recent graduates of the program include their perception of preparedness for practice in all core areas of the urologic residency curriculum, proficiency of surgical skills, readiness to engage in practice management, professional development, interpersonal communication, and adaptation to their new practice environment post-graduation [1]. When targeting the current residents of the program, a well-designed focus group setting led by a curriculum planner may be a very time-efficient way to evaluate this cohort as all parties are proximately located on numerous occasions during the educational period of residency. The content can be similar to that sought from the recent graduate cohort, keeping in mind that at different levels of training, the feedback will vary from inexperience. Currently practicing physicians should also be surveyed for their perspective. Other considerations to consider in curriculum development include the requirements of the residency review committee (RRC) and in-service exam results. Communication with other program directors who have gone through the same process can be invaluable in planning and implementing changes.

Once the needs assessment is completed, reviewed, and analyzed, the assessment should be validated for accuracy to make sure identified needs are the actual needs. If the needs assessment was well designed and carried out, validation is a cursory exercise, and the gaps are sound and clearly identified, which leads to the next step in the process: constructing precise in-depth program goals and objectives. The composition of a concise mission statement can help define the program and help planners prepare to write thoughtful goals and objectives. A well-written mission statement defines the focus of the program and the educational philosophy behind it. Goals and objectives are not synonymous [2]. Program goals are global phrases that are written to include all components of the program and define who will be affected and what will change. Goals provide direction, do not have a deadline, and often are not precisely measurable. In contrast, objectives are more precise. Their purpose is to provide structure to attaining goals through individual measurable benchmarks or standards that must be met in a defined period of time. Objectives can be thought of as a connection between the items identified in the needs assessment and the performance desired. Unfortunately, many curriculum goals and objectives are not well written, are not reviewed yearly, are rarely used or referred to, and may not match what is taught by the faculty. Benefits of well-written goals and objectives include learning prioritization, standardization of the curriculum, justification of resources, and in solidifying organization and expectations of the educators. Drawbacks of poorly written objectives include they are time consuming and hard to do well and to update frequently; many are often too broad and only teach to minimum competencies and are usually not reviewed by faculty or learners. Thus, for the program goals and objectives to be useful, they must accurately provide the framework that supports the curriculum based on the identified needs defined in the needs assessment.

There are three types of goals in surgical learning which include knowledge acquisition, skill set and procedural development, and behavioral attitudes, values, and professionalism [3]. Knowledge base includes cognitive aptitude and ranges from factual knowledge to problem-solving and clinical decision-making. Skill set includes history taking and performing a physical exam and procedure skills. Behavioral attitudes, values, and professionalism are very important aspects of medical training, and good skills in this area are essential to a successful career.

Example of a well-written goal:

Residents will work well on a team to enhance patient safety awareness.

Note the two basic components of a well-written goal are present, that is, who is affected (i.e., residents) and what is supposed to change (i.e., work well on a team to enhance patient safety awareness.)

Good objectives should reflect clarity, state the accomplishment expected, and be measurable [2]. To ensure usefulness, the objective should include the following four components:

1. The outcome to be attained (or what specifically is expected to change):
   (a) Usually the verb (the action) of the objective.
   (b) Some verbs are more appropriate than others (e.g., "list" is a good outcome word for an awareness level objective, but "explain" would be better for a knowledge level objective).
2. The conditions under which the outcome will be observed or when a change will happen:
   (a) This could be a date of completion, such as by the end of PGY −1; or, as a result of participation, the resident will….

3. The benchmark to decide whether the outcome has been met:
   (a) The measurable component which may be a qualitative threshold (e.g., always or never, yes or no) or a quantifiable measurement (e.g., 75% of the time, at least 300 cases).
4. The population for which the objective is intended:
   (a) The residents, students, educators, administration, institution

Example of a well-written objective:

The resident applies structured communication techniques and tools (e.g., *SBAR*) *during handoffs and in changes in patient condition 100% of the time to enhance patient safety.*

Note all the elements of a well-written objective are present: the outcome to be achieved (applies structured communication techniques to enhance patient safety), conditions under which the outcome will be observed (during handoffs and changes in patient condition), the criterion or benchmark for deciding whether the outcome has been achieved (uses the tool 100% of the time), and the priority population (the resident).

There are many resources that can be helpful in development of educational objectives. These include the educational literature, professional societies and ACGME, data from the needs assessment, and personal experience.

Once the needs assessment is done and the goals and objectives are written and reviewed, they need to be shared with educators as well as learners. This will allow the educators to develop specific content that will meet the objectives and fill the gaps in knowledge that were identified from the needs assessment. Teaching methods are greatly variable and may include textbooks, web-based resources, weekly conferences and quizzes, bedside rounds, SIM lab sessions, observation and increasing responsibilities in the operating room as operative skills develop, M&M conferences, literature reviews, and research projects.

Educators should be given feedback on their performance in a timely and consistent manner and provided with adequate resources to improve their instruction skills. When excellent educators are identified, appropriate recognition should be given. This will provide a positive environment and promote advancement of educational skills proficiency throughout the department. Regular feedback should also be provided to the learners to be certain that milestones are being met, that high achievers are encouraged and given growth opportunities, and that those struggling are supported and inspired to improve [4].

Finally, the curriculum needs to continually be reviewed and modified to allow the program to adapt [4] to the changing practice environment and advances in the science of surgery. A strong curriculum is a living document and must be actively tended to provide the best support and outcomes for the program. Although the effort is time consuming, the work of conducting a complete needs assessment and developing clear goals and objectives will allow your educators and learners to know what is expected of them and in turn allow them to excel as outstanding educators and surgeons.

References

1. Homboe ES, Batalden P. Achieving the desired transformation: thoughts on next steps for outcomes- based medical education. Acad Med. 2015;90(9):1215–23.
2. McKenzie JF, Neiger BL, Thackeray R. Planning, implementing, & evaluating health promotion programs a primer. 5th ed. San Francisco: Pearson Education Inc. Copyright; 2009.
3. Accreditation Council for Graduate Medical Education. http://www.acgme.org/Portals/0/PDFs/Milestones/UrologyMilestones.pdf. Accessed 1 June 2017.
4. Posavac EJ, Carey RG. Program evaluation methods and case studies. 7th ed. New York: Pearson Education Inc. Copyright; 2007.

Curriculum Development

3

Elspeth M. McDougall and Bradley Schwartz

Most surgeons affiliated with an academic institution and thereby involved in medical student, resident, and fellowship teaching have never had any formal training to be an educator. The demands of both clinical practice and educational needs of the learners are constantly increasing and changing requiring these educators to teach more in less time [1]. The key element to the presentation of an efficient and effective educational program or course is the methodical and constructive development of the curriculum. This chapter will outline the six key steps to curriculum development which address the components constituting the effective creation and maintenance of the training curriculum for any level of learner. Following these guidelines will ensure that the educator understands the needs of the learners, and the learners have a clear knowledge of what is expected of them in achieving proficiency in acquiring the necessary skills to provide excellence in patient care.

A curriculum is a planned educational experience, and the word is derived from the Latin word for "racecourse" [2]. Curriculum development is defined as a planned, purposeful, progressive, and systematic process in order to create positive improvements in an educational system [3]. John Dewey advocated that a curriculum should teach concepts not just facts and teach for desired patient outcomes thereby linking the curriculum to health-care needs. A logical and systematic approach to curriculum development will help achieve the desired aims and goals of an educational program. David Kerns has written extensively on

E.M. McDougall, MD, FRCSC, MHPE (✉)
University of British Columbia,Gordon & Leslie Diamond Health Care Centre,
11th Floor – 2775 Laurel Street, Vancouver, BC V5Z 1M9, Canada
e-mail: elspeth.m@ubc.ca

B. Schwartz, DO, FACS
Department of Surgery, Urology, Southern Illinois University School of Medicine,
Springfield, IL, USA

T.S. Köhler, B. Schwartz (eds.), *Surgeons as Educators*,
https://doi.org/10.1007/978-3-319-64728-9_3

curriculum development and considers this process within six main areas of focus [4]. Each area is important in its own development, but all six areas must be constructed from and within the perspective of the other areas to establish a robust and comprehensive curriculum:

1. General needs assessment
2. Targeted needs assessment
3. Goals and objectives
4. Educational strategies
5. Implementation
6. Evaluation and feedback

General Needs Assessment

A curriculum must address the needs of the learner in order to be relevant and sustainable. Therefore it is critical to identify the focus of the teaching program and the general needs of the participant. The difference between how the problem is currently being addressed and how it should ideally be addressed is the general needs assessment. This characterization of the problem can be accomplished by assessing the existing educational program and soliciting feedback from the learners and educators as to perceived deficiencies in knowledge and/or skills related to this learning method. Also, soliciting and utilizing input and guidelines established by certifying and credentialing boards and associations are important to this general process.

The current approach to the curriculum or program should be analyzed in detail to highlight strengths and weaknesses. It is important to maintain the successful components of the educational program or activity while addressing needed changes or revisions to the less helpful aspects of the curriculum. Developing an outline of the ideal curriculum or educational program can be a good initial step, recognizing that some of these objectives may not be attainable or realistic due to educational equipment, educator, and financial resources. However, from this framework, gaps between the ideal educational program and the reality of the available resources allow development of best options for teaching strategies and methods.

Other groups may also have a vested interest in the development of an appropriate educational curriculum and thereby contribute to the needs assessment process. For example, there is a perceived need for formal urology training guidelines by the Accreditation Council of Graduate Medical Education (ACGME), and they in turn look to the Urology Residency Review Committee (RRC) to create these training parameters. This has led to the development of the Urology Milestones project which is a joint initiative between the ACGME and the American Board of Urology (ABU) [5]. Ultimately the ABU defines the specific competencies required for subspecialty training in urology and sets qualifying examinations to determine if candidates achieve proficiency in these areas of knowledge and skill. It is the required competencies which provide a basic road map for urology curriculum development. The Urology Milestones project considers the education of the urologist in five categorical levels.

Level 1	The resident demonstrates milestones expected of an incoming resident
Level 2	The resident is advancing and demonstrates additional milestones
Level 3	The resident continues to advance and demonstrate additional milestones; the resident demonstrates the majority of milestones targeted for residency in this sub-competency
Level 4	The resident has advanced so that he or she now substantially demonstrates the milestones targeted for residency. This level is designed as the graduation target
Level 5	The resident has advanced beyond performance targets set for residency and is demonstrating "aspirational" goals which might describe the performance of someone who has been in practice for several years. It is expected that only a few exceptional residents will reach this level

While this pertains to the national urology curriculum, it can be applied to any proposed program or curriculum being assessed.

The first step starts with the identification and analysis of a health-care need or other problem that is to be addressed by the curriculum. A clear definition of the problem helps to focus a curriculum's goals and objectives which in turn will focus on the curriculum's educational and evaluation strategies. Clarification of the health-care problem to be addressed and the current and ideal approaches to addressing the problem is required to focus the education intervention toward solving the problem. Conclusions from this step may or may not apply to a particular group of learners so the next step is to perform an explicit assessment of the specific needs of the targeted learners.

Targeted Needs Assessment

It is critical that the curriculum be pertinent to the specific learner, and so it is important to identify and clearly define the learner. A medical student will have very separate educational needs compared to a junior resident, and similarly the junior resident needs are unique from the senior resident or fellow in training. Postgraduate clinicians and surgeons will also have very discrete educational needs that are relevant to their clinical practice. At times, especially as the result of rapidly advancing technologies and new techniques in surgery, there may be overlap of learner groups such that resident and postgraduate learners have similar educational needs as has been seen with introduction of laparoscopic and robot-assisted laparoscopic surgery. However, each learner group should be considered separately and a curriculum devised that meets each unique need of the specific group.

Methods for performing learner needs assessment include:

- Informal discussions/formal interviews
- Focus group discussions
- Questionnaires
- Direct observation of skills
- Examinations
- Audits of current performance
- Strategic planning session

Junior trainees and medical students cannot be expected to understand what they necessarily need to know about a specific area of medicine or surgical discipline. It therefore must fall to the expert educators to determine the baseline needs of these novice groups of learners. Considering the educational needs of junior trainees may necessitate the utilization of the Delphi technique to determine the content of the curriculum.

The Delphi technique is a structured communication process or method which was originally developed as a systematic interactive forecasting method which relies on a panel of experts [6]. It is designed as a group communication process which aims to achieve a convergence of opinion on a specific real-world issue. It has been applied to various aspects of educational program development including surgical training programs. Surgical experts review and suggest materials that they consider critical to the comprehensive training of specific surgical trainees. A facilitator, often one of the key surgical experts, provides anonymous summaries of the expert's feedback and reasons for their judgments during the process. Thus, experts are encouraged to revise their earlier contributions in light of the replies and suggestions of other expert members of the panel. During this deliberative process, the range of suggestions and decisions on educational content will decrease, and the group will converge toward an agreed consensus. It is important that these same experts determine not only the content of the curriculum but delineate what is expected performance or proficiency levels and identify specific errors or unacceptable performance and how this should be remediated.

More advanced learners such as senior residents, fellows, and postgraduate surgeons should be included in the needs assessment process of curriculum development. In this way the specific educational needs of these learners can be identified and addressed in the development process. Input from these groups can be solicited with survey questionnaires, small group discussions, and from curriculum evaluation of existing educational programs or courses. Addressing the specific educational needs of these more advanced groups of learners will ensure that they will be fully engaged in the curriculum and complete the learning material or skills training.

Residency training programs themselves may identify specific educational needs for their residents and tailor their training programs accordingly. Continual feedback from residents will assist in creating a relevant educational curriculum and identify specific areas within the learning program that may require special attention or new learning material. Finally the public and patients can provide a valuable mechanism for creating curriculum revision or change. It is this area of educational need that results in the development of best practice statements and guidelines by organizations such as the American Urological Association (AUA) [7]. However, patient survey feedback on resident encounters in the hospital or outpatient setting can give valuable information to educators and help address specific educational needs, particularly pertaining to nontechnical skills such as communication and professionalism.

Less resource intensive options for teaching may allow for equally effective learning by the learners and actually stimulate them to become more active self-directed learners. As an example, a cadaveric hands-on, robotic surgery teaching laboratory experience may not be within the budgetary constraints of a residency training program. However, a live animal hands-on, robotic surgery teaching laboratory offers a less costly experience and allows more residents to participate in learning opportunities with a single model that provides the valuable teaching environment of pulsatile tissue handling and management. Important basic robotic surgery skills can be taught effectively with both the cadaveric and live animal models. More detailed discussion on simulation and skills lab is addressed in another chapter.

Once the educational issue has been clearly identified, it is next important to determine what finite resources can be directed toward developing and implementing an applicable solution or developing a curriculum. Demonstrating the feasibility of the curriculum development will then lead to the establishment of goals and objectives specific to the curriculum.

Goals and Objectives

An educational goal describes the "real-world" performance the learners can expect to exhibit once they have completed the curriculum. Educational goals describe the overall learning outcome. Subsequent objectives, methods, and evaluation procedures are directed toward achieving the goals. Broad educational goals communicate the overall purposes of a curriculum and establish criteria for various components of the program.

Ideally goals should describe overall outcomes and be stated in terms that clearly define the expected learner outcomes of the curriculum. It is intuitive, but important to ensure, that the goals are realistically attainable by the completion of the curriculum. Goals are usually stated in terms of the knowledge, behavior, and/or attitudes the learner will acquire by completing the course of training. They describe the real-world behaviors that are expected to be used by the learner.

Some examples of goals that could be associated with a urology curriculum include:

- Perform a thorough urological history and physical examination.
- Recognize the presenting symptoms of pyelonephritis.
- Articulate the staging and associated treatment options for bladder cancer.

While goals are often expressed in somewhat vague terms, curriculum objectives must be very specific. Educational objectives are descriptive statements that are precise and measurable in terms of what the learner will be able to do at the end of the instructional sequence within the curriculum. The well-written objective delineates the audience for whom the objective is intended, outlines the observed and/or recorded behavior of the learner, and defines the conditions of the observed behavior and the degree to which a behavior must be performed. It is often best to consider how the learner will be tested to determine if they have actually achieved the knowledge, behavior(s), and/or attitudes that are expected from completing the curriculum when writing objectives. It is the objectives that would let any group of educators adopt the curriculum and know how to complete the necessary educational program. It is also the objectives that provide the framework on which learner and curriculum evaluation will be constructed.

Objectives relate to a curriculum goal but they are designed to determine exactly what the learners will be able to do at the end of the curriculum. Objectives are stated in terms of precise, observable, and measurable parameters. They must be realistically attainable during the curriculum. As a guide to creating curriculum objectives, five basic elements should be considered:

1. Who
2. Will do
3. How much or how well
4. Of what
5. By when

Some examples of objectives that could be associated with a urology curriculum include:

- A first year urology resident will be able to demonstrate a testicular and digital rectal examination of a male patient, meeting criteria on a checklist as judged by a trained observer by the end of their first 6 months of training
- A second year urology resident will be able to perform a cystoscopy, place a ureteral guidewire into the upper urinary tract, and insert an indwelling ureteral stent satisfactorily by evaluation of at least two urology faculty observing the resident in two separate clinical cases

Specific measurable objectives permit refinement of curricular content and guide the selection of appropriate educational and evaluation methods. Goals and objectives should be determined by specialty experts or dictated by required competency metrics established by certifying bodies. Objectives usually fall within three major domains including knowledge, affective or attitudinal, and motor or psychomotor skills. Knowledge can encompass factual knowledge to higher levels of function such as problem solving and clinical decision-making. Attitudes, values, beliefs, biases, emotions, and role expectations are also important components of medical and surgical training objectives. Surgeons' technical skills and procedural objectives are paramount to our daily clinical practice, but equally important are behavioral objectives such as history taking, physical examination, interpersonal communication, professionalism, and record keeping.

Bloom's taxonomy defines the cognitive domain by level of complexity and abstraction. It is clear that advancing cognitively requires movement from the broad base of these skills to the more discriminatory peak of the triangle.

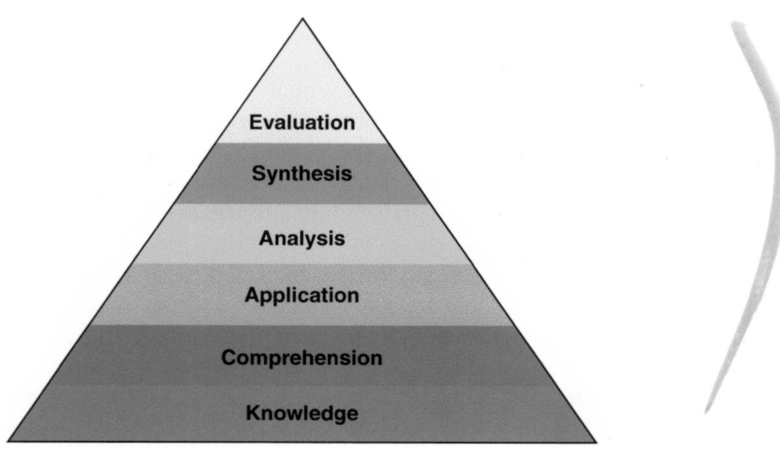

When writing curriculum objectives, especially those pertaining to behavioral skills, it is important to use active verbs because these imply measurability. Within Bloom's taxonomy there are numerous active verbs which are useful for the construction of objectives.

Skill	Vague	More specific
Knowledge objectives	Know or understand	List Recite Present Distinguish Define, describe, give an example of
Skill objectives	Be able or know how	Demonstrate (as measured by), use or incorporate into performance (as measured by)
Attitudinal objectives	Appreciate, grasp the significance of, believe, enjoy, learn, teach	Rank as valuable, rank as important, identify, rate or rank as a belief or opinion, rate as enjoyable

While careful development of the curricular objectives is a primary focus of the development process, it is important to remember that most educational experiences are much more than a list of preestablished objectives. Also considerable learning occurs from unanticipated learning experiences within the curriculum and during the pursuit of skill development as other learning needs are often identified by the learner as a result of these experiences [8, 9]. So while a list of learning objectives is important to the development of a curriculum, it should not be overwhelming, limit creativity, or limit learning related to individual learner needs and experiences.

Educational Strategies

The clearly defined and measurable learning objectives of the curriculum will then allow specific teaching techniques or educational strategies to be developed for each of the objectives. After selecting the learning objectives and assessments for the course, it is important to consider the various instructional activities that could be used to engage students with the material and enable them to meet the objectives. Of course, the key is to align instructional strategies with the objectives and assessment tools. Many instructional strategies are flexible and can be used to address several learning objectives, but some of them are better suited for a particular set of objectives.

Educational strategies can be considered within two broad categories related to content and methods of the teaching. Content is the specific material to be included in the curriculum and this flows directly from the specific measurable objectives. Methods are the ways in which the curricular content can be presented and should be selected appropriately for cognitive, affective, and psychomotor learning objectives. It is important to maintain congruence between objectives and methods when developing these components of the curriculum. To meet different learning styles and motivations, maintain learner interest, and reinforce the learning process to deepen understanding and promote retention, it is important to use multiple educational methods. These educational strategies should be chosen because of their feasibility in the terms of available resources but also for their effectiveness in learning the skill.

The methods to address cognitive learning are well understood and developed by educators and include readings, lectures, audiovisual materials, discussion, problem-solving exercises, programmed or online learning, and assigned learning projects.

Examples of cognitive learning strategies for urology training

Cognitive learning strategies	Urology specific cognitive learning strategy
Readings	*Campbell's Urology* text AUA Core Curriculum
Lectures	Grand rounds lectures Visiting professorships to department
Audiovisual materials	AUA laparoscopic and robotic surgery teaching videos Webcast programs available through AUA and other urology specific organizations
Discussion	Morbidity and mortality rounds Formal teaching sessions with expert faculty GU oncology rounds, especially with interprofessional participation
Problem-solving exercises	GU oncology rounds – multidisciplinary review and discussion of specific clinical cases Review of specific patient cases – during outpatient clinical work, ward rounds on operative patients, and review of complications during morbidity and mortality rounds AUA clinical problem solving protocols Morbidity and mortality rounds
Programmed or online learning	AUA clinical guidelines AUA clinical problem solving protocols with built-in evaluation AUA Core Curriculum with built-in self-assessment testing
Assigned learning projects	Resident assigned grand rounds presentations Required resident research and/or manuscript development

The methods for achieving affective objectives within a curriculum require exposure to knowledge, experiences, or the views of respected experts and faculty that either contradict undesired or confirm desired attitudes. Selection of well-respected, reliable faculty with a commitment to clinical excellence and constructive educational participation in a training program are instrumental to the success of affective learning for urology trainees. Trainee exposure to affective objectives can be through readings, discussion, and clinical experiences. Facilitation of openness, introspection, and reflection are key to these encounters and usually need to be overseen by faculty to ensure a constructive process. All personnel and faculty with whom residents train are role models, and it is critical that these educational encounters are consistent and reflect the caring and professional attitudes we desire in our next generation of urologists. It is important that senior and chief residents recognize that they serve as important role models for medical students and junior residents and as such are very visible attitudinal instructors within training programs.

Motor and psychomotor skill objectives are a salient aspect of any surgical training program. Kern and colleagues have similarly developed a model that integrates the six-step principles of curriculum development and simulation design that is applicable across surgical specialties [10]. Its use could lead to high-quality simulation courses that integrate efficiently into an overall curriculum.

A variety of educational strategies can be used to teach the critical skill sets to multiple specialties in surgery and medicine. Methods for achieving psychomotor learning objectives include supervised clinical experiences, simulated learning and practice sessions with artificial materials models, animal models, cadaveric models, standardized patients, and role-playing sessions. In addition, audio and visual reviews, such as video libraries for specific surgical procedures and techniques available within the AUA Core Curriculum, can be very helpful for trainees developing their surgical skills and judgments. These help them identify good surgical techniques and performance proficiency levels when developed by reliable expert educators and have been shown to improve resident trainee operative task performance [11].

Research has shown that repetitive distribution of motor skills learning is superior to single concentrated skills learning [12, 13]. The development of neural patterns for long-term establishment of motor skills is facilitated by the cycle of repetitive simulated practice to prescribed proficiency criteria [14]. Introduction to skills learning is usually done through didactic presentations, demonstrations, and discussion. On this framework of skills knowledge, it is then important to build opportunities to practice the skills, experience errors or complications including management of these undesired outcomes, and then reflect upon the entire learning process and determine how to better address the skill practice at a subsequent learning session. Constructive, facilitative feedback from an expert to the learner is very valuable in this process and is best administered during or immediately following the learning experience. In this way the trainee can repeat the motor skill learning cycle until they have mastered the skill to the predetermined proficiency level. This is best accomplished in a safe and supportive learning environment. Structured simulation is an ideal platform for this type of learning because it allows for repetitive practice of skills, to a prescribed and objectively measurable proficiency level, away from the patient. Immediate feedback and re-practice with learned information from errors or complications experienced during the skills practice are the hallmarks of simulation. Of critical importance, the simulated learning is completely learner-focused rather than a patient-centered encounter where the learner is of secondary importance to the naturally clinical demands of a patient. Also, it appears that providing a preoperative surgical warm-up with instructor feedback can improve operative performance compared to either a warm-up or feedback alone [15].

One of the key objectives of any curriculum is to foster or promote the learner to become committed to self-directed learning. However, training the learner in the skills relevant to self-directed learning is critical and sometimes difficult. This can be achieved through self-assessment, information searching, critical appraisal, and clinical decision-making. Surgeons are notoriously poor at self-assessment so this process of learning self-directed learning must be overseen by educators providing concrete feedback in the information searching, critical appraisal, and clinical decision-making processes [11]. Independent learning projects and personal learning plans or contracts can also be useful strategies to promote self-directed learning. Through this process, trainees can eventually formulate and answer their own questions which is the definition of self-directed learning. Once again role modeling, as provided by educators and faculty, is an additional method by which the next generation of urologists will understand the importance of self-directed learning.

The clinical work in urology is dependent on effective teamwork as it pertains to the operating room and multidisciplinary delivery of comprehensive care to complex urologic patients such as those with oncologic diseases. As such, it is important that the curriculum focuses on educational strategies for promoting teamwork. These strategies can include collaborative learning experiences as experienced in team-based learning, creating work environments that model effective teamwork, regular review and assessment of team function in which the trainee is included, and dedicated simulated training in team skills and functions [16]. Several researchers have demonstrated that team-simulated practice of communication and technical skills significantly improve these parameters in all team members and makes teamwork more efficient and effective. This type of training can be performed in situ thereby assisting in the identification of institutional or environmental factors that may directly impact on the effectiveness of the team.

Implementation

While the challenging initial work of creating a curriculum determines the learner needs and establishes the learning objectives and teaching strategies, it is equally important to plan an efficient and calculated implementation of the curriculum. To accomplish this step of curriculum development, it is important to clearly identify the resources that will be required to introduce and maintain the curriculum. These resources include personnel, time, facilities, and funding costs. Personnel factors will encompass not only educators and faculty but secretarial and administrative support for the maintenance and evaluation of the curriculum. It is also important to consider patients within this personnel support and how they will be impacted as well as interact with, and provide feedback for, the trainees. Patients need to be fully informed of their participation in the training program so they are prepared for encounters with trainees and providing assessment of the trainees and the training program.

It takes time to enact an educational curriculum both in its development and implementation. These time implications need to be defined for faculty, support or administrative staff, and the learners and should be calculated in hours per week or hours per month. In some groups of personnel, such as administrative staff, this will translate into financial remuneration either directly or as part of their job description. Faculty will unlikely have financial remuneration directly for their involvement in the implementation of the curriculum but must be prepared to dedicate time to teaching responsibilities and have a clear understanding of how this impacts their academic status within the department and institution. Much of the learning in a curriculum occurs in physical space such as lecture halls, small group discussion rooms, or simulation/education centers. The required times and locations must be accurately determined and then reserved for specific education sessions. When teaching occurs in clinical sites, it is important that the facility can accommodate all the learners, educators, potential patients, and staff involved in both the educational activity and the clinical process. Time allotments for patient encounters usually need to be modified in the situation of a concurrent educational activity as these have been shown to take more time than patient encounters not involving students. Having an "educational culture" within your department is crucial for the successful implementation of any curriculum. It takes the endorsement and affirmed valuation of the educational program by the leader or head of the department to neutralize the "naysayers" and pessimists to ensure implementation and successful execution of the curriculum.

Determining funding costs of an educational curriculum can often be challenging as there are many variables in the component of implementation. The funding costs may be directly calculable from facility and equipment requirements to administrative staff hours of support. However, many costs are hidden or opportunistic and these can be very specific for individual institutions. For example, when developing an animal model skills training laboratory session, the costs of technicians to handle, anesthetize, and euthanize the animals may be built into the overall facility fee for the event, whereas for other institutions these costs may be separate charges within the activity. Having a clear understanding of the institution's policies and requirements for educational space, equipment, and support is important at the initiation of a specific educational curriculum. There are also very specific regulations as to where funding, even as educational grants, may be procured to support various educational programs and activities nationally, locally, and institutionally. It is the responsibility of the curriculum developer to be fully aware of these requirements and restrictions.

Educational programs and curricula will have associated financial costs which must be met in order to implement the educational activities determined to be necessary for effective learning. This support may be obtained internally from administrative authorities such as the dean's office, hospital administration, and directly from departmental allocated educational funding. Occasionally financial support may be available from outside sources such as government agencies, professional societies, managed care, philanthropic donors for funding, and political groups. Funding from industry should always be procured as an educational grant to the department, institution, or education center.

Type of educational support	Internal	External
Personnel	Faculty Administrative support Residents as educators	Faculty educators outside department Administrative support outside department Patients
Time	Faculty Administrative support Residents as educators	Faculty educators outside department Administrative support outside department Patients
Facilities and equipment	Specific spaces for educational activities Specific equipment for educational activities	Space for educational activities outside department Equipment for educational activities outside department Online access to educational programs outside department
Financial	Departmental Philanthropic Institutional curricular or faculty development resources	Dean's office Hospital administration Government agencies Professional societies Managed care Philanthropic donors Political groups Curricular or faculty development resources Industry

Prior to the implementation process of curriculum development and preferably early in the course of this initiative, it is important to anticipate and thereby address potential barriers to implementation. The most obvious barrier is pertaining to financial resources, and this is often the primary reason why a curriculum or specific components of a curriculum are not obtainable. However, in addition there may be substantial competing demands on personnel and time as defined by the curriculum. Finding solutions for the personnel and the time they are required to dedicate to the curriculum can be challenging especially if it is not a clear mandate of their job description or academic mandate. Also at play are attitudes and the sense of power that people may perceive within and as a result of the curriculum implementation. It may be critical to engage the departmental lead or dean's office early in the curriculum development process to ensure buy-in by all stakeholders in the delivery of the educational program. Being able to provide assurance of specific personnel roles and job security may be necessary in establishing long-term administrative support for a program.

Evaluation and Feedback

When introducing a new curriculum or major curricular reform to a program, it will be important to consider the process of this introduction. It is often prudent to make the initial introduction of the curriculum a pilot experience or study and provide ample opportunity for faculty, administrators, and learners to provide anonymous feedback. Once there appears to be general acceptance or minimal required revisions of the curriculum, it can then be phased-in over a specified period of time or across variable years of the entire curriculum. Again in this phase-in process, there should be ample opportunity to obtain constructive feedback and evaluation of the curriculum. With successful acceptance of the curriculum, it can then be fully implemented. Even after full implementation, it is imperative that continued evaluation and feedback continue for the maintenance and sustainability of the curriculum.

A curriculum is a dynamic process which is continually developing based on a closed loop including evaluation and feedback. It is this ongoing acquisition of information from educators, learners, and administrators that provides a guide to improvement of components, and even, of the entire curriculum. In addition, evaluation results can be utilized to seek continued or additional support for a curriculum, assess individual achievements within the program, satisfy external requirements such as those from ACGME, and serve as a basis for scholarly activity in the development of presentations and publications.

The evaluation process should identify users, uses, and resources utilized by the curriculum. It should also identify specific evaluation questions and designs and choose measurement methods and construct instruments of assessment. Ethical concerns within the curriculum should be addressed and the accurate collection, analyzing, and reporting of the data must be insured in this process. These evaluations may be formative, or internal to the curriculum, and are a method for judging the worth of a program while the program activities are forming or in progress. Equally important is summative evaluation of the curriculum where the focus is on the outcome of a program to determine if the overriding goals of the educational program are being achieved. An example of formative program evaluation is: After each didactic lecture of the ambulatory urology rotation, learners completed an evaluation form. It was discovered that students had already learned about UTIs in the AUA online clinical problem solving on this topic, so the lecture was replaced with one on STDs. As an example of summative evaluation: The final evaluation for the pilot basic ultrasound skills training program showed residents had a high level of satisfaction and learner proficiency, so additional educational grant funding was sought to ensure continued resources and time to maintain and expand this program.

Most of the evaluation questions should relate to specific measurable curricular objectives for the learner, the process or outcome of the curriculum. It is helpful if questionnaires include items that do not relate to specific objectives and are open-ended in nature or seek a short answer response in order to detect unexpected strengths and weaknesses within the curriculum. Providing space and opportunities for generalized comments or observations by learners and educators can be very illuminating.

A successful curriculum is constantly developing and changing ideally based on a 360 degree feedback process. Understanding this process by sustaining and managing the strength of the curriculum, changing or realigning the weaknesses, and promoting further improvements will result in an educational program that successfully meets the needs of the learners and readily engages enthusiastic participation by faculty.

References

1. Collins JP, Gough IR. An academy of surgical educators: sustaining education--enhancing innovation and scholarship ANZ. J Dermatol Surg. 2010;80(1–2):13–7.
2. www.etymonline.com/index.php?term=curriculum.
3. Alvior M. The meaning and importance of curriculum development. http://simplyeducate.me/2014/12/13/the-meaning-and-importance-of-curriculum-development/.
4. Kern DE, Thomas PA, Hughes MT. Curriculum development for medical education: a six-step approach. Baltimore: Johns Hopkins University Press; 2009.
5. http://www.acgme.org/acgmeweb/Portals/0/MilestonesFAQ.pdf.
6. Hsu C-C, Sandford BA. The Delphi technique: making sense of consensus. Pract Assess, Res Eval. 2007;12(10):1–8.
7. https://www.auanet.org/education/aua-guidelines.cfm.
8. White C, Bradley E, Martindale J, Roy P, Patel K, Yoon M, Worden MK. Why are medical students 'checking out' of active learning in a new curriculum? Med Educ. 2014;48(3):315–24.
9. LaVelle BA, McLaughlin JJ. Simulation-based education improves patient safety in ambulatory care. In: Henriksen K, Battles JB, Keyes MA, Grady ML, editors. Source advances in patient safety: new directions and alternative approaches (Vol. 3: performance and tools). Rockville: Agency for Healthcare Research and Quality (US); 2008.
10. Khamis NN, Satava RM, Alnassar SA, Kern DE. A stepwise model for simulation-based curriculum development for clinical skills, a modification of the six-step approach. Surg Endosc. 2016;30:279–87.
11. Vyasa P, Willis RE, Dunkin BJ, Gardner AK. Are general surgery residents accurate assessors of their own flexible endoscopy skills? J Surg Educ. 2017;74(1):23–9.
12. Gallagher AG, Jordan-Black JA, O'Sullivan GC. Prospective, randomized assessment of the acquisition, maintenance, and loss of laparoscopic skills. Ann Surg. 2012;256(2):387–93.
13. Mitchell EL, Lee DY, Sevdalis N, Partsafas AW, Landry GJ, Liem TK, Moneta GL. Evaluation of distributed practice schedules on retention of a newly acquired surgical skill: a randomized trial. Am J Surg. 2011;201(1):31–9.
14. Ziemann U, Muellbacher W, Hallett M, Cohen LG. Modulation of practice-dependent plasticity in human motor cortex. Brain. 2001;124(Pt 6):1171–81.
15. Kroft J, Ordon M, Po L, Zwingerman N, Lee JY, Pittini R. Can surgical "warm-up" with instructor feedback improve operative performance of surgical trainees? J Minim Invasive Gynecol. 2015;22(6S):S17–8.
16. Fung L, Boet S, Bould MD, Qosa H, Perrier L, Tricco A, Tavares W, Reeves S. Impact of crisis resource management simulation-based training for interprofessional and interdisciplinary teams: a systematic review. J Interprof Care. 2015;29(5):433–44.

4 Measurement in Education: A Primer on Designing Assessments

Collin Hitt

So you want to assess students on their attitudes and beliefs, on their surgical skills, or on their knowledge and reasoning. This chapter will help you to find, or even design, the right assessment tool.

Your choice of tool will depend on what you want to measure. You might use a survey questionnaire, a third-party rating of surgical performance, or a multiple-choice test. No matter what kind of assessment tool you use and no matter what you're trying to assess, take the following advice. Before you ever use a tool to assess students, first use it to assess yourself.

If you're giving students a survey questionnaire, fill it out for yourself. If you're rating their surgical performance, rate your own recent performance in the same way, or have a colleague do so. If you're giving students a test, take that test. In doing so, you will gain a greater understanding of what you're actually measuring.

Measuring skills and attitudes and knowledge is messy. Healthcare professionals are accustomed to working with concrete numbers – blood pressure, oxygen levels, and so forth. Surveys and tests and rating forms are designed to give us numerical scores, and the numbers they produce have the appearance of being precise. For example, a student may score a 3.88 on the Duckworth Grit scale, or a resident may receive a 5.11 mean score on an operative performance rating during a laparoscopic cholecystectomy. But these scores are not like vital signs. They are not precise measures. There's no better reminder of this than to take an assessment for yourself.

In order to assess skills well, we must accept this uncomfortable fact. Even when using the best tools available, the numbers we collect do not perfectly capture the skills we're trying to measure. Substantial "measurement error" is always involved, and because such error is involved even in the best of circumstances, we have little

C. Hitt, PhD
Department of Medical Education, Southern Illinois University School of Medicine, Springfield, IL, USA
e-mail: chitt47@siumed.edu

T.S. Köhler, B. Schwartz (eds.), *Surgeons as Educators*,
https://doi.org/10.1007/978-3-319-64728-9_4

room for other errors in the assessment process. This is why it is crucial to follow a strict process when choosing or developing an assessment tool.

If we select a measurement tool that is not right for our purpose or if we design a tool with bad questions, it will only make a messy situation worse. Mistakes are easy to make when choosing and designing an assessment. If we make too many of them, the numbers we collect will be useless.

This chapter is an introduction to the basics of developing a specific type of assessment – ratings that use a multiple-choice format. These tools are by no means the only way to assess skills, but they have distinct advantages. They can be efficiently given to a large number of people. They are transparent and can easily be shared with other researchers. And the results can be compared across different settings and across separate studies.

The discussion in the chapter will alternate between two main types of multiple-question assessments: self-reported questionnaires and third-party reports. Below are examples of each from the surgical education literature:

Self-reported survey questionnaires:

Researchers at Stanford University examined whether having "grit" was an important predictor of mental well-being for general surgery residents [13]. Grit – defined as perseverance and a passion to pursue long-term goals – was measured by giving each resident an eight-item questionnaire previously developed by psychologist Angela Duckworth [6]. Each item on the questionnaire contained a statement (e.g., "I am diligent" and "I finish whatever I begin") with response choices ranging from "not like me at all" to "very much like me." Responses to each item are scored from 1 to 5, using a simple rubric, and the average score across all items provides a Grit score.

Later in residency, the study participants were given questionnaires on burnout and psychological well-being. These questions followed a similar format. The authors found that the association between grit and mental well-being was significant. Residents who reported higher levels of grit reported lower levels of burnout and higher levels of mental well-being.

Third-party reports:

Third-party reports can be used to collect measures on soft skills or personality traits such as grit – observers rate subjects using questionnaires similar to those used to collect self-reports. For example, teachers can be surveyed on individual student attitudes and behaviors (e.g., [11]).

Third-party reports have another key use: performance ratings. For example, researchers at Southern Illinois University have developed a series of operative performance ratings that are available via the American Board of Surgery [10]. Residents (or any surgeon) can be monitored (either live or via video) during surgery (real or simulated) and have their performance rated using a standard scoring sheet that follows the steps of the surgery.

This chapter draws heavily on the literature surrounding the design of self-reported measures. However, the principles discussed – regarding the selection and design of an assessment – apply just as well to third-party reports.

There is an important type of assessment that we will *not* explore in great detail: standardized tests of knowledge and reasoning. The design principles we discuss apply to tests as well, but standardized tests have a series of other properties that make them considerably more complicated to create than surveys. That said, even if your interest is in the kind of knowledge captured by a test such as the American Board of Surgery In-Training Examination, the lessons of this chapter should prove useful.

This chapter poses nine key questions. These questions follow a sequence. They lay out a step-by-step process for choosing and designing an assessment. If you commit to finding clear and convincing answers to each of these questions, you will be following a rigorous process that is used by leading researchers from social psychology to medical education.

This chapter is introductory and intentionally nontechnical. It will steer you to more detailed guides and resources. As you search for answers to these nine key questions, you'll also discover additional resources on your own. You'll find none more helpful than the work of Hunter Gehlbach, Anthony Artino, and colleagues (e.g., [1, 2, 9]). Their work heavily influences the structure of this chapter, and their research again and again points to a common theme. Designing an assessment is a social endeavor. It cannot be done alone. You will need to rely heavily on colleagues, experts, and your target audience for feedback and advice. You may need to find a statistician to work with, once data is collected. And you will rely on peers to review your findings, should you attempt to publish research based on the data you collect.

Nine Key Questions of Assessment

The process of designing assessments and collecting data can be long and complicated. But each step comes down to very basic principles:

1. Who do you want to assess?
   Define your target audience. Where are they in the learning process; what is their professional status; what are their demographics and educational backgrounds, etc.*?*
2. What are you trying to measure?
   Define the attitude or skill or competency that you want to assess. This is called your "construct." It is likely complex, which means it has many components. Give it a clear name, and clearly spell out the components that make up the construct.
3. How have other researchers measured what you're trying to measure?
   Conduct a thorough literature review. Identify tools that others have used, and draw upon previous research to improve how you define your construct.
4. What does your target audience think about what you're trying to measure?
   Assemble a focus group of people who resemble your target audience. Provide them with the name of your construct. Ask them how they would define it. Note how your definition of the construct differs from theirs.

5. Once you start writing questions for your assessment, do your questions ask what you mean for them to ask?
   Choose your words very carefully. Make questions as straightforward as possible. The quality of your data depends on it.
6. What do the experts think about the questions you've written?
   Find experts in the area you're focused on. Ask them for feedback on your assessment items. Determine if any additional questions are needed and if all of the questions you've written are relevant.
7. What does your target audience think about the questions you've written?
   Again collect the thoughts of people who resemble your audience. Let them see the items and questions you've developed.
8. It's time to pilot your assessment: do the numbers come back as expected?
   Check the variance, consistency, and validity of your data. This requires some statistical skills. Just as importantly, it requires intuition regarding the statistical tests needed.
9. Is your assessment interesting and useful to other researchers?
   Make your assessment available to other educators and researchers. Present your results at professional and academic conferences. Attempt to publish your results in an academic journal.

Question 1: Who Do You Want to Assess?

Who are the learners you want to assess? A simple answer might be "residents" or "surgical teams" or "nurses" or "surgeons." Provide as much detail as possible. The more information you have about your learners' backgrounds, the better.

At this stage in the process, you may not have available all of the background information you hope to eventually have. Make an educated guess about the characteristics of your audience – this will be important later. Also, take notes of background information you'd like to have. When you assess your students, you can include a form that gathers background information.

The level of background information you'll want to collect is going to be determined by the skills you're attempting to assess. There is some information, however, that you'll almost certainly want to collect no matter what the context: educational background, job title, and professional experience.

Question 2: What Are You Trying to Measure?

No matter what we're trying to assess – skills or knowledge or attitudes – we have the same problem. We are trying to measure something we can't directly see, something that is complex.

In assessment terminology, the thing you are trying to measure is called the "construct." It's a bland word but it fits. Consider a simple definition: a construct is an object made of multiple components. In surgical education, you are trying to measure something complex – a skill or attitude or body of knowledge made up of many parts. Measuring that construct means you must define its component parts.

In the clearest terms possible, you must be able to answer the question, "What are you trying to measure?" The following are a few examples of how your assessment will be shaped by how you answer that question. An assessment of a construct is, in essence, an assessment of its component parts:

Operative performance: The American Board of Surgery (ABS) requires that general surgery residents be rated on their performance during operative procedures. Rating tools for several different procedures are available on the ABS website, developed by researchers at Southern Illinois University School of Medicine [10]. Using these tools, evaluators observe a resident during an operation and rate the performance on a standardized form.

The construct being measured is "performance during an operative procedure." This is a complex construct – because operations are complex procedures – made up of several key components. The rating form for a laparoscopic cholecystectomy, for example, asks evaluators to score residents on incision and port placement, exposure, cystic duct dissection, cystic artery dissection, and gallbladder dissection. Residents are also scored on more general criteria: instrument handling, respect for tissue, time and motion, and operation flow.

Performance in the operating room is, in many ways, an ideal example of a complex construct. Performance in this context cannot be reduced to a single question. The same is usually true when measuring attitudes or psychological traits.

Grit: The concept of "grit" has gained a great deal of attention. Developed and popularized by personality psychologist Angela Duckworth, grit is defined a "perseverance and passion for long term goals" [5, 6]. Take notice of the word "and" – grit has two components. In order to measure grit, one must measure both perseverance *and* passion for long-term goals.

An eight-item "short grit scale" is publicly available on the Duckworth Lab website. Four of the items focus on perseverance. Four focus on long-term goals. The items use a "Likert-type" format, meaning that response options are aligned along a continuum, in this case from "very much like me" to "not like me at all." This format allows items to be scored numerically, from 1 to 5 in this instance. Scores across all items can be averaged to form an overall Grit score.

The Grit scale has multiple items because grit is a multifaceted construct. But there is another reason why the Grit scale and other scales like it ask multiple questions, because no single question perfectly captures a construct. Language is messy. And since no single question is perfect, researchers ask about the same construct in several different ways, with the hope that a common pattern will emerge across answers.

Self-esteem: The Rosenberg self-esteem scale is designed to measure a person's sense of self-worth. The concept of self-esteem has a singular component (or to use the technical language of assessment, it is "unidimensional"). Grit, you'll recall, was two dimensional: perseverance *and* passion. Even so, measuring self-esteem still requires several questions.

The United States Department of Education has used a version of the self-esteem scale in surveys of tens of thousands of American schoolchildren. Students can respond "strongly agree," "agree," "disagree," or "strongly disagree" to a series of seven items:

- *I feel good about myself.*
- *I feel I am a person of worth, the equal of other people.*
- *I am able to do things as well as most other people.*
- *On the whole, I am satisfied with myself.*
- *I certainly feel useless at times.*
- *At times I think I am no good at all.*
- *I feel I do not have much to be proud of.*

In this case, items can be scored from 1 to 4, since four response options were given. For the top four items, "strongly agree" is scored 4, while "strongly disagree" is scored 1. The bottom four items are known as reverse-coded items, where "strongly agree" is scored 1, while "strongly disagree" is scored 4. In the reverse coded items, the construct is framed in negative terms, which is why the scores run in the reverse order. Scores across all items can be combined to form a self-esteem score.

These examples show how the structure of an assessment flows directly from the definition of the construct. In defining our construct, we list its component parts, and each component part forms the basis of a question that we ask.

Question 3: How Have Other Researchers Measured What You're Trying to Measure?

After you have defined what you want to measure, the next step is to review the scholarly literature on the topic. Has someone in the past tried to measure your construct or any of its component parts? The only way to answer this question is to do a thorough review of the literature.

A literature review can be tedious. Embrace it. This is not simply a perfunctory step, something boring to be done before you begin the real work of writing questions and collecting data. It is the foundation of your entire project.

If you've reached this step, you have already developed a clear definition of the construct you hope to assess – which means you've built a list of the construct's component parts. When doing a literature review, you'll want to search by name for articles covering your construct – and you'll also want to search for studies covering the component parts.

Your literature review will yield one of three results:

The right assessment tools already exist. It's possible that your literature review will turn up a tool that measures *exactly* what you are trying to measure. If you are attempting to measure "grit," for example, you'd be in luck – your literature review would reveal several publicly available, high-quality surveys on grit. Likewise, if you are hoping to assess operative performance on a laparoscopic cholecystectomy, you can find a validated tool online.

Some helpful tools exist, but they're not an exact fit. At the very least, you probably will find tools that partly cover what you hope to measure – you may be able to use some items from those tools – but will need to write additional questions that suit your needs. For example, a team of researchers at Southern Illinois University School of Medicine sought to assess skill in urological operative procedures. The operative performance rating forms available through the American Board of Surgery formed the basis for a rating tool, but new items needed to be developed for urological procedures [3].

No tools exist. This is the least likely outcome. It is *possible* that the construct you hope to measure has never been empirically measured, even partly. This makes the following steps more difficult, as you'll be designing a tool from scratch. But it also signals an opportunity: you're covering a topic that is entirely new in the scholarly literature.

A literature review will take time, but it will be one of the best uses of your time. This chapter outlines how to build an assessment – a several-step process that requires a great deal of work. It's tempting to skip the literature review to begin work on those steps. In reality, however, skipping the literature review would almost certainly create more work than it would save. It would be a waste to build an assessment tool if all along an adequate tool already existed.

When searching the literature, you will probably discover that others have attempted to measure the skills, attitudes, or knowledge that you are trying to measure. Whenever this is the case, recall the advice that was given at the beginning of this chapter. Find the assessment tool used, and *take it for yourself.*

After examining a particular assessment tool, you may feel that it suits your needs. However, if you find a tool that you think works, be sure to ask yourself whether it measures *exactly* what you want to measure. A common pitfall in assessment – and in survey-based work more generally – is when researchers use tools that seem "good enough." If you're reading this textbook, it is likely because you have *specific* educational goals and concerns about your learners. Your assessment should be aligned to those goals and concerns as closely as possible.

Reviewing the literature will accomplish at least two goals: you will learn how people have tried to measure your construct in the past, and at the same time, you will gain greater knowledge about how researchers think about the construct. After conducting a literature review, it's important to consider updating the definition of your construct – adding components that other authors identified and perhaps eliminating components that seem at odds with the literature.

Question 4: How Does Your Target Audience Think About What You're Trying to Measure?

Designing an assessment tool is a social exercise. Question 1 asked, "Who is your audience?" Your answer to this question is now the key.

At this stage, you've defined your construct and its component parts. You've reviewed the literature to see how other researchers have tried to measure that construct. You've likely come to the following place: you found some helpful tools that you think you can adapt and improve upon, for your purposes. Or perhaps you found nothing. In either case, it's going to be necessary to write new items for your assessment. But before you do that, it is beneficial to gather the thoughts of a group of people who resemble your target audience.

This is not a step taken by all survey researchers. It is inspired directly by the work of Hunter Gehlbach, Anthony Artino, and colleagues [1, 9]. They recommend forming a focus group: "researchers need to hear how participants talk about the construct in their own words, with little or no prompting from the researcher." It is important to give members of the focus group the chance to speak. In essence, members of the focus group should be allowed to form their own definition of your construct. What does it mean to them? What do they see as its component parts?

Face-to-face interactions are extremely valuable. Technology offers other options. If done seriously, interviews with a focus group will provide nuanced feedback.

If you've developed careful answers to Questions 1, 2, and 3, your construct should resonate at least partly with your target audience. Their definition of the construct should overlap with yours. But in reality you'll never know what a focus group is going to say, until you form one. It's possible that your audience thinks about your construct completely differently than you do.

If you follow the remaining steps, you're going to build and refine an assessment. One way or another, your audience's understanding of your construct is going to make its way into your assessment – either through specific feedback in the early stages or through confused and unclear answers on the assessment itself. A consistent theme throughout the assessment design process is this: it's better to catch problems early than to collect bad data later. A focus group can help you prevent later missteps.

A literature review can help you refine the definition of your construct to fit with previous research. A focus group can help you refine the definition of your construct to fit with the ideas of your audience.

Question 5: It's Time to Start Writing Questions for Your Assessment, But Do Your Questions Ask What You Mean for Them to Ask?

You've developed an initial definition of your construct. You've conducted a literature review to see how others have defined and measured that construct, and you've gathered information of how your target audience defines the construct. You've updated your definition based on that feedback. So now you have a list of components that make up your construct, and you should develop (or refine) a question for every single one of them.

It's easy to write a bad question. Writing a good question requires work. Bad questions will yield bad data, and, for this reason, it is important to scrutinize every part of every question you write.

To paraphrase the late Jacques Barzun, the writing of a sentence isn't finished until its meaning is clear, until it means just one thing. The same rule should be applied when writing assessment questions: a question isn't finished until its answer means just one thing. If a question is unclear or confusing, then so will be the data you collect.

Consider the following survey item:

My peers are conscientious and caring:

- *Always*
- *Sometimes*
- *Never*

There is nothing wrong with the grammar of this item. It seems clear enough – one could imagine it placed in a survey on workplace morale. And yet, in nine words, there are no fewer than six serious errors.

There are many rules to writing assessment items. Not all of them can be covered here, but we can cover common and completely avoidable errors.

Avoid conjunctions: No word has a simpler meaning than *and*. Yet *and* is perhaps the most problematic word in the example item above. In assessment jargon, this is called a "double-barreled" question, because it asks the respondent to consider two ideas at once: "my peers are conscientious" and "my peers are caring." This creates confusion. If, for example, a person's peers are always conscientious and sometimes caring, the correct answer is unclear.

The simplest way to avoid double-barreled items is to break the question into separate items. Two items – "My peers are conscientious" and "My peers are caring" – work far better than the confusing single item.

When writing a survey question, you must scrutinize every word. Conjunctions are easy to spot. It's more difficult to check one's vocabulary: are you using words that your readers understand?

Avoid big words, rare words, and jargon: If your reader doesn't know what a word means, then you can't know what her answer means. Consider our example item: "my peers are conscientious." One word should stand out – *conscientious*. You may know what the word means, but is it a word that your readers know so well that they would be comfortable using it themselves? If your answer to that question is anything other than "definitely yes," then you need to find another, simpler word.

Avoid jargon and technical language whenever possible: Avoid long words in general (like "conscientious"). This is a common rule for writing. Rules have exceptions: you are reading this chapter because you are interested in assessing the skills of people who are doing surgery. If asking questions about a laparoscopic cholecystectomy, some medical terminology may be necessary, but this is not a license to use big words at will. Your readers will know certain terms and jargon, as part of their profession. However, just because members of a surgical team probably know words like "pneumoperitoneum," it doesn't mean that they know what "conscientiousness" means.

"Conscientious" is a big and relatively rare word. So is "pneumoperitoneum." But there's also a major difference. "Pneumoperitoneum" is very specific in meaning. "Conscientious" is much more complex.

Avoid complex words: What does it mean to be *conscientious*? The word brings to mind a certain person: hardworking, responsible, orderly, honest, punctual, decisive, and with a respect for the rules [12]. *Conscientious,* is a single word that captures a complex idea. So when your reader answers that his peers are "sometimes" conscientious, what are you to make of it? Does it mean that his peers are all of these things sometimes, some of these things sometimes, some of these things always but others never? The complexity of the word conscientiousness creates numerous ways to interpret the same answer.

In lieu of using a complex word, two easy alternatives exist.

One, you can break apart the complex concept and ask questions about its various parts. Several clear and simple questions are better than one unclear, complicated question. Rather than using an unclear and complicated phrase like "my peers are conscientious," it is better to break the question into simpler items like "my peers are hardworking," "my peers are responsible," "my peers are orderly," and so on.

Two, if you want to stick to a single question, you can focus on the part of the concept best suits your purpose. Let's continue with the example of the word "conscientious." Including seven items about the different facets, conscientiousness may be overkill. Perhaps your main interest is in whether members of the surgical team are "hardworking." In this case, the lone item of "my peers are hardworking" is preferable to "my peers are conscientious."

Complex words make your data messy. Vague words have the same effect – even if they are short, simple, and common.

Avoid vagueness: In our example, the word *conscientious* stands out, but there is another problematic word hiding ahead of it – *peers.* It is a simple and common word, but, without context, *peers* is vague. Imagine you asked the above question to every member of a surgical team, as part of an assessment of team morale. How might, say, a general surgery resident interpret the word *peers*? Would she answer with the whole operating room team in mind or with respect only to other surgeons? to other surgeons? Perhaps she would be thinking about her fellow residents or her friends outside of work. The item above gives no guidance at all on this issue. Unless you know what your reader has in mind with respect to her peers, you do not know how to interpret her answer.

One solution to this problem is to replace "my peers" with a more specific term, such as "my co-workers in the operating room." Our items would then read, "My co-workers in the operating room are caring," "My peers in the operating room are hardworking," and so on.

Another alternative is to offer a prompt before the series of items that ask about one's peers: "Please answer questions about your co-workers in the operating room. The questions below refer to them as your *peers*." A problem with prompts and vignettes is that readers sometimes don't read or remember them. Nevertheless, it's better to include a prompt at the top of the page than to leave readers on their own to interpret a vague word like "peers."

We must also scrutinize syntax. The general rules of writing apply. Survey items should be simple and direct. As sentences get longer, they get harder to follow. Shorter isn't always better, but words should be added only when necessary. Adding words, like we did above when replacing "my peers" with "my co-workers in the operating room," comes at a cost.

Avoid questions that are too wordy for your audience: When building an assessment for schoolchildren, an unofficial rule is that a question should be readable to students three–five grade levels below the target audience. There are methods for calculating readability. Word processing software can provide readability statistics for highlighted text, or formulas for calculating readability can be found online. The first sentence in this paragraph, for example, is written at a 12th grade level, according to its score on the Flesch-Kincaid readability test. Knowing your audience is key when writing items (see Question 1). If writing a survey for a college-educated audience, a 12th grade reading level is about the right readability target, if possible. The item "My co-workers in the operating room are hardworking" is written at 9th grade reading level.

So far, we have adjusted almost every word of our survey item. We haven't yet discussed how to structure response options.

Avoid answer choices that are too narrow: Our example item offers the response options "always," "sometimes," and "never." Two of those words are very clear, and one is very vague. When using Likert-type items, a certain amount of ambiguity is unavoidable. The consensus in the literature is that a Likert-type item should offer at least five response options (e.g. [1, 2, 8, 9]). For our example item, a considerable improvement would be "always," "most of the time," "sometimes," "rarely," and "never."

We started with a simple item:
My peers are conscientious and caring:

- *Always*
- *Sometimes*
- *Never*

And following a few simple rules of item design, our initial item has expanded into at least two longer but clearer items:
My co-workers in the operating room are hardworking:

- *Always*
- *Most of the time*
- *Sometimes*
- *Rarely*
- *Never*

My co-workers in the operating room are caring:

- *Always*
- *Most of the time*
- *Sometimes*
- *Rarely*
- *Never*

The differences between our initial item and this pair of revised items may appear small, but the difference in quality is substantial. Writing the initial item was easy. Editing and refining the item was much more difficult. And the editing work might not be done yet.

The number rules and bits of advice for creating survey items are more numerous than we can explore here. For example, some research suggests that items should be written as questions not statements (e.g., "Are your co-workers in the operating room hardworking?"). Related research suggests that response options be written as complete thoughts, rather than as single words (e.g., "My co-workers always work hard" as opposed to "Always"). There is no definitive rule for such decisions, but it is important to consider every alternative (e.g., [2, 8]).

Question 6: What Do the Experts Think About the Questions You've Written?

In your literature review, you likely identified researchers who are experts in the concepts covered by your questions. Moreover, if you are focused on a particular procedure in surgery, you may know experts in that procedure. Attempt to build a panel of experts to review the items you've written.

You should provide reviewers with the definition of your construct and the full list of items you've developed. It is best to provide them with a standard reviewer form, different versions of which are readily available.

Questions to ask your reviewers fall along the following lines. Is each question clearly written? Is each question relevant to the construct? Are there other relevant questions I should be asking?

Question 7: What Does Your Target Audience Think About the Questions You've Written?

In response to Question 4, you assembled a focus group that resembled your target audience. Do this again, but on a one-on-one basis. Earlier in the process, you gathered thoughts on the construct. Here you want to gather thoughts on the questions you've written. This process has been called "cognitive interviewing" – you want respondents who resemble your target audience to fill out your questionnaire and then provide details about what they think the question *means*. This essentially is an opportunity for your audience to answer Question 5, in their own words: do your questions ask what you mean for them to ask?

There are various approaches and guides to conducting cognitive interviews. Here again the work of Artino and colleagues is the most useful in medical education [1, 14].

Question 8: It's Time to Pilot Your Assessment; Do the Numbers Come Back as Expected?

The first time you administer your assessment should be considered a pilot run. You're assessing real learners in the actual setting you're interested in.

After we have fielded our assessment and collected pilot data, it is time to analyze the numbers. This will require some expertise in statistics, as well as special software. In this chapter, we won't focus on the formulas for calculating various test statistics. It's more important to understand the intuition behind each step in your data analysis.

The key property that we will examine in our data, time and again, is *variation*. Is there variation in the data we collect? How does our data vary?

We began this exercise because we were interested in a certain construct – a set of skills or attitudes that we believe *varies* from person to person. We believe that measuring this construct is important because we believe the construct correlates with other important, measurable factors. What explains the variation in our construct? What does variation in our construct help us to explain? Questions like these can only be answered if the data we collect meets certain conditions.

Do Answers to Each Question Vary?

Our initial data analysis should examine one question at a time. Each question is designed to help us tell people *apart* in terms of a given concept. Therefore we are interested in the *variation* in responses that we get to our questions.

There are many measures of variation (e.g., variance, standard deviations). Simple tabulations are the safest place to start: what is the frequency of each response to each question? The goal for each question should be that it returns a variety of responses.

A lack of variation is a problem. If every respondent gives the same answer to a given question, the item will not help us distinguish between people on a given concept – because every answer is *the same*. Likewise, if nearly everyone returns the same answer, the item's usefulness in distinguishing between people is very limited.

However, the opposite is not true. Just because there is variation in responses to a given item, it doesn't mean that the variation is meaningful. Recall our conversation above: a badly written item can produce a wide variety of answers simply because your readers are confused.

Here, intuition plays a role. Does the spread of answers resemble what you would expect? This is not a statistical question, but a conceptual one, based on how you've defined the concept that you're attempting to measure with that question.

Then there is the question of whether our items fit together. When examining a single question, we want responses to vary. When looking across several questions, we examine whether they *covary*.

Are Answer Patterns Consistent?

This chapter has focused on the development of multiple-question assessments. We might combine the answers into a single composite score. This is somewhat strange exercise, taking answers to *qualitative* questions and averaging them into a single, *quantitative* score. After all, we couldn't take answers to any two random questions (e.g., "My co-workers in the operating room are hardworking" and "My co-workers in the operating room are fans of major league baseball") and combine them to into a meaningful measure. So what justifies our doing so with the data we've collected? Psychometric tests are needed.

We ask multiple questions for two main reasons, when trying to measure a single construct. The first is that our construct is complex – it has many parts – and we need different questions to cover different parts of our construct. The second is that language is messy – there is no perfect way of asking about a given thing, so we sometimes ask redundant questions, with the hope that the common theme across several answers will be more accurate than the answer to any single question.

Put more simply: in a multi-item assessment, each question is really just a different way of asking about the same construct. Therefore, we would expect a person's answer to one question to resemble her answers to other questions on the same assessment. That is, throughout our data, we would expect answers across items to be *correlated* with one another.

Consider a hypothetical two-item assessment. If answers to the first item were completely unrelated to answers to the second, it would be difficult to argue that the items were measuring *the same thing*.

This intuition is the basis for what in psychometrics is called "internal consistency and reliability." Various statistical tests of reliability exist. When analyzing individual items, an "item-rest" correlation is one of the most popular tests. This straightforward statistic simply tells us the correlation between answers to a given item and the average score for all other items on the assessment (see [7]).

Overall, answers to each item in a given assessment should be correlated with answers on the remaining items. We should be able to reasonably predict the answer to any single item using answers given to the other items on the assessment. If answers to an item are weakly correlated with answers to other items, this probably means that the item shouldn't be grouped with all of the others.

A measure called Cronbach's alpha is the most common test of internal consistency and reliability. It provides an overall estimate of how closely correlated our items are with one another. If we find that our items are weakly correlated, it means that all of our items are not measuring the same thing – and therefore our items are not all measuring our construct. A low level on internal consistency does not, however, mean that *none* of our items are capturing our construct. It is possible that a few items are weakly correlated with most of the others and are dragging down the overall consistency levels. Virtually every statistics package that calculates Cronbach's alpha would help to spot such items.

Another popular, related measure explores the relationship in answers to our assessment: factor analysis. Factor analysis can be used to explore internal consistency, but it can also be used to explore dimensionality. Exploratory factor analysis, in layman's terms, can examine whether a subset of your items are intercorrelated to a stronger (or weaker) degree than all of the items together.

Cronbach's alpha and factor analysis are powerful tools. They are surprisingly easy to conduct using everyday statistics software. Too easy perhaps. You should not proceed with these tests without studying them more closely than we have done here. The purpose of this section is to highlight the *intuition* behind these psychometric procedures – not the mathematical mechanics or the deeper theoretical underpinnings, which are important. If you've never used these procedures before, work with someone who has. Again, assessment is a social enterprise.

Our goal has been to create a measure that is drawn from a *composite* of answers to multiple questions. Our data must pass certain tests in order for us to combine answers into an average score (which can be raw or weighted). However, simply passing tests of internal consistency is only a step. It means that our questions have the appearance of measuring something in common. But it does not yet mean that our questions measure what we think they measure.

Does Your Measure Predict Other Outcomes?

You are developing an assessment because you want to measure a skill (i.e., construct) that you believe is *important to the real world of surgery*. Scores on your assessment should be measurably related to outcomes in the real world – this is the intuition behind a concept called *predictive validity*.

We have mentioned the example of "grit" throughout this chapter. Grit was defined by Duckworth and colleagues as perseverance and passion for long-term goals. Therefore scores on the Grit scale should be *predictive* of outcomes in instances where these traits are important. In a now seminal article, Duckworth and colleagues demonstrated that grit scores predicted retention among cadets at West Point, as well as success among contestants in the Scripps National Spelling Bee [5].

Throughout this chapter, we've also discussed operative performance ratings. Presumably, operative performance ratings are predictive of patient outcomes in future operations – but such data are scarcely available to researchers. However, another real-world factor is absolutely measurable: experience. Multiple studies have found that the year of residency is strongly related to operative performance ratings – greater experience predicts higher performance, exactly as one would expect [3, 10].

Another test of validity is called *concurrent validity* – are scores on your assessment correlated with scores on other assessments that measure a similar construct? Grit has been shown in repeated studies to be related to self-reports of *conscientiousness*, as one would expect (e.g., [15]). A validation study of an operative performance rating system in urology showed that performance during a kidney stone procedure was correlated with performance during other urological operations. These are examples of concurrent validity.

When piloting your assessment, it might be desirable to assess your students using other tools found in the literature review. This might seem odd. Presumably, you developed a new assessment tool because you believed it was different than what was available. However, if *similar* measures exist to your own, it is worthwhile to deploy them during your pilot testing. This has two benefits. It allows you to test for concurrent validity, and it allows you to test whether your assessment has *greater predictive validity* than other assessments.

Beyond *predictive* and *concurrent* validity, there are other concepts of whether a measure is "valid" (e.g., divergent validity and curricular validity). These should be examined too, if relevant.

But more importantly, we must remind ourselves that no amount of evidence can *prove* that our assessment measures what it purports to measure. We are trying to measure something that we can't see, and so we can never know for certain whether our assessment is truly valid. Stephen M. Downing puts it nicely: "Assessments are not valid or invalid; rather, the scores or outcomes of assessments have more or less evidence to support (or refute) a specific interpretation." [4]

Question 9: Is Your Assessment Interesting and Useful to Other Researchers?

If you have found satisfactory answers to Question 1 through 8, you have produced an assessment tool that you should be proud of. It can be the basis for a publishable paper. You have followed the same process used by leading researchers in assessment research. Don't let your effort end there.

A final test of your assessment can come through peer review. And by peers, we mean "your co-researchers in surgical education." If you can clearly answer Questions 1 through 8, then you have the clear framework for an academic publication. Present the work at conferences, and submit it to a journal. The feedback you receive will sharpen your work further, and publication of your work will allow others to consider using the tool you've developed. There's no measure of validity that quite compares to seeing other teachers use your tool to assess their students.

References and Further Reading

1. Artino AR Jr, La Rochelle JS, Dezee KJ, Gehlbach H. Developing questionnaires for educational research: AMEE guide no. 87. Med Teach. 2014;36(6):463–74.
2. Artino AR Jr, Gehlbach H, Durning SJ. AM last page: avoiding five common pitfalls of survey design. Acad Med. 2011;86(10):1327.
3. Benson A, Markwell S, Kohler TS, Tarter TH. An operative performance rating system for urology residents. J Urol. 2012;188(5):1877–82.
4. Downing SM. Validity: on the meaningful interpretation of assessment data. Med Educ. 2003;37(9):830–7.
5. Duckworth AL, Peterson C, Matthews MD, Kelly DR. Grit: perseverance and passion for long-term goals. J Pers Soc Psychol. 2007;92(6):1087.
6. Duckworth AL, Quinn PD. Development and validation of the short grit scale (GRIT–S). J Pers Assess. 2009;91(2):166–74.
7. Hitt CE. Just filling in the bubbles: using careless answer patterns on surveys as a proxy measure of noncognitive skills. Chapter in Doctoral Dissertation (Character Assessment: Three Essays). Fayetteville: Department of Education Reform, University of Arkansas; 2016.
8. Gehlbach H. Seven survey sins. The Journal of Early Adolescence. 2015;35(5–6):883–97.
9. Gehlbach H, Brinkworth ME. Measure twice, cut down error: a process for enhancing the validity of survey scales. Rev Gen Psychol. 2011;15(4):380.
10. Larson JL, Williams RG, Ketchum J, Boehler ML, Dunnington GL. Feasibility, reliability and validity of an operative performance rating system for evaluating surgery residents. Surgery. 2005;138(4):640–9.
11. Poropat AE. Other-rated personality and academic performance: evidence and implications. Learn Individ Differ. 2014;34:24–32.
12. Roberts BW, Lejuez C, Krueger RF, Richards JM, Hill PL. What is conscientiousness and how can it be assessed? Dev Psychol. 2014;50(5):1315.
13. Salles A, Cohen GL, Mueller CM. The relationship between grit and resident well-being. Am J Surg. 2014;207(2):251–4.
14. Willis GB, Artino AR Jr. What do our respondents think We're asking? Using cognitive interviewing to improve medical education surveys. J Grad Med Educ. 2013;5(3):353–6.
15. Zamarro GE, Cheng A, Shakeel M, Hitt C. Comparing and validating measures of character skills: Findings from a nationally representative sample, 4th coming, J Behav Exp Econ.

Performance Assessment in Minimally Invasive Surgery

5

Evalyn I. George, Anna Skinner, Carla M. Pugh, and Timothy C. Brand

Introduction

Since the mid-1980s, the method of choice for the most high-volume surgical procedures has shifted from traditional open surgery to laparoscopic surgery, also referred to as minimally invasive surgery (MIS). This form of surgery reduces the risk of infection, shortens postoperative hospitalization and recovery time, and decreases postoperative pain and scarring [1].

The benefits are abundant, but there is a cost, and one that falls particularly heavily onto the surgeon: MIS techniques are difficult to master. Laparoscopy involves the use of long and often awkward instruments operating through an unintuitive fulcrum. The length of the instruments exacerbates any tremor from the surgeon's hands as the surgeon performs delicate, dexterous tasks within small spaces. Traditional laparoscopy also requires the surgeon to work within a 3-dimensional space while relying primarily on visual feedback in the form of a 2-dimentional video feed on a screen.

Robot-assisted laparoscopic surgery (RALS) reduces issues of tremor through the use of robotic arms controlled by the surgeon from a surgical console, which also provides the surgeon with better depth perception via stereoscopic vision. However, the stereoscopic (3-dimentional) vision must be used to overcome the

E.I. George, BS
Henry M. Jackson Foundation/Madigan Army Medical Center, Tacoma, WA, USA

A. Skinner, PhD
Black Moon, LLC, Washington, DC, USA

C.M. Pugh, MD, PhD, FACS
Department of Surgery, University of Wisconsin School of Medicine and Public Health, Madison, WI, USA

T.C. Brand, MD, FACS (✉)
Madigan Army Medical Center, Tacoma, WA, USA
e-mail: timothy.c.brand.mil@mail.mil

T.S. Köhler, B. Schwartz (eds.), *Surgeons as Educators*,
https://doi.org/10.1007/978-3-319-64728-9_5

lack of haptic feedback a surgeon receives when directly controlling laparoscopic instruments. Furthermore, RALS necessitates training with millions of dollars of equipment that is often tied to the operating room (OR) and therefore is available in only a limited capacity for initial skill acquisition and rehearsal. As a result, these techniques require specialized training and assessment beyond the scope of traditional methods.

This chapter provides an overview of current assessment methods for both laparoscopic and RALS skills, both during simulation and operative procedures. Some of the most exciting means of doing so are virtual reality simulators that automatically output scores, but they are far from the only option. Laparoscopic surgery features an extensively accepted testing and certification process, called the Fundamentals of Laparoscopic Surgery. This multistep curriculum later became the basis for a similar program in RALS, the Fundamentals of Robotic Surgery. As MIS continues to grow, the importance of specialty-specific and indeed procedure-specific simulation and testing has been highlighted. Further development of these curriculums is ongoing.

Smaller scale and more individualized means of assessment are also available, including global rating scales, motion tracking devices and software, technology-based data export, idle time analysis, and combined analysis of technical and non-technical skills.

Validation and Training

Past models of medical training revolved around students rehearsing skills on actual patients – a questionable process that has since been largely jettisoned. The Halsteadian model of medical education was introduced in the early twentieth century as a way for experience to be gradually gained from patients under the supervision of experienced physicians. The advent of medical simulation presents a viable alternative to this practice. Suturing can be rehearsed with artificial tissue models, intubation can be practiced on life sized manikins, and entire surgical procedures can be simulated in virtual reality. The patient can thus be safely removed from the technical aspect of training.

Specifically for minimally invasive surgery, there are countless training options ranging from homemade box trainers adapted from a shoebox to six-figure virtual reality simulators. With such a wide range, surgical educators must determine how best to train and assess students based on a variety of factors, not the least of which is cost. Traditionally, options are set as the "gold standard," a broadly accepted and validated objective that can be reproduced at most sites. Validation includes several factors. Face validity, how realistic, or how a method feels, and content validity, how applicable of an instructional tool it is, are both subjective – meaning that they are at mercy to the assessor's opinions and beliefs. Commercial simulators often rely heavily on face validity, using the realism of their product as a selling point.

In the old dictum, objective measures of validity which are those independent of personal influence, were defined as construct, concurrent, and predictive. Research in surgical education focused on demonstrating construct validity, with this form of validity typically being one of the first to be cited in the research literature once a new method of training became available. It was defined as the ability to distinguish between experts and novices and can be easily tested in a variety of settings. Following traditional assessments of construct validity, new curriculums, simulators, and trainers are then compared to the gold standard to establish concurrent validity. Predictive validity remained the most elusive. In order to be established, one needs to show how the teaching tool can estimate future performance and necessitating long-term studies without participant attrition.

These definitions were based on the American Psychological Association (APA) and American Educational Research Association (AERA) 1985 *Standards for Educational and Psychological Testing* [2]. The *Standards* were revised in 1999, which presented validity as a unitary concept, rather than a tripartite approach of content, criterion, and construct validity [3]. The unitary view places construct validity as the keystone and other forms of validity falling beneath it [4]. The 1999 *Standards* have since been widely supported but have yet to make their way into the majority of MIS literature.

Both subjective and objective assessments aid in a trainees' learning; however, a wealth of technological tools now exist that can make subjective assessment less central to a training regimen. Subjective assessment isn't inherently bad, but is less dependable between raters as well as expensive in terms of monetary cost and time. Minimally invasive surgery is a growing field but populated by only a limited number of expert surgeons. Even with the small pool, there can be large discrepancies as to what critical skills should look like or even which skills should be critical to progression.

Objective measures allow for higher accountability and precise measurement of skills, with the goal of a higher standard of patient safety; however, more research is needed to link assessment of skills to increase in skill level. Being told where on a scale one is can stimulate self-evaluation and targeted practice; however there is a paucity of literature supporting one objective measure over another. In order to practice both safe and efficient medical training, the medical community needs to advance currently used and antiquated educational methods.

Laparoscopic Training and Assessment Platforms

MISTELS/FLS

Some standards have been established for MIS training and evaluation, including standardized credentialing requirements. Within laparoscopic surgery, the McGill Inanimate System for Training and Evaluation of Laparoscopic Skills (MISTELS), a physical video box simulator was developed in an effort to provide a standardized method for training and assessing fundamental technical skills associated with performance of laparoscopic procedures. The five MISTELS manual skills tasks have shown to be reliable, valid and to provide a useful educational tool [5], which has been incorporated into the manual skills training practicum portion of the Society of American Gastrointestinal and Endoscopic Surgeons (SAGES) Fundamentals of Laparoscopic Surgery (FLS) training program. SAGES began development of the FLS curriculum back in the late 1990s with four goals in mind; to improve cognitive and psychomotor skills, to focus on uniquely laparoscopic material, to avoid anatomic specificity, and to both assess and instruct MIS skills [22]. Completion of the FLS curriculum requires completion of didactic material, originally via CD-ROM and now via online courseware/assessment in addition to training and testing of the five manual skills on the MISTELS portable pelvic video box trainer. MISTELS was purposefully selected over VR simulation options to keep site costs low as well as the fact that the system is easily transported and reproduced. MISTELS includes an opaque box trainer, optical system, and laparoscopic instruments that resemble those found in the OR. FLS box trainer scores have been shown to be independently predictive of intra-operative laparoscopic performance as measured by the Global Operative Assessment of Laparoscopic Skills (GOALS), described in more detail below. This lead the FLS training program to be recognized as the current "gold standard" in laparoscopic training and resulting in its rapid adoption as a primary component of many general surgery residency programs [6–8]. Furthermore, recently SAGES has developed a technical skills curriculum specifically designed for use in residency training programs, which can be found at http://www.flsprogram.org/index/fls-program-description/.

Before trainees begin the psychomotor skills training component, they must first complete the didactic curriculum, which divides laparoscopic skills across five modules, listed below in Fig. 5.1 [6–8].

Manual skills training includes exercises done with the current version of the MISTELS box trainer, which is referred to as the FLS box trainer. Each exercise has

Module I – Preoperative Considerations

- § Laparoscopic Equipment
- § Energy Sources
- § OR Set Up
- § Patient Selection / Preoperative Assessment
- § Preoperative Assessment

Module II – Intraoperative Considerations

- § Anesthesia & Patient Positioning
- § Pneumoperitoneum Establishment & Trocar Placement
- § Physiology of Pneumoperitoneum
- § Exiting the Abdomen

Module III – Basic Laparoscopic Procedures

- § Current laparoscopic procedures
- § Diagnostic Laparoscopy
- § Biopsy
- § Laparoscopic Suturing
- § Hemorrhage & Hemostasis

Module IV – Postoperative Care and Complications

- § Postoperative Care
- § Postoperative Complications

Module V – Manual Skills Training

Fig. 5.1 FLS skill module progression

been set to a nationalized and validated standard. The curriculum is proficiency-based, whereby trainees are oriented to the materials and self-practice until expert-derived performance levels are reached.

The following provides a description of each of the FLS manual skills tasks, including the recommended proficiency requirements for each task.

Recommended proficiency requirements for each task:

The peg transfer exercise requires the trainee to lift six objects (shown in Fig. 5.2) with a grasper first in his or her nondominant (i.e., left) hand and to transfer the object midair to the dominant hand. Each object is then placed on a peg on the right side of a peg board. There is no importance placed on the color of the objects or the order in which they are placed. Once all six pegs have been transferred, the process is reversed. Each peg is lifted using the dominant (i.e., right) hand from the right side of the pegboard, transferred midair to the left hand and placed on the pegs on the left side of the board. The required proficiency score is 48 s with no pegs dropped out of the field of view. Proficiency scores must be achieved on 2 consecutive repetitions and on 10 additional (nonconsecutive is acceptable) repetitions.

This exercise requires trainees to cut out a circle from a square piece of gauze suspended between alligator clips, as shown in Fig. 5.3. The required proficiency score is 98 s with all cuts within 2 mm of the line (either side) Proficiency scores must be achieved on 2 consecutive repetitions only.

In this task trainees are required to place a pre-tied ligating loop or endoloop around a tubular foam appendage on a provided mark as seen in Fig. 5.4. Once they have positioned the endoloop properly, they must break off the end of the plastic pusher at the scored mark on the outside of the box and secure the knot on the mark near the base of the foam appendage by sliding the pusher rod down. A penalty is assessed if the knot is not secure and for any distance that the tie misses the mark. The required proficiency score is 53 s with up to 1 mm accuracy error; no knot security errors (slippage) are allowed. Proficiency scores must be achieved on two consecutive repetitions only.

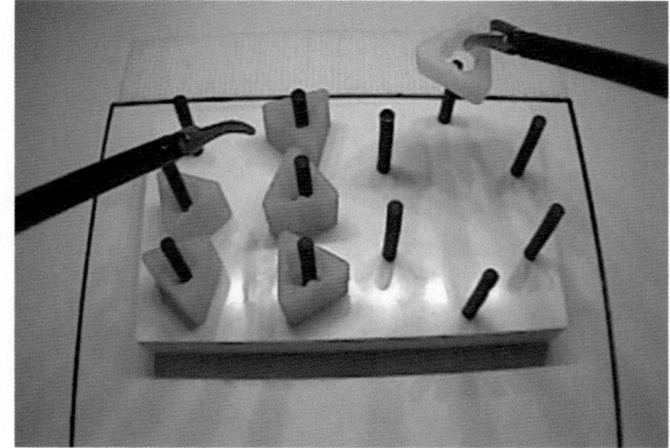

Fig. 5.2 Task 1: Peg transfer (Fundamentals of Laparoscopic Surgery® (FLS) Program is owned by Society of American Gastrointestinal and Endoscopic Surgeons and American College of Surgeons. Images used with permission)

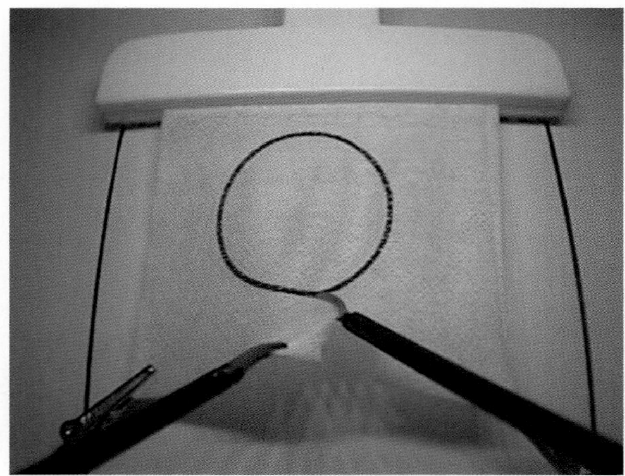

Fig. 5.3 Task 2: Pattern cut (Fundamentals of Laparoscopic Surgery® (FLS) Program is owned by Society of American Gastrointestinal and Endoscopic Surgeons and American College of Surgeons. Images used with permission)

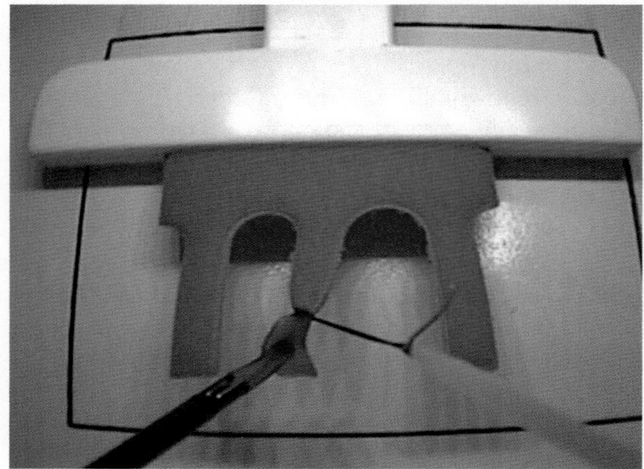

Fig. 5.4 Task 3: Placement and securing of ligating loop (endoloop) (Fundamentals of Laparoscopic Surgery® (FLS) Program is owned by Society of American Gastrointestinal and Endoscopic Surgeons and American College of Surgeons. Images used with permission)

This suturing task requires trainees to place a simple stitch through two marks in a longitudinally slit Penrose drain as shown in Fig. 5.5. Trainees are then required to tie the suture extra corporeally, using a knot-pushing device to slide the knot down. They must tie the knot tightly enough to close the slit in the drain, being careful not to avulse the drain off the foam block. At least three square throws are required to ensure that the knot will not slip under tension. The required proficiency score is 136 s with up to 1 mm accuracy error; no knot security errors (slippage) are allowed. Proficiency scores must be achieved on 2 consecutive repetitions and on 10 additional (nonconsecutive is acceptable) repetitions.

This suturing task requires trainees to place a suture precisely through two marks on a Penrose drain that has been slit along its long axis as shown in Fig. 5.6. Trainees are then required to tie the knot using an intracorporeal knot. They must place at least three throws that must include one double throw and two single throws on the suture and must also ensure the knots are square and won't slip. Between each throw

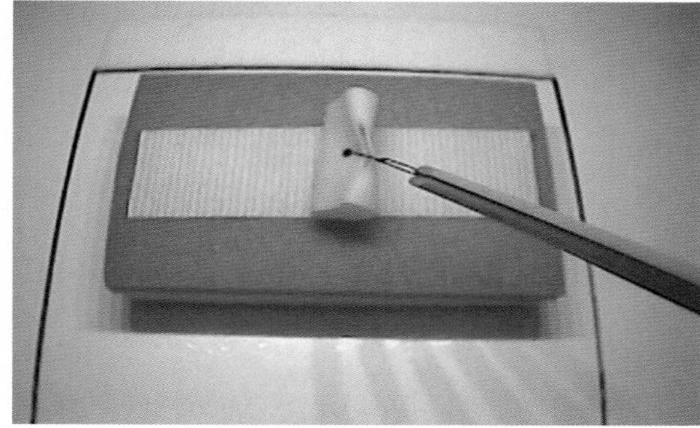

Fig. 5.5 Task 4: Simple suture with extracorporeal knot (Fundamentals of Laparoscopic Surgery® (FLS) Program is owned by Society of American Gastrointestinal and Endoscopic Surgeons and American College of Surgeons. Images used with permission)

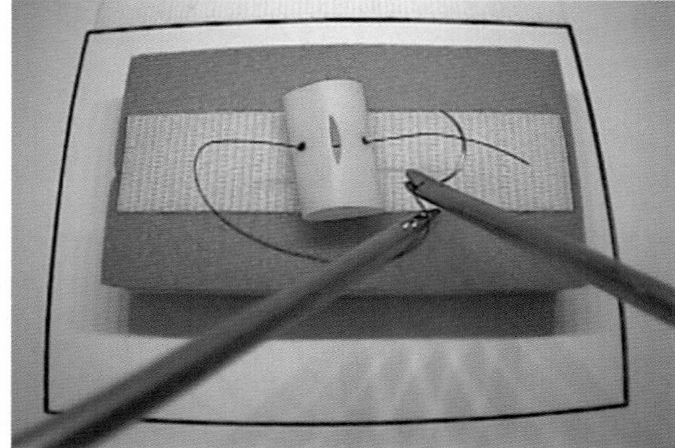

Fig. 5.6 Task 5: Simple suture with intracorporeal knot Fundamentals of Laparoscopic Surgery® (FLS) Program is owned by Society of American Gastrointestinal and Endoscopic Surgeons and American College of Surgeons. Images used with permission

trainees must transfer the needle to their other hand. Skills required include proper placement of the needle in the needle holder, needle transferring, suturing skills, and knot tying. A penalty is applied for any deviation of the needle from the marks, for any gap in the longitudinal slit in the drain and for a knot that slips when tension is applied to it. If the drain is avulsed from the block to which it is secured by VelcroTM, a score of zero will be applied. The required proficiency score is 112 s with up to 1 mm accuracy error; no knot security errors (slippage) allowed. Proficiency scores must be achieved on 2 consecutive repetitions and on 10 additional (nonconsecutive is acceptable) repetitions.

BLUS

The American Urological Association (AUA) stood on the shoulders of FLS to create BLUS, the Basics of Laparoscopic Urologic Surgery. As FLS was created to apply to all specialties who might utilize laparoscopic surgery, it purposefully avoids anatomic specificity. BLUS simply adds to FLS to make it more appropriate

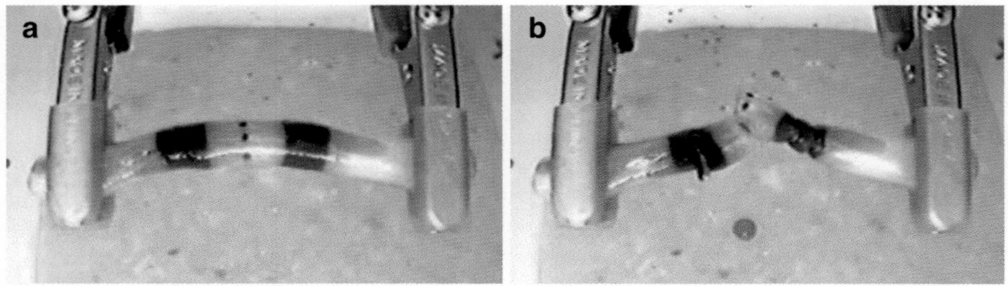

Fig. 5.7 BLUS renal artery clipping exercise before (**a**) and after (**b**) clipping

as a urologic training model by removing endoloop and extracorporeal knot-tying procedures, adding didactic material, and clip-applying exercise as well [9]. BLUS was designed by the Laparoscopic, Robotic, and New Surgical Technology (LRNST) Committee, with the renal artery model developed by the University of Minnesota Center for Research in Education and Simulation Technologies (CREST).

The renal artery module was made from organosilicate materials from CREST's human tissue database. Each 6 cm artery, pictured in Fig. 5.7, is filled with artificial blood and marked with two black lines for clip placement, then attached to a machine that simulates arterial pulsing. Surgeons were tasked with placing to clips on each side of the artery and cutting between the marks. Scores were decreased for improper clip placement, crossing clips, and leaking from the clips. The exercise illustrated evidence for face, content, concurrent, and convergent validity by Sweet et al. [9].

A later BLUS study found that all tasks showed evidence for construct validity when based on skill categories from their demographic survey, but only the peg transfer and suturing skill tasks earned construct validity when based on established objective metrics [10]. This discrepancy in construct validity, or how well a test can distinguish between skill levels, emphasizes how self- reporting values (as in the demographics questionnaire researchers presented consented subjects with) may be disappointingly inaccurate. The authors noted that some of the values reported were simply impossible (it isn't possible to do 2 procedures every week while simultaneously reporting 2 procedures per month). This analysis led them to a larger and even more concerning question: if subjects can't even accurately describe the number of cases they've done, will their reported performance benchmarks be any more reliable?

While the renal artery clipping exercise showed evidence for validity, it is not yet commercially available and must be assembled by hand. The proposed urology-specific didactic material is still currently being developed. As of yet, BLUS has yet to be implemented, but does look promising, and may serve as a model for other laparoscopic specialties to implement their own specific FLS-based training curricula.

Simulation

In order to enable rehearsal of the psychomotor skills unique to laparoscopic surgery, so-called box trainers, which consist of an inanimate physical task, placed inside an enclosed box with a lighted camera and instruments inserted from outside, have commonly been used. A variety of box trainers have been developed over the years, running a wide spectrum of technological complexity. The simplest can be constructed with a smartphone, a box, a video display screen, and some non-sterile or expired laparoscopic instruments (YouTube provides numerous demonstrations and instructions for building these), while the more advanced have sophisticated integrated cameras and realistic mimetic tissue models for procedural practice.

Virtual reality (VR) simulators have integrated metrics that grade each performance, whereas "dry lab" rehearsal relies on either self-evaluation or that of a proctor. Herein lies the problem – what is the basis of this assessment? Time to complete a task, as well as many overt errors such as instrument collisions, suture breakage, and drops, can be immediately and easily identified and quantified; however, detection and analysis of more subtle errors and techniques is increasingly difficult. With the addition of a trained observer, further skills such as keeping instruments in view of the camera, dissection and suturing patterns, and proper handoff techniques can be gauged. However, without extra hardware and software, box trainers lack the ability to track and analyze motion-based metrics such as path length and economy of motion, among other metrics important for successful surgery.

For laparoscopic surgery there are a multitude of VR trainers available, but not all record metrics of assessment in the same way. As one of the first medical simulators that recorded objective measures, the Minimally Invasive Surgical Trainer, Virtual Reality by Mentice Medical Simulation, MIST-VR emerged in the late 1990s as the forerunner of what would soon be a highly competitive and technologically advanced market. MIST-VR functioned with handles mimicking laparoscopic instruments attached to gimbals with motion information transferred to an adjacent computer and the monitor displaying relative VR instrument tips. Foot pedals could also be operated for simulated energy application.

Unlike the advanced modules seen on simulators today, MIST-VR made no attempt to create simulated tissues or surgical materials, like suture. Instead, MIST-VR required trainees to perform hand to hand transitions and object manipulation with a virtual ball. This could include instrument exchanges, diathermy application, and highly specific object placement tasks. The computer would log time duration of the exercise, any designated errors that occurred, and overall accuracy of the performance [11]. MIST-VR was intentionally not representative of a surgical environment as it was intended to be used for assessment rather than training [11].

Since MIST-VR, the medical industry has seen a surge in VR technology, producers of simulators, and growth in laparoscopic procedures. As a result, there are numerous laparoscopic VR simulators on the market with the ability to focus on both training and assessment. Only two will be discussed here; however a variety of other reputable options exist.

The LAP Mentor, by 3D systems (formerly Simbionix) is one such example. The latest iteration includes an adjustable height tower housing a 24″ touch screen monitor, PC with processor, and foot pedals. Operative tools include exchangeable instrument handles with haptic feedback and five degrees of freedom and a multi-angle endoscope. The LAP Mentor can be connected to other devices for team training, such as the LAP Express, a portable laparoscopic simulator, or the RobotiX Mentor, discussed below.

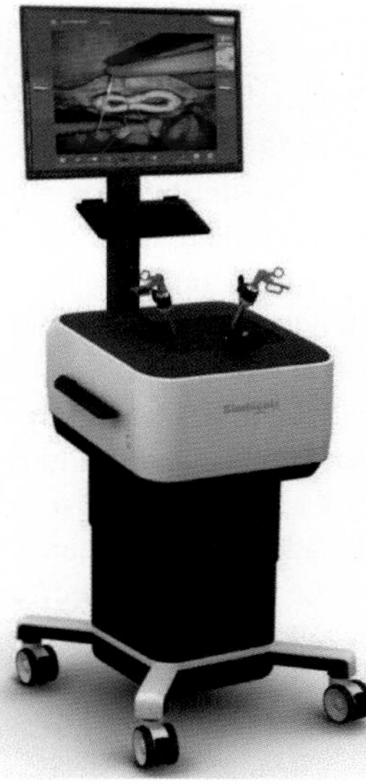

Fig. 5.8 LAP Mentor virtual reality simulator (Image courtesy of 3D Systems, formerly Simbionix)

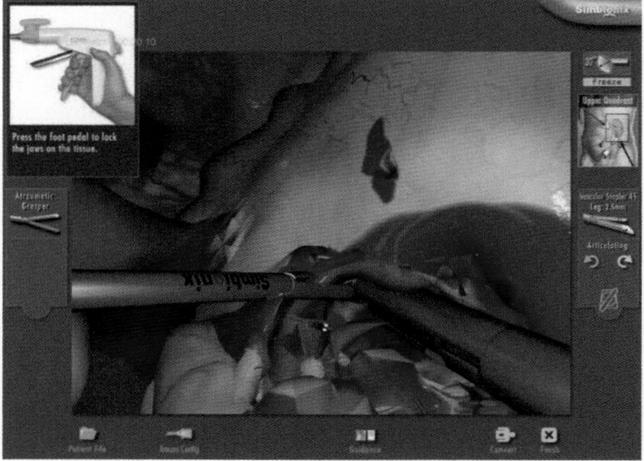

Fig. 5.9 Lap Mentor simulation illustrating use of unique instrumentation (Image courtesy of 3D systems, formerly Simbionix)

LAP Mentor, shown in Fig. 5.8, houses a wide panel of modules, from basic orientation tasks to simulated laparoscopic cases for multiple surgical specialties. Basic tasks include orientation, various levels of suturing practice, as well as tasks based on FLS modules such as peg transfer and circle cutting. More complex are the procedural exercises, cholecystectomy, cholangiography, appendectomy, incisional hernia, gastric bypass, sigmoidectomy, hysterectomy, vaginal cuff closure, and lobectomy. For gynecology, there are additional "essential" tasks, including tubal sterilization, salpingostomy, salpingectomy, and salpingo-oophorectomy. Figure 5.9 shows a sample screen for using a new tool in a procedure.

Once a module has been completed, an automatically generated performance report appears, illustrated in Figs. 5.10a, b. Metrics are defined for particular

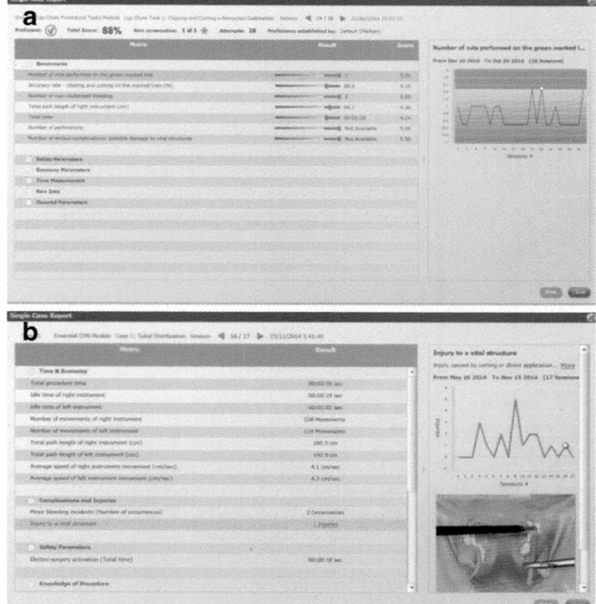

Fig. 5.10 Representative general (**a**) and detailed (**b**) metrics from Lap Mentor score sheet. Image courtesy of 3D systems, formerly Simbionix

simulations but include measures such as total procedure time, idle time in seconds, number of movements, total path length, and average speed individually for left and right instruments. Any task complications, such as bleeding or tissue damage, are also reported. Task-specific metrics would be seen for energy application, correct knots, etc. An attempt can be compared to those previously completed using the displayed learning curve.

The proficiency score board marks a check mark if the task reached proficient levels, as well as indicating the best score measured as a percentage, a star if the required number of consecutive or nonconsecutive attempts was made (this quantity is set by an administrator), total count of attempts, and the required skill level. Clicking on this reveals more refined information, such as total time, path length, accuracy, and additional task-specific metrics.

Benchmarks are set on a scale from 1 to 5. Less than 2 is noted as poor, between 2 and 4 average, with a 4 being the set proficient mark. Greater than 4 yields an expert, or even superior level when over 4.5. Benchmarks are only seen when metrics have a defined skill level. The scale is color coordinated, with poor and average scores being red and yellow, respectively, while scoring a 4 or higher shows green. Scores can be viewed and exported to a CSV file.

Another laparoscopic VR simulator that has demonstrated validity is the LapVR, created by CAE Healthcare of Sarasota, Florida. LapVR, similar to the Lap Mentor, is a single tower unit, with an internal computer, flat screen monitor, foot pedals, and exchangeable instrument grips. The simulated camera and instruments provide haptic feedback to the trainee.

LapVR has many modules available, catering to various skill levels. Most basic are the essential skills, with camera navigation, clip application, cutting, peg transfer, knot tying, and needle-driving exercises, each having several skill levels available. Trainees can then progress to procedural skills, rehearsing adhesiolysis, running the bowel, and varying suturing and knot-tying tasks.

Lap VR also has a number of full-length procedures catering to general and obstetrics/gynecology surgery, such as appendectomy, cholecystectomy, bilateral tubal occlusion, tubal ectopic pregnancy, and salpingo-oophorectomy. Each procedure has multiple cases available, with and individual patient histories, as well as notes on procedural perpetration and aftercare.

Once an exercise or case is complete, users can view the results tab. Results are tailored to the task at hand and are highly detailed. For example, completion of one of the appendectomy cases will be evaluated based on groupings of time, proficiency, dexterity, and use of virtual aid. Each of these contains detailed results. The time header carries information on the duration of the total procedure and energy application. The proficiency group details cc's of blood lost, number of clips placed, length of appendix stump, and adhesion removal, among others. Dexterity remarks on left- and right-hand path lengths, as well as errors like excessive force on tissue. Each result is directly compared to an acceptable score. If the two correlate, the user earns a green check mark adjacent to their result. If ever metric has a check, the result is labeled a successful completion. Reports can be viewed after completion and printed for external evaluation.

Several studies have demonstrated that virtual reality training translates to improved laparoscopic skills in the operating room [12–15]. However, the primary methods of assessment include supervision by trained instructors and documentation of the time required to perform standardized drills. Supervision by instructors is an inherently subjective method of assessment. It has also been demonstrated that time to completion is a poor metric for the objective assessment of laparoscopic task performance compared to analysis of accuracy [6, 16].

While early results suggest that VR simulators and video trainers such as the FLS have an important role to play in the determination of what constitutes surgical skill proficiency and how it is to be objectively assessed within training, further validation of the specific metrics used within these training systems is needed, particularly with respect to objectivity, and novel objective metrics are needed to enable accurate and reliable assessment of laparoscopic surgical skills training, proficiency, and decay/retention [17]. These metrics must demonstrate reliability, validity, practicality, and consistency with measures of high-quality surgery in the operating room in order to provide the basis for proficiency-based learning programs. [5] Proficiency-based training has been shown to result in laparoscopic skills that are durable up to 11 months and retention of such skills was also shown by Hiemstra, Kolkman, Van de Put, and Jansen (2009) to be durable for up to 1 year for three MIS-related tasks, similar to FLS tasks [18, 19]. However, these studies have relied primarily on subjective metrics for assessment.

Robotic-Assisted Laparoscopic Surgery Training and Assessment Platforms

Simulators

The da Vinci surgical robot (Intuitive Surgical, Sunnyvale, CA) is currently the most widely used surgical robot and is the only surgical robot approved for use in the United States by the Food and Drug Administration (FDA).

Intuitive Surgical Inc. (ISI) provides a four-step training pathway for the da Vinci. The first phase includes an online course, procedural video review, and robotic system in service guided by an ISI representative [20]. Prospective surgeons then proceed with skill development during phase two. Here, surgeons work to develop proficiency on critical skills, using multiple forms of simulation [20].Phase three works to introduce more advanced techniques and instrumentation to the developing robotic surgeon, as well as gaining experience as the bedside assistant in surgical cases [20]. By the fourth phase, surgeons will take on the role of console surgeon [20]. Each step has recommended time commitments, ideal scoring ranges, and case involvement.

Many hospitals and simulation centers also offer both wet and dry surgical training labs, which may be supported by personnel from ISI or external simulation companies and also by in-house simulation technicians. The majority of facilities will only house one simulator, but institutions specializing in training MIS techniques have the capacity to train in a group setting, demonstrated in Fig. 5.11.

Additionally, as with open surgery and laparoscopic surgery, junior robotic surgeons often perform partial procedures, with a senior surgeon observing and the option of performing more difficult parts of the procedure. The dual console

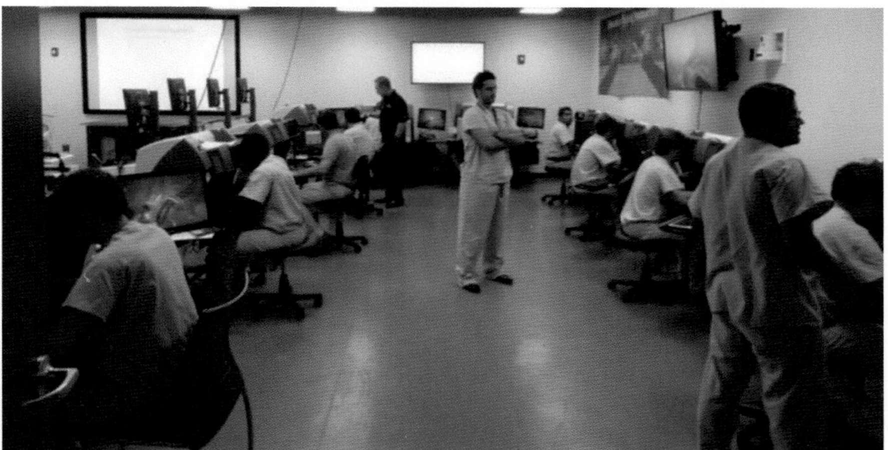

Fig. 5.11 Group simulation with Mimic dV-Trainer

capacity of the da Vinci offers unique opportunities of training while in the OR. When two consoles are available, both show the same image visualized by the patient cart's endoscope. Instruments can be handed back and forth between consoles, either one at a time or all three arms at once. The operative field can also be visualized from the surgical tower's 2D touchscreen. Any guiding telestration on the touchscreen will be visible in both consoles.

Mimic Technologies was the first to produce a robotic-specific box trainer, shown in Fig. 5.12. MLabs features three physical dry lab training modules, which are also replicated in VR on the dV-Trainer and dVSS VR simulators (described below): the Pick & Place, Matchboard1, and Pegboard1 tasks. All three represent basic robotic skills.

As with laparoscopic skills, assessing RALS dry labs can be difficult. Traditional laparoscopic box trainers may be better than nothing for low-fidelity simulation but lack the ability to judge and test depth perception that robotic surgery necessitates. The MLabs trainer has been successfully evaluated evidence in several validity constructs including usability (face), content, known-groups (construct), and concurrent validity by Ramos et al. [21] This trainer provides an objective and low-cost way to rehearse and assess robotic skills. This particular study was unique in that it assessed validity evidence not only for the physical tool for training but a broader evaluative one as well, discussed below.

There are several VR robotic simulators available on the market, each with their own charms and detriments, and numerous others on the fringes of entering the scene. So far, four simulators, each presented in Fig. 5.13, have demonstrated validity evidence as training tools for robotic surgery; the dV-Trainer by Mimic Technologies out of Seattle, WA; the da Vinci Skills Simulator from Intuitive in Sunnyvale, CA; the Robotic Skills Simulator through Simulated Surgical Skills LLC, Williamsville, NY; and the RobotiX mentor by 3D Systems in Littleton, CO. Each system has its own graded metrics, grading scale, and presentation of score.

The da Vinci Skills Simulator (dVSS or "backpack") is made by the same company that produces the da Vinci robot. Unlike other simulators, the dVSS is

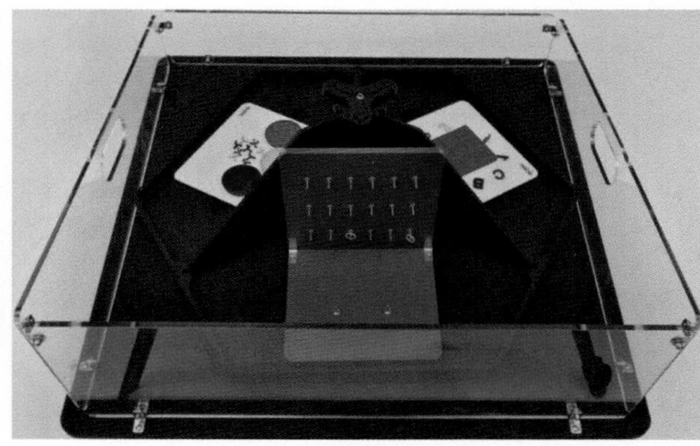

Fig. 5.12 MLabs box trainer

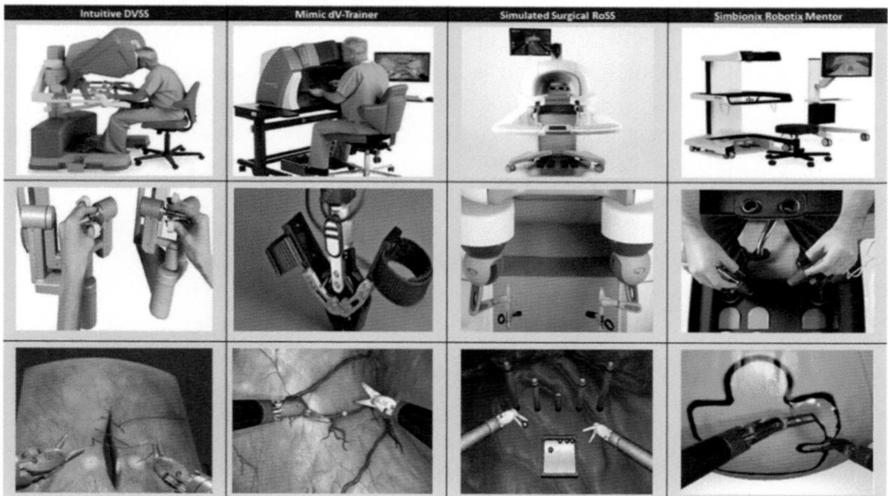

Fig. 5.13 Four robotic simulators, their controllers, and representative simulation

integrated into the robot's surgeon console, utilizing the master controllers, stereoscopic viewer, and foot pedals. The dVSS simply hooks onto the back of the console and connects to the console with the same cables used for integrating the robot in the OR.

Mimic developed most of the software available on the dVSS; as such the grading metrics are very similar to those found on the dV-Trainer. Originally they looked nearly identical, but upgrades to both simulators have caused them to diverge over time. The majority of exercises found on the dVSS target improvement of robotic handling and basic surgical skills, like transferring shapes from one hand to another, moving a ring along a wire, retracting a panel using the third arm, needle driving, and energy application.

Each attempt garners an overall percentage score, which is the summation of numerous weighted metrics, such as completion time, economy of motion, instrument collisions, excessive force, instruments out of view, master of workspace range, and additional exercise specific values, such as drops, broken vessels, blood loss, or misapplied energy. The majority of these scores are self- explanatory, but the economy of motion and master of workspace range earn some confusion. Economy of motion references instrument tip path length within the simulation, in centimeters. Master of workspace range is the radius of the master controller's motion from user manipulation in the physical environment. The distinction appears subtle but in reality can assess how effectively trainees are clutching their instruments and making hesitating or unnecessary movements. Clicking on each metric reveals a brief explanation of the score and weight.

The dVSS also houses a set of suturing exercises created by 3D systems. Each task is graded on time to complete, time efficiency, knot tying, and needle handling. Instead of a percentage score, for each metric, the trainee receives a green or red dot or a gold star. Clicking on each score opens a secondary score sheet with a more detailed explanation and key. These detailed reports can also be expanded to show descriptions of each metric as well as a color-coded scale marking the range of results.

Once the score sheet has been exited, it can be viewed again, upon any other exercise's completion. Metrics can also be compared over time by a bar graph on each score report.

Data can also be drawn from the dVSS using a USB memory drive and viewed on an external computer. With the skills simulator software, the drive must be wiped of data and prepared for data upload. Once the drive is plugged into the simulator, user data will automatically be copied over. Another method is to simply plug a blank drive into the simulator and under the administrator login and export user reports. This method will only show the number of attempts and highest score for each module.

Mimic Technologies has made their own simulator as well, featuring many of the same modules as the dVSS. The dV-Trainer is a standalone device that sits on an adjustable table with a panel of foot pedals below. Processing and navigation occur through an adjacent PC and monitor. Scores are automatically presented upon completion of a task. Each completion generates an overall percentage of success, which is a summation of individual metrics described above for the dVSS. The metrics graded are still dependent on the task (i.e., needle drops is a redundant score when there was no needle present). The dV-Trainer has a plethora of additional exercises not found on the dVSS, including full-length procedures with their Maestro-AR augmented reality software. Trainees can perform partial nephrectomies, inguinal hernia repairs, hysterectomies, and prostatectomies with VR instrumentation layered over actual 3D surgical video.

The Robotic Skills Simulator (RoSS) is also a standalone device. It looks similar to the surgeon console for the actual da Vinci but is slightly smaller. Whereas the dV-Trainer has utilized a tension-based system, RoSS uses standard linkage connections that simulate the master controller robotic arms. Simulated exercises for RoSS are independent from the dVSS or dV-Trainer and range from basic coordinating skills to full-length procedures. RoSS presents scores as a bar for each metric, which starts out red, but turns green when a certain level is reached.

RoSS was also designed to perform more holistic evaluations using Fundamental Skills of Robotic Surgery (FSRS) metrics. Four FSRS tasks are performed, with the safety in operative field, critical error, economy, bimanual dexterity, and time metrics weighted and averaged [22]. In general, metrics are scored as an amalgamation of camera movement, left and right tool grasps and number of times out of view, and any instrument collisions or drops. RoSS also allows for data export under the administrator login.

The final robotic simulator is also the most recently released. The RobotiX Mentor by is a standalone device that has several unique features. Most obviously, the simulated master controllers aren't under any tension – they're basically free floating – and are only connected by a cord on each side. Each metric is scored on a percentage, as with the dV-Trainer and most of the dVSS.

RobotiX Mentor metrics are in some ways more detailed than the other simulators, offering kinematic results such as left and right instrument as well as camera path length, the path length of instruments that traveled out of view, as well as total time, number of movements per right and left instrument, instrument collisions, and clutch usage.

Working at any of these simulators, it is usually clear if an attempt at a particular exercise went successfully or if it went poorly. It is not clear, unfortunately, what that success necessarily entailed or how that success correlates to success on a similar exercise on a different simulator.

Fundamentals of Robotic Surgery

The Fundamentals of Robotic Surgery (FRS) is a robotic surgical skills training and assessment program that was developed through a consensus conference involving subject matter experts from varied backgrounds including surgeons, medical educators, behavioral psychologists, and cognitive scientists. The goal of the development process for FRS was to develop a proficiency-based curriculum of basic technical skills on which surgeons could be trained and assessed in order to ensure that they have acquired the basic technical skills in robotic surgery before beginning training in RALS procedures across a wide range of specialties. The FRS curriculum in its current form is divided into four modules, including an introduction to surgical robotic systems, didactic instructions, psychomotor skills curriculum, and team training.

Training begins with a rigorous four-course online curriculum which focuses upon skills needed for performing surgical procedures. Although it does include some pre- and postoperative care beyond manual skills once the patient is in the confines of the operating floor, the main focus is upon all the technical skills from the time the patient enters the operating room until the patient leaves. In addition, it includes information on the physical robot component vernacular and identification, as well as emergency protocols and communication skills. The didactic component does not include basic surgical knowledge such as indications and contraindications, importance of comorbidities, postoperative complications, and nonsurgical complications; the training begins and ends at the operating room door.

Processes such as operating room arrangement, port and robotic arm placement, docking and undocking, and instrument operation are all presented. Each psychomotor exercise is introduced. The seven tasks that need to be completed and potential errors are presented. Each of the four courses is followed by a short quiz which requires a minimum of 70% correct to proceed. The entire curriculum has a larger, cumulative, cognitive test as well upon module completion.

FRS validation testing was done with both VR simulation using the dVSS and dV-Trainer, as well as a physical dome model, which was created using the identical VR exercises which are on both simulators. Each study group included the same seven psychomotor skill exercises; docking and instrument insertion, ring and rail transfer, knot tying, suturing, fourth arm cutting, puzzle piece dissection,

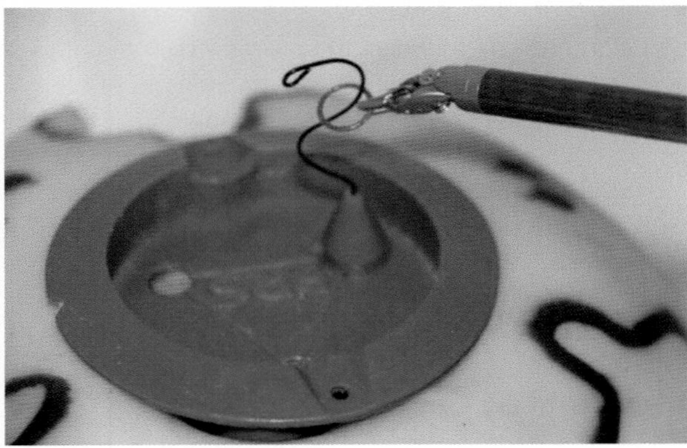

Fig. 5.14 FRS Task 1: Ring tower transfer. The trainee removes a ring from the top right middle tower and places it on the lower left side tower. Then the ring from the top left middle tower is removed and placed on the lower right side tower. *Primary skills*: eye-hand instrument coordination, camera navigation, use of camera pedal, and wristed instrument maneuvering. *Secondary skills*: wrist articulation and ambidexterity

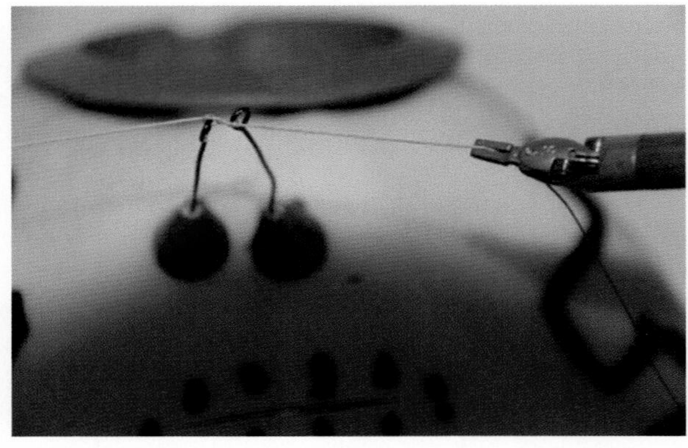

Fig. 5.15 FRS Task 2: Knot tying. The trainee ties a surgeon's knot to approximate the two eyelets such that they touch each other and then back up the knot with two more throws. *Primary skills*: appropriate handling of suture material and tying secure knots. *Secondary Skills***:** Wrist articulation, hand-eye instrument coordination, and ambidexterity

and vessel energy dissection. Six of the psychomotor skill tasks are described in Figs. 5.14, 5.15, 5.16, 5.17, 5.18, and 5.19 below. Each task had to be completed two consecutive times to the proficiency benchmark level. Proficiency was set to benchmark performances by expert surgeons, which were determined independently for each task of each simulator (i.e., the number of errors that were the benchmark score on VR simulators and the physical dome varied for each exercise, as per the expert performances). Visual representations of the same six exercises are seen in Fig. 5.20.

The validation trial of the psychomotor skills included pre- and post-tests with avian tissue models, evaluated with both a numeric metric checklist by the proctor and a video analysis of both the checklist and a GEARS scoring. In the future, an advanced fundamentals of specialty-specific basic skills have been (and others will be) developed by the 12 participating specialties.

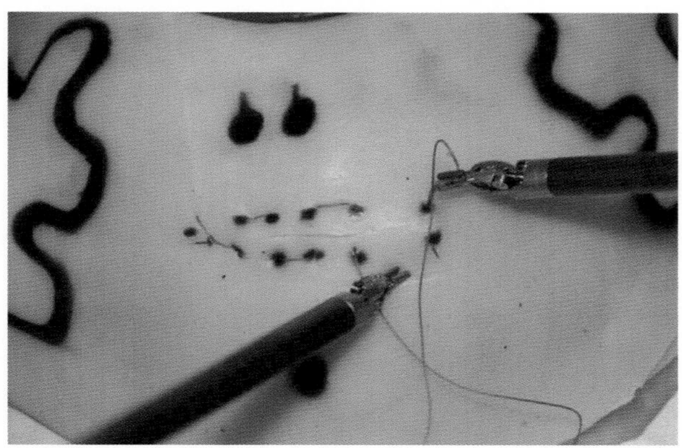

Fig. 5.16 FRS Task 3: Railroad track. The trainee must perform horizontal mattress suturing through a series of target points to approximate the tissue, followed by anchoring the needle by passing it through the final two target points twice. *Primary skills*: holding and manipulation of the needle, following the curve of the needle, utilizing the full range of motion of the endowrist, and using graspers. *Secondary skills*: eye-hand instrument coordination, passing objects between instruments, appropriate handling of suture material, and running suture

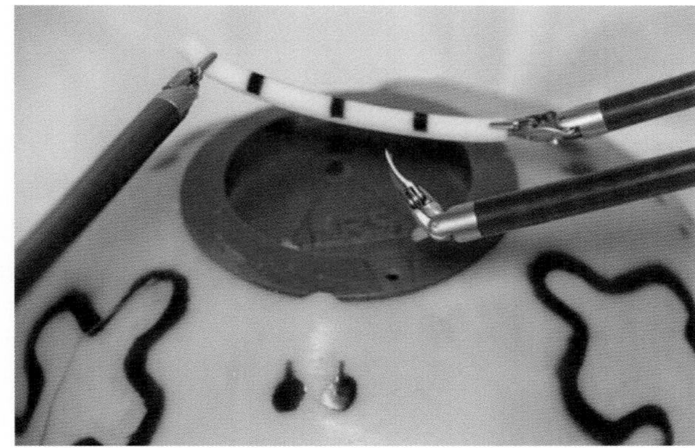

Fig. 5.17 FRS Task 4: Third arm cutting. The trainee must switch control between different instruments to use the monopolar scissors to cut the vein transversely at the hash marks. *Primary skills*: switching between and controlling multiple arms and cutting. *Secondary skills*: atraumatic handling of tissue and eye-hand instrument coordination

FRS was designed with the agreement of the various surgical specialties that each specialty would develop an advanced, specialty-specific FRS which emphasized the basic skills unique to their specialty that was not common to all specialties (and therefore not included in the FRS) – for example, clipping and stapling were not included in FRS because all of the specialties did not use surgical clips or staples.

Development within the gynecologic branch, FRGS has already been completed and that for thoracic surgeons is under development. While many of the skills critical to safe and effective robotic handling are constant across different specialties, the actual procedures vary widely. Proposed additions to FRGS include VR simulation-based training on the dissection of the bladder flap, the colpotomy incisions, the closure of the vaginal cuff, and the dissection of the ureter.

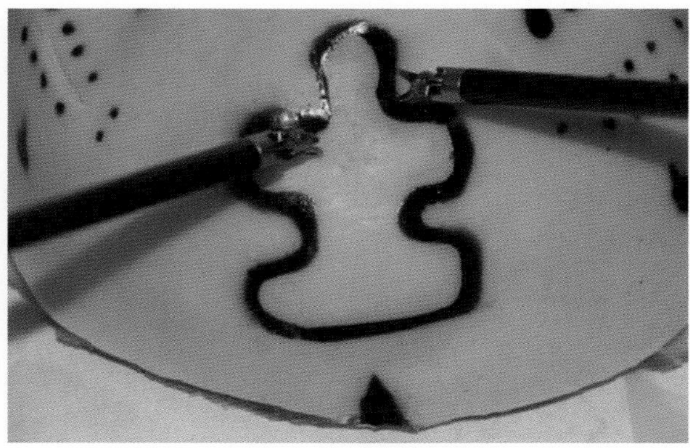

Fig. 5.18 FRS Task 5: Puzzle piece dissection. In this task, the trainee must cut the puzzle piece pattern between the lines without incising the underlying tissue or cutting outside of the lines. *Primary skills*: dissection, cutting, atraumatic tissue handling, and sharp and blunt dissection. *Secondary skills*: eye-hand instrument coordination and wrist articulation

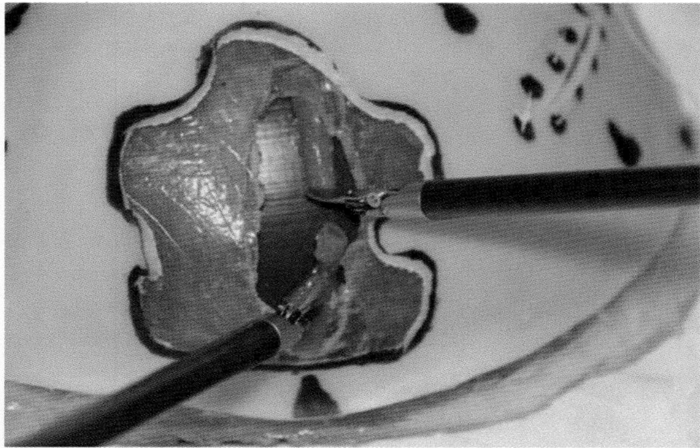

Fig. 5.19 FRS Task 6: Vessel energy dissection. The trainee must dissect through the fat layer to expose the vessel then coagulate the vessel at two points and finally cut the vessel between the two coagulated points. *Primary skills*: accurate activation and use of energy sources, dissection of vessels and tissues, cutting and coagulation of vessels, and multiple arm control. *Secondary skills*: atraumatic tissue handling and eye-hand instrument coordination

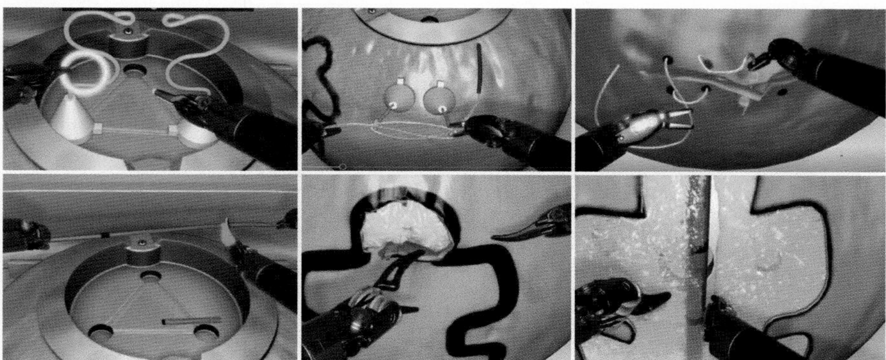

Fig. 5.20 FRS modules from dVSS

MIS Assessment Methods and Metrics

Da Vinci Application Programming Interface

The da Vinci robot stores vast amount of user information, but in a "black box" of proprietary algorithms and inaccessible data, both raw and processed. There is currently no way, as with the simulators, to download operative data to an external drive.

The da Vinci's application programming interface (API) is a bridge between this data and the outside world. Live information can be streamed through an Ethernet connection to another computer containing kinematic data of the user. This data includes how the patient cart joint angles were set up, how the master controllers are positioned and moved, Cartesian positions of the master controllers, patient side instruments and endoscope, and velocity of the master controllers and patient side joints. Any actions taken by the surgeon at the console are also saved, including data from the head sensor trigger, and standby and ready button usage, as well as master clutch, camera control, and arm swap pedals.

API data is not openly available. Those who are interested in using it must first enter a legal agreement with ISI. The agreement defines liability and intellectual property rights and is only awarded if specific conditions are met. Intuitive requires that research is designed for long-term results that is cohesive with current internal research, that the researchers have experience with the tasks at hand and work in a supportive clinical environment, and that the researchers and clinic can communicate effectively [23]. Only then will the API interface be activated, and onsite training by intuitive on how to best utilize the resource can proceed.

API motion data is transferred over a frequency ranging from 10 to 100 Hz at 334 different data measurements. This massive amount of information can be utilized in a number of ways for skills analysis [23].

Kumar et al. employed the API to quantify expert proficiency and differentiation from nonexpert task completion by measuring master controller movement while instruments were clutched [24]. In doing so, they measured only operative skills. Operative skills are those involved with how the operator (surgeon) interacts with the machine (robot). Typical Halsteadian training focuses instead on procedural skills (like suturing) or the surgical technique. By eliminating measurement of other skills, they were able to directly assess how a person was utilizing the technology, rather than their overall adeptness at surgery.

The data measured from master movement during clutching were translated into a vector with a Cartesian position plot. Analysis of the vectors led to 87–100% accuracy in identifying expert and nonexpert trainees [24]. Setting thresholds on the vector values noted at expert values for trainees would ensure an objective and quantifiable means of assessment for robotic operational skills. The assessment could even take place without interfering with other training or clinical schedules, as the API is integrated into the da Vinci system with minimal additional hardware.

Da Vinci's API can do more than assess proficiency. Several teams have used the technology to analyze what movements define a particular task. Lin et al. asked what discrete and fundamental motions (or "surgemes") make up a simple vertical suturing task [25]. They found eight surgemes for each throw with the needle, but not all of the eight were utilized by every surgeon [25]. For example, a surgeon would not need to tighten the suture after a throw with their left hand and their right hand. Knowing which surgemes are distinctive to training level would help to model a truly proficient surgeon. As this study only tested one expert and one intermediate surgeon (albeit over a number of trials), the definition cannot be made yet.

An important note is that the API's data stream is only one way. Data moves from the robot to an external computer, never the opposite direction.

ProMIS

ProMIS is a surgical simulator with known validity evidence for laparoscopy but can be adapted for assessing robotic performance by punching an extra hole in the simulated abdomen and adding tracking tape to da Vinci instruments [26]. Already equipped with optical tracking software and objective performance metrics, ProMIS proved readily adaptable to robotic applications. ProMIS had already been documented to show validity evidence as a laparoscopic training tool, and as such was a useful benchmark in assessing how VR simulators (like the dV-Trainer or da Vinci Skill Simulator) can train surgeons.

A primary challenge in RALS training as it currently exists is that there is not yet an established "gold standard." Therefore, VR simulators may be useful devices, but without a baseline to which their progress can be compared, data showing user improvements isn't as elucidating as it could be. McDonough et al. sought to resolve this problem using ProMIS, pictured docked to the da Vinci below in Fig. 5.21. They were able to confirm evidence for face, content, and construct validity for the

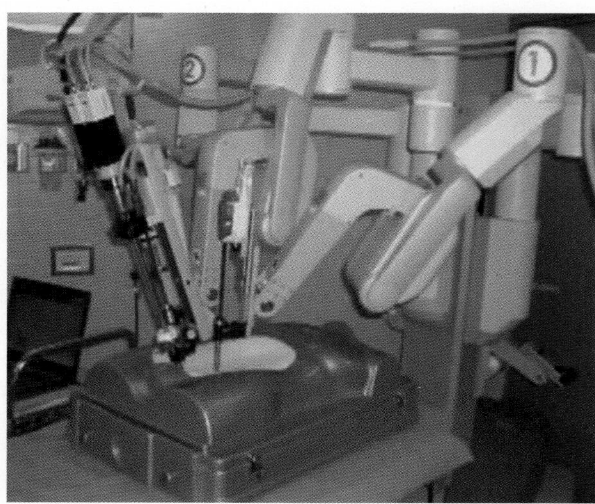

Fig. 5.21 ProMIS simulator with docked da Vinci [27]

da Vinci-ProMIS interface as well as proposing that ProMIS be instated as a regular form of robotic training at the institution [26].

ProMIS was found to have known-groups validity again by Jonsson et al., by comparison of novice and experts during four tasks [28]. Required exercises included stretching rubber bands, dissecting a shape, suturing and knot tying, and an anastomosis. Researchers compared path length, duration, and evenness in movement. Path length did not exhibit statistical significance, but the other two factors did [28].

ProMIS is advantageous to box trainers in that it generates objectively measured metrics such as time, efficiency of motion, and path length. Blatant errors, such as instrument collisions or incorrect cuts, were added in as a penalty by an observer. Together, these metrics cover most of what is assessed using a VR simulator.

Motion Tracking Sensors

Another means of collecting data on tool paths and economy of motion includes the use of electromagnetic or optical monitoring systems. Generally, a small marker is placed on the tool tip that needs to be monitored, while a larger device generates an electromagnetic field. There are several brands available.

One such device is the trakSTAR Tool Tip Trackers, by Ascension Technology Corporation in Burlington, VT, visualized in Fig. 5.22. Utilization of three-dimensional electromagnetic transponder and trackers allows for generation of a complete Cartesian position. Tausch et al. showed that novice, and expert surgeon's

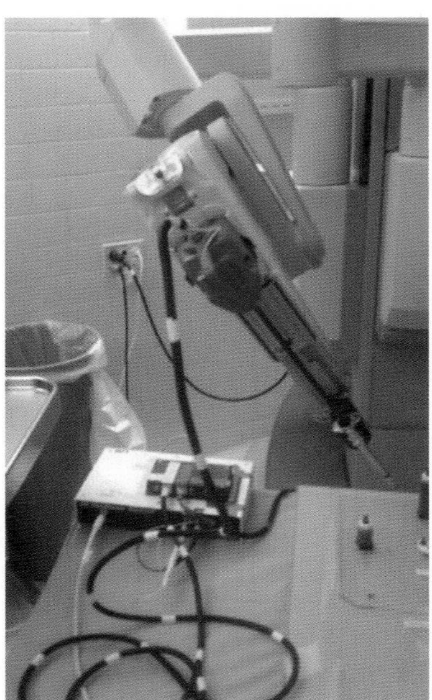

Fig. 5.22 da Vinci training instrument fitted with trakSTAR tool tip tracker [27]

plots look remarkably different, in that the expert surgeon has condensed and concise movements, whereas the novice generates an amorphous heap of unnecessary motion [29]. The trakSTAR system costs around $4000 and is easily attached to da Vinci tools or other laparoscopic instruments.

Using the FLS block transfer and intracorporeal suturing tasks as well as a novel ring tower exercise, time (s), path length (cm), and economy of motion (cm/s) were tested using trakSTAR technology. In all areas the experienced surgeon scored better than the novices, and the generated position plots demonstrated why. Graphs plotting instrument tip paths in Fig. 5.23a, b illustrate how the expert surgeon can distinguish left- and right-hand motions to their respective sides of the given task, as well as minimizing excessive or unnecessary motions. The expert was shown to have clean, distinct motion depictions, while novices have a cloud of extraneous movement. Experts also utilize less three-dimensional space than the novices are able to, marking greater precision with their instruments [29].

Other trackers that have been utilized for laparoscopic techniques include AURORA from Northern Digital Inc., Ontario, Canada, which functions with an electromagnetic field like trakSTAR but is a smaller system, and TrENDO, from Delft University of Technology, Delft, the Netherlands, which is only an optical tracker. TrENDO is a two-axis three-sensor gimbal device [30]. The instrument is inserted through the sensors, which can then measure four degrees of freedom. Information about the motions is transferred across 100 Hz. The setup is bulkier than other options and is integrated into the box trainer itself.

Data from tracker systems such as these is useful but requires some vector analysis for the information to have any meaning. They also can only be used on a box trainer, never applied to a clinical setting, severely limiting when assessment can occur. Trackers also fail to grade the quality of the surgeon's work. Things like incorrect knots, broken suture, missed cuts, and instrument collisions must either be counted by an observer or forsaken.

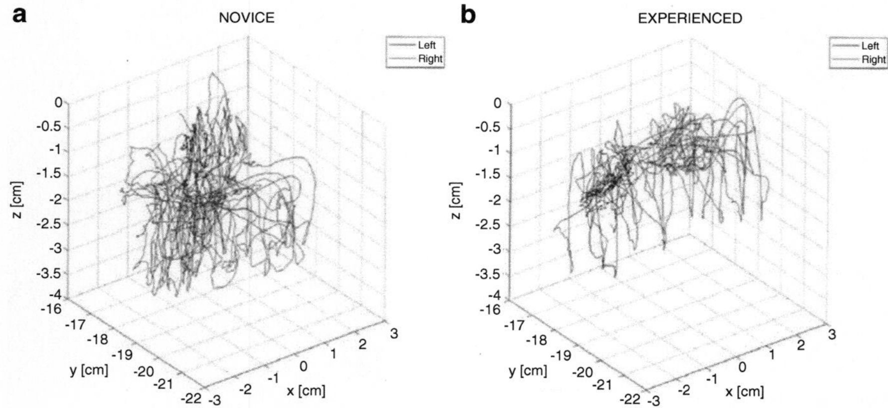

Fig. 5.23 3D Cartesian coordinates of novice (**a**) and expert (**b**) robotic tool tips during FLS block transfer task plotted from trakSTAR system [29]

Some simulators have integrated tracking capabilities, such as the Electronic Data Generation for Evaluation (EDGE) device by the Simulab Corporation out of Seattle, WA, shown with the FLS peg transfer task in Fig. 5.24a, b. EDGE utilizes six sensors to measure exercise duration, path length, rotation, and force used on the instruments in reality-based simulation. Depending on the goal of a particular training session, different tasks can be placed in the trainer. Comparison of expert and novice tool tip paths with EDGE in Fig. 5.25a, b appears similarly to those measured with trakSTAR; dominating features are left- and right-hand distinctions as well as discrete instrument paths traveled [10, 17].

The haptic forces measured by EDGE can also distinguish between experts and novices. The plots below (Fig. 5.26a, b clearly illustrate that novice surgeons use more force and more frequently. This data is inherently valuable, as excessive force can cause irreparable tissue damage during operative procedures).

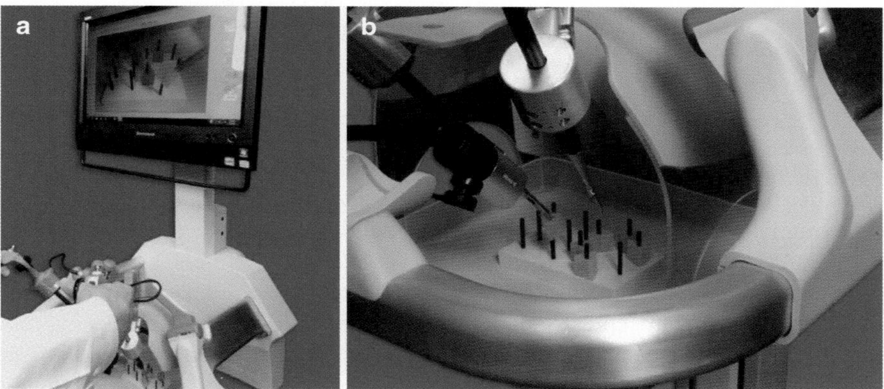

Fig. 5.24 (**a**, **b**) Simulab EDGE laparoscopic simulator

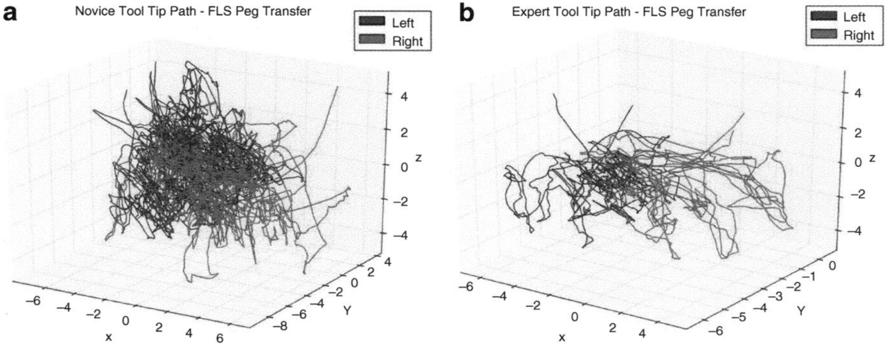

Fig. 5.25 Novice (**a**) and expert (**b**) instrument tip path during FLS peg transfer [27]

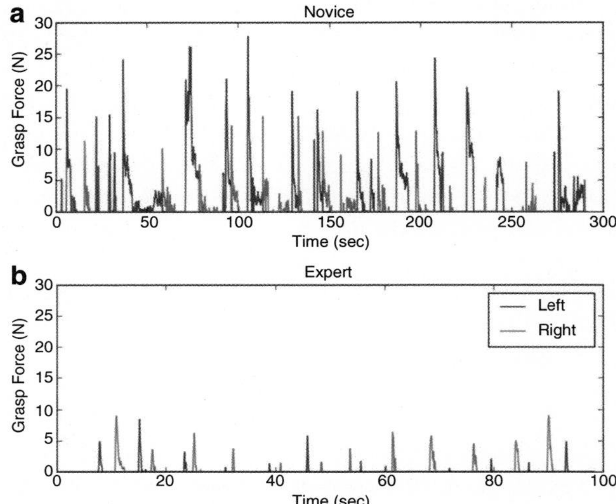

Fig. 5.26 Novice (**a**) and expert (**b**) grasp force over time during FLS peg transfer [27]

Idle Time

While previous work has demonstrated that motion-based metrics provide reliable and objective measures of surgical skill components [4], periods of nonmovement (idle time) have been largely ignored. Recent surgical skills research has identified a novel metric that focuses on periods during surgical task performance in which the hands are not moving: idle time. Idle time is characterized as, "a lack of movement of both hands and may represent periods of motor planning or decision making that can be used to differentiate performance" [31]. Specifically, idle time may reflect momentary pauses in task performance related to underlying cognitive, perceptual, and psychomotor skill components. Preliminary analyses applying idle time as a metric to existing data sets have revealed promising correlations between idle time characteristics and independent variables such as level of expertise and task difficulty.

Idle time as a metric of surgical assessment was initially defined through a conference-based consensus effort of surgical trainers who were members of the crucial surgical societies and boards responsible for the education, training, and certification of surgeons [10]. Subsequently, this metric has been quantified using tool/hand motion data and has been used to stratify surgical skills [5, 11–15]. This metric has been successfully used in analysis of performance on a suturing board [5] dataset and assessment of performance in 5 of 10 needle insertion during subclavian central line placement [15]. With these intriguing, preliminary results, further exploration of "idle time" within surgeon speech is warranted as this potentially may indicate cognitive overload, particularly in the case of novices.

More recently, Crochet et al. included a measure of idle time as one of several metrics in an evaluation of the validity of a laparoscopic hysterectomy (LH) module using the Lap Mentor VR simulator [32]. However, Crochet et al. refer to idle time as being "nonproductive" time, and, specifically, "total time the movements of the instruments do not make tissue contact" [32]. While this study only assessed total idle time and did not examine the temporal location or duration of each idle event, it succeeded in demonstrating initial construct validity of the idle time metric. Significant (p=0.0001) differences in idle time were reported for each of the three experience levels 8 experienced (M = 357 s), 8 intermediate (M = 654 s), and 24 inexperienced surgeons (M = 747 s) [32]. It is worth noting that idle time is a relatively new metric that appears on few of the currently available VR simulators.

Global Rating Scales

OSATS

The objective structured assessment of technical skill (OSATS) was one of the first assessments to utilize a global rating scale, which became widely accepted for evaluating surgical residents during open procedures. Along with a global rating scale represented in Table 5.1, OSATS also includes a detailed checklist. Checklists are procedure specific and individually validated for each additional evaluated surgery.

The global rating scale was first validated for an inferior vena cava repair necessitated by a stab wound, on both a bench trainer and live porcine model [33]. The global ratings scale outperformed the checklist in consistency between models (box trainer and animate porcine tissue) [33]. An outcome of this is that MIS-specific objective assessment tools are based on the global ratings scale portion of OSATS, to be discussed later.

However, more recent research shows that the checklist may be a more valuable tool than initially thought. Checklists have defined yes or no answers and are thus designed to have low ambiguity, making it easier for studies to establish interrater reliability [34]. Direct comparison of checklists and global rating scales shows that interrater reliability was significantly higher for the checklist evaluations, though this study was disadvantaged by having only two raters [34].

Presented above is the global ratings scale from OSATS. Each metric is graded with a numeric anchored Likert scale. Rensis Likert, a psychologist at the University of Michigan in the mid-1900s, developed the Likert scale as a way to uniformly test people's attitudes toward a subject. There are several qualifications to being a Likert scale. Firstly, they must have multiple metrics that are being graded. A Likert scale is said to be anchored by using labeled integers as the score for each item. Descriptions of the score must be arranged symmetrically and evenly. Summing the scores generates the overall score, though they can be averaged. OSATS, and the other global ratings scales we'll discuss here, only anchor points 1, 3, and 5, which does give the assessor slightly more freedom.

Note that use of assistants metric is not critical, or even relevant in some procedures, and thus this metric is frequently absent. Depending on the task at hand, assessors add in metrics such as suture handling or scales of overall performance and quality of final product, which are not found on the original global ratings scale [35]. Martin's original scale also included a final pass/fail question, though this was lost in later versions due to poor reliability [33].

Table 5.1 OSATS

Respect for time	1 Frequently used unnecessary force on tissue or caused damage by inappropriate use of instruments	2	3 Careful handling of tissue but occasionally caused inadvertent damage	4	5 Consistently handled tissues appropriately with minimal damage
Time and motion	1 Many unnecessary moves	2	3 Competent use of instruments although occasionally appeared stiff or awkward	4	5 Economy of movement and maximum efficiency
Instrument handling	1 Repeatedly makes tentative or awkward moves with instruments	2	3 Competent use of instruments although occasionally appeared stiff or awkward	4	5 Fluid moves with instruments and no awkwardness
Knowledge of instruments	1 Frequently asked for the wrong instrument or used an inappropriate instrument	2	3 Knew the names of most instruments and used appropriate instrument for the task	4	5 Obviously familiar with the instruments required and their names
Use of assistants	1 Consistently placed assistants or failed to use assistants	2	3 Good use of assistants most of the time	4	5 Strategically used assistant to the best advantage at all times
Flow of operation and forward planning	1 Frequently stopped operating or needed to discuss next move	2	3 Demonstrated ability for forward planning with steady progression of operative process	4	5 Obviously planned course of operation with effortless flow from one move to the next
Knowledge of specific procedure	1 Deficient knowledge. Needed specific instruction at most operative steps	2	3 Knew all important aspects of the operation	4	5 Demonstrated familiarity with all aspects of the operation

Adapted from Martin et al. [33]

OSATS is thorough but demands extensive time and resources from both the examiners and examinees. The question changed from how to evaluate technical skills to how to efficiently evaluate technical skills. Issues also arise from potential examiner bias. Instructors grading their own students are motivated to give students higher scores in order to reflect well on themselves, even inadvertently. Blinding is impossible unless the procedure is recorded and evaluated later (see section "C-SATS").

OSATS was created with open surgical skills in mind but served as a platform for later MIS-specific objective measures.

GOALS

For the most part, OSATS has held up well for evaluating technical skills in open procedures but needed adaption for minimally invasive procedures. There are any number of global rating scales for MIS but few that could be used universally for the huge variety of surgical skills and presentations seen in MIS. Take, for example, ORCS, the objective component rating scale for a Nissen fundoplication. It is a validated and reliable tool, but only for one particular surgery, and only during operative procedures [36].

The result was Global Operative Assessment of Laparoscopic Skills (GOALS) [37]. While similar to OSATS with different metrics graded on Likert scale from 1 to 5, GOALS clearly tests different factors, confirmed in Table 5.2. Depth perception is certainly an aspect in open procedures but is compounded and vastly more complicated when viewing an image generated by a monocular endoscope. OSTATS tested time and motion, and in GOALS this is more clearly outlined under the "efficiency" metric while blended with the original "flow of operation." Bimanual dexterity is critical to MIS – and as such has earned its own metric. OSATS's "respect for tissue" translates to "tissue handling" but is asking the same question. Similarly, "knowledge of specific procedure" becomes the similar "autonomy" grade, which inquires how well the procedure was performed without outside aid [37].

To test GOALS, researchers compared the prospective global scale against a procedure-specific ten-item checklist and two 10 cm visual analogue scales (VAS). The VAS asked raters to place a mark on the line for the degree of difficulty, ranging from "extremely easy" to "extremely difficult" and overall competence extending from "maximum guidance" to "fully competent" [37]. The checklist could not differentiate skill level, was only applicable to a laparoscopic cholecystectomy, and had poor interrater reliability. The VAS similarly failed between proctors but did have construct validity. Overall, there was no added benefit to adding in the checklist or VAS, as such they were excluded from the final version of GEARS. Vassilou suggested that the VASs were too lenient, and the checklists too rigid, but that the global ratings scale fell somewhere in the middle [37].

The transition from OSATS to GOALS has proven to be a consistent one. Dual analysis of novice laparoscopic surgeons reveals high correlation between OSATS and GOALS scores [38].

GOALS have achieved evidence for construct validity several times over. Gumbs et al. showed that novice and experienced residents can accurately be differentiated from each other using GOALS during laparoscopic cholecystectomy and laparoscopic appendectomy procedures [39]. Experienced surgeons (PGY 5–6) consistently outperformed novice surgeons (PGY 1–3) with statistical significance during laparoscopic cholecystectomy and laparoscopic appendectomy procedures [39]. On a finer scale, GOALS could distinguish even between novice and graduating surgical fellows [40].

In the Gumbs study, attending surgeons completed GOALS as part of each case's operative note, with the scale automatically generated. This method not only

Table 5.2 GOALS

Depth perception	1 Constantly overshoots target, wide swings, slow to correct	2	3 Some overshooting or missing of target but quick to correct	4	5 Accurately directs instruments in the correct plane to target
Bimanual dexterity	1 Uses only one hand, ignores nondominant hand, poor coordination between hands	2	3 Uses both hands but does not optimize interaction between hands	4	5 Expertly uses both hands in a complimentary manner to provide optimal exposure
Efficiency	1 Uncertain, inefficient efforts; many tentative movements; constantly changing focus or persisting without progress	2	3 Slow but planned movements are reasonably organized	4	5 Confident, efficient, and safe conduct; maintains focus on task until it is better performed by the way of an alternative approach
Tissue handling	1 Rough movements, tears tissue, injures adjacent structures, poor grasper control, grasper frequently slips	2	3 Handles tissues reasonably well, minor trauma to adjacent tissue (i.e., occasional unnecessary bleeding or slipping of the grasper)	4	5 Handles tissues well, applies appropriate traction, negligible injury to adjacent structures
Autonomy	1 Unable to complete entire task, even with verbal guidance	2	3 Able to complete task safely with moderate guidance	4	5 Able to complete task independently without prompting

Adapted from Vassilou et al. [37]

contributed to a large number of cases to evaluate (51 laparoscopic cholecystectomies and 43 laparoscopic appendectomies) but is an easily sustainable way for an institution to collect GOALS.

One potential flaw with this method of assessment is lack of blinding. Attending surgeons completing GOALS for their residents would certainly know who they were and be subject to their own biases about both the person and procedure in question. Particularly in situations where remediation is being considered, unbiased and objective assessment could be a valuable tool. A solution is blinded video review by high-performing laparoscopic surgeons. In a direct comparison of blinded video review and direct observation, studies established that it is possible but have highlighted the necessity of evaluator training [41, 42].

An interesting question, and one that presented itself uniquely for GOALS though is likely evident in other global ratings scales, was if any of the metrics were more discriminating than the others. Watanabe et al. found that by utilizing item response theory, they were able to calculate which aspects of GOALS are more difficult over an impressive 12-year time period with a total of 396 evaluations [43]. These metrics included the bimanual dexterity, efficiency, and autonomy items and were also found to show nonlinear regression in achieving marks on the higher side of the scales. This means that not only are certain aspects more difficult but that it is increasingly more difficult to earn a higher score the further to the right on the global rating scale one goes [43].

GEARS

Robotic-assisted surgery comes with new challenges for robotic-assisted surgery and thus for assessment. At the present, there isn't technology to support haptic feedback during robotic-assisted surgery, though this will likely be changing shortly. As a consequence, gaining skill in force sensitivity and robotic handling are critical, yet tricky, businesses that differentiate robotic from laparoscopic surgery. Another distinguishing skill is addition of 3D stereoscopic visualization, compared to laparoscopies 2D endoscopes.

To generate the means of assessing these differences, Goh and his team based a global ratings scale off of GOALS that measured robotic-specific skills, pictured below in Table 5.3 [44].

Since GEARS' development it has undergone extensive validation. Evidence of construct validity has been shown many times over by various studies [21, 44–47], as well as face, content, and concurrent validity [21]. The majority of GEARS research has been done with in vivo cases, though construct validity has also extended to dry lab simulation [21]. Interrater reliability has also been illustrated, across a number of different grading groups.

Nabhani et al. took GEARS further with evaluations on surgeons immediately after robotic prostatectomies and robotic partial nephrectomies [48]. They took a slightly different approach to completing evaluations, using faculty, fellows, residents, and surgical technicians. The findings were not surprising; surgeons with higher levels of experience had better correlation than the other groups, particularly resident self-evaluations and the surgical technicians. Overall though, GEARS performed well as an assessment for live surgery [48].

GEARS not only can be utilized for evaluating skills acquisition during surgery or dry lab rehearsal but also for assessing progress during dry lab or VR robotic simulation and for full-length procedures [46, 49]. All VR simulators utilize varying metrics to grade performance, but GEARS can be used as a baseline score generator to compare viability as a training tool for the different devices.

C-SATS

Crowd sourcing is a plausible solution to the notoriously long wait times for expert review. In a study evaluating possible means of scoring BLUS tasks and earlier robotic attempts at FLS modules, researchers found that Amazon.com's Mechanical Turks could rate exercises as well as both expert reviewers and motion capture technology [50, 51]. (Why Turks? The story goes the Napoleon Bonaparte, brilliant

Table 5.3 GEARS

Depth perception	1 Constantly overshoots target, wide swings, slow to correct	2	3 Some overshooting or missing of target but quick to correct	4	5 Accurately directs instruments in the correct plane to the target
Bimanual dexterity	1 Uses only one hand, ignores nondominant hand, poor coordination	2	3 Uses both hands but does not optimize interaction between hands	4	5 Expertly uses both hands in a complementary way to provide best exposure
Efficiency	1 Inefficient efforts; many uncertain movement constantly changing focus or persisting without progress	2	3 Slow but planned movements are reasonably organized	4	5 Confident, efficient, and safe conduct; maintains focus on task, fluid progression
Force Sensitivity	1 Rough moves, tears tissue, injuries nearby structures, poor control frequent suture breakage	2	3 Handles tissues reasonably well, minor trauma to adjacent tissue, rare suture breakage	4	5 Applies appropriate tension, negligible injury to adjacent structures, no suture breakage
Autonomy	1 Unable to complete entire task, even with verbal guidance	2	3 Able to complete task safely with moderate guidance	4	5 Able to complete task independently without prompting
Robotic Control	1 Consistently does not optimize view, hand position, or repeated collisions even with guidance	2	3 View is sometimes not optimal. Occasionally needs to relocate arms; occasional collisions and obstruction of assistant	4	5 Controls camera and hand position optimally and independently. Minimal collisions or obstruction of assistant

Adapted from Goh et al [44].

strategist and chess player, was beaten at the game by an 1800s version of a robot, painted and dressed to look Turkish. The defeat was of course not from artificial intelligence but from man, one who would puppeteer the device while hidden inside).

Mechanical Turks complete Human Intelligence Tasks (HITs) for pay; some are very simple and only earn a few pennies, and others require specific skill and can earn several dollars. HITS are approved by the agency requesting the task, and each workers approval rating can be viewed before they are hired for a task.

Crowd-sourcing videos of surgeons performing dry lab or operative procedures is becoming an increasingly popular means of evaluating training regimes. The first to do so, Chen et al. took videos from a previous study, which filmed surgeons performing Fundamentals of Laparoscopic Surgery tasks using the da Vinci robot [52]. 501 Amazon.com crowd workers and 110 Facebook users were selected as the crowdsourced reviewers, and ten expert robotic surgeons were recruited for the control group. All participants reviewed the same video and completed only three domains of GEARS to grade: depth perception, bimanual dexterity, and efficiency. Facebook users and experts received no compensation; the Mechanical Turks received $1.00 per HIT.

Crowed sourced scores that did not fall within a 95% confidence interval of the gold standard set by the expert reviewers as a benchmark were excluded. This eliminated one expert, 92 of the Mechanical Turks, and 43 of the Facebook users (90%, 82%, and 63% retained, respectively) [51]. Response times were also highly variable. Whereas it took expert surgeons 24 days to review the video, it took Mechanical Turks only 5. Facebook users took the longest, at 25 days. Chen's study was limited to only one video, but it was able to show that the Mechanical Turks were efficient and reliable assessors than social media in general.

Kowalewski et al. advanced C-SATS further, beginning with 24 videos taken from the BLUS validation study of the pegboard and suturing exercises [10, 50]. Each was reviewed approximately 60 times by individual crowd – workers, who had first been evaluated for calibration and attention. This involved discontinuation of participation with workers who failed to notice a trick question or whose answers strayed too far from the norm [50]. 1,438 reviews passing the exclusion tests arrived within 48 hours, far surpassing the 10-day period it took to get a mere 120 ratings from the expert reviewers [50]. The crowd workers were also more discriminating than the expert reviewers, marking 10 videos as failing versus the experts' 8. Out of what the experts designated passing and failing videos, the crowd workers passed no failing performers and failed 89% of what experts claimed was only "questionably good" [50]. Direct comparison of expert and crowd worker scores yielded between a 1.16 and 1.57 line of best fit, illustrated in Fig. 5.27 for the suturing and pegboard tasks, again showing that the experts gave slightly higher scores than crowd workers [50].

In the Turks evaluation against EDGE tracking devices, the crowd workers were equally reliable and advantageous in terms of cost. Each Turk earned $0.67 per video, costing a total of around $1200. EDGE itself costs several times that number and cannot evaluate every possible metric, as some do not include tool movement [10].

The goal of a global ratings scale is to have a universal and objective model for scoring. However, even with anchored points along the Likert scale, there is a measure of objectivity. A human is still required for the test and thus introduces their biases, perceptions, and potential for error. Some researchers consider global rating scales to be subjective means, while only computer-generated scores can be truly objective [53].

All of these methods have been extensively validated by a multitude of different sites and teams. However, there is some evidence that this kind of assessment may fail to accurately assess the end result – the actual surgery done on a patient.

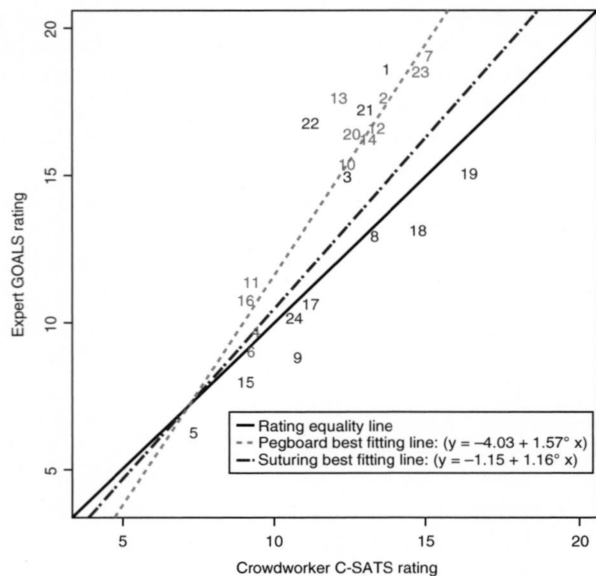

Fig. 5.27 Expert GOALS rating compared to crowd worker C-SATS ratings [50]

Anderson et al. assessed residents with OSATS during articular fracture reductions and found that higher OSATS scores did not correlate with restoring articular congruity [54]. They concluded that OSATS may overestimate surgical skills, at least for orthopedics. No such studies have been conducted evaluating GOALS or GEARS.

Combined Metrics: Epistemic Network Analysis

Global rating scales, such as OSATS, do not include generalizable metrics for nontechnical skills and fail to include any metrics on errors and procedural outcomes [33]. During a skills assessment comparing OSATS ratings with task-specific checklist ratings and final product analysis, results have shown that OSATS did not correlate with multiple task-related errors or predict final product quality [31]. Current assessment metrics for nontechnical skills, including teamwork, leadership, communication, situational awareness, and decision-making, focus on these skills in isolation of technical skills [55]. As such, performance feedback is usually one-dimensional and fails to elucidate the connection between technical and nontechnical skills or how these skills relate to procedural errors and outcomes. Consequently, the use of checklists and global rating scales as isolated assessment tools limits the type of feedback trainees receive and increases the risk of rating clinicians as competent despite the possibility of having critical performance deficits.

Surgical competency requires mastery of numerous, widely diverse, technical, and nontechnical skills that must be integrated seamlessly in fast-paced, stressful environments. Technical competency represents a highly complex class of skills requiring integration of psychomotor, cognitive, and perceptual skill components within the context of operative procedures with multiple steps and decision points [56–58]. Problem: Technical skills have traditionally been the primary focus of surgical training and performance assessments, for which the gold standard metrics comprise procedure-specific checklists and global rating scales completed by experienced observers [33, 59]. The emphasis on technical skills fails to appreciate the importance of critical nontechnical aspects of surgical performance such as leadership, teamwork, error recognition and management, and communication. While there has been increasing emphasis on nontechnical skills, and development of multiple evaluation techniques, these skills are largely assessed in an isolated fashion away from technical skills [55, 60–66]. Moreover, while technical and nontechnical skills metrics have shown validity and application to clinical care, there is still a lack of appreciation for how these metrics relate to one another [62, 63, 67, 68]. Solution: As the concept of workplace-based assessment draws attention to assessing clinical skills, they are actually used – in a complex, integrated fashion, a way to achieve the goal of integrated and holistic assessments must be found [69–71].

Preliminary research using epistemic network analysis (ENA), a sophisticated mathematical modeling technique, has shown promise in the ability to (1) integrate performance metrics from a variety of data sources and (2) generate holistic assessment models that reveal the complex interactions between performance metrics. ENA has been used in multiple domains to model complex thinking and problem-solving [72]. Recently, preliminary data analysis using ENA revealed significant correlations between procedural outcomes (quality and errors) and how surgeons talk during a simulated surgical procedure [73–75]. One of the most significant findings of preliminary work using ENA is the discovery of a relationship between procedural outcomes and how surgeons talk during a simulated surgical procedure [73–75].

Conclusion

In a recent review of surgical assessment methods, 202 individual research papers documented 567 different metrics of analysis; yet time was by far the most prevalent, appearing in 69.8% of the reviewed material. [76] Task time can correlate with objective skill, in some cases to near perfection [77]. However, the peril with using a stopwatch to gauge surgical skill is immeasurable. How can areas of improvement be identified without analysis of errors? In the same review, laparoscopic and MIS were the most predominant skills setting and the most frequently occurring skills cited overall. [76] Clearly this is a time where the continued development and appraisal of MIS should foster a culture of incentivized learning and analysis.

An estimated 48,000–90,000 people died in the year 2000 due to medical errors [78]. How many of those deaths were due to errors because of poorly earned or maintained MIS skill isn't known or likely even calculable; however, there are several recognizable truths. Surgical skill correlates to surgical outcome, and training improves operating room performance [8, 67]. The final key is that training becomes more meaningful when used alongside an equally meaningful assessment. A number can have no meaning out of context, and a percentage is useless without comparison. Assessment is the context for learning, while "learning is a euphemism for potentially avoidable harm" [79].

In this dynamic, fast-paced field of surgery, it is unacceptable to allow experience, or learning in any form, to come from clinical mistakes. Some harm is horribly unavoidable but is the duty of medical professionals to strive for excellence. Excellence needs to mean more than the best at one's institution or a flashy new technique. It needs to be defined and continually refined by measureable standards. Only through assessment methods as advanced as the techniques they aim to evaluate can these standards can be set.

References

1. Fuchs KH. Minimally invasive surgery. Endoscopy. 2002;34(2):154–9.
2. American Educational Research Association.; American Psychological Association.; National Council on Measurement in Education.; Joint Committee on Standards for Educational and Psychological Testing (U.S.). Standards for educational and psychological testing. Washington, DC: American Educational Research Association; 1985.
3. American Educational Research Association.; American Psychological Association, et al. Standards for educational and psychological testing. Washington, DC: American Educational Research Association; 1999.
4. Brown T. Construct validity: A unitary concept for occupational therapy assessment and measurement. Hong Kong J Occup Ther. 2010;20(1):30–42.
5. Fried GM, et al. Proving the value of simulation in laparoscopic surgery. Ann Surg. 2004;240(3):518–25; discussion 525–8
6. McCluney AL, et al. FLS simulator performance predicts intraoperative laparoscopic skill. Surg Endosc. 2007;21(11):1991–5.
7. Soper NJ, Fried GM. The fundamentals of laparoscopic surgery: its time has come. Bull Am Coll Surg. 2008;93(9):30–2.
8. Sroka G, et al. Fundamentals of laparoscopic surgery simulator training to proficiency improves laparoscopic performance in the operating room-a randomized controlled trial. Am J Surg. 2010;199(1):115–20.
9. Sweet RM, et al. Introduction and validation of the American Urological Association Basic Laparoscopic Urologic Surgery skills curriculum. J Endourol. 2012;26(2):190–6.
10. Kowalewski TM, et al. Validation of the AUA BLUS tasks. J Urol. 2016;195(4 Pt 1):998–1005.
11. Wilson M, et al. MIST VR: a virtual reality trainer for laparoscopic surgery assesses performance. Ann R Coll Surg Engl. 1997;79(6):403.
12. Ahlberg G, et al. Proficiency-based virtual reality training significantly reduces the error rate for residents during their first 10 laparoscopic cholecystectomies. Am J Surg. 2007;193(6):797–804.
13. Rosser JC, Rosser LE, Savalgi RS. Skill acquisition and assessment for laparoscopic surgery. Arch Surg. 1997;132(2):200–4.
14. Korndorffer JR, et al. Simulator training for laparoscopic suturing using performance goals translates to the operating room. J Am Coll Surg. 2005;201(1):23–9.
15. Van Sickle KR, et al. Prospective, randomized, double-blind trial of curriculum-based training for intracorporeal suturing and knot tying. J Am Coll Surg. 2008;207(4):560–8.
16. Smith CD, et al. Assessing laparoscopic manipulative skills. Am J Surg. 2001;181(6):547–50.
17. Cosman PH, et al. Virtual reality simulators: current status in acquisition and assessment of surgical skills. ANZ J Surg. 2002;72(1):30–4.

18. Stefanidis D, et al. Skill retention following proficiency-based laparoscopic simulator training. Surgery. 2005;138(2):165–70.
19. Hiemstra E, et al. Retention of basic laparoscopic skills after a structured training program. Gynecol Surg. 2009;6(3):229–35.
20. Intuitive Surgical Inc. da Vinci Residency & Fellowship Training Program. 2016. 12 Oct 2016.
21. Ramos P, et al. Face, content, construct and concurrent validity of dry laboratory exercises for robotic training using a global assessment tool. BJU Int. 2014;113(5):836–42.
22. Simulated Surgical Systems LLC. RoSS II robotic surgery simulator; 2017. 3/14/2017.
23. DiMaio S, Hasser C. The da Vinci research interface. In: MICCAI Workshop on Systems and Arch. for Computer Assisted Interventions, Midas Journal; 2008.
24. Kumar R, et al. Assessing system operation skills in robotic surgery trainees. Int J Med Robot. 2012;8(1):118–24.
25. Lin HC, et al. Towards automatic skill evaluation: detection and segmentation of robot-assisted surgical motions. Comput Aided Surg. 2006;11(5):220–30.
26. McDonough PS, et al. Initial validation of the ProMIS surgical simulator as an objective measure of robotic task performance. J Robot Surg. 2011;5(3):195–9.
27. Brand TC. Educational curricula, simulation, and skills assessment for the da Vinci platform, in Society of Government Service Urologists, San Diego. 2015.
28. Jonsson MN, et al. ProMIS can serve as a da Vinci(R) simulator – a construct validity study. J Endourol. 2011;25(2):345–50.
29. Tausch TJ, et al. Content and construct validation of a robotic surgery curriculum using an electromagnetic instrument tracker. J Urol. 2012;188(3):919–23.
30. Chmarra MK, et al. The influence of experience and camera holding on laparoscopic instrument movements measured with the TrEndo tracking system. Surg Endosc. 2007;21(11):2069–75.
31. D'Angelo A-LD, et al. Idle time: an underdeveloped performance metric for assessing surgical skill. Am J Surg. 2015;209(4):645–51.
32. Crochet P, et al. Development of an evidence-based training program for laparoscopic hysterectomy on a virtual reality simulator. Surg Endosc. 2017; 31(6):2474-2482.
33. Martin JA, et al. Objective structured assessment of technical skill (OSATS) for surgical residents. Br J Surg. 1997;84:273–8.
34. Gallagher AG, et al. Objective structured assessment of technical skills and checklist scales reliability compared for high stakes assessments. ANZ J Surg. 2014;84(7–8):568–73.
35. Datta V, et al. The surgical efficiency score: a feasible, reliable, and valid method of skills assessment. Am J Surg. 2006;192(3):372–8.
36. Dath D, et al. Toward reliable operative assessment: the reliability and feasibility of videotaped assessment of laparoscopic technical skills. Surg Endosc. 2004;18(12):1800–4.
37. Vassiliou MC, et al. A global assessment tool for evaluation of intraoperative laparoscopic skills. Am J Surg. 2005;190(1):107–13.
38. Kramp KH, et al. Validity and reliability of global operative assessment of laparoscopic skills (GOALS) in novice trainees performing a laparoscopic cholecystectomy. J Surg Educ. 2015;72(2):351–8.
39. Gumbs AA, Hogle NJ, Fowler DL. Evaluation of resident laparoscopic performance using global operative assessment of laparoscopic skills. J Am Coll Surg. 2007;204(2):308–13.
40. Hogle NJ, et al. Evaluation of surgical fellows' laparoscopic performance using Global Operative Assessment of Laparoscopic Skills (GOALS). Surg Endosc. 2014;28(4):1284–90.
41. Vassiliou MC, et al. Evaluating intraoperative laparoscopic skill: direct observation versus blinded videotaped performances. Surg Innov. 2007;14(3):211–6.
42. Chang L, et al. Reliable assessment of laparoscopic performance in the operating room using videotape analysis. Surg Innov. 2007;14(2):122–6.
43. Watanabe Y, et al. Psychometric properties of the Global Operative Assessment of Laparoscopic Skills (GOALS) using item response theory. Am J Surg. 2016;213(2):273–6.
44. Goh AC, et al. Global evaluative assessment of robotic skills: validation of a clinical assessment tool to measure robotic surgical skills. J Urol. 2012;187(1):247–52.
45. Hung AJ, et al. Comparative assessment of three standardized robotic surgery training methods. BJU Int. 2013;112(6):864–71.

46. Aghazadeh MA, et al. External validation of Global Evaluative Assessment of Robotic Skills (GEARS). Surg Endosc. 2015;29(11):3261–6.
47. Sánchez R, et al. Robotic surgery training: construct validity of Global Evaluative Assessment of Robotic Skills (GEARS). J Robot Surg. 2016;10(3):227–31.
48. Nabhani J, et al. MP11-11 analysis of Global Evaluative Assessment Of Robotic Surgery (GEARS) as an immediate assessment tool in robotic surgery curriculum. J Urol. 2016;195(4):e115–6.
49. Ghani KR, et al. Measuring to improve: peer and crowd-sourced assessments of technical skill with robot-assisted radical prostatectomy. Eur Urol. 2016;69(4):547–50.
50. Kowalewski TM, et al. Crowd-sourced assessment of technical skills for validation of basic laparoscopic urologic skills tasks. J Urol. 2016;195(6):1859–65.
51. Chen C, et al. Crowd-sourced assessment of technical skills: a novel method to evaluate surgical performance. J Surg Res. 2014;187(1):65–71.
52. Lendvay TS, et al. Virtual reality robotic surgery warm-up improves task performance in a dry laboratory environment: a prospective randomized controlled study. J Am Coll Surg. 2013;216(6):1181–92.
53. van Empel PJ, et al. Objective versus subjective assessment of laparoscopic skill. ISRN Minim Invasive Surg. 2013;1–6
54. Anderson DD, et al. Objective Structured Assessments of Technical Skills (OSATS) does not assess the quality of the surgical result effectively. Clin Orthop Relat Res. 2016;474(4):874–81.
55. Yule S, et al. Surgeons' non-technical skills in the operating room: reliability testing of the NOTSS behavior rating system. World J Surg. 2008;32(4):548–56.
56. Pugh CM, et al. Intra-operative decision making: more than meets the eye. J Biomed Inform. 2011;44(3):486–96.
57. Skinner A. Retention and retraining of integrated cognitive and psychomotor skills. Proceedings of the Interservice/Industry Training Systems & Education Conference, 2014, Orlando; 2014.
58. Skinner A, Lathan C, Meadors M, Sevrechts M. Training and retention of medical skills. Proceedings of the Interservice/Industry Training Systems & Education Conference, 2012, Orlando; 2012.
59. Pugh C, et al. Outcome measures for surgical simulators: is the focus on technical skills the best approach? Surgery. 2010;147(5):646–54.
60. Parker SH, et al. The Surgeons' Leadership Inventory (SLI): a taxonomy and rating system for surgeons' intraoperative leadership skills. Am J Surg. 2013;205(6):745–51.
61. Mishra A, Catchpole K, McCulloch P. The Oxford NOTECHS System: reliability and validity of a tool for measuring teamwork behaviour in the operating theatre. Qual Saf Health Care. 2009;18(2):104–8.
62. Hull L, et al. Observational teamwork assessment for surgery: content validation and tool refinement. J Am Coll Surg. 2011;212(2):234–43.e5.
63. Nathwani JN, et al. Relationship between technical errors and decision-making skills in the junior resident. J Surg Educ. 2016;73(6):e84–90.
64. DaRosa D, et al. Impact of a structured skills laboratory curriculum on surgery residents' intraoperative decision-making and technical skills. Acad Med. 2008;83(10):S68–71.
65. D'Angelo A-LD, et al. Use of decision-based simulations to assess resident readiness for operative independence. Am J Surg. 2015;209(1):132–9.
66. Dedy NJ, et al. Teaching nontechnical skills in surgical residency: a systematic review of current approaches and outcomes. Surgery. 2013;154(5):1000–8.
67. Birkmeyer JD, et al. Surgical skill and complication rates after bariatric surgery. N Engl J Med. 2013;369(15):1434–42.
68. Hull L, et al. The impact of nontechnical skills on technical performance in surgery: a systematic review. J Am Coll Surg. 2012;214(2):214–30.
69. Miller A, Archer J. Impact of workplace based assessment on doctors' education and performance: a systematic review. BMJ. 2010;341:c5064.
70. Norcini J, et al. Criteria for good assessment: consensus statement and recommendations from the Ottawa 2010 Conference. Med Teach. 2011;33(3):206–14.

71. Norcini J, Burch V. Workplace-based assessment as an educational tool: AMEE Guide No. 31. Med Teach. 2007;29(9–10):855–71.
72. Shaffer DW, Collier W, Ruis A. A tutorial on epistemic network analysis: analyzing the structure of connections in cognitive, social, and interaction data. J Learn Analytics. 2016;3(3):9–45.
73. D'Angelo A. Evaluating operative performance through the lens of epistemic frame theory. University of Wisconsin–Madison; 2015.
74. Ruis A, et al. Modeling operating thinking in a simulation- based continuing medical education course on laparoscopic hernia repair. Presented at the American College of Surgeons, 2017.
75. Ruis A, et al. The hands and heads of a surgeon: modeling operative competency with multimodal epistemic network analysis. Presented at the American College of Surgeons, 2017.
76. Schmitz CC, et al. Development and verification of a taxonomy of assessment metrics for surgical technical skills. Acad Med. 2014;89(1):153–61.
77. Kowalewski TM. Real-time quantitative assessment of surgical skill. Thesis from university of washington 2012.
78. Donaldson MS, Corrigan JM, Kohn LT. To err is human: building a safer health system. National Academies Press; 2000.
79. Dimick, Justin (jdimick1). "Learning- euphemism for potentially avoidable harm." 2016. Tweet.

Crowdsourcing and Large-Scale Evaluation

6

Jessica C. Dai and Mathew D. Sorensen

Abbreviations

ACGME	Accreditation Council for Graduate Medical Education
GEARS	Global Evaluative Assessment of Robotic Skills
GOALS	Global Operative Assessment of Laparoscopic Skills
MUSIC	Michigan Urological Surgery Improvement Collaborative
OSATS	Objective Structured Assessment of Technical Skills
RACE	Robotic Anastomosis and Competency Evaluation

Current Paradigms of Surgical Education

The teaching of surgeons is unique in that surgical trainees must not only acquire fundamental specialty-specific knowledge and sound clinical judgment outside of the operating room but also achieve mastery of technical surgical skills within it. Though still largely based on the Halsteadian model of graduated responsibility with progression through residency training, the current model of surgical education has been shaped by advances in educational theory, the rise of cost-conscious care, and national concerns regarding patient safety and litigation, as well as novel developments in surgical technology [1, 2]. Though surgical competency was traditionally believed to be accomplished by sheer volume of clinical exposure, changes in the modern clinical practice of surgery, including increasing patient complexity, burgeoning administrative burdens, and work-hour limits, have led surgical training

J.C. Dai • M.D. Sorensen (✉)
University of Washington, Department of Urology,
1959 NE Pacific St, HSB BB 1121 Seattle, WA, USA
e-mail: jcdai@uw.edu; mathews@uw.edu

T.S. Köhler, B. Schwartz (eds.), *Surgeons as Educators*,
https://doi.org/10.1007/978-3-319-64728-9_6

programs to reexamine and restructure their educational approach to training residents. Furthermore, volume-based advancement ensures that patients will be exposed to surgeons in their learning curves which may be negatively correlated with outcomes. Given the rapid pace of new technological developments within surgery over the past few decades, similar challenges are also being faced by graduated surgeons already in practice trying to master new surgical techniques and skills not learned in residency.

Several other factors have contributed to renewed interest in how to foster mastery of technical skills within the current training paradigm. National patient safety concerns have drawn attention to the role of healthcare systems and practitioners in preventable medical errors and spurred quality initiatives throughout the healthcare system [3–5]. National malpractice claims have demonstrated that overall 41% of errors in surgical and perioperative care resulting in patient injury are due to errors in technical competence; of those cases, a trainee's lack of technical competence was implicated 40% of the time [6]. In this context, surgical skills development takes on implications beyond simply training individual residents, as developing technical competence directly impacts patient outcomes [7].

Cost is also a significant consideration in the current model of surgical education. Resident involvement in operative cases decreases efficiency. Multiple studies of general surgical procedures have demonstrated that resident involvement increases operative time in almost all cases [8–10]. Given the high cost of operating room time, which has been estimated at $900–1200 per hour, the annual cost burden attributed to extra operating room time for resident education has been estimated at $53 million [8, 11]. The efficient development of surgical proficiency both within and beyond the operating is therefore paramount.

To appropriately address the need for more efficient development of technical skills, it is critical to understand the current educational theory surrounding the acquisition and mastery of procedural skills. Much of the foundation for mechanical and surgical learning theory is based on the classic three-stage theory of motor skills acquisition proposed by Fitts and Posner in 1967. This separates learning into cognitive, associative, and autonomous stages (Table 6.1). In the cognitive stage, the task and its mechanics are largely intellectualized; the procedure is carried out in a series of small steps, and the task performance is often erratic and inefficient. In the associative phase, knowledge about how to perform the task is translated into task performance. With deliberate practice and feedback, task performance becomes more efficient. In the final autonomous stage, task performance becomes fluid and continuous through continued feedback and refinement of performance, with minimal dependence on conscious cognitive thought [12]. As applied to surgical training, it is this autonomous mastery of basic skills such as knot tying or suturing that allows trainees to focus on the more complex technical and nontechnical aspects of operating and to grow as surgeons. Thus, it has been suggested by some that the cognitive and associative stages should be practiced by trainees largely outside of the operating room to maximize the utility of intraoperative time [1]. Such calls have paralleled the increasing use of simulation in surgical training.

Table 6.1 The Fitts-Posner three-stage theory of motor skills acquisition

Stage	Goals	Method	Characteristics
Cognitive	Establish task goals Determine appropriate sequence of actions to achieve desired goal	Explicit knowledge	Slow, inconsistent, interrupted movements
Associative	Understand and perform mechanics Attention to specific subparts and transitions within the sequence	Exploration of details Deliberate practice Feedback	More fluid and efficient
Autonomous	Task performance is honed Development of automatized routine	Continued feedback Repetition	Accurate, consistent, fluid, continuous

Adapted, Fitts and Posner [12]

Ericsson's theories on the development of expertise further inform current models of surgical education. Experts are those individuals whose performance of a particular task is identified as reproducibly superior to that of their peers. For these individuals, continued improvement in performance occurs gradually and over extended periods of time. Indeed, 10 years or 10,000 h is generally regarded as the time investment required to attain expert levels of performance. Mastery of a task requires motivation on the part of the trainee, detailed, immediate feedback on their task performance, and repeated practice. This concept has been termed "deliberate practice" [13]. In contrast with previous theories by Sir Francis Dalton implicating innate ability as the primary factor for expert performance, the idea of deliberate practice suggests that expertise is attainable primarily through motivated and focused practice.

A critical component of deliberate practice and attainment of expert performance is both the quantity and nature of feedback. Within the education literature, there remains disagreement as to the optimal timing and quantity of feedback to maximize procedural mastery. Across several studies, frequent, intermittent, and immediate feedback appears to be most effective in improving procedural performance, decreasing error, and improving learning curves among cohorts of novice trainees [14, 15]. However, other studies have demonstrated that too intense feedback during the early stages of learning may actually hinder learning [16]. Regardless, the role of feedback is central to the development of expert performance and plays a critical role in the education of surgical residents in the current training paradigm.

Current methods of surgical skills evaluation are limited in scope, timing, and objectivity. Accreditation Council for Graduate Medical Education (ACGME) operative case logs serve as an overall surrogate for a trainee's surgical exposure and, by extrapolation, the development of their surgical skills. However, this remains an imprecise marker for technical skill, as it does not completely capture the extent of a trainee's involvement in the case, their innate surgical ability and clinical judgment, or technical progress. Moreover, it depends on accurate and appropriate logging of cases by the trainee and is therefore prone to a degree of subjectivity. Surveys examining the perceptions of surgical residents and faculty regarding the degree of resident involvement in operative cases have demonstrated that there is poor agreement between faculty and residents regarding the role and percent of the case performed by the resident; in only 47–58% of cases was there good correlation [17, 18]. Though ACGME operative case logs provide a general assessment of operative case volume, their use to assess the overall surgical skill of trainees carries obvious limitations.

Day to day, most trainees receive constructive feedback on specific operative performances and technique from their attending surgeons to refine operative skills. Such feedback may be provided informally and directly in the moment within the operating room or more commonly may be presented indirectly in aggregate as part of a formalized feedback mechanism at the conclusion of a rotation. However, the quality, quantity, and formative values of this feedback may be highly variable. Such feedback represents a single surgeon view, may carry a significant degree of bias, and usually applies to a limited repertoire of observed surgical procedures [19, 20]. Moreover, the timing of such feedback may be significantly delayed. In one survey conducted at a large academic orthopedic surgery program, 58% of residents reported that end-of-rotation evaluations were rarely or never completed in a timely fashion, with more than 30% of such evaluations completed over 1 month after a rotation's end. Moreover, the majority of residents and faculty members felt that such end-of-rotation evaluations were inadequate for surgical skills feedback [21].

In practice, patient outcomes might provide an additional indirect measure of a surgeon's technical skills, as this has previously been linked to postoperative complications [7]. However, as trainees operate under the supervision of more experienced attending surgeons, their technical missteps are often immediately corrected and therefore may not necessarily be reflected in a patient's clinical course. Moreover, postoperative outcomes are influenced by many other nonoperative variables such as patient disease, ancillary therapies, and post-hospitalization care that limit direct correlation between outcomes and specific surgical techniques. The delayed nature of such feedback also makes it challenging to directly link specific technical aspects of the operation to the overall patient outcome. Lastly, the rotation-based nature of surgical training programs does not always ensure the continuity of care for trainees necessary for this to be a consistently useful form of feedback.

In an attempt to minimize the variability and subjectivity inherent in standard evaluative mechanisms, more structured assessment tools have been developed to help standardize and formalize feedback for specific surgical tasks (Table 6.2). These include the validated Objective Structured Assessment of Technical Skills (OSATS), the Global Operative Assessment of Laparoscopic Skills (GOALS), and the Global Evaluative Assessment of Robotic Skills (GEARS) [22–24]. These assessment tools have been largely used in evaluating videotaped performance in simulation tasks but have also been used to assess intraoperative skills and have been correlated to patient surgical complications and outcomes [7, 25]. While these tools allow evaluators to provide uniform and more objective feedback for a surgical

Table 6.2 Validated surgical technical skills assessment instruments

(a) Objective Structured Assessment of Technical Skills (OSATS) [22]					
Respect for tissue	1 Frequently used unnecessary force on tissue or caused damage by inappropriate use of instruments	2	3 Careful handling of tissue but occasionally caused inadvertent damage	4	5 Consistently handled tissue appropriately with minimal damage
Time and motion	1 Many unnecessary moves	2	3 Efficient time/motion but some unnecessary moves	4	5 Economy of movement and maximum efficiency
Instrument handling	1 Repeatedly makes tentative or awkward moves with instruments	2	3 Competent use of instruments although occasionally appeared stiff or awkward	4	5 Fluid moves with instruments and no awkwardness
Knowledge of instruments	1 Frequently asked for the wrong instrument or used an inappropriate instrument	2	3 Knew the names of most instruments and used appropriate instrument for the task	4	5 Obviously familiar with the instruments required and their names
Use of assistants	1 Consistently placed assistants poorly or failed to use assistants	2	3 Good use of assistants most of the time	4	5 Strategically used assistant to the best advantage at all times
Flow of operation and forward planning	1 Frequently stopped operating or needed to discuss next move	2	3 Demonstrated ability for forward planning with steady progression of operative procedure	4	5 Obviously planned course of operation with effortless flow from one move to the next
Knowledge of specific procedure	1 Deficient knowledge. Needed specific instruction at most operative stages	2	3 Knew all important aspects of the operation	4	5 Demonstrated familiarity with all aspects of the operation
Overall on this task, should this candidate: □ Pass □ Fail					

(b) Global Operative Assessment of Laparoscopic Skills (GOALS) [23]					
Depth perception	1 Constantly overshoots target, wide swings, slow to correct	2	3 Some overshooting or missing of target, but quick to correct	4	5 Accurately directs instruments in correct plane to target

(continued)

Table 6.2 (continued)

(b) Global Operative Assessment of Laparoscopic Skills (GOALS) [23]					
Bimanual dexterity	1 Uses only one hand, ignores non-dominant hand, poor coordination between hands	2	3 Uses both hands but does not optimize interaction between hands	4	5 Expertly uses both hands in a complimentary manner to provide optimal exposure
Efficiency	1 Uncertain, inefficient efforts, many tentative movements, constantly changing focus or persisting without progress	2	3 Slow but planned movements are reasonably organized	4	5 Confident, efficient, and safe conduct, maintains focus on task until it is better performed by way of an alternative approach
Tissue handling	1 Rough movements, tears tissue, injures adjacent structures, poor grasper control, grasper frequently slips	2	3 Handles tissue reasonably well, minor trauma to adjacent tissue (i.e., occasional unnecessary bleeding or slipping of the grasper)	4	5 Handles tissues well, applies appropriate traction, negligible injury to adjacent structures
Autonomy	1 Unable to complete entire task, even with verbal guidance	2	3 Able to complete task safely with moderate guidance	4	5 Able to complete task independently without prompting

(c) Global Evaluative Assessment of Robotic Skills (GEARS) [24]					
Depth perception	1 Constantly overshoots target, wide swings, slow to correct	2	3 Some overshooting or missing of target, but quick to correct	4	5 Accurately directs instruments in correct plane to target
Bimanual dexterity	1 Uses only one hand, ignores non-dominant hand, poor coordination	2	3 Uses both hands, but does not optimize interaction between hands	4	5 Expertly uses both hands in a complimentary manner to provide best exposure
Efficiency	1 Inefficient efforts, many uncertain movements, constantly changing focus or persisting without progress	2	3 Slow but planned movements are reasonably organized	4	5 Confident, efficient, and safe conduct, maintains focus on task, fluid progression

Table 6.2 (continued)

Force sensitivity	1 Rough moves, tears tissue, injures nearby structures, poor control, frequent suture breakage	2	3 Handles tissues reasonably well, minor trauma to adjacent tissue, rare suture breakage	4	5 Applies appropriate tension, negligible injury to adjacent structures, no suture breakage
Autonomy	1 Unable to complete entire task, even with verbal guidance	2	3 Able to complete task safely with moderate guidance	4	5 Able to complete task independently without prompting
Robotic control	1 Consistently does not optimize view, hand position, or repeated collisions even with guidance	2	3 View is sometimes not optimal. Occasionally needs to relocate arms. Occasional collisions and obstruction of assistant	4	5 Controls camera and hand position optimally and independently. Minimal collisions or obstruction of assistant

task, they remain imperfect. The resources required to record trainees' task performances, as well as the time investment and associated cost required on the part of each surgeon to watch and assess each task performance, limit the scalability of this means of evaluation across a large cohort of residents [26, 27]. Indeed, the limitations of our current surgical feedback mechanisms have become so significant that a recent consensus of the Association for Surgical Education has prioritized the determination of the best methods and metrics for assessment of technical and non-technical surgical performances as a top ten research priority for twenty-first-century surgical simulation research [28].

One proposed means to better foster mastery of surgical skills is the use of surgical coaches. Work by Greenberg and colleagues from the University of Wisconsin has provided a framework by which peer-based surgical coaching might be integrated into a program for surgical skills development, both for surgeons in training and experienced surgeons in practice. Surgical coaches are poised to optimize "deliberate practice" by setting goals, providing motivation and encouragement, and providing guidance within the context of a collegial relationship [29]. Such an approach could address not only the technical aspects of surgical skills development but also cognitive and nontechnical areas as well. With the increasing volume of laparoscopic and minimally invasive approaches in surgery, video-based peer surgical coaching has also been introduced as a potential alternative to traditional feedback mechanisms [30]. However, even with such innovative approaches, the challenges of scalability and time investment remain, as these frameworks continue to rely on the expertise of a limited number of expert surgeons to advance the skills of numerous residents and peer surgeons.

Crowdsourcing Technology: Definitions and Evolution

In the context of such constraints in our current surgical training paradigm, increasing interest in crowdsourcing has developed. This term refers to a large-scale approach to accomplishing a task by opening it to a broad population of decentralized individuals who may complete the task more effectively in aggregate than any single individual or group of individuals [31]. Despite its recent rise in popularity, such a large-scale approach to problem-solving dates back as far as 1714, with the British Parliament's establishment of the Longitude Act. This declaration offered up to £20,000 to any individual who could provide a simple, practical, and accurate method of determining the longitude of a ship at sea. It has since been applied across multiple fields from astronomy to ornithology, with the advantages of efficiency, scalability, flexibility, and diversity to solving the particular problem at hand [32]. The success of crowdsourcing lies in aggregating the collective intelligence of all participants, such that the distributed wisdom of the group surpasses that of any single individual [33].

Over the past few decades, the widespread integration of the Internet has further helped to shape the evolution of crowd-based wisdom. The aggregate value of crowds networked through the Internet has been termed by some as "collective intelligence," an entity that is constantly changing, growing, and evolving in real time [34]. The Internet has not only allowed for the rapid connection of individuals in the pursuit of a single problem's solution but has also facilitated the formal organization of such virtual individuals into an easily accessible entity that can solve a wide range of problems, from straightforward tasks to complex problems requiring critical intellectual input.

The Amazon Mechanical Turk is one example of this phenomenon. This marketplace service provides access to more than 500,000 "Turker" crowdworkers from over 190 countries who perform a range of "human intelligence tasks," including data processing, information categorization, business feedback, and content moderation. Such tasks are generally deemed too challenging or inefficient for current artificial intelligence algorithms to complete. For each completed task, workers are paid a small sum. One survey of these workers actually found that monetary incentive was the primary reason for their participation in such tasks, particularly for those not based in the United States [35].

Such organization of crowdworkers has allowed for the recent rapid and widespread adoption of crowdsourcing across a multitude of fields. Within the business realm, several corporations have been built around crowd-based wisdom, capitalizing on their collective intelligence to sell merchandise, amass repositories of photographs, and develop innovative research and development solutions [33]. The reach of crowdsourcing also extends into the healthcare realm, where it has served a myriad of roles in the areas of molecular biology, comparative genetics, pathology, and epidemiology [36]. Challenges in computational molecular biology have been readily addressed by large-scale problem-solving, which has been used to discover tertiary protein folding patterns [37] and to generate phylogenetic arrangements of genetic promoter regions from vast numbers of nucleotides [38]. Crowdsourcing has also been demonstrated to be a powerful resource in diagnostic challenges involving high volume data processing, with crowdworkers successfully able to identify colonic polyps [39] and red blood cells infected with malaria [40]. Crowdsourcing has even been used to generate epidemiologic symptom maps for the flu, which have corresponded well to the Centers for Disease Control and Prevention data [41].

Within the realm of clinical medicine, there has been significant interest in crowdsourcing technology in the diagnosis and discrimination of disease processes. In urology, large-scale evaluation has been used to help validate confocal laser endomicroscopy as a potential technology for the diagnosis of urothelial carcinoma, with crowdworkers able to correctly diagnose urothelial carcinoma of the bladder 92% of the time [42]. Within the field of ophthalmology, crowdworkers have been used to identify abnormal fundi among diabetic patients and glaucomatous optic disks, though sensitivity was high for both tasks, ranging from 83 to 100%, specificity remained limited at 31–71% [43, 44]. Additional refinement of crowdsourcing for clinical diagnosis applications is clearly warranted, but this technology carries enormous potential in the future of clinical medicine.

Recent research in medical education has also explored the potential of collective crowd wisdom to teach future generations of medical providers. A crowd-based approach has been used to generate curricular content for trainees at both the pre-medical and graduate medical education levels with initial success [45, 46]. However, one of the most promising applications of crowdsourcing technology lies in optimizing technical skills development for surgical trainees, which has been demonstrated to be an area in particular need of innovation and adaptation for the current training environment.

Crowdsourcing and Surgical Evaluation

One of the primary challenges in the current paradigm of surgical training is in providing, individualized, timely, and cost-efficient, feedback to trainees regarding their technical skills. Moreover, the widespread trend toward simulation in surgical education further generates a need for objective, formative feedback on a large scale [1]. Indeed, simulation without feedback has been demonstrated to result in more errors among trainees [14], suggesting that feedback is a critical part of simulation-based learning. Given these demands, reliance on surgeon feedback alone becomes difficult to sustain. The application of crowdsourcing to surgical skills evaluation addresses these issues of efficiency, cost, and scalability.

In 2014, Chen and colleagues performed an initial study demonstrating the added value of crowdsourced evaluation, which has provided a methodology upon which most subsequent research on large-scale technical skills evaluation has been based. Three groups were recruited to evaluate recorded robotic knot tying performance: 409 Amazon.com Mechanical Turk users, 67 Facebook users, and 9 faculty surgeons. Subjects first answered a qualification question by rating side-by-side videos of Fundamentals of Laparoscopic Surgery peg transfer task performed by high-skilled and intermediate-skilled surgeons. Then, they were asked to rate a videotaped robotic suturing task on three GEARS domains. Embedded within this task was an attention question. Ratings from the expert surgeons served as a "gold standard" for the true quality of the task performance. Mean scores among the groups were markedly similar; the mean surgeon rating was 12.22 (95% CI 11.11–13.11) as compared to 12.21 (95% CI 11.98–12.43) and 12.06 (95% CI 11.57–12.55) for Amazon Mechanical Turk workers and Facebook users, respectively. Notably, responses were obtained from all Amazon Mechanical Turk users within just 5 days, as compared to 25 days for Facebook users and 24 days for the faculty surgeons. Moreover, more complex feedback from the crowdworkers appeared to correlate with the expert ratings, suggesting that it might also be possible to identify higher-quality responses to optimize this form of feedback [47]. This study was the first to suggest that inexperienced crowdworkers could evaluate surgical simulation task performance in a manner consistent to expert surgeons and in a markedly more expeditious fashion.

One of the most important aspects of crowd-based feedback is its apparent equivalency to feedback provided by surgical experts for specific technical tasks. Published studies in the literature using well-established objective scoring systems have demonstrated good correlation between crowdsourced ratings and expert surgeon ratings for technical tasks across a wide range of specialties (Table 6.3). Several studies have demonstrated a strong linear relationship between the two groups, with Pearson's coefficients ranging from 0.74 to 0.89 [48–54] and r^2 values for such correlations ranging between 0.70 and 0.93 [27, 49, 55]. Others have quantified this relationship by comparing mean composite rating scores between crowdworkers and surgical experts using Cronbach's α scores, with scores greater than 0.9 indicating "excellent agreement," 0.9–0.7 indicating "good agreement," and scores below 0.5 indicating "poor and unacceptable" levels of agreement. Multiple studies using this analysis have demonstrated Cronbach's α from 0.79 to 0.92 across a wide range of tasks, including robotic and laparoscopic pegboard transfer and suturing, as well as a simulated cricothyroidotomy exercise [49, 50, 56].

It is notable that in one study examining medical student performance on a variety of surgical skills tasks, poor correlation has been described. Twenty-five medical students performed four simulation-based tasks for open knot tying, robotic suturing, laparoscopic peg transfer, and a fulguration skills tasks on the LAP Mentor ©, a commercially available virtual reality laparoscopic simulator. For the first three tasks, videos were assessed both by faculty experts and crowds using the C-SATS platform employing OSATS, GEARS, and GOALS, respectively. For the fulguration task, candidates were evaluated using a proprietary ranking score generated by the LAP Mentor ©, in lieu of expert evaluation. There was fair agreement of crowd assessments for the knot tying task (Cronbach's $\alpha = 0.62$), good agreement for the robotic suturing task (Cronbach's $\alpha = 0.86$), and excellent agreement for the laparoscopic peg transfer (Cronbach's $\alpha = 0.92$). However, the proprietary assessments generated by the LAP Mentor © had poor agreement with crowd assessments with Cronbach's α of 0.32 [56]. Given the consistent agreement between crowds and experts for the other simulation tasks, the authors attributed such poor correlation to

Table 6.3 Summary of current studies evaluating the application of crowd-based evaluation of surgical skills

First author	Year	Task performers	Task	Evaluation mechanism	Average time to feedback	Rating agreement between crowds and experts	Compensation
Chen	2014	1 "above average" performer	Robotic knot tying	GEARS[a] Depth perception Bimanual dexterity Efficiency Global domain Verbal comments	Turk workers: 5 days Facebook users: 25 days Surgeons: 24 days	Similar ratings among 409 Turk workers, 67 Facebook users, and 9 teaching surgeons	\$1.00/HIT[d]
Holst	2015a	3 urology residents (PGY2, PGY4, PGY5) 2 urology faculty	Fundamentals of laparoscopic surgery (FLS) intracorporeal suturing	GEARS[a] Depth perception Bimanual dexterity Efficiency	Turk workers: 2 h, 50 min Surgeons: 26 h	Cronbach's $\alpha = 0.91$ $r^2 = 0.93$	\$0.50/ HIT[d]
Holst	2015b	12 surgeons of varying robotic surgical experience	Live porcine robotic-assisted urinary bladder closures	GEARS[a] Bimanual dexterity Depth perception Efficiency Force sensitivity Robotic control	Turk workers: 4 h, 28 min Surgeons: 14 days	Cronbach's $\alpha = 0.93$ $r^2 = 0.91$	\$0.75/HIT[d]
White	2015	49 surgeons 25 urology general surgery and obstetrics and gynecology PGY1–PGY6 trainees 24 faculty surgeons	Robotic pegboard transfer and suturing task	GEARS[a] Depth perception Bimanual dexterity Efficiency	Turk workers: 8 h, 52 min for suturing task; 108 h, 48 min for pegboard task	Pegboard task: Cronbach's $\alpha = 0.84$ Suturing task: Cronbach's $\alpha = 0.92$	\$0.25/pegboard task \$0.50/ suturing task

(continued)

Table 6.3 (continued)

First author	Year	Task performers	Task	Evaluation mechanism	Average time to feedback	Rating agreement between crowds and experts	Compensation
Malpani	2015	4 expert surgeons and 14 trainee surgeons	Robotic suturing and knot tying	Anonymous survey of preference for superior task segment performance between paired videos distributed to Johns Hopkins community Computed percentile scores for segment performance using preferences Predicted task-level scores using segment-level percentile scores	Inexperienced survey respondents: < 72 h Experts: ~672 h	83% agreement between inexperienced survey respondents and experts Segment score: Spearman's $\rho \geq 0.86$ Task score: Pearson's $\rho \geq 0.84$	$10 gift card/survey

Aghdasi	2015	26 participants Medical students Residents Attending physicians	Simulated cricothyroidotomy procedure	OSATS[b]-like tool Respect for tissue Time/motion Instrument handling Knowledge of instruments Flow of operation Knowledge of procedure	Turk workers: 10 h Surgeons: 60 days	Pearson's $r = 0.83$ $r^2 = 0.7$ Cronbach's $\alpha = 0.83$	\$0.50/ HIT[d]
Polin	2016	105 obstetrics/ gynecology, urology, general surgery trainees, fellows, and surgeons	Dry lab robotic surgical drills Tower transfer Roller coaster Big dipper Train tracks Figure of eight	Robotic-OSATS[b] Depth perception/ accuracy of movements Force/tissue handling Dexterity Efficiency of movements	Turk workers: 16 h	Tower transfer: Pearson's $r = 0.75$ Roller coaster: Pearson's r = 0.91 Big dipper: Pearson's $r = 0.86$ Train tracks: Pearson's r = 0.76 Figure of eight: Pearson's $r = 0.87$	N/A

(continued)

Table 6.3 (continued)

First author	Year	Task performers	Task	Evaluation mechanism	Average time to feedback	Rating agreement between crowds and experts	Compensation
Vernez	2016	25 medical student urology residency interviewees	Open square knot tying Laparoscopic peg transfer Robotic suturing Skill task eight on LAP mentor	OSATS[b] GEARS[a] GOALS[C]	Turk workers: <3.5 h Surgeons: 22 days	Open knot tying: Cronbach's $\alpha = 0.62$ Laparoscopic peg transfer: Cronbach's $\alpha = 0.92$ Robotic suturing: Cronbach's $\alpha = 0.86$ LAP mentor skill eight: Cronbach's $\alpha = 0.32$	\$0.44/ HIT[d]
Lee	2016	99 trainees Canadian medical students urology applicants Urology trainees (PGY3 and PGY5) 6 attending urologists	American urological association basic laparoscopic urologic skills curriculum tasks Peg transfer Pattern cutting Suturing/knot tying Vascular clip application	GOALS[c]	N/A	Peg transfer: Pearson's $r = 0.87$ Pattern cutting: Pearson's $r = 0.75$ Suturing/knot tying: Pearson's $r = 0.89$ Vascular clip applying: Pearson's $r = 0.59$	N/A

Powers	2016	5 surgeons PGY3 and PGY 4 urology residents Attending surgeons	Intraoperative renal artery and vein dissection during live robotic partial nephrectomy	GEARS[a] Novel five-point scale for hilar dissection	Turk workers: 11 h, 33 min Surgeons: 13 days	Surgeon-level GEARS ratings: Pearson's $r = 0.84$ Video-level GEARS ratings: Pearson's $r = 0.82$ Force sensitivity domain: Pearson's $r = 0.35$ Pearson's r for remainder of GEARS domains = 0.76–0.83 Renal artery specific rating: Pearson's $r = 0.83$	N/A
Ghani	2016	Practicing urologists in the state of Michigan, enrolled in Michigan Urological Surgery Improvement Collaborative (MUSIC)	Live video from nerve-sparing robotic-assisted laparoscopic radical prostatectomy Bladder neck dissection Apical dissection Nerve sparing Urethrovesical anastomosis	GEARS[a] Robotic Anastomosis and Competency Evaluation (RACE) for anastomosis performance Summary pass/fail	Turk workers: 21 h for GEARS; 38 h for RACE Surgeons: 15 days for both ratings	GEARS: Pearson's $r = 0.78$ RACE: Pearson's $r = 0.74$ Identical evaluation of relative passing rate for each surgeon	N/A

(continued)

Table 6.3 (continued)

First author	Year	Task performers	Task	Evaluation mechanism	Average time to feedback	Rating agreement between crowds and experts	Compensation
Deal	2016	7 general surgery intern volunteers	Fundamentals of laparoscopic surgery tasks Peg transfer Precision cutting Intracorporeal knot tying	GOALS[c] Depth perception Bimanual dexterity Efficiency Tissue handling Overall pass/fail Verbal comments	Turk workers: 19 h Surgeons: 10 days	GEARS: Pearson's $r = 0.78$ Pass/fail evaluation: Pearson's $r = 0.80$ Qualitative examination of comment content: similar between two groups	N/A

[a]*GEARS* Global Evaluative Assessment of Robotic Skills
[b]*OSATS* Objective Structured Assessment of Technical Skills
[c]*GOALS* Global Operative Assessment of Laparoscopic Skills
[d]*HIT* human intelligence task

the different criteria used by crowdworkers and the simulation software to generate their respective assessments. Given the existing literature regarding crowd-based feedback, this suggests that perhaps this form of surgical evaluation may actually be superior to current artificial intelligence-based models, in that it more closely approximates the assessments of expert human surgeons.

Large-scale evaluation using crowdworkers has also been shown to be economically efficient. Across multiple published studies, crowdworkers such as Amazon Mechanical Turks are compensated small monetary sums ranging from \$0.50 to \$1.00 per task [27, 47, 49, 50, 55]. For crowdworkers, the amount of remuneration has been linked to the rapidity of feedback, which may provide further opportunities to improve the efficiency of this method of technical assessment [47]. In contrast, the cost for an expert surgeon assessment of a 5–10-min video is estimated to range from \$54 to \$108 or about \$10 per minute, assuming an annual surgeon salary of \$340,000 per year and a 2000-h work year [50]. Aggregate calculations based on the available data in the literature estimate that the cost of feedback provided by surgeons ranges from 1.15 to 8.38 times more expensive than that provided by crowds for the same task [57]. Thus, crowd-based evaluation of surgical task performance videos is consistently more cost-effective, particularly when scaled to multiple videos for an entire group of residents.

A 2016 systematic review highlighted that crowdworkers consistently completed evaluation tasks significantly faster than experts, ranging from 9 to 144 times faster [57]. In the current published literature, the time required for crowdworkers to return feedback for a specific task ranges from 5 days to as little as 2 h and 50 min, with variation depending on the length of task video and complexity of the task. In contrast, the time for expert surgeons to return feedback for the same tasks ranges from 26 h to 60 days [27, 47, 49, 51, 52, 54–56].

Though the value of crowd-based evaluation in dry lab simulation settings has been repeatedly validated, the impact of crowdsourced feedback on live intraoperative performance has been less extensively studied. Systematic reviews investigating skills transfer for laparoscopic and endoscopic simulation tasks suggest that such training improves operative performance [58], but there has been limited data on skills transfer from robotic simulation tasks [59]. Unlike simulation tasks, intraoperative performance is not limited to a single skill or task segment, with successful performance requiring nuanced surgical judgment in addition to basic technical fluency. Thus, equivalency between crowd-based evaluation and expert evaluation for the performance of a narrow scope of simulation tasks may not be maintained for more complex operative procedures performed in real time.

To address this issue, several groups have investigated the use of crowd-based feedback in the assessment of live operative video. Powers and colleagues generated 14 10-min video clips of renal hilar dissection performed at varying skill levels by 5 postgraduate year 3 or 4 urology residents and surgical attendings. Using the validated GEARS tool plus a novel renal artery dissection question, the videos were assessed by Amazon Mechanical Turk workers and urologic surgeons with expertise in robotic-assisted laparoscopic surgery and robotic partial nephrectomy. Complete ratings were returned by 14 expert surgeons in 13 days, as compared to

11 h and 33 min for the crowdworkers. Interestingly, the internal consistency of videos rated by experts was low, with an intra-class correlation coefficient of 0.38; this variability again highlights one of the limitations of our current system of feedback for surgical trainees. There was consistent correlation between the expert and crowdsourced ratings of video in aggregate ($R = 0.82$, $p < 0.001$), when separated by surgeon level ($R = 0.84$, $p < 0.001$), and for task-specific assessment ($R = 0.83$, $p < 0.001$). Though there were several limitations to this study, it suggests that large-scale evaluation may indeed be generalizable beyond dry lab simulation tasks to live human surgical procedures [51].

The increasing body of literature on the efficiency, cost-effectiveness, and parity of large-scale feedback to expert feedback for a wide range of technical tasks and surgical procedures has garnered the interest of the entrepreneurial world. Emerging companies such as C-SATS, Inc. (Seattle, WA) have capitalized on crowd-based wisdom to provide online platforms for surgical skills evaluation. Such technology is becoming increasingly utilized for a multitude of surgical procedures across the fields of gynecology, urology, general surgery, orthopedics, and reconstructive and plastic surgery. The promise of such large-scale evaluation is also beginning to become recognized by educational leaders across surgical subspecialties, such that it is starting to be explored in the development of nationally standardized technical skills curricula as a means of validating new educational material [60]. Though several barriers remain to the widespread adoption of crowdsourcing for technical skills evaluation, including surgeon "buy-in," requirement for intraoperative video capabilities, and a need for a cultural shift in residency education [61], the current body of literature suggests that it carries great potential for rapid and widespread use across surgical training programs.

Models for the Integration of Crowd-Based Evaluation in Surgical Skills Education

The early application of crowdsourced technology to surgical skills development has largely utilized Amazon Mechanical Turk workers and examined surgical task performance videos in a dry lab simulation setting using a variety of predefined laparoscopic, robotic, and procedural tasks, including laparoscopic and robotic peg transfer, suturing, and intracorporeal knot tying [27, 47, 50, 52, 54]. In the simulation setting, the primary value of large-scale feedback lies in its objective, prompt, and cost-effective assessment of trainees' technical skills. Crowdsourcing has been proposed as a mechanism to allow training programs to more efficiently identify those trainees who lag behind in basic technical skills early in their training and provide a consistent means of feedback to facilitate rapid remediation [27]. For other trainees, feedback from crowds may facilitate the acquisition and mastery of basic technical skills by providing the necessary feedback critical to successful motor learning and deliberate practice [12, 13].

One of the limitations of the feedback provided by crowdworkers is that it is largely reflective rather than formative. Most of the published studies on crowdsourced feedback for technical skills asked crowds to evaluate the performance of a specific task using an objective numeric scoring system, rather than to provide a subjective critique. In contrast, subjective feedback from expert surgeons might be not only reflective but also corrective, thereby facilitating refinement in surgical technique. Even in studies where subjective feedback was solicited from crowdworkers, the potential utilization of such comments to generate subtle improvements in technique was not specifically examined [47, 54]. It is notable, however, that subjective evaluation of expert and crowd comments regarding the same task performance reveal that the two encompass similar content, suggesting that perhaps either form of feedback might be of similar value to the trainee [54]. Moreover, there is evidence to suggest that specific and individualized feedback may not be as critical for adequate technical skills development as previously believed, particularly among novice learners [62].

Though most of the literature on crowdsourced feedback focuses on refining the technical skills of surgical trainees, emerging work has suggested that this technology might be further applied to refine the skills of those already considered to be "expert surgeons." Even attending surgeons and surgeons in practice are not impervious to error. Indeed in a study of national malpractice claims, 58% of technical errors resulting in patient harm involved a surgeon practicing within his or her own specialty but lacking in technical expertise [6]. Moreover, whether it is to maintain a pre-existing skill set or to become proficient with new surgical technology, even experienced surgeons will need to develop and hone their surgical skills throughout the course of their careers.

Ghani and colleagues studied the use of crowd-based evaluation through the lens of quality improvement in a population of practicing urologists through the Michigan Urological Surgery Improvement Collaborative (MUSIC). Overall, 76 video clips of technically challenging portions of nerve-sparing robotic-assisted laparoscopic prostatectomy from 12 surgeons within the consortium were selected for evaluation by at least 4 surgical experts and at least 30–55 Amazon Mechanical Turk workers per clip using the GEARS assessment and the Robotic Anastomosis and Competency Evaluation (RACE) for urethrovesical anastomosis video segments. Both GEARS and RACE scores between the two groups were strongly and significantly correlated (Pearson's correlation = 0.78 and 0.74, respectively; $p < 0.001$). There was significantly greater intra-peer variability in ratings from expert surgeons ($p < 0.001$). Expert peer reviewers took 15 days to return both global skills and anastomosis ratings, whereas crowdworkers returned global ratings on average in 21 h and anastomosis ratings in 38 h. Moreover, both the crowdworkers and experts were able to identify the bottom five surgeons ranked by technical skill for this procedure [53]. The use of crowdsourced feedback may therefore be valuable for experienced surgeons as well, as it may provide a model for continued surgical skills refinement, facilitate future peer evaluation of currently practicing surgeons, and lend itself to quality improvement initiatives in practice.

Future Applications of Crowd-Based Evaluation

Crowdsourced technology can identify those trainees requiring additional surgical skills improvement and might also provide the potential to prospectively identify those trainees who may be surgically precocious. Indeed, there is evidence to suggest that in addition to deliberate practice, individual factors and ability play a significant role in the acquisition of expertise, particularly in situations where the tasks are unfamiliar or particularly complex [63]. In the surgical arena, where even commonly performed procedures remain unique, challenging, and complex due to individual patient factors, anatomy, and clinical context, trainees with innate ability might therefore be more apt to efficiently develop expertise.

This is particularly germane in the context of residency trainee selection, as prior research has demonstrated that completing a surgical residency program alone does not ensure competence. One longitudinal study suggested that about 5–10% of trainees in a 5-year surgical training program did not reach technical proficiency by the completion of their residency program [64]. Another survey of North American fellowship directors revealed that 21% of fellows were deemed unprepared for the operating room, with 66% unable to operate independently for more than 30 consecutive minutes [65]. In this setting, identifying those future trainees with the strongest potential for technical aptitude is critical, given the large time and financial investments in the surgical training of residents. Despite a large body of work investigating the predictive value of personal questionnaires and tests of innate aptitude, manual dexterity, visual-spatial ability, and basic performance resource tests, no single test or combination of tests has yet been identified to reliably and accurately predict technical aptitude [66].

Among surgical residency program directors, there has been growing interest in including technical skills as a factor when considering applications from future surgery trainee [66]. Long-term correlation between pretraining skills assessments and the final performance of these applicants within their respective training programs remains to be elucidated, though there is evidence from the otolaryngology field to suggest that such a relationship may indeed exist [67]. Crowd-based feedback on directly observed technical tasks might provide a means to efficiently accomplish this assessment during the residency recruitment process. Such application of crowdsourcing technology would potentially have significant implications on the identification and selection of future cohorts of surgeons particularly suited to high-risk or complex surgery.

In 2016, Vernez and colleagues at the University of California, Irvine, explored this idea by applying crowdsourcing technology to a group of 25 medical students applying into a urologic residency program. Applicants were asked to perform a series of surgical simulation tasks and were then ranked in order of desired match by both expert surgeons and crowds based on task performance scores alone. Interestingly, the final submitted residency match rank list had poor concordance with both match lists generated solely on crowd scores and on expert scores (Cronbach's $\alpha = 0.46$ and 0.48, respectively). However, among those ranked in the bottom five on the match rank list, three of the five were identified by crowds, and two of the five were identified by faculty to be among the bottom five performers in these simulation tasks [56]. These findings suggest that technical performance alone is not the primary predictor of success within surgical training. Indeed, there are multiple other intangible factors assessed during an interview, such as tenacity, flexibility, creativity, discipline, and emotional intelligence, which contribute to success in residency training. However, this study further suggests that crowd-based skills assessment may be particularly useful to identify those who are weak in surgical skills and provides a framework by which crowdsourced evaluation could be used to incorporate technical skills assessments into the complex process of resident recruitment.

Though a critical component of surgical competency, excellent technical skill alone clearly does not define excellent surgical care. This also involves complex preoperative and intraoperative decision-making, surgical knowledge, and interpersonal patient care skills. These are more challenging to develop but are equally essential parts of a comprehensive surgical education. With the recent adoption of milestone-based competency for surgical training, there is increased focus on helping trainees achieve competency in not only technical performance but also in the realms of professionalism and communication, which are more difficult to objectively measure. Surgical curricula directed toward these proficiencies have historically been evaluated using standardized patient interactions and the Objective Structured Clinical Examination [68, 69]. However, such evaluative measures carry the same challenges of cost, time investment, and subjectivity inherent to surgical skills feedback. To date, large-scale evaluation of such competencies has not yet been explored, but integration with these existing assessment tools might be a novel application of this technology. The use of crowdsourcing to enhance such nontechnical aspects of surgical education remains a potential area of new research.

Conclusions

The use of crowd-based evaluation in the realm of surgical education remains relatively novel, but the present literature has demonstrated that this technology may address a significant challenge in the current paradigm of surgical education. The consistency, economics, and rapidity of crowd-based feedback may be one means by which the attainment of technical proficiency among surgical trainees can be facilitated in the face of current work-hour limitations, administrative burdens, and inconsistent feedback mechanisms that constrain residency training programs across multiple surgical specialties. As new surgical technologies and techniques continue to develop, crowdsourcing may also prove to be an integral part of continuing medical education and skills development for those surgeons already in practice. Moreover, given the initial promise of this technology within the realm of technical skills development, crowd-based evaluation may soon become even more broadly used to help trainees develop nontechnical skills, validate national surgical curricula, and inform the selection of future surgical trainees.

Additional research is warranted to more directly define the relationship between crowdsourced evaluation and surgical development among trainees. Particularly in the areas of live operative feedback, individualized formative feedback, and assessment of nontechnical competencies, the role of large-scale evaluation platforms is yet to be explored. The efficacy of this technology as part of a formalized surgical skills curriculum remains to be fully assessed. However, given the initial promise of crowdsourcing as an emerging technology in surgical education, this has already begun to be introduced into surgical training curricula across a few institutions. As the value of large-scale feedback becomes further established, this platform is poised to become more widely adopted across surgical training programs and practices and has the potential to become an integral component of our model of surgical skills development in the future.

References

1. Reznick RK, MacRae H. Teaching surgical skills – changes in the wind. N Engl J Med. 2006;355(25):2664–9.
2. Polavarapu HV, Kulaylat AN, Sun SHO. 100 years of surgical education: the past, present, and future. Bull Am Coll Surg. 2013;98(7):22–7.
3. Kohn LT, Corrigan JM, Donaldson MS. To err is human: building a safer health system. Washington, D.C.: National Academy Press; 2000. 360 p.
4. Altman DE, Clancy C, Blendon RJ. Improving patient safety — five years after the IOM report. N Engl J Med. 2004;351(20):2041–3.
5. Leape LL, Berwick DM. Five years after to err is human what have we learned? JAMA. 2005;293(19):2384–90.
6. Rogers SO Jr, Gawande AA, Kwaan M, Puopolo AL, Yoon C, Brennan TA, et al. Analysis of surgical errors in closed malpractice claims at 4 liability insurers. Surgery. 2006;140(1): 25–33.
7. Birkmeyer JD, Finks JF, O'Reilly A, Oerline M, Carlin AM, Nunn AR, et al. Surgical skill and complication rates after bariatric surgery. N Engl J Med. 2013;369(15):1434–42.
8. Bridges M, Diamond DL. The financial impact of teaching surgical residents in the operating room. Am J Surg. 1999;177(1):28–32.
9. Babineau TJ, Becker J, Gibbons G, Sentovich S, Hess D, Robertson S, et al. The "cost" of operative training for surgical residents. Arch Surg. 2004;139(4):366–70.
10. Papandria D, Rhee D, Ortega G, Zhang Y, Gorgy A, Makary MA, et al. Assessing trainee impact on operative time for common general surgical procedures in ACS-NSQIP. J Surg Educ. 2012;69(2):149–55.
11. Macario A. What does one minute of operating room time cost? J Clin Anesth. 2010;22(4): 233–6.
12. Fitts PM, Posner MI. Human performance. Belmont: Brooks/Cole; 1967. p. 469–98.
13. Ericsson KAK, Krampe RRT, Tesch-Romer C, Ashworth C, Carey G, Grassia J, et al. The role of deliberate practice in the Acquisition of Expert Performance. Psychol Rev. 1993;100(3):363–406.
14. Boyle E, Al-Akash M, Gallagher AG, Traynor O, Hill ADNP. Optimising surgical training: use of feedback to reduce errors during a simulated surgical procedure. Postgr Med J. 2011;87(1030):524–8.
15. Bosse HM, Mohr J, Buss B, Krautter M, Weyrich P, Herzog W, et al. The benefit of repetitive skills training and frequency of expert feedback in the early acquisition of procedural skills. BMC Med Educ [Internet]. 2015;15(1):22. Available from: http://www.pubmedcentral.nih.gov/articlerender.fcgi?artid=4339240&tool=pmcentrez&rendertype=abstract.

16. Stefanidis D, Korndorffer JJ, Heniford B, Scott D. Limited feedback and video tutorials optimize learning and resource utilization during laparoscopic simulator training. Surgery. 2007;142(2):202–6.
17. Perone J, Fankhauser G, Adhikari D, Mehta H, Woods M, Strohmeyer J, et al. Who did the case? Perceptions on resident operative participation. Am J Surg. 2017;213(4):821–6.
18. Morgan R, Kauffman DF, Doherty G, Sachs T. Resident and attending perceptions of resident involvement: an analysis of ACGME reporting guidelines. J Surg Educ. 2016;74(3):415–22.
19. Reznick RK. Teaching and testing technical skills. Am J Surg. 1993;165(3):358–61.
20. Williams RG, Klamen DA, McGaghie WC. Cognitive, social and environmental sources of bias in clinical performance ratings. Teach Learn Med. 2003;15(4):270–92.
21. Gundle K, Mickelson D, Hanel D. Reflections in a time of transition: orthopaedic faculty and resident understanding of accreditation schemes and opinions on surgical skills feedback. Med Educ Online. 2016;21(1):30584.
22. Martin JA, Regehr G, Reznick R, Macrae H, Murnaghan J, Hutchison C, et al. Objective structured assessment of technical skill (OSATS) for surgical residents. Br J Surg. 1997;84(2):273–8.
23. Vassiliou MC, Feldman LS, Andrew CG, Bergman S, Leffondré K, Stanbridge D, et al. A global assessment tool for evaluation of intraoperative laparoscopic skills. Am J Surg. 2005;190(1):107–13.
24. Goh AC, Goldfarb DW, Sander JC, Miles BJ, Dunkin BJ. Global evaluative assessment of robotic skills: validation of a clinical assessment tool to measure robotic surgical skills. J Urol. 2012;187(1):247–52.
25. Hogg M, Zenati M, Novak S, Chen Y, Jun Y, Steve J, et al. Grading of surgeon technical performance predicts postoperative pancreatic fistula for Pancreaticoduodenectomy independent of patient-related variables. Ann Surg. 2016;264(3):482–91.
26. Shah J, Darzi A. Surgical skills assessment: an ongoing debate. BJU Int. 2001;88(7):655–60.
27. Holst D, Kowalewski TM, White LW, Brand TC, Harper JD, Sorensen MD, et al. Crowd-sourced assessment of technical skills: differentiating animate surgical skill through the wisdom of crowds. J Endourol. 2015;29(10):1183–8. 150413093359007
28. Stefanidis D, Arora S, Parrack DM, Hamad GG, Capella J, Grantcharov T, et al. Research priorities in surgical simulation for the 21st century. Am J Surg. 2012;203(1):49–53.
29. Greenberg CC, Ghousseini HN, Pavuluri Quamme SR, Beasley HL, Wiegmann DA. Surgical coaching for individual performance improvement. Ann Surg [Internet]. 2015;261(1). Available from: http://journals.lww.com/annalsofsurgery/Fulltext/2015/01000/Surgical_Coaching_for_Individual_Performance.8.aspx.
30. Greenberg C, Dombrowski J, Dimick J. Video-based surgical coaching: an emerging approach to performance improvement. JAMA Surg [Internet]. 2016;151(3):282–3. Available from: https://doi.org/10.1001/jamasurg.2015.4442.
31. Howe J. The rise of crowdsourcing. Wired Mag [Internet]. 2006;14(6):1–5. Available from: http://www.clickadvisor.com/downloads/Howe_The_Rise_of_Crowdsourcing.pdf.
32. Garrigos-Simon FJ, Gil-Pechuán I, Estelles-Miguel S. Advances in crowdsourcing. Cham: Springer; 2015. p. 1–183.
33. Brabham DC. Crowdsourcing as a model for problem solving: an introduction and cases. Converg Int J Res into New Media Technol. 2008;14(1):75–90.
34. Lévy P. Collective intelligence: Mankind's emerging world in cyberspace [internet]. Challenges. 1997:277 p. Available from: http://portal.acm.org/citation.cfm?id=550283
35. Ipeirotis P. Demographics of mechanical turk. Working Paper CeDER-10-01. 2010. http://hdl.handle.net/2451/29585
36. Ranard BL, Ha YP, Meisel ZF, Asch DA, Hill SS, Becker LB, et al. Crowdsourcing – harnessing the masses to advance health and medicine, a systematic review. J Gen Intern Med. 2014;29:187–203.
37. Cooper S, Khatib F, Treuille A, Barbero J, Lee J, Beenen M, et al. Predicting protein structures with a multiplayer online game. Nature. 2010;466:756–60.
38. Kawrykow A, Roumanis G, Kam A, Kwak D, Leung C, Wu C, et al. Phylo: a citizen science approach for improving multiple sequence alignment. PLoS One. 2012;7(3):e31362.

39. Nguyen TB, Wang S, Anugu V, Rose N, McKenna M, Petrick N, et al. Distributed human intelligence for colonic polyp classification in computer-aided detection for CT colonography. Radiology. 2012;262(3):824–33.
40. Mavandadi S, Dimitrov S, Feng S, Yu F, Sikora U, Yaglidere O, et al. Distributed medical image analysis and diagnosis through crowd-sourced games: a malaria case study. PLoS One. 2012;7(5):e37245.
41. Freifeld CC, Chunara R, Mekaru SR, Chan EH, Kass-Hout T, Iacucci AA, et al. Participatory epidemiology: use of mobile phones for community-based health reporting. PLoS Med. 2010;7(12):e1000376.
42. Chen SP, Kirsch S, Zlatev DV, Chang TC, Comstock B, Lendvay TS, et al. Optical biopsy of bladder cancer using crowd-sourced assessment. JAMA Surg. 2016;151(1):90–2.
43. Brady CJ, Villanti AC, Pearson JL, Kirchner TR, Gupta OP, Shah CP. Rapid grading of fundus photographs for diabetic retinopathy using crowdsourcing. J Med Internet Res. 2014;16(10):e233.
44. Mitry D, Peto T, Hayat S, Blows P, Morgan J, Khaw KT, et al. Crowdsourcing as a screening tool to detect clinical features of glaucomatous optic neuropathy from digital photography. PLoS One. 2015;10(2):e0117401.
45. Bow HC, Dattilo JR, Jonas AM, Lehmann CU. A crowdsourcing model for creating preclinical medical education study tools. Acad Med. 2013;88(6):766–70.
46. Blackwell KA, Travis MJ, Arbuckle MR, Ross DA. Crowdsourcing medical education. Med Educ. 2016;50(5):576.
47. Chen C, White L, Kowalewski T, Aggarwal R, Lintott C, Comstock B, et al. Crowd-sourced assessment of technical skills: a novel method to evaluate surgical performance. J Surg Res. 2014;187(1):65–71.
48. Malpani A, Vedula SS, Chen CCG, Hager GD. A study of crowdsourced segment-level surgical skill assessment using pairwise rankings. Int J Comput Assist Radiol Surg. 2015;10(9):1435–47.
49. Aghdasi N, Bly R, White LW, Hannaford B, Moe K, Lendvay TS. Crowd-sourced assessment of surgical skills in cricothyrotomy procedure. J Surg Res. 2015;196(2):302–6.
50. White LW, Kowalewski TM, Dockter RL, Comstock B, Hannaford B, Lendvay TS. Crowd-sourced assessment of technical skill: a valid method for discriminating basic robotic surgery skills. J Endourol. 2015;29(11):1295–301.
51. Powers MK, Boonjindasup A, Pinsky M, Dorsey P, Maddox M, Su L-M, et al. Crowdsourcing assessment of surgeon dissection of renal artery and vein during robotic partial nephrectomy: a novel approach for quantitative assessment of surgical performance. J Endourol. 2016;30(4):447–52.
52. Polin MR, Siddiqui NY, Comstock BA, Hesham H, Brown C, Lendvay TS, et al. Crowdsourcing: a valid alternative to expert evaluation of robotic surgery skills. Am J Obstet Gynecol. 2016;215:644.e1–7.
53. Ghani KR, Miller DC, Linsell S, Brachulis A, Lane B, Sarle R, et al. Measuring to improve: peer and crowd-sourced assessments of technical skill with robot-assisted radical prostatectomy. Am J Obstet Gynecol. 2016;69:547–50.
54. Deal SB, Lendvay TS, Haque MI, Brand T, Comstock B, Warren J, et al. Crowd-sourced assessment of technical skills: an opportunity for improvement in the assessment of laparoscopic surgical skills. Am J Surg. 2016;211(2):398–404.
55. Holst D, Kowalewski TM, White LW, Brand TC, Harper JD, Sorenson MD, et al. Crowd-sourced assessment of technical skills: an adjunct to urology resident surgical simulation training. J Endourol. 2015;29(5):604–9.
56. Vernez SL, Huynh V, Osann K, Okhunov Z, Landman J, Clayman R V. C-SATS: assessing surgical skills among urology residency applicants. J Endourol. 2016;31(S1):S-95-S-100. doi: https://doi.org/10.1089/end.2016.0569.
57. Katz AJ. The role of crowdsourcing in assessing surgical skills. Surg Laparosc Endosc Percutan Tech. 2016;26(4):271–7.

58. Sturm LP, Windsor JA, Cosman PH, Cregan PC, Hewett PJ, Maddern GJ. A systematic review of surgical skills transfer after simulation-based training. Ann Surg. 2008;248(2):166–79.
59. Moglia A, Ferrari V, Morelli L, Ferrari M, Mosca F, Cuschieri A. A systematic review of virtual reality simulators for robot-assisted surgery. Eur Urol. 2016;69(2):1065–80.
60. Lee JY, Andonian S, Pace KT, Grober E. Basic laparoscopic skills assessment study – validation and standard setting among Canadian urology trainees. Eur Urol. 2017;197(6):1539–44.
61. Lendvay TS, White L, Kowalewski T. Crowdsourcing to assess surgical skill. JAMA Surg. 2015;150(11):1086–7.
62. Phillips A, Matthan J, Bookless L, Whitehead I, Madhavan A, Rodham P, et al. Individualised expert feedback is not essential for improving basic clinical skills performance in novice learners: a randomized trial. J Surg Educ. 2017;74(4):612–20.
63. Kulasegaram KM, Grierson LEM, Norman GR. The roles of deliberate practice and innate ability in developing expertise: evidence and implications. Med Educ [Internet]. 2013;47(10):979–89. Available from: https://doi.org/10.1111/medu.12260.
64. Cuschieri A. Lest we forget the surgeon. Semin Laparosc Surg. 2003;10(3):141–8.
65. Mattar SG, Alseidi AA, Jones DB, Jeyarajah DR, Swanstrom LL, Aye RW, et al. General surgery residency inadequately prepares trainees for fellowship: results of a survey of fellowship program directors. Ann Surg [Internet]. 2013;258(3):440–9. Available from: http://www.ncbi.nlm.nih.gov/pubmed/24022436.
66. Louridas M, Szasz P, de Montbrun S, Harris KA, Grantcharov TP. Original reports: optimizing the selection of general surgery residents: a national consensus. J Surg Educ [Internet]. 2017; Available from: http://10.0.3.248/j.jsurg.2016.06.015%5Cnhttps://ezp.lib.unimelb.edu.au/login?url=https://search.ebscohost.com/login.aspx?direct=true&db=edselp&AN=S1931720416300915&site=eds-live&scope=site.
67. Moore EJ, Price DL, Van Abel KM, Carlson ML. Still under the microscope: can a surgical aptitude test predict otolaryngology resident performance? Laryngoscope. 2015;125(2):E57–61.
68. Iramaneerat C. Instruction and assessment of professionalism for surgery residents. J Surg Educ. 2009;66(3):158–62.
69. Hochberg MS, Kalet A, Zabar S, Kachur E, Gillespie C, Berman RS. Can professionalism be taught? Encouraging evidence. Am J Surg. 2010;199(1):86–93.

Teaching Residents to Teach: Why and How

7

James Feimster, Alexandria D. McDow, and John D. Mellinger

Teaching Residents to Teach: Why and How

The teaching role of a resident is a fundamental aspect of modern surgical training and education. Not only are surgical residents themselves training for a career that requires a strong knowledge base and refined technical skills, but they also play critical roles in educating more junior residents and medical students at their institutions. In this chapter, we will outline why teaching residents to teach is both challenging and essential to contemporary surgical education, review current memory and learning science theory, and detail how residents can apply clinical teaching models to enhance the surgical knowledge and skills of their students and colleagues.

Importance of Residents as Teachers

Contemporary surgery has become a complex team-based exercise that involves multidisciplinary workgroups in which residents and medical students are together embedded. In the social context of such activities, studies have shown that residents have a greater summative influence on not only the knowledge but also the attitudes and behavioral standards adopted by medical students, given their intimate involvement in the students' learning environment [1, 2]. Medical students also rate the

J. Feimster, MD • A.D. McDow, MD
General Surgery, Southern Illinois University School of Medicine, Springfield, IL, USA

J.D. Mellinger, MD (✉)
Department of Surgery, Southern Illinois University School of Medicine, PO Box 19638, 701 N. First St., Springfield, IL, USA, 62794-9638
e-mail: jmellinger@siumed.edu

T.S. Köhler, B. Schwartz (eds.), *Surgeons as Educators*,
https://doi.org/10.1007/978-3-319-64728-9_7

percentage of knowledge gained from residents as equal to or greater than that gleaned from faculty, second only to what is gathered from their own independent study efforts [1, 3–5].

Challenges Encountered in Preparing Residents to Teach

In order for surgical residents to teach junior house staff and medical students, the resident must first themselves develop the technical skills and clinical knowledge required to perform operative tasks and manage complex patients. The increasing demands of documentation and electronic health records, alongside the pressures of duty hour reform, have created a challenging environment for such development. Recent studies have shown that there is a gap between the amount of experience US general surgery graduates receive while in residency and what is expected [6]. Bell et al. performed a study which categorized operative procedures that graduating residents were expected to be able to perform independently. This study identified a large variation of experience between residents nationwide and many cases in which residents had limited or no experience yet were expected to achieve competence. Accordingly, many graduating residents do not feel confident to enter independent general surgery practice following residency, and this may be a significant factor in motivating them to pursue further training in fellowship [7]. Finally, Pugh et al. reported that surgical faculty and residents have significantly different perceptions of residents' learning needs, especially as pertained to learning goals and priorities in the operating room [8]. All these factors represent significant challenges facing residents seeking to develop their own competence as a requisite foundation for teaching and instructing junior residents and students.

There are many factors contributing to this decrease in experience and lack of confidence in the current training paradigm. Kairys et al. evaluated operative experience among general surgery residents since the implementation of the 80-h work duty restrictions [9]. They observed a decrease in total major cases, cases performed as a chief resident, and, most significantly, cases logged as both first assistant and teaching assistant. This decrease in teaching assistant cases and first assistant cases represents a significant loss of educational opportunities, not only for the junior resident but also for the chief resident practicing and refining his or her ability to teach. Additionally, there has been a shift in the degree of autonomy allotted to a resident in many programs due to the general public's expectations and supervision requirements. Whereas in the past, many programs offered a "chief-run" service in which the chief resident performed cases not directly supervised by the attending physician, this experience is now lacking in many programs. With increased supervision requirements and expectations, and decreased operative case volume, graduating residents may feel inadequately prepared to commence the independent practice of general surgery, as well as to give their time and personal experience opportunity to teach more junior learners.

Recognizing these challenges, there are conversely some very important reasons why residents may be the most effective teachers for junior colleagues and students. We will now turn to detailing some of these.

Reasons Why Residents May Be Advantaged as Teachers

A number of theories have been put forth regarding why residents may have such a strong influence on the education of more junior house staff and medical students. These include theories related to skill development and deconstructive skill, peer relationship and social theory, and time pressure considerations related to alternative teachers, notably surgical faculty.

Conscious vs. Unconscious Performance

One commonly held theory suggests that surgical residents, who themselves are still in a training environment, require ongoing conscious thought to perform most of their skills and daily activities. In contrast, attending surgeons, by virtue of their larger volume of experience, have become less cognizant of the steps and processing required in performing a particular skill. That is, in terms of the four stages of competence described by Burch in the 1970s, the resident is still engaged in the "consciously competent" phase of their own development, in which understanding and decision making are detached, whereas many attendings function in the "unconsciously competent" sphere in which responses are intuitive based on experience [10, 11]. Accordingly, the resident's proximity in relation to their student learner's zone of skill acquisition allows them to more readily deconstruct and verbalize to junior learners the individual steps of a process, particularly with reference to performing technical skills [5].

For example, a junior resident teaching a medical student how to tie square knots would be more likely to go through each individual step, as the resident would still themselves be progressing toward automaticity. Conversely, an attending surgeon who has tied thousands of surgical knots in their career is more removed from such sequencing and deconstructive analysis and may struggle more with teaching individual steps and sequencing to a novice learner. While skilled teachers learn to develop such deconstructive skills even after achieving personal mastery, resident teachers typically have a shorter bridge to the level of the novice or junior learner and cross that gap more instinctively.

"Near-Peer" Relationship

Another theory is based on the relative age difference between the learner and the teacher. Surgical residents are closer in age and generational status to other residents and medical students than are the attending surgeons. Attending surgeons typically come from the baby boomer era and Generation X, while most residents come from the millennial generation. The relative closeness in age between a medical student and a resident allows for a "near-peer" relationship that enables understanding of generational norms and contributes to open conversations and questions from the student [5, 12]. A question that a student might not feel comfortable asking an attending surgeon because it might seem unintelligent would be more easily asked of a resident due to this near-peer relationship [3]. Being in generational proximity may accordingly promote educational dialog for the resident educator and serve as an advantage in comparison to a faculty teacher.

Faculty Time Pressure

Changes in modern healthcare including pressures for efficiency, cost control, volume production, duty hour reform as referenced above, and quality have fostered an environment in which attending surgeons manage their workflow priorities in a fashion often counterproductive to the teaching of novice learners. Critics state that with medical school budgets becoming tighter and more reliant on clinical volume and related revenue, attending surgeons are obligated to spend more time in patient care and less time in traditional and more pure or focused teaching venues [5, 13]. These forces may cause attendings to spend more of their time in direct clinical and administrative pursuits, limiting their availability and flexibility for teaching especially more junior learners and increasing the scenarios in which residents are the sole or predominant remaining educators available for medical students.

Summary

Recognizing that for all these reasons, residents may be better suited and/or available for student education, it is clear that resident teaching of students and more junior house staff is a vital component of contemporary surgical education. Many residents enjoy and embrace the opportunity of this teaching role and would like to become better educators themselves during their training years [1]. Accordingly, a number of surgical programs around the nation have developed, or begun to develop, curricula that incorporate teaching skills into the fabric of residency training. Morrison et al. have shown that a teaching skills curriculum improves teaching effectiveness of residents when compared to residents with no teaching guidance [5, 14].

Beyond the importance of residents in teaching junior learners, it is also recognized that educational skill is fundamental to a resident's long-term career activities even in nonacademic settings. This is apparent when one considers the fundamental role of a professional as an educator for those whom they serve as patients, colleagues, or clients. Given the strategic importance of educational development as part of a resident's training, the remainder of this chapter will focus on some of the tools and strategies which can be used to equip resident teachers for these purposes. Pertinent to this theme, we will review current cognitive science regarding learning and retention and then review specific strategies which may be used in the clinical setting to facilitate teaching effectiveness.

How Residents Learn: An Update on Cognition Science

For residents to become excellent teachers, it is useful for them to understand the current literature on cognition, as well as related theories on how people learn and store information in memory. Numerous theories have been described. Until recently, it has been assumed that learning is primarily facilitated from repetitive exposure through studying and resulting encoding of information in memory [15]. However recent data has shown the benefit of test-enhanced learning in long-term memory and retrieval.

Test-Enhanced Learning

Test-enhanced learning is a model that has been developed over the past decade; it states that repeated retrieval of information through testing increases retention and long-term memory [16]. Testing has long been thought to be a neutral event in the process of memory and not a determinant of learning itself [15, 16]. Yet, recent studies have redefined how testing affects the process of long-term memory acquisition and how it produces results superior to studying over the long term.

Karpicke and Roediger in 2008 performed a study evaluating college students and their ability to remember word pairs from a foreign language and their native tongue as a function of whether they studied and/or were tested in the interval from initial learning to evaluation of performance on a final delayed test [15]. The first group of students was allowed to study and engaged in interval testing (ST). The second group was simply tested (S_NT), but did not study. The third group was allowed to study, but was not tested (ST_N). Finally, the fourth group was not allowed to study or test once they had initially learned the word pairs (S_NT_N). The results demonstrated that students who were tested only performed just as well as students who both studied and tested and students who studied but did not undergo interval testing performed almost as poorly as those who neither studied nor tested (ST 80% on final test, S_NT 80%, ST_N 36%, S_NT_N 33%).

In other words, interval testing, and not the conventional studying, was the important operative determinant of how well the students performed as reflected by long-term recall. The process of repeated retrieval of the information (i.e., testing) allowed the students to correctly recall approximately 80% of the foreign language word pairs regardless of whether they studied or not, while the students who were not repeatedly tested (even if engaged in study) recalled around 35%, similar to those who engaged in neither studying nor testing in the interval from initial learning to final testing.

These results have been reproduced in numerous other studies. Larsen et al. in 2015 studied a group of neurologists that were participating in continuing medical education (CME) courses. Groups were divided into no additional exposure after the initial CME course, repeated study after the CME course, and repeated retrieval/quizzing after the CME course. The results showed that neurologists that were repeatedly tested had a higher portion of correct answers on final delayed testing (55%) when compared to both the no additional exposure (44%) and repeated studying groups (46%), who performed similarly on the delayed recall examination [16].

Test-enhanced learning has lead surgical residency programs to introduce weekly quizzes and mock exams. The Surgical Council on Resident Education (SCORE), an almost universally used general surgery residency curriculum developed by multiple surgical societies under the auspices of the American Board of Surgery, has incorporated weekly quizzes in its comprehensive curricular outline. The American Board of Surgery In-Service Training Examination (ABSITE) is a yearly exam that predicts resident performance on the ABS Qualifying Examination. In one study, introduction of the test-enhanced learning model by incorporating regular quizzing alongside other academic development strategies has been shown in the authors' own residency program to increase ABSITE mean percentile scores by as much as 34% [17].

Spacing

Not only does repeated testing and retrieval of information enhance long-term memory, but the spacing between testing events has an effect as well. Many curricula for incoming surgical interns and continuing medical education sessions offer short demanding courses that typically last anywhere from 1 day to 1 week. This is known as *massed practice* [18–21]. Afterward there is often no delayed follow-up on knowledge or skill performance, and deterioration of retention and/or performance over time is observed. Therefore spacing (also known as *distributed practice*) has become an important concept in terms of retrieval of information from long-term memory [18].

One such study that shows the importance of spacing involved a surgical skills laboratory and junior residents' ability to perform a microvascular anastomosis on anesthetized rats. Moulton et al. divided the residents into a massed group, which received all four instructional sessions in a single day, and a spaced group, which received the four sessions once per week over a period of 4 weeks. At the end of the month, the two groups were tested on performance of a microvascular anastomosis. The results showed that the spaced group completed the surgery in less time, with fewer hand movements, and had 100% success at performing the anastomosis when compared to the massed group. Additionally, the massed group had 16% of residents damage the anastomosis beyond repair [18].

Spacing has been shown to be superior to massed practice in promoting longer-term retention and allows for easier transfer of surgical skills to real-life situations. It is thought that spacing activates differing regions of the brain during the learning session and between sessions. This activation allows for the consolidation and more enduring retention of the learned material. Spacing also stimulates the learner to mentally rehearse and prepare for key aspects of each session or segment of material [18, 22–24].

Interleaving

Another concept that has developed over the past decade is the concept of interleaving. Interleaving is defined by the mixing of topics during learning sessions, instead of a single topic in isolation being taught at each learning session [25, 26]. This can be diagrammed by the interleaving group having one session consisting of topics ABCD, another session BADC, etc. with each letter corresponding to a different topic. The standard, traditional blocked learning would accordingly look like AAAA, BBBB, CCCC, etc.

Studies have shown that the traditional blocked learning may provide superior immediate retention of information, but in the acquisition of long-term memory, interleaving is superior [25]. Rohrer and Taylor studied math students that were placed in a blocked group or mixed group and evaluated their performance on subsequent tests. The blocked group (traditional) performed well on the immediate practice test, averaging 89%, with the mixed group behind at 60%. However, once it came to the final retention test several weeks later, the mixed group averaged 63%, much higher than the blocked group's average of 20% [25].

It is thought that interleaving improves long-term memory by allowing the learner to discriminate between different topics when asked about them in the future. Blocked learners have difficulty discriminating between topics and are therefore unable to move on to the correct solution that may involve more complex or varied tasks or combinations thereof [26, 27].

Feedback-Enhanced Testing

Test-enhanced learning has brought on the use of quizzing as a tool to enhance learning and long-term memory. Question banks and practice tests that involve multiple choice questions are readily available to residents and cover many medical and surgical topics. Although these quizzes have been shown to improve retrieval and long-term memory, studies have shown that quizzes with multiple choice questions can lead to negative effects with incorrect information. For example, a resident is stumped on a multiple choice question and takes an educated guess. That guess could be based off of false information, leading the learner to misinterpret key concepts. This is why feedback is imperative with test-enhanced learning [28, 29].

Feedback allows students to correct mistakes and misinterpreted concepts and then solidify correct concepts in their memory. Types of feedback include a simple one-line response to the correct answer, detailed explanations of correct responses, or study materials to help delineate the correct response [28]. Karpicke and Roediger have shown that feedback during repeated testing enhances retrieval and long-term memory by 25% or more when compared to no feedback [30].

Feedback is typically presented immediately after the test to ensure effective retention. This can be done after each individual question or at the end of the quiz. Recent literature has even shown that delayed feedback may have more benefit. It is thought that delayed feedback that is fully processed by the learner leads to better retrieval because it leads to an additional spaced exposure to the material. One limitation to delayed feedback, experts point out, is that students may not be motivated to review feedback in the delayed setting, not guaranteeing full processing of the feedback material [28].

Summary

Test-enhanced learning allows for greater retrieval of information and retention in long-term memory than study alone. To maximize the effect of testing, the literature supports five principles that should be followed [16]:

- Tests should be developed from the educational objectives in the program's curriculum.
- Questions should allow for the production of answers instead of simple recognition of answers.
- Tests should allow for repeated retrieval practice.
- Repeated tests should be spaced and interleaved to necessitate effortful retrieval of information.
- Feedback should be given after each test.

Understanding these principles in regard to human learning and memory provides a critical foundation for exploring the specific strategies residents can employ in the clinical setting to become more effective teachers.

Feedback in the Clinical Arena

Feedback is a critical component of all education, not only in the testing realm but also in the clinical teaching and learning environment, and has a pronounced effect on the success of surgical residents. Feedback incorporates an interaction between the learner and teacher that provides accurate information on the learner's performance and behavior. This interaction is a learning opportunity to provide guidance for future activities and performances [31, 32]. It is important for feedback to be a two-way conversation that allows the learners to self-reflect and assess their performance [33].

Residents have rated feedback as exceedingly important in their overall training. In prior studies, the process of giving feedback has been rated second only to the clinical competence of the attending surgeon in describing the characteristics of effective clinical teaching [34]. Feedback, positive or constructive, gives residents a learning opportunity to reinforce good skills and abandon mistakes or undesirable habits. If feedback is not given at regular intervals, habits that are deemed desirable might be abandoned, and conversely, undesirable habits retained [35].

Many studies have shown the relative infrequency in which feedback is given in medical education. Hewson et al. stated in a survey of residents that 8% were satisfied with the feedback they received. Approximately 80% of residents never or seldom received corrective feedback from their attendings [33]. Studies in the operating room have shown approximately 18% of residents reported attendings identifying operative goals in the preoperative period. Additionally, only 37% of surgical attendings discussed areas of improvement with the residents [36].

Barriers to Feedback

There appear to be several barriers to providing appropriate feedback. These barriers can be broadly categorized into two groups: educator/teacher barriers and learner barriers. Barriers that affect the educator/teacher include:

- Time constraints
- Lack of observation of the behavior or activity
- Desire to avoid upsetting the learner
- Feedback focus on person and personal qualities, rather than skill/task

With the contemporary time-intense focus on clinical responsibilities for teachers, feedback for more junior residents is often left out or truncated. The teacher needs to be present and observe the learner to accurately provide appropriate feedback. Additionally, constructive feedback might not be given due to the possibility of creating an upsetting emotional response from the learner. Once the feedback is given by the teacher, there is a dysfunctional tendency for the feedback to be focused on the learner's personal characteristics instead on the procedural skill performed [32].

Barriers that affect the learner include insecurity, lack of growth mindset, and insufficient foundational knowledge. Constructive feedback to the insecure resident may be misinterpreted as being perceived as a bad resident. A resident that lacks the mindset of growth or feels like they have no weaknesses is not receptive to receiving feedback. Finally, a sufficient knowledge base in the area of knowledge or procedural skill being demonstrated is necessary to comprehend the feedback given by the teacher [32].

Giving Appropriate Feedback

To give appropriate feedback, a conducive environment must be first established. This nonjudgmental environment should provide a relaxing, respectful atmosphere for the learner to feel comfortable and fully engaged in the conversation. The learner should also be notified ahead of time that he or she will be receiving feedback. It is important for feedback to start with a self-assessment by the learner. This helps create an open two-way conversation and allows the teacher to assess the resident's mindset and insight [33].

Feedback should be based on direct observations in order to provide the most realistic assessment for the learner. This allows the educator to discuss specific events that were appropriate or needed improvement. When feedback focuses on generalities, it leaves the learner with an incomplete assessment and with little direction for improvement [32, 33]. Furthermore, the quantity of feedback given should be limited to one or two topics in order to not overwhelm the learner in the context of any given interaction [32]. Feedback is most effective when it occurs in a respectful environment, is based on direct observation rather than hearsay, is non-judgmental, is specific rather than general, is focused on limited elements rather than a wide range of topics, is oriented to behavior and skills rather than personality traits, is goal or objective based, is accomplished in the context of dialog, and includes suggestions for improvement [33].

Each feedback session concludes with the development of goals for future experiences. Goals for improvement should include strategies and input from both the educator and the learner. Strategies might include further reading of the literature, working in the skills lab, or new approaches to procedures. At the conclusion, the educator and learner agree upon the goals, and then the learner reviews his or her understanding of the feedback [33].

Having reviewed the critical nature of feedback as an essential skill in all learning settings and environments, we will now turn to reviewing specific strategies residents can use and develop as part of their learning and teaching repertoire to enhance their effectiveness. In the following sections, we will identify several specific teaching models and strategies useful in framing and developing educational competency and the journey toward independent practice, both clinically and pedagogically.

Teaching Models

There are many models in the current medical education literature proposed to help faculty teach residents and to assess a resident's level of competency. Although many residency programs offer a "Residents as Teachers" course to develop senior residents' leadership skill acquisition, there is relatively little focused scholarship in the current medical education literature describing specific techniques for senior residents to employ in teaching junior learners. In the following section, we will describe several models that may be adapted in training residents as teachers.

Dreyfus Model and Learner-Focused Teaching

The Dreyfus model of skill acquisition lays a framework for skill acquisition by describing developmental stages beginning with novice and progressing through advanced beginner, competent, proficient, expert, and master [37]. The progression is one in which the learner progresses from following rules based on limited experience without comprehension of context, toward intuitive decision making based on analysis and ultimately intuition as experience grows. As the learner progresses, they also progress from detached commitment to involved commitment based on progressive understanding. It is paramount that the teachers recognize, or "diagnose," the learner's current stage in order to employ techniques that both reinforce the learner's existing knowledge base and empower the learner to grow [38]. This model of teaching can be used in the clinic, hospital wards, or in the operating room.

Through surgical residency, these early skills are most likely acquired with the help of a senior resident's leadership based on the "near-peer" relationship as described above. It is crucial for the senior resident to see one of his or her primary duties as teaching the more junior residents on his or her team. The teacher of a novice learner aids by helping the learner organize their clinical knowledge by pointing out meaningful diagnostic information in the history and physical exam, eliminating irrelevant information, and encouraging learners to read about the clinical scenario. A new intern can find the amount of work involved in developing these skills alongside performing even relatively simple tasks overwhelmingly. At this novice stage, it is difficult to discern what information is relevant to a patient's care and what is extraneous. The senior resident can teach the junior resident strategies to remain organized and methods to gain efficiency. This can be taught both by instruction and role modeling.

As the learner progresses to an advanced beginner, the teacher encourages him or her to formulate and articulate their own differential diagnosis and treatment plan. In the midst of a busy day with many time constraints, it is often more efficient for the more senior resident to formulate a patient care plan. However, it is crucial for the junior residents to develop a plan prior to hearing the senior's assessment and to be given the opportunity to synthesize and articulate the plan. The senior resident should ask, "What is your plan?" This promotes synthesis of information, application, and reinforcement of already existing medical knowledge, prioritization and decision-making skill, and the development of ownership and responsibility in the patient's care.

In the Dreyfus model, the teacher of a competent learner must balance supervision with autonomy in order to allow the learner to become accountable for their decisions. This balance is found by elucidating what tasks the learner can be trusted to perform well independently and what tasks need guidance. Lev Vygotsky introduced a concept called the "zone of proximal development," which defines tasks that the learner cannot do unaided, but can be completed with guidance [39]. An attending or senior resident must discern which tasks the junior resident can be entrusted to perform independently versus those that require instruction or close supervision, as well as those beyond the learner's capabilities even with assistance. Teachers should strive to teach in this zone of proximal development, where the benefit of the teacher's assistance is neither superfluous nor facilitates danger, but enabling. Here lies the balance required between autonomy and guidance, which leads to the most growth and progression—defining the point of maximal teaching impact for the learner. Further influences on developing resident autonomy will be discussed below.

The last two stages of the Dreyfus model place much of the responsibility on the learner. At the stage of proficiency, the learner must trust his or her instincts while also being aware of his or her limitations and the point in which additional help is needed. At this stage the teacher must follow Barbara Lourie Sand's astute observation that she describes in her book *Teaching Genius*. Here she states that the secret of success teaching is to train "pupils to think, and to trust their ability to do so effectively [40, 41]." As the learner reaches the stage of expert or master, he or she gains increasing experience and exposure to complex and difficulty cases and continues to grow through continued self-directed learning.

Granting Autonomy

Traditionally, surgical residents' education occurred through a graduated system of increased responsibility and awarded autonomy. As described above, recent studies have provided evidence that many surgical graduates are not prepared to enter fellowship or independent practice or at a minimum are not confident in their ability to do so. Teman et al. [42] identified factors that influence attending surgeons' decision to entrust the resident with increased autonomy. The most important factors were the observed clinical skill of the resident, the attending surgeon's confidence level with the procedure, and the ease of the operation. The greatest barrier preventing entrustment of responsibility was the increased focus on patient outcomes followed by a desire for increased efficiency and the patient's or institution's expectation of attending involvement. The same likely holds true for chief residents and other senior residents teaching junior residents and medical students. As a chief resident, one feels a great responsibility for not only the care and successful outcome of his or her patients but also to meet the expectation placed on him or her by the faculty. Recognizing these barriers, the authors recommended that the focus be placed on entrustment of responsibilities by defining and measuring entrustable professional activities (EPAs).

Entrustable Professional Activities

Entrustable professional activities are defined, concrete tasks that can be observed and assessed by the teacher [43, 44], for example, consenting a patient for a laparoscopic appendectomy or placing a central venous line. Unlike the ACGME's core competencies which can be abstract ideas that are difficult to measure, EPAs are distinct tasks identified in the learner's regular workflow that can be evaluated. They are "units of professional activity." Using an EPA model, one can determine when the learner is prepared for increased responsibility, greater complexity of tasks, and further independence.

This is not only true for how attending surgeons approach teaching residents but also how a chief resident should teach the other members of his or her team. For example, at the beginning of one's first year in residency, the resident learner typically may not know how to accomplish relatively simple tasks such as writing a progress note or inserting orders into the electronic medical record. The intern learns how to perform these duties from his or her senior resident. Initially, this requires close monitoring and frequent help from the senior resident to ensure appropriate task completion and learning. As the intern develops experience and demonstrates trustworthiness in reliable completion of the task under direct observation, the senior resident should give further independence to the intern and begin teaching the intern more complex tasks ideally while maintaining intermittent ongoing monitoring of tasks already entrusted to ensure continued appropriate execution.

BID Model

Another model specifically designed for teaching surgical residents in the operating room, the BID model, was introduced by Roberts et al. [45]. The briefing, intraoperative teaching, and debriefing model allows the learner and the teacher to set specific objectives prior to beginning an operation in order to deliberately focus on a particular aspect of the learner's performance as the point for improvement and growth. This model is easy to remember and fits well into the busy schedule of an attending surgeon's practice. During *briefing*, the teacher asks the learner what he or she would like to focus on during the procedure, or with very inexperienced learners, the suggested focus may be provided by the teacher. This interaction, which can occur with a succinct conversation at the scrub sink, assesses the needs of the learner while also deliberately setting an objective for educational focus and improvement during the case. The objective set during the briefing allows for focused *intraoperative teaching*. During the procedure, the teacher may coach the learner through the operation but pays particular attention to instruction which applies to the outlined objective. Purposeful slowing down at this point can help provide an optimal context for learning at the point of maximal impact while allowing for required operative efficiencies during the less educationally productive portions of the case. Finally, during closing the teacher and learner debrief together. *Debriefing* consists of four elements, namely, reflection, rule, reinforcement, and correction. It is a time to allow the resident to reflect on his or her overall performance while assimilating a "rule" to guide future practices. The teacher should inquire on what the learner recognized and would do differently in the future, and ask why, and reinforce aspects of the resident's performance that were done well while correcting mistakes. Reinforcement not only encourages the learner during his or her development, it also emphasizes portions of the performance that should be repeated in the future. Correcting mistakes is also crucial for the learner to improve his or her skill level but should always be addressed in a way to avoid embarrassment or degradation. The BID model allows the teacher and the learner to intentionally focus on one learning objective which then guides the intraoperative teaching and is further solidified during debriefing. The learner not only receives immediate constructive feedback, it occurs in a way that is conducive to the demanding schedule of a busy attending surgeon.

Let's use an inguinal hernia repair as an example. At an intern level, the resident is learning the anatomy and memorizing the steps of the procedure. The defined objective set at the "briefing" may be simply closing the incision or properly injecting local anesthetic. The senior resident can teach the junior resident proper suturing techniques and principles of inguinal nerve anatomy and analgesia. As the learner progresses, focus may be changed to elements such as nerve identification, cord mobilization, sac dissection, prosthesis placement, and so forth. Ultimately, special situations and their management such as persistent incarceration, sliding defects, rarer hernia types, and non-prosthetic repairs become suitable foci of teaching effort.

With more experienced residents, such as a chief resident, and under the supervision of an attending surgeon, it is an excellent learning opportunity for both residents to have the chief resident walk a junior resident through a case. The chief resident must have extensive knowledge about the patient, disease process, anatomy, and operative steps. In some ways, this gives the senior resident the greatest degree of autonomy allotted in our current training paradigm. It develops both the junior resident and senior resident's operative skills while also developing the senior resident's ability to teach. Using this model, the attending, senior resident, and junior resident can define a particular objective to focus on through the case. The attending and senior resident should give feedback to the junior resident regarding his or her technical performance. In addition, the senior resident can receive feedback from the attending and junior resident regarding his or her teaching style.

Striving for Excellence as a Resident Teacher

As a resident matures becoming a mid-level and on to a chief resident, the mindset must change to not only growing in one's own medical knowledge, clinical judgment, and technical skills but also to one of teaching and leading a team. Leadership, emotional intelligence, and both self- and team management skills become more critical and represent transitional skills in the progression from graduate to postgraduate lifelong learning. Over the next few paragraphs, we will outline strategies senior residents can use to begin to incorporate some of these skills in their most common and high-stakes learning environment, the operating room.

Developing Intraoperative Teaching Skills

Cox and Swanson described five key elements that characterized outstanding operative instructors, which include (1) demonstration of awareness and sensitivity to resident learning needs, (2) provision of direct and ongoing feedback regarding resident progress, (3) possession of technical expertise and up-to-date knowledge, (4) encouragement of resident participation, and (5) maintenance of a respectful and supportive learning environment [46, 47]. As outlined above, in many ways, senior residents can be the best teachers of junior residents. Senior residents may often be more aware of junior residents' learning needs as they have many of the same needs or recent experiences. Furthermore, residents often feel more comfortable giving and receiving feedback from a close colleague.

When learning to teach, senior residents should keep in mind the seven principles reported by Skoczylas et al. of effective operative teaching [47, 48]:

- Emphasis of anatomical landmarks
- Instruction of both visual and tactile procedural elements
- Encouragement of repetition
- Promotion of early independence
- Demonstration of confident competence
- Maintenance of calm demeanor
- Willingness to accept responsibility for mistakes and consequences

Developing the Nontechnical Teaching Skills

As is clear from several of the elements outlined in the above principles, being a good teacher means not only giving instruction in or out of the operating room but also leading a team effectively. As John Maxwell states in his book *Developing the Leader Within You*, leadership is defined as "casting vision and motiving people [49]." Good leadership is accomplished through displaying integrity and communicating effectively. An effective leader, as Kouzes and Posner describe it, models the way [50]. If a senior resident leads by example and acts in accordance to the greater good of the team rather than for himself or herself, trust is built.

Once one gains trust, learners are more likely to listen and feel comfortable asking questions. When residents change services, senior residents should take time to set goals and define expectations with his or her junior residents. It is vital for the senior resident to not only ask questions but also to welcome questions along the way. Midway through a rotation, senior residents should give and receive both positive and constructive feedback with their junior residents. This facilitates educational accountability, allows time for correction or remediation, and aids in reorienting to key goals and objectives.

As the resident moves toward maturity both in terms of their personal professional identity and their effectiveness as an educator, continued self-development through reading, focused mentorship, and coursework, formal or informal, becomes critical in preparing them for lifelong practice-based learning. This is no less true in the realm of educational maturation than it is in the clinical or technical skill realm. Continuing to develop attitudes and interpersonal skills alongside knowledge and technical prowess will lead the senior resident into areas such as advanced time management, conflict resolution, patterns promoting resilience, and expanding influence through strategic investment in the lives of others. Harkening back to where we began the chapter, residents may find this new set of skills daunting, but also exhilarating and fulfilling to pursue, and will often find themselves in an advantageous position to share the lessons they learn with more junior learners. Developing these skills and a community of learning that celebrates them can change an educational culture and stimulate the expanding influence to the benefit of many that is the goal of all educational endeavor.

Conclusion

Teaching residents to teach junior residents and medical students is fundamental to the mission of surgical education. As Deborah Ball, Dean of the School of Education at the University of Michigan, said, "Good teachers aren't born, they're trained" [51]. Just as one trains a resident to perform complex surgical skills, one must also coach and encourage residents to act as teachers to their junior colleagues. There are many challenges facing the current surgical training paradigm including resident preparedness for independent practice. Senior residents should keep the teaching mindset as a top priority, for as the Roman philosopher Seneca said, "While we teach, we learn." We hope that applying the theories of modern memory science and educational principles reviewed will help the interested reader enhance their own personal surgical competency and skill and their impact on the progression of all around them.

References

1. Sheets KJ, Hankin FM, Schwenk TL. Preparing surgery house officers for their teaching role. Am J Surg. 1991;161:443–9.
2. Patel VL, Dauophinee WD. The clinical learning environments in medicine, pediatrics, and surgery clerkships. Med Educ. 1985;19:54–60.
3. Barrow MV. The house officer as a medical educator. J Med Educ. 1965;40:712–4.
4. Barrow MV. Medical student opinions of the house officer as a medical educator. J Med Educ. 1966;41:807–10.
5. Wilson FC. Teaching by residents. Clin Ortho & Related Res. 2006;454:247–50.
6. Bell RH Jr, Biester TW, Tabuenca A, Rhodes RS, Cofer JB, Britt LD, Lewis FR Jr. Operative experience in US general surgery programs: a gap between expectation and experience. Ann Surg. 2009;249(5):719–24.
7. Bucholz EM, Sue GR, Yeo H, Roman SA, Bell RH Jr, Sosa JA. Our trainees' confidence results from a national survey of 4136 US general surgery residents. Arch Surg. 2011;146(8):907–14.
8. Pugh CM, DaRosa DA, Glenn D, Bell RH Jr. A comparison of faculty and resident perception of resident learning needs in the operating room. J Surg Educ. 2007;64(5):250–5.
9. Kairys JC, McGuire K, Crawford AG, Yeo CJ. Cumulative operative experience is decreasing during general surgery residency: a worrisome trend for surgical trainees? J Am Coll Surg. 2008;206(5):804–11.
10. Dreyfus SE. The five-stage model of adult skill acquisition. Bull Sci Technol Soc. 2004;24(3):177–81.
11. Adams L. Learning a new skill is easier said than done. http://www.gordontraining.com/free-workplace-articles/learning-a-new-skill-is-easier-said-than-done/
12. Wall J. Millennium generation poses new implications for surgical resident education. https://www.facs.org/education/resources/rap/millennium-generation-poses-new-implications-for-surgical-resident-education.
13. Pardes H. The perilous state of academic medicine. JAMA. 2000;283:2427–9.
14. Morrison EH, Rucker L, Boker JR, Gabbert CC, Hubbell FA, Hitchcock MA, Prislin MD. The effect of a 13-hour curriculum to improve residents' teaching skills: a randomized trial. Ann Intern Med. 2004;141:257–63.

15. Karpicke JD, Roediger HL. The critical importance of retrieval for learning. Science. 2008;319:966–8.
16. Larsen DP, Bulter AC, Aung WY, Corboy JR, Friedman DI, Sperling MR. The effects of test-enhanced learning on long-term retention in AAN annual meeting courses. Neurology. 2015;84:748–54.
17. Buckley EJ, Markwell S, Farr D, Sanfey H, Mellinger JD. Improving resident performance on standardized assessments of medical knowledge: a retrospective analysis of interventions correlated to American Board of Surgery in-Service Training Examination performance. Am J Surg. 2015;210:734–8.
18. Muolton CE, Dubrowski A, MacRae H, Graham B, Grober E, Reznick R. Teaching surgical skills: what kind of practice makes perfect? A randomized controlled trial. Ann Surg. 2006;244:400–9.
19. Lee TD, Genovese ED. Distribution of practice in motor skill acquisition: learning and performance effects reconsidered. Res Q Exerc Sport. 1988;59:277–87.
20. Schmidt RA, Bjork RA. New conceptualization of practice. Psychol Sci. 1992;3:207–17.
21. Donovan JJ, Radosevich DJ. A meta-analytic review of the distribution of practice effect: now you see it, now you don't. J Appl Psychol. 1999;84:795–805.
22. Hall JC. Imagery practice and the development of surgical skills. Am J Surg. 2002;184:465–70.
23. Bohan M, Pharmer JA, Stokes A. When does imagery practice enhance performance on a motor task? Percept Mot Skills. 1999;88:651–8.
24. Whitley JD. Effects of practice distribution on learning a fine motor task. Restor Q. 1970;41:576–83.
25. Rohrer D, Taylor K. The shuffling of mathematics problems improves learning. Instr Sci. 2007;35:481–98.
26. Birnbaum MS, Kronell N, Bjork EL, Bjork RA. Why interleaving enhances inductive learning: the roles of discrimination and retrieval. Mem Cogn. 2013;41:392–402.
27. Taylor K, Rohrer D. The effects of interleaved practice. Appl Cogn Psychol. 2010;24:907–12.
28. Bulter AC, Roediger HL. Feedback enhances the positive effects and reduces the negative effects of multiple-choice testing. Mem Cogn. 2008;36:604–16.
29. Toppino TC, Luipersbeck SM. Generality of the negative suggestion effect in objective tests. J Ed Psych. 1993;86:357–62.
30. Karpicke JD, Roediger HL. Is expanding retrieval a superior method for learning text materials? Mem Cogn. 2010;38:116–24.
31. Ende J. Feedback in clinical medical education. JAMA. 1983;250(6):777–81.
32. Anderson P. Giving feedback on clinical skills: are we starving our young? J Grad Med Educ. 2012;4(2):154–8.
33. Hewson MG, Little ML. Giving feedback in medical education. J Gen Intern Med. 1998;13:111–6.
34. Wolverton ST, Bosworth MF. A survey of resident perceptions of effective teaching behaviors. Fam Med. 1985;17(3):106–8.
35. Glenn JK, Reid JC, Mahaffy J, Shurtleff H. Teaching behaviors in the attending-resident interaction. J Fam Med. 1984;18(2):297–304.
36. Snyder RA, Tarpley MJ, Tarpley JL, Davidson M, Brophy C, Dattilo JB. Teaching in the operating room: results of a national survey. J Surg Educ. 2012;69:643–9.
37. Batalden P, Leach D, Swing S, Dreyfus H, Dreyfus S. General competencies and accreditation in graduate medical education. Health Aff (Millwood). 2002;21:103–11.
38. Carraccio CL, Benson BJ, Nixon LJ, Derstine PL. From the educational bench to the clinical bedside: translating the Dreyfus developmental model to the learning of clinical skills. Acad Med. 2008;83(8):761–7.
39. Dunphy BC, Dunphy SL. Assisted performance and the zone of proximal development (ZPD); a potential framework for providing surgical education. Aust J Educ Dev Psychol. 2003;3:48–58.
40. Gawande A. Personal Best. Top athletes and singers have coaches. Should you? *The New Yorker*. October 3, 2011.

41. Sand BL. Teaching genius: Dorothy delay and the making of a musician. Portland: Amadeus Press; 2000. Print.
42. Teman NR, Gauger PG, Mullan PB, Tarpley JL, Minter RB. Entrustment of general surgery residents in the operating room: factors contributing to provision of resident autonomy. J Am Coll Surg. 2014;219(4):778–87.
43. ten Cate O. Entrustability of professional activities and competency-based training. Med Educ. 2005;39(12):1176–7.
44. ten Cate O, Scheele F. Competency-based postgraduate-training: can we bridge the gap between theory and clinical practice? Acad Med. 2007;82(6):542–7.
45. Roberts NK, Williams RG, Kim MJ, Dunnington GL. The briefing, intraoperative teaching, debriefing model for teaching in the operating room. J Am Coll Surg. 2009;208(2):299–303.
46. Cox SS, Swanson MS. Identification of teaching excellence in operating room and clinic settings. Am J Surg. 2002;183:251–5.
47. Timberlake MD, Mayo HG, Scott L, Weis J, Gardner AK. What do we know about intraoperative teaching? A systematic review. Ann Surg. 2017;266(2):251–9. Epub ahead of print
48. Skoczylas LC, Littleton EB, Kanter SL, et al. Teaching techniques in the operating room: the importance of perceptual motor teaching. Acad Med. 2012;87:364–71.
49. Maxwell JC. Developing the leader within you. Nashville: T. Nelson; 1993. Print.
50. Kouzes JM, Posner BZ. The leadership challenge. San Francisco: Jossey-Bass; 2007. Print.
51. Hulett S. Teaching teachers to teach: It's not so elementary. NPR Illinois. 2015. http://www.npr.org/sections/ed/2015/10/24/437555944/teaching-teachers-to-teach-its-not-so-elementary. Accessed 31 Mar 2017.

Teaching in the Operating Room

8

Moben Mirza and Joel F. Koenig

Introduction

Medicine has evolved dramatically during the last century to the extent that much of what goes on in modern medical care would be unrecognizable to a physician at the turn of the twentieth century. The impact of novel therapies, surgical techniques, and diagnostic technologies over the last 30 years alone is staggering. Education in the operating room, the cornerstone of surgical training, however has made little substantive progress since the days of surgical apprenticeships. The institution of surgical residencies in the early twentieth century provided structure to research and didactic curriculums, but operative training is still primarily based on individual observation and mentorship with limited objective standards and oversight. The demands of our modern medical era, from duty hour restrictions to financial pressures, as well as a heightened sense of public accountability and transparency highlight the need to harness every available resource to maximize operating room education for teachers, trainees, and ultimately for patients.

Historical Context

Prior to the twentieth century, the training of surgeons was primarily a one-on-one apprenticeship model in which young trainees would spend several years observing and imitating a mentor surgeon giving rise to the well-known dictum "watch one, do one, teach one." The quality of training within this system by its nature varied greatly with the quality of the individual mentor and the lacked central organization

M. Mirza, MD
University of Kansas Medical Center, Kansas City, MO, USA

J.F. Koenig, MD (✉)
Children's Mercy Hospital, Kansas City, MO, USA
e-mail: jfkoenig@cmh.edu

T.S. Köhler, B. Schwartz (eds.), *Surgeons as Educators*,
https://doi.org/10.1007/978-3-319-64728-9_8

or standards. Like any apprenticeship, learning was heavily restricted to what the trainee could directly observe, and progress and innovation were difficult.

Beginning in the early twentieth century, surgical training in the United States began to acquire structure. As medical education reform was shaped by William Osler, the Flexner Report of 1910 and the American Medical Association (AMA), William Halsted laid the groundwork for our modern surgical residencies with the triad of research, basic science knowledge, and graduated patient responsibility. From the time of its inception in 1913, the American College of Surgeons (ACS) has played a vital role in developing, maintaining, and refining surgical standards. The AMA published the "Essentials of Approved Residencies and Fellowships" in 1928, and shortly after in 1939, the ACS issued their first Fundamental Requirements for Graduate Training in Surgery [1].

As the medical care delivery and payment continued to evolve throughout the twentieth century, so too did medical education oversight, and in 1981 the ACGME was formed to create a unifying force over the various medical specialty and subspecialty resident review committees. The medical education landscape has changed dramatically over the last 20 years with duty hour restrictions, the Next Accreditation System (NAS), and the current Milestones project. For surgical specialties, greater emphasis has been put on demonstration of competence including progression of skill in the operating room. The actual task of teaching in the operating room each day however is still remarkably similar to the old apprenticeship model. Residents and fellows participate in surgical cases with varying degrees of autonomy and oversight from their mentors often with minimal structured feedback to know specifically what they did well and what needs improvement. Summative, infrequent evaluations, which are still the basis for ACGME review, do little to foster the kind of continual improvement cycle needed to guide trainees through the most critical time in the development of their surgical skills. Fortunately, the last several decades have also seen an increase in psychological research and technological advances that can be used to make the most of time spent educating in the operating room.

The Case for Better Teaching in the Operating Room

Some may think the old adage "if it isn't broken, don't fix it" may apply to operative training. After all modern medicine, including surgical medicine, has seen many great achievements, and surgeons who complete years of training want to think they are adequately prepared. There are however several factors that highlight the need to continuously assess and improve our teaching in the operating room.

While the amount of medical knowledge and number and complexity of surgical cases has increased across all disciplines, time pressure on learners, particularly residents, has also increased. The most obvious of these pressures is the restriction of resident duty hours. While this limitation affects residents in all specialties, it is felt most acutely in surgical disciplines in which textbooks, didactics, or simulation cannot wholly take the place of real operative experience. Several recent studies illustrate this effect on current surgical residencies. Surgical residents completing training in 2010 and 2011 performed one-third of essential common operations as defined in the Surgical Council on Resident Education (SCORE) curriculum a median of less than five times and four of these a median of zero times [2]. The effects of these increased demands compared to available time can be seen in the fact that over one-quarter of surgery residents worry about their confidence to perform procedures independently upon graduation [3]. A recent survey of surgery fellowship program directors found that 21% felt that new fellows were unprepared for the operating room with 30% unable to independently perform a laparoscopic cholecystectomy and 66% unable to operate on their own for 30 min unsupervised in a major operation [4]. Although this survey was based on the opinion of program directors and is not a scientific assessment of actual operating skills, the findings are concerning given the amount of time and effort that goes into training residents and the great responsibilities they have after graduation.

The pressures on teaching physicians and the landscape of the modern academic medical center have also changed dramatically in the last century. Although we would like to separate the financial and educational aspects of teaching hospitals and medical schools, they are inextricably joined. In decades past, only a small fraction of the operating costs of medical schools was directly derived from clinical revenue. Through 1965 a typical medical school relied on faculty practice for only about 6% of their budget, while 60% came from federal research spending [5]. After the advent of Medicaid and Medicare in 1965 and through the fee-for-service era, the clinical revenue of academic hospitals grew, and by 1980 approximately half of a typical medical school's budget came from its clinical practice [5]. Within our current managed care era, influence from insurance companies has shortened hospital stays, decreased payments, and increased demands on clinicians to see more patients in less time which in turn decreases time for clinical teaching. These pressures along with increased concerns over patient safety and public accountability have led to decreased time and freedom for resident education and autonomy in the operating room. Faculty teaching in the operating room must therefore adapt to maximize the time available.

The educational environment in which we are teaching in the operating room has also changed over the last several decades. New research has provided insights into education that can be utilized to make the most of the time we do have to teach in the operating room. We would not ignore clinical research in our field that guided us to better patient care, and we should not ignore education research that benefits our residents. We must also factor in generational differences between current residents and their teaching faculty and how these differences affect learning and teaching in the operating room. Although there are many timeless principles regarding operative education, the way in which these principles are applied to different learners in different situations can have a great impact on their effectiveness. A more detailed discussion of generational differences is covered elsewhere in this book, but the current millennial generation's desire for more direct constant feedback, assimilative learning style, and technological prowess should be harnessed if we are to make the most of educational time in the operating room. As stated by Ian Jukes, "We must prepare students for their future, not our past" [6].

The Purpose of Operating Room Education

The two primary purposes of the education in the operating room are assessing current surgical proficiency (knowledge, skill, judgment, professionalism) and facilitating continual advancement of this proficiency toward the ultimate goal of safe, independent, competent surgical practice. Although a precise definition of "surgical competence" may be difficult to articulate bringing to mind Justice Potter Stewart's description of obscenity, "I know it when I see it [7]," a reasonable working definition may be that upon graduation we would recommend our residents to friends and family in need of medical care. It is important to have this framework in mind when thinking about resident assessment and improvement. Evaluating how well a resident *did*, whether addressing a single operation, time spent on a particular rotation, or their entire residency tenure, is not as important and extrapolating how well a resident *will do* in their future independent practice. The decisions to allow residents to progress at each step of their training and ultimately graduate are high-stakes decisions and as such should not be made only on hunches and intuition.

Our patients understand this and the public demand for better accountability is increasing. Historically most patients have placed tremendous trust in their physicians and their training without looking for much to support their trust other than a diploma on the wall. Public trust in physicians however has been declining, and recently third-party groups such as Propublica [8] have been collecting and reporting available data on information such as surgical outcomes. Undoubtedly a similar trend for increased public accountability of competence in medical and surgical education will follow. For the sake of the public trust and our own conscience as educators, we as teachers should be able to provide, "defensible, dependable, and trustworthy operative performance information" [9] to support these high-stakes decisions regarding our support of a trainee's license to practice medicine. In the era of evidence-based practice, medical decision-making relies on ample and accurate data that has been collected and reported with clarity. Medical education decisions should require similar stringent support.

Clearly it is impossible to have perfectly complete and accurate knowledge of a resident's operative competency or predict how he or she will perform in every possible scenario, but we should have as our goal when teaching in the operating room an assessment system that provides a true picture of the resident's competency trajectory and can explain deviation from this trajectory due to factors such as changes in operative environment or faculty variation. We must then also have the proper training and knowledge to use the information we gain from this assessment to guide our residents to be the best surgeons they can be.

Assessment of Operative Performance

Education in the operating room, in terms of both validation of competence and guiding improvement, begins with a thorough and accurate assessment of surgical skill. Both the quality of the individual evaluations and the total number of evaluations are important factors in generating such an assessment. Mellinger and his colleagues compared educational assessment to work done by early astronomers in which the accuracy of each individual measurement was of course important, but only by combining multiple measurements from multiple observes over time could a more true and complete picture of the universe and accurate extrapolations of the future be made [9]. Although this is not a perfect analogy, important comparisons can be instructive. Every individual measurement of any kind is hindered by a variety of factors that prevent perfect accuracy. In the case of astronomy, these factors included the instruments used, atmospheric conditions, and human error on the part of the astronomer among others. Similarly, in the operating room, human factors (outside stressors, fatigue), the environment (case complexity), and assessment instruments will affect the accuracy of each assessment performed. Fortunately, there is a growing body of research to help refine the practice of assessment to provide high-quality data efficiently in the midst of a busy practice.

Historically, there may have been variable feedback and coaching within the operating room, but recorded assessments happened infrequently, typically as annual or semiannual evaluations asking each faculty member to reflect on their time with the resident. The individual evaluations were then grouped into a single report for each resident. Using the framework above, this method has several inherent problems. In regard to the quality of the assessment itself, summarizing 6 months of operative performance into a single account limits its ability to differentiate among many variable operations and surgical skills. Recall bias will typically bring to mind either the most recent experiences with a resident or particularly positive or negative experiences, and previous research has demonstrated the negative impact of delay in completion of operative assessments [10]. As much as these flaws affect each individual evaluation, the small number of assessments generated by this method is probably a more important limitation. By providing only a handful of assessments across a resident's tenure, it is much more difficult to determine whether the evaluations truly represent their surgical competence or outlying measurements. Whenever measurements of any kind are recorded, the more data points there are, the easier it is to accurately determine the true normal distribution and the outliers. This will also allow determining what led to outlying measurements and refining of the measurement tool. Having more data points is especially important when trying to extrapolate future performance which is the ultimate goal of operative assessment. Research has demonstrated the importance of collecting a sufficient number of evaluations to accurately portray a resident's operative performance [11]. Infrequent evaluations by their nature also minimize the ability of the assessment to identify struggling residents or act as a tool for residents to guide their own improvement. These infrequent summative assessments have served as records of residents meeting minimum requirements, but not much more. For all of the potential benefit offered by more frequent evaluations, actually implementing these evaluations and collecting and processing their data have been difficult without applying more recent technological advances. In the midst of a busy surgical practice, the time and inconvenience required by paper evaluations would be difficult obstacles to overcome for many training programs. Fortunately, smartphones and internet-based programs can greatly increase the ease and efficiency of frequent evaluations of individual operative performances.

To try and conceptualize the various assessment tools already in use and any in the future, it may be helpful to understand them in terms of their final product. Each assessment produces an account of the operative performance based on the parameters set forth in its design. This account or characterization is most often a numerical score due to the fact that they are simple and quick to complete and have the advantages of being easy to quantify, combine, and analyze. What the numerical score actually represents will depend on the design of the assessment. The most commonly used design involves a generic assessment that can be applied to all procedures and asks the rater to provide a numerical score, for various aspects of the operative performance. Examples include the objective assessment of technical skills (0SATS) system [12], the nontechnical skills for surgeons system [13], and the O-SCORE system [14]. In an effort to make the assessment thorough and descriptive, as many as eight separate elements of surgical performance will be rated on a scale with five to nine levels. Similar systems have also been developed with procedure-specific metrics or a combination of universal and specific parameters such as global operative assessment of laparoscopic skills (GOALS) [15] and OPRS [16]. Procedure-specific evaluations may provide more detailed data or identify particular techniques that a resident needs to improve but yield fewer comparable data points to analyze.

Whichever of these two approaches is chosen, however, there is a growing body of research highlighting some important drawbacks. It may seem straightforward to assign a numerical value along a Likert-type scale to metrics such as preoperative planning or tissue handling, particularly when clear descriptions of the metrics and numerical values are given. However, raters appear to largely ignore the prescribed categories and rankings and instead view the performance in terms of one or two broad characterizations that are applied to all the metrics used in the assessment [17, 18]. This at least partially explains why many assessments used in medical teaching tend to show more correlation among a single assessor's ratings of multiple different trainees than they do among different assessors' ratings of the same trainee or performance [17]. The other main drawback to assessments based around multiple categories with detailed descriptions is that they take more time to read, understand, and complete. Although more experience with a given system and utilization of technology such as smart phones may expedite the process, more questions will always equal more time to complete. And the more time it takes to complete an evaluation, the more likely that fewer evaluations will be completed.

We then seemingly have to choose between fewer evaluations with more detailed, although possibly flawed, data or more evaluations with less detailed data. There is a growing body of research suggesting that a greater number of completed evaluations, even if they are comprised of only one or two questions, may be more valuable. Williams and colleagues reported that increasing the number of evaluations had a greater impact on reliability than did increasing the number of items assessed [11]. They later compared a single-item global assessment of operative performance to the standard OPRS evaluation of approximately ten items and found nearly identical reliability coefficients and again highlighted in need for an adequate number of evaluations for reliability [19]. The most widely used application that approaches this idea of a single global evaluation of a resident's performance is the SIMPL smartphone-based application [20]. This tool asks for a global assessment of overall performance in a case and a score for the degree of autonomy and case complexity. With the small number of questions and smartphone-based platform, the evaluation can be completed in very little time with minimal interruption to normal work flow [21].

Another approach to operative performance assessment could eschew numeric ratings altogether and rely on a verbal narrative. These verbal narratives can potentially convey a greater amount of information more efficiently than numeric ratings. This is particularly true when accounting for the types of factors such as case complexity or other unusual circumstances that may be difficult to adequately capture in a predetermined numerical score. Instead of the rater wondering whether they should give the resident a lower score when struggling through a difficult case or a higher score after factoring in unusual circumstances, the rater simply describes what happened. Schwind et al. found that written comments were particularly helpful at identifying performance deficits compared to numerical scores [22]. This attribute would be particularly useful for a system of immediate operative assessments since one of its main goals is to recognize and help struggling residents earlier. The difficulty with verbal narratives, of course, is that they can be more time-consuming to create, tabulate, and report out in an organized fashion. However, we probably should not favor a numerical system simply because its numbers seem more precise and easier to understand if what is actually conveyed by those numbers is misleading. Fortunately, technology can help with verbal narrative-based systems as well. With voice recognition software, a faculty member could dictate a short narrative after a case just as quickly as they could fill out a set of predetermined numerical scores, and software could similarly help to synthesize the various narratives into a cohesive report. If an assessment of operative performance has twin goals of recording how well the trainee did and also guiding improvement, it may make more sense to simply keep the entire discussion as a verbal narrative. Giving a resident a simple numerical score does little to tell them how to improve. If a verbal narrative can accomplish both goals efficiently, we may not need to bother taking the extra time to try to assign an arbitrary numerical rating. Ideally this would be done as both a verbal, two-way discussion between the resident and faculty member and recorded narrative to document the assessment.

Guiding Improvement in Operative Competency

Effective education in any setting, including the operating room, requires of course not just evaluation and assessment but also guidance to help the learner improve and reach their ultimate goal. Learning will always be most effective when there is a high level of self-direction, but teachers have a great impact on how far that self-direction will carry a student. Becoming a skilled clinician in any field and maintaining that skill over a career require physicians to be lifelong self-motivated learners, but lack of adequate expert guidance will foster education that is inefficient at best and develops harmful improper patterns at worst. To provide the most efficient and effective guidance in the operating room setting requires teaching faculty to overcome the unique challenges of operating room education so that residents and students can make timely measurable improvement in both technical and non-technical clinical operative skills.

Feedback

To foster resident development, faculty must move beyond simply evaluating an operative performance and provide the resident with feedback that will help him or her improve. Although the precise words used to describe what we are doing when we give feedback may change, this is not a matter of mere semantics. There are important differences between evaluating a person and providing them with feedback. Providing good feedback to residents will help both faculty and residents get the most of their educational experience in the operating room, and the importance of feedback to both faculty and residents has previously been demonstrated [23, 24]. Ende does an excellent job of outlining exactly why feedback is so important to medical training and how we can draw on lessons learned from medical training and other disciplines to provide good-quality feedback [23]. He first helps us to understand the importance of feedback by explaining the consequences of inadequate or ineffective feedback. When a learner such as a medical student or resident enters a new environment, they are seeking feedback, and when this is not given, they develop their own internal system of validation. In the case of residents, this internal validation system tends to develop along with an increasing sense of their own competence. As time goes on, they become increasingly resistant to outside criticism which may continue on after graduation from residency [25]. Without a model of constructive feedback, they do not seek out or respond to even well-intentioned outside evaluations of their performance. Perhaps this is part of the explanation for the limited use of third-party coaching by practicing surgeons despite its ubiquitous presence in other fields such as music or athletics. In the absence of a better model, they may fill in the gap and see themselves as their own best judges. The lack of quality feedback has previously been demonstrated in surveys of residents with only 8% being highly satisfied with the feedback they receive and 80% receiving no feedback [26]. Correspondingly faculty frequently report learning how to give effective feedback as one of their greatest needs [24].

To understand how to give effective feedback, it is helpful to first define it and distinguish it from evaluation. Feedback uses information gleaned about a system and reinserts that information back into the system and in the context of education or learning has as its goal, the improvement of the learner. It is important to keep this ultimate goal of improvement in mind, particularly when trying to change human behavior. There are many ways that we can provide a learner with information about a performance or offer guidance for improvement that may not be optimal for improvement. Feedback is formative; it helps the learner achieve their goals and looks forward to continued improvement. This is best done with neutral descriptions about what occurred and what could be improved. Evaluations are summative and look backward, reflecting the past performance and providing judgment about how well a learner compared to a standard or their peers [23]. An evaluation of a poor performance, although informative, will not be nearly as helpful as a formative feedback session that provides guidance on how to perform better next time.

Within this general framework, several specific characteristics of effective feedback have been drawn from medical education and other fields such as personnel management and validated for use by medical educators [23, 24]. The characteristics summarized in Fig. 8.1 can be broadly divided into those apply to setting up the environment for feedback and specific techniques for the feedback itself and can be applied to both positive reinforcement and negative constructive feedback. For the context of this textbook, we will focus on feedback from the perspective of the educator for two reasons: (1) this book is primarily written for educators, and (2) in medical education in general and in the operating room in particular, the educator or attending faculty member has tremendous influence on establishing the environment and leading educational objectives. In this context, directing our efforts toward teachers will likely offer important gains in educational outcomes and may be a necessary prerequisite before turning our attention to learners [27].

Because we are dealing with human learners, the complex dynamics of emotions and interpersonal relationships have a tremendous impact on the success or failure of any educational endeavor including operative performance feedback with its high-stress, high-stakes decisions and close relationship with the faculty. Humans have a natural defensive mechanism against negative emotions defined by Gilbert

Setting up the feedback environment

- Based on direct first-hand observation
- Timely: as soon as possible after the observed task, not more than 72 hours
- Self-directed by the learner
- Respectful unthreatening climate
- Non-judgmental
- Based on well defined pre-negotiated goals

Feedback techniques

- Eliciting thoughts and feelings before giving feedback
- Focusing on behaviors not personality
- Basing feedback on specific observed facts
- Providing the correct amount of feedback (not too much or too little)
- Providing specific suggestions for improvement
- Works with the learner to establish an action plan for continued development

Fig. 8.1 Characteristics of effective feedback

and Wilson [28] as the psychological immune system which may limit the extent to which feedback is sought or implemented by a learner. Learners first require a certain amount of internal confidence in order to be prepared for feedback. This will allow them to seek out feedback and deal with the inevitable negative constructive assessments necessary for improvement [29]. Much of a resident's internal confidence will have been established prior to beginning residency, but it is important for us as educators to recognize where they are starting and do what we can to develop an appropriate level of confidence in our learners. This is also good to keep this in mind regarding all of our interactions with younger learners such as medical students or undergraduates and understand how much influence we can have on their future. After the internal confidence of the resident has been taken into account, the feedback will be most effective if the learner perceives the feedback to be truthful and delivered with their best interests in mind [29]. Accurate feedback will best be given by a direct observer of the evaluated task, and learners are more likely to trust and incorporate feedback from direct observation as opposed to second- or third-hand reports [24]. The timing of feedback also has an impact on its accuracy and precision. Williams and colleagues have demonstrated that a delay of greater than 72 h was associated with a significant decrease in the quality of the operative assessment as demonstrated by a loss in detail and nuance in favor of broad generalizations [10]. These aspects of effective feedback highlight the weaknesses of the standard semiannual evaluation in which feedback may be based on direct observations of multiple faculty members but is typically relayed to the resident months later by a single person (i.e., the program director) who only observed a fraction of the operative performances.

Of course, simply providing an accurate assessment is not enough if our goal is incorporation of the feedback to change behavior and improve performance. For a resident or any other learner, to translate feedback into behavior modification requires motivation. This begins with the resident understanding that they have to be the one actually doing the learning and implementing the changes. They must have an understanding on the target performance, how their performance differs, and how they can narrow that difference. A teacher simply prescribing specific actions to take will not be as effective as the learner working toward a clear understanding of the final goal and how those actions fit into that goal [27, 30] and further developing their sense of autonomy (i.e., the learner has ultimate control over future changes to their performance) [27]. This self-directed learning will be further supported by fostering a healthy relationship between the teacher and the learner. This allows for the feedback to be a collaborative process sought by the learner in which the learners work toward a set of clear predetermined objectives as opposed to one imposed by the teacher with an arbitrary standard of the teacher's choosing. This, combined with a neutral, objective, nonjudgmental tone, moves the experience from a performance focus to a learning focus [23, 27].

Within the actual feedback session, certain techniques will both increase the effectiveness of the feedback given and further improve the relationship between the teacher and learner for future sessions. First the teacher should ask for the resident's own thoughts and feelings about the case. This will allow the faculty member to evaluate the resident's self-assessment skills which are invaluable in developing trust between the faculty and resident and for the resident's lifelong learning. It will also allow the faculty to gage the resident's current emotional state which, as stated previously, can have a significant impact on the feedback. The time immediately after a difficult strenuous case with a negative outcome may not be the best time to go over the fine points of particular surgical techniques. The feedback should be based on specific observed behaviors ("you could improve on appropriate tissue handling techniques") and not on personality traits ("why are you so careless?"). Similarly, suggestions for improvement should be specific and limited to an appropriate amount for the feedback session. Based on theories of cognitive load, this would probably only be one or two well-defined objectives for after an assessment of a single operative performance.

Entrustability

An area that deserves special mention in any medical education context and is vital to operative training is that of entrustability. Entrustment is the act of confiding the care of a person or thing or the execution of a task to an individual [31]. In the operating room, as in all of medicine, entrusting someone else with an aspect of patient care has a measured degree of risk. This measured risk is viewed in the setting of all the other various measured risks we take when caring for patients [9, 32]. Any decision we make or intervention we perform or chose not to perform has possible risks and benefits that we weigh against the odds of helping or harming our patients.

Entrustment is a constantly evolving process that is at work from very simple tasks (i.e., entrusting someone else to cut a suture without cutting the knot) to the entrustment of complex operations or difficult clinical decisions or ethical dilemmas. Much of what goes in the development of entrustment during a resident's education is unspoken and poorly defined. We have the sense of trusting some residents more than others, and hopefully entrustability increases over the course of a resident's tenure, but defining specific goals or objectives and assessing completion of those goals in a way that guides residents toward high levels of entrustability can be difficult. As with skill competence, however, clear definitions of entrustability will lead to more efficient progression toward the ultimate goal of independent practice.

The entrustable professional activity (EPA) concept gives a conceptual framework to help guide appropriate increasing entrustment of trainees. EPAs are "units of professional practice, defined as tasks or responsibilities to be entrusted to the unsupervised execution by a trainee once he or she has attained sufficient specific competence" and are "independently executable, observable, and measurable in their process and outcome, and therefore, suitable for entrustment decisions" [33]. The EPA model does not replace competency, but rather helps to break down a particular competency and translate it into clinical practice [33]. In fact, keeping the end competency goals in mind can help direct assessment of individual EPAs along the road to independent clinical practice. The ACGME Milestones project [34] provides help to guide faculty assessment of EPAs (i.e., safe performance of percutaneous nephrolithotomy) and waypoints along the path to those goals that are both technical (i.e., demonstration of correct assembly and handling of endoscopic equipment or safely achieving percutaneous access) and nontechnical (i.e., deciding what imaging to order in the workup of a patient suspected to have a kidney stone). A single EPA will typically include multiple core competencies such as medical knowledge, patient care, and system-based practice and therefore is a useful model for the integration of the competencies in clinical practice.

Fostering the increasing entrustability that is necessary for resident growth from new intern to independent clinician is a delicate balance. It may be more difficult to define and assess than medical knowledge of technical skill but is arguably of equal, if not greater, importance to medical education. Because entrustability is more difficult to define, the chasm that must be crossed to reach the goal of independent practice seems especially wide. Vygotsky's concept of the zone of proximal development (ZPD) may be helpful in this context because it breaks down the discrepancy between a trainee's starting point and eventual goal by more narrowly defining the space between their current status and their next level in development [35, 36]. The real work of teaching then is safely and efficiently helping residents move along each transition point. Doing this requires the appropriate interplay between the teacher's guidance and expectations and the learner's efforts to meet those expectations and openness to honest feedback. If faculty provide too little room for resident autonomy, growth will be hindered. If this continues over years, there is a risk that residents will not be ready for independent practice. Alternatively, if given too much autonomy too soon, there is a risk to patient safety as well as the possibility for a significant setback in the entrustability relationship between the faculty and the resident that may slow progress in the long term. As the one controlling the teaching relationship and the operating room, the faculty member has the most important role in establishing the entrustability framework for the resident. The resident, however, must then reciprocate by demonstrating their trustworthiness by preparing for tasks assigned, independently seeking learning opportunities, and being open to correction from faculty. As residents move across each individual ZPD, there will be a gradual shift from their role as observer to participant, to semiautonomous surgeon, and to independent clinician. The faculty will have a reciprocal shift from instructor to advisor and to active observer. This means that as a resident moves through training, it will be important for the faculty member not merely to correct mistakes but eventually observe how the resident self-corrects during a case and problem solves without the aid of faculty input. This will help ensure that when we graduate residents, we can say with confidence not only that we can vouch for what they have done but what they will do in the future.

Learning Environment

The operating room can be an intimidating and busy environment. Depending on the level of the resident, this can be a very fresh or very familiar space. We often don't recognize that our first year and second year residents have limited experiences in the operating room, while our senior residents have learned to negotiate the intricacies of the operating room quite well.

All educators can agree without references and science that an environment conducive to learning will produce better-trained residents. The body of surgical educational literature focuses on surgeons and teachers and more recently toward residents as learners. However, we have not addressed the learning environment of the operating room and how it can be optimized.

The challenges of the learning environment can be divided into these domains [37]:

- The physical environment
- Emotional impact of surgery as work
- Challenge of the educational task
- Managing social relationships

Learners must learn to negotiate the physical environment of the operating room. There are appropriate etiquette and protocols as learners familiarize themselves with the operating room culture [38]. The nuisances, complexity, and particulars of a surgical procedure determine the allocation and sequence of all work and interaction, including when and how the teaching takes place. For example, a resident can become completely detached from teaching during a case where a faculty member is performing an independent task. This can also occur during a really complex case where two faculty members are working together. Surgery is serious work, and there is clear element of risk. During periods of intense concentration and teamwork, teaching material cannot be distilled easily to extract only the most interesting, useful, or critical bits.

The operating room environment can be counterproductive to learning. Residents can have the fear of appearing foolish as questions they ask and can be repeated to them as questions they should know the answer to rather than questions that lead to inquiry and teaching. Of course, there is a balance in expectations based on the level of the learner, but the teaching value of the case may change based on the enabling of inquiry allowed by the team members.

Managing the educational task is different for the level of the resident and is also very different for other learners present like medical students. For example, the focus of a medical student would be to gain exposure and the requisite knowledge to be able to pass an exam or achieve competence for future career goals. Relevance and utility of the learning is a significant driver. The residents' educational task is not only to achieve evaluable competency for progression and promotion but more importantly to gain the skill and knowledge to practice independently upon graduation. This goal is often unrecognized and becomes more urgent toward the end of training. Regardless, learners are worried about lack of clear objectives and feedback in the learning environment to properly manage the educational task [37].

Patricia Lyon developed an interpretive model of learning and teaching based on her study of medical students as learners in the surgical environment [39]. Although her study does not include residents, it does drive home very important points about managing the relationship of a teacher and learner.

The central concept of her model is a process called "sizing up." Surgeons and learners are engaged in a continuous dynamic of observation of each other's behaviors. Surgeons have to consider the task at hand, manage the operating room team, as well as teach technical skills and meaningful concepts. They "size up" the learner and gage the level of motivation and commitment, which in turn translates to how they respond as teachers. Levels of motivation and commitment can be demonstrated by preparedness, inquisitiveness, engagement, attitude, and demeanor. Legitimacy and trust are central to the processes of teaching and learning in the operating room.

The learning environment of the operating room starts with a commitment in the training program that teaching and learning are essential components of the daily activity. Faculty need to engage the learner and have clear learning objectives as the surgical day begins. Residents need to come in prepared and motivated so when they are "sized up," their teachers sense the commitment and reciprocate via an engaged process in which they constantly look for opportunities to meet the objectives and advance the training of the resident.

Needs Assessment to Set the Stage of the Learning Environment

Teaching in the operating room rarely starts with a needs assessment. Residents are assigned to cases based on some internal institutional culture. These could be assignments based on service models, mentorship models, or chief residents assigning cases based on seniority and perceived level appropriateness. Busy academic practices challenge these models greatly since operative opportunities and learning are more numerous than the available resident compliments.

Surgical faculty and residents have different perceptions regarding the residents' learning needs. The disparity between faculty and resident perception of residents' learning needs in the operating room was demonstrated by Pugh et al. in a study designed to evaluate learning resources utilized by residents when preparing for surgical cases [40]. This underscores the importance of residents to be included in needs assessments relating to surgical training.

Residents come to the operating room with differing learning needs that are dependent on expectations, learning styles, skill level, knowledge, and experience. Their self-assessment and preparation for a case may start with the case assignment. There is minimal faculty input at this level. Residents will utilize variable resources including surgical atlases, surgical texts, advice from colleagues, web resources, videos, as well as previous operative reports [41].

More often than not, the faculty surgeon sees the assisting resident in the operating room as the patient is being prepared for surgery. Although the time from patient setup to beginning of procedure is short, a conversation around needs assessment is a very integral part of establishing the learning environment. It may include the following:

- Have you done this case before and how many?

Advantage	Disadvantage
Identifies if resident has participated in a similar case	Previous participation does not guarantee retention of concepts/skills demonstrated or taught
Can serve as a rough marker for resident familiarity and comfort with case	Number of cases scrubbed may not be a metric of familiarity and comfort

- What are the indications, potential approaches, positioning, and preparatory considerations?

Advantage	Disadvantage
Identifies if resident has reviewed patient chart	Having reviewed patient chart may not give the resident insight into alternatives and decision-making
Identifies if resident has reviewed available resources like surgical texts and videos. Faculty can assess if resources being utilized are appropriate. For more advanced teaching environments, this can lead to standardization in case preparation resources	Surgical approaches are not tailor-made, and preparatory considerations involve higher level of thinking like potential for blood loss, postoperative pain control, etc.

- Outline the steps of the case

Advantage	Disadvantage
Identifies if resident has reviewed surgical atlas, texts, and videos	Previous participation does not guarantee retention of concepts/skills demonstrated or taught
Enables resident to demonstrate being able to articulate steps of a case in discrete and anatomical terms. For advanced residents, selection of instruments and surgical technique can be incorporated into this approach	May not translate into surgical skill, comfort with technique, as well as instrument selection. Being able to identify surgical tasks may not lead to accomplishing surgical goals

- Which parts of the case are you comfortable performing and which require additional coaching?

Advantage	Disadvantage
Identifies if resident has engaged in self-assessment	Subjective assessment of residents' own skills may not be accurate

Resident training in the operating room tends to be highly focused on operative techniques, as the goal is to successfully complete the technical aspects of a surgical procedure. Performing a needs assessment with the residents cannot be limited to technical aspects and speaks to a larger need for a comprehensive curriculum-based focus on both technical and nontechnical competencies. Although popular didactic conferences like "indications conference" can serve these goals, they are not individualized to the learner. If surgical teaching is to incorporate a needs assessment, then the teaching and assessment need to begin well before the patient is being prepared for surgery. Needs assessment of surgical education has many opportunities for training programs in patient-centered communication, learning models, training in interprofessional/interdisciplinary team communication, and teamwork [42].

Learning Model

The first part of the chapter covers limitations of the current assessment methods. There is evidence that observational assessment of technical skills is valid and supported, but the majority of studies don't achieve a comprehensive analysis as judged on a systematic review [43]. Additionally, most checklist forms demonstrate poorer evidence of validity and reliability.

Many evaluation tools use scale systems and numbered scores. Narrative evaluations are also picking up much attraction and being more effective. Experienced teaching faculty often find scales and scoring methods cumbersome and use experience to teach and often teach very well. Standardized vocabulary, framework, and articulating descriptive operating room teaching and assessment can help establish teaching practices that not only help teachers evaluate learners but also track their performance from a task orientation and goal orientation.

DaRosa et al. have reported on the "Zwisch model" which seeks to accomplish a standardization in the conceptualization of the learning model [44]. The model proposes four stages of supervision and divides faculty and resident behaviors for each stage. These are summarized in Table 8.1 and adopted from the referenced article. Again, these may seem intuitive to experienced teachers. However, it can give faculty and residents a common language for expectations and needs assessments. Additionally, it may at some point translate into mapping milestones of surgical technique.

Show and Tell Stage [44]

In the needs assessment, the faculty and resident will establish that the resident is not experienced at the case and will be a focused observer and assistant. The resident should come into the case prepared having consulted the appropriate surgical texts and/or videos and have reviewed the patient's chart thoroughly. The faculty has to be an active teacher in this environment. The attending "shows" and "tells" the resident key aspects of the case in a "thinking aloud" method. There should be a running commentary during the case that imparts the important technical points and

Table 8.1 Model for teaching and assessment in the operating room [44]

Zwisch stage of supervision	Attending behaviors	Resident behavior
Show and tell	Performs majority of surgery Narrates and articulates steps of the case Demonstrates key concepts, anatomy, and skills	Engages as focused and active learner First assists and observes Opens and closes
Graduating step		Actively assists and anticipates surgeon's needs
Smart help	Shifts between surgeon and assistant Leads resident as first assistant when resident in surgeon role Obtains and optimizes exposure and identifies anatomical landmark Demonstrates planes and structures Coaches technical skills, next steps	Shifts between surgeon and assistant Knowledgeable about all the component technical skills Demonstrates increasing ability to perform key parts with attending assistance
Graduating step		Able to perform majority of steps with attending assistance
Dumb help	Assists and commits to follow the lead of the resident Coaches refining of techniques	Able to stage, set up, and accomplish next step with increasing efficiency Recognized critical transition points
Graduating step		Can transition between all steps with passive assistance
No help	Monitor progress and patient safety Very little unsolicited advice	Can work with inexperienced first assist Safely complete procedure without attending help Can recover most errors Recognizes when to seek help/advice

decision-making points of the procedure. The resident should be engaged in focused observation and assists as the attending teaches:

- Instrument handling
- Exposure of pertinent anatomy and tissue planes
- Hand positioning with hand bracing and demonstration
- Tips and techniques

The resident should assist and anticipate the next steps of the procedure, verbalize understanding, answer questions, and ask questions that demonstrate a higher level of understanding.

In order to graduate to the next step, the resident must demonstrate:

- Having done the homework
- Understanding of indications and approach
- Understanding of anatomy and pathophysiology
- Being able to articulate procedural steps
- Understanding of the key decision-making parts of the case
- Understanding of potential errors/complications

The focus in this stage is priming the resident for task-oriented steps, and the learning environment is very active. The attending must be invested to teach and find the learner motivated and committed as "sizing up" happens.

Smart Help Stage [44]

The resident at this stage will assume the role of surgeon for parts of the surgery. In the needs assessment, the attending will review expectations and judge patient complexity, and then based on the resident's level, the resident and attending will decide the expectations regarding which parts of the surgery the resident will perform. The understanding is that the role of surgeon and assistant is fluid between the faculty and residents. The attending taking over as surgeon is not a criticism of the resident but rather part and parcel of the instructional strategy in which the surgeon role is "fair play." Residents perceive faculty takeovers negatively as unfair and indicative of poor teaching [45]. The negative perception can be curtailed in an active learning environment where expectations are reviewed in advance. When the resident is performing as the surgeon, the faculty is engaged in instruction, constructive criticism, and encouragement toward independence. The resident can be very task oriented in the beginning levels of this stage and become more goal oriented in the advanced levels of this stage.

The graduating steps are:

- Resident is technically capable.
- Resident can safely perform the major and key portions of the case with minimal correction or direction.
- Resident knows all the steps of the operation.

Dumb Help Stage [44]

In the needs assessment, the resident and attending agree that although the resident can technically perform most major components of the surgery, the resident still requires attending's help in providing anatomical exposure as well as first assistance from the attending or from someone with a higher level of understanding of the surgery. The attending should assume the first assist role with the expectation that the surgeon's role is for the resident unless the attending can anticipate the development of a problem. The coaching from the attending is fine adjustments of techniques, alternative techniques, and taking note of teaching points and feedback.

The resident at the beginning levels of this stage that is goal oriented however still relies on the passive actions of a skilled assistant in the attending. The resident needs to lead the case, ask for appropriate instruments, set up adequate exposure, anticipate needs, and communicate with operating room team regarding specimen, medications, etc. In order for residents to take full advantage of the learning in this stage, the attending needs to fight the temptation of continuous verbal and technical feedback. The residents should be allowed to safely struggle, refine their techniques, and practice their problem-solving skills to gain confidence in their abilities.

The resident need not only complete the requisite tasks but also be able to critically think through key transition points and guide the progress of the surgery. When the resident is able to accomplish this with minimal input from attending, then the graduating step has been reached.

No Help Stage [44]

The needs assessment of a resident at this stage would indicate that the resident is able to perform the procedure independently without help. The resident may at this stage advance into a teaching role for a junior resident. The attending does not need to actively participate but be present. The coaching would be limited to refining technique and reviewing higher levels of understanding, generating hypothesis, and advanced treatment planning.

Limitations here would be that the no help stage may not be applicable to some major operative cases. For example, we would not expect nor allow our residents to perform a radical nephrectomy and caval thrombectomy independently. These types of surgeries may incorporate various stages at different phases of the procedure. The resident may be in "no help" phase during exposure of the retroperitoneum, "dumb help" for lateral and inferior mobilization, "smart help" for hilar dissection, and maybe "show and tell" for caval thrombectomy. Obviously, these can vary.

Expectations in the operating rooms are often not stated. There is data that supports that often expectations of residents don't match with expectations of attending surgeons [46]. Residents often feel they don't get enough feedback or that their attendings "hog" the case so they don't get enough independence to advance. Attendings feel residents are too indifferent, come ill prepared, and don't understand the value of learning by observation and in stages.

An approach that assesses needs, sets expectations, follows an instructional model which is clear, standardizes the vocabulary, and values the learning environment can align all involved toward patient safety and excellent training.

Nontechnical Skills

The learning model can incorporate nontechnical skills, which are often harder to teach and even harder to assess. Since the technical aspect of the learning often comes first, teaching and evaluation of nontechnical skills assume some level of independence. Evaluation and teaching of nontechnical skills are best suited for more senior residents. However, the learning environment can encourage observation and identification of nontechnical skills for junior residents especially in an active learning environment, which points out these essential skills. Examples of nontechnical skills include:

- Forward planning: the ability to anticipate needs and think ahead to set up the operative field in an optimum fashion [47]
- Self-direction: refers to the demeanor of the trainee
- Professional conduct
- Staying focused
- Slow down when appropriate
  Expert surgeons are able to slow down and transition from fast and rote tasks toward more focused and analytic behavior [48]. Fatigue, distractions, lack of experience, failing to recognize critical information, overconfidence, and favoring speed can compromise this ability:
- Accept and respond to feedback
- Recognizes when to seek help/advice
- Judgment and patient safety: the ability to recognize and solve problems and to avoid and recover from errors and unexpected events [49]
- Assess and interpret cues and provide team leadership: best practice, resource usage, and time management

The assessment of these abilities can be made by direct observations in the operating room or also in simulation exercises. These skills incorporate into a learning model, which encourages the resident to articulate the steps of the case in a needs assessment exercise and also during the operation. Facilitating steps can be taken. For example, attendings should also allow pauses so the resident is prompted to think of the next step. Often as residents are completing a part of the case, the attending physician is preparing for the next step.

The attending can also prompt the forward progress by asking "what should you be thinking of next as you finish…?" or "what if you were not able to identify the ureter as the peritoneum is incised…?" By allowing responding to prompts, the resident can demonstrate critical slowing down. Additionally, the attending can discern lack of confidence or tameness from a fundamental knowledge gap or lack of experience.

Response to feedback is very insightful for all level of learners. This has been covered in the earlier section of the chapter. Feedback needs to be constructive from the teacher. The acceptance of feedback shows a willingness to improve and also regard for the teacher, which helps in the "sizing up" and helps the teacher be more committed to the learning environment.

Mental rehearsal can also play a role in promoting resident learning as regards to nontechnical training. Rehearsal of tasks is well studied in sports and music and also supported as an effective strategy in surgery [50]. Residents can again focus on needs assessment exercises, which rehearse critical oversteps in their mind without physical movement or equipment.

There are definite difficulties in carrying nontechnical skills from an operating room to a simulated environment. In other words, deconstructing a task or a set of steps can be challenging when it is not real. Cognitive psychology research teaches us that it is hard to capture critical decision-making steps because experts rely on knowledge that has become automated and is no longer accessible to consciousness and therefore difficult to recall [51]. Tackling a task like life-threatening bleeding from the vena cava results in an expert surgeon following a series of steps like holding pressure, clamping, asking for sutures, looking at monitors, communicating with anesthesia, asking for blood, and requesting backup just to name a few. Expert surgeons have somehow learned these tasks and can negotiate difficult situations while maintain patient safety. The attending may not be able to impart similar knowledge in a mental rehearsal or simulation exercise. Steps can be taken to forward the cause using cognitive task analysis in which automated skills are deconstructed to create a checklist of critical decision-making steps and options to avoid error and teach decision-making. Incorporating cognitive task analysis has proven to be an effective tool in improving insertion of percutaneous tracheostomy [52]. Creating a checklist for more complex surgery can be cumbersome; it can be a focused effort on critical aspect of a case, for example, control of the dorsal venous complex during a radical prostatectomy.

Briefing, intraoperative teaching, and debriefing:

- Briefing: needs assessment and setting specific performance targets
  - Can be one or multiple objectives
  - Could be based on stage of learning
- Intraoperative teaching
  - Attending teaches to the objective
  - Redefines objectives as needed
  - Provides coaching to accomplish objective
- Debriefing
  - Feedback after the case which addresses the objective(s)
  - Create learning plan
  - Review progress on stages within learning model

Conclusion

Teaching in the operating room is a complex task with many challenges. It is clear that improvements need to be made on how residents are taught, evaluated, assessed, and graduated to be able to not only perform safe and effective procedures but also manage difficult situations and the operating room environment. The concepts of creating a learning environment, thoughtful assessments, needs assessment, clear expectations, commitment and preparedness, entrustability, learning model, feedback, needs assessment, acquiring technical and nontechnical skills, and debriefing are central to effective teaching in the operating room and need be embraced. There are several evaluation tools, smart apps, checklists, narrative evaluations, milestones, and learning models that can be incorporated into teaching in the operating room. The most effective method will continue to evolve. Until then, teachers and residents need to fully commit to teaching and learning in the operating room.

References

1. Evans CH, Schenarts KD. Evolving educational techniques in surgical training. Surg Clin North Am. 2016;96:71–88. https://doi.org/10.1016/j.suc.2015.09.005.
2. Malangoni MA, Biester TW, Jones AT, Klingensmith ME, Lewis FR. Operative experience of surgery residents: trends and challenges. J Surg Educ. 2013;70:783–8. https://doi.org/10.1016/j.jsurg.2013.09.015.
3. Yeo H, Viola K, Berg D, Lin Z, Nunez-Smith M, Cammann C, et al. Attitudes, training experiences, and professional expectations of US general surgery residents. JAMA. 2009;302:1301. https://doi.org/10.1001/jama.2009.1386.
4. Mattar SG, Alseidi AA, Jones DB, Jeyarajah DR, Swanstrom LL, Aye RW, et al. General surgery residency inadequately prepares trainees for fellowship. Ann Surg. 2013;258:440–9. https://doi.org/10.1097/SLA.0b013e3182a191ca.
5. Ludmerer KM. The development of American medical education from the turn of the century to the era of managed care. Clin Orthop Relat Res. 2004;(422):256–62.
6. Daniels M. 10 Inspirational quotes for EdTech-friendly teachers 2011. https://www.knewton.com/resources/blog/teacher-tools/10-inspirational-quotes-for-edtech-friendly-teachers/.
7. Supreme Court-Jacobellis v. Ohio. Leagal Inf Institute-Cornell Univ Law Sch n.d. https://www.law.cornell.edu/supremecourt/text/378/184. Accessed 1 Jan 2017.
8. Propublica Surgeon Scorecard. Propublica n.d. https://projects.propublica.org/surgeons/. Accessed 1 Jan 2017.
9. Mellinger JD, Williams RG, Sanfey H, Fryer JP, DaRosa D, George BC, et al. Teaching and assessing operative skills: from theory to practice. Curr Probl Surg. 2017;54:44–81. https://doi.org/10.1067/j.cpsurg.2016.11.007.
10. Williams RG, Chen X, Sanfey H, Markwell SJ, Mellinger JD, Dunnington GL. The measured effect of delay in completing operative performance ratings on clarity and detail of ratings assigned. J Surg Educ. 2014;71:e132–8. https://doi.org/10.1016/j.jsurg.2014.06.015.
11. Williams RG, Verhulst S, Colliver JA, Dunnington GL. Assuring the reliability of resident performance appraisals: more items or more observations? Surgery. 2005;137:141–7. https://doi.org/10.1016/j.surg.2004.06.011.
12. Martin JA, Regehr G, Reznick R, MacRae H, Murnaghan J, Hutchison C, et al. Objective structured assessment of technical skill (OSATS) for surgical residents. Br J Surg. 1997;84:273–8.
13. Yule S, Flin R, Paterson-Brown S, Maran N, Rowley D. Development of a rating system for surgeons' non-technical skills. Med Educ. 2006;40:1098–104. https://doi.org/10.1111/j.1365-2929.2006.02610.x.
14. Gofton WT, Dudek NL, Wood TJ, Balaa F, Hamstra SJ. The Ottawa surgical competency operating room evaluation (O-SCORE). Acad Med. 2012;87:1401–7. https://doi.org/10.1097/ACM.0b013e3182677805.
15. Kramp KH, van Det MJ, Hoff C, Lamme B, Veeger NJGM, Pierie J-PEN. Validity and reliability of global operative assessment of laparoscopic skills (GOALS) in novice trainees performing a laparoscopic cholecystectomy. J Surg Educ. 2015;72:351–8. https://doi.org/10.1016/j.jsurg.2014.08.006.
16. Larson JL, Williams RG, Ketchum J, Boehler ML, Dunnington GL. Feasibility, reliability and validity of an operative performance rating system for evaluating surgery residents. Surgery. 2005;138:640–9. https://doi.org/10.1016/j.surg.2005.07.017.

17. Gingerich A, Regehr G, Eva KW. Rater-based assessments as social judgments: rethinking the etiology of rater errors. Acad Med. 2011;86:S1–7. https://doi.org/10.1097/ACM.0b013e31822a6cf8.
18. Weber DE, Mavin TJ, Roth W-M, Henriqson E, Dekker SWA. Exploring the use of categories in the assessment of airline pilots' performance as a potential source of examiners' disagreement. J Cogn Eng Decis Mak. 2014;8:248–64. https://doi.org/10.1177/1555343414532813.
19. Williams RG, Verhulst S, Mellinger JD, Dunnington GL. Is a single-item operative performance rating sufficient? J Surg Educ. 2015;72:e212–7. https://doi.org/10.1016/j.jsurg.2015.05.002.
20. SIMPL n.d. http://www.procedurallearning.org/simpl.
21. Bohnen JD, George BC, Williams RG, Schuller MC, DaRosa DA, Torbeck L, et al. The feasibility of real-time intraoperative performance assessment with SIMPL (system for improving and measuring procedural learning): early experience from a multi-institutional trial. J Surg Educ. 2016;73:e118–30. https://doi.org/10.1016/j.jsurg.2016.08.010.
22. Schwind CJ, Williams RG, Boehler ML, Dunnington GL. Do individual attendings' post-rotation performance ratings detect residents' clinical performance deficiencies? Acad Med. 2004;79:453–7.
23. Ende J. Feedback in clinical medical education. J Am Med Assoc. 1983;250:777–81. https://doi.org/10.1001/jama.1983.03340060055026.
24. Hewson MG, Little ML. Giving feedback in medical education: verification of recommended techniques. J Gen Intern Med. 1998;13:111–6. https://doi.org/10.1046/j.1525-1497.1998.00027.x.
25. Freidson E. Preface in becoming professional. Beverly Hills/ Los Angeles: SAGE PublicationsSage; 1977.
26. Isaacson J, Posk L, Litaker D, Halperin A. Resident perceptions of the evaluation process. J Gen Intern Med. 1995;10(suppl):89.
27. Johnson CE, Keating JL, Boud DJ, Dalton M, Kiegaldie D, Hay M, et al. Identifying educator behaviours for high quality verbal feedback in health professions education: literature review and expert refinement. BMC Med Educ. 2016;16:96. https://doi.org/10.1186/s12909-016-0613-5.
28. Gilber D, Wilson T. Miswanting. In: Forgas J, editor. Think. Feel. role Affect Soc. Cogn. Cambridge: Cambridge University Press; 2000. p. 178–97.
29. Eva KW, Armson H, Holmboe E, Lockyer J, Loney E, Mann K, et al. Factors influencing responsiveness to feedback: on the interplay between fear, confidence, and reasoning processes. Adv Health Sci Educ. 2012;17:15–26. https://doi.org/10.1007/s10459-011-9290-7.
30. Locke EA, Latham GP. Building a practically useful theory of goal setting and task motivation. A 35-year odyssey. Am Psychol. 2002;57:705–17.
31. Ten Cate O, Hart D, Ankel F, Busari J, Englander R, Glasgow N, et al. Entrustment decision making in clinical training. Acad Med. 2016;91:191–8. https://doi.org/10.1097/ACM.0000000000001044.
32. Han PKJ, Klein WMP, Arora NK, Eddy–david. Varieties of uncertainty in health care: a conceptual taxonomy. Med Decis Mak. 2011;31(6):828–38. https://doi.org/10.1177/0272989X11393976.
33. Ten Cate O. Nuts and bolts of Entrustable professional activities. J Gr Med Educ. 2013;5:157–8. https://doi.org/10.4300/JGME-D-12-00380.1.
34. Holmboe ES, Edgar L, Hamstra SJ. Milestone overview. Chicago: ACGME; 2016.
35. Vygostky L, Hanfmann E, Vakar G, Kozulin A. Thought and language. Cambridge, MA: MIT Press; 2012.
36. ten Cate O, Snell L, Mann K, Vermunt J. Orienting teaching toward the learning process. Acad Med. 2004;79:219–28.
37. Lyon P. Med Educ. 2003;37(8):680–8.
38. Lingard L, et al. Team communications in the operating room: talk patterns, sites of tension, and implications for novices. Acad Med. 2002;77:232–7.
39. Lyon P. A model of teaching and learning in the operating theatre. Med Educ. 2004 Dec;38(12):1278–87.
40. Pugh J, et al. A comparison of faculty and resident perception of resident learning needs in the operating room. J Surg Educ. 2013;64:250–5.

41. Pugh J, et al. Am J Surg. 2010;199(4):562–5.
42. Kim S, et al. Surg. 2014;156(3):707–17.
43. Aggarwal R, Grantcharov T, Moorthy K, et al. Toward feasible, valid, and reliable video-based assessments of technical surgical skills in the operating room. Ann Surg. 2008;247:372–9.
44. DaRosa, et al. J Surg Edu. 2013;70(1):24–30.
45. Ko CY, Escarce JJ, Baker L, et al. Predictors of surgery resident satisfaction with teaching by attendings: a national survey. Ann Surg. 2005;241:373–80.
46. Rose JS, Waibel BH, Schenarts PJ. Disparity between resident and faculty surgeons' perceptions of preoperative preparation, intraoperative teaching, and postoperative feedback. J Surg Educ. 2011;68:459–64.
47. Sanfey H, Williams RG, Chen X, et al. Evaluating resident operative performance: a qualitative analysis of expert opinions. Surgery. 2011;150(4):759–70.
48. Moulton CA, Regehr G, Mylopoulos M, et al. Slowing down when you should: a new model of expert judgment. Acad Med. 2007;82(Suppl):S109–16.
49. Sanfey H, Williams R, Dunnington G. Recognizing residents with a deficiency in operative performance as a step closer to effective remediation. J Am Coll Surg. 2012;216(1):114–22.
50. Moulton C, Regehr G, Lingard L, et al. Operating from the other side of the table: control dynamics and the surgeon educator. J Am Coll Surg. 2010;210:79–86.
51. Mellinger JD, Williams RG. Sanfey H, et al. Curr Probl Surg. 2017;54:44–81.
52. Sullivan ME, Brown CVR, Peyre SE, et al. The use of cognitive task analysis to improve the learning of percutaneous tracheostomy placement. Am J Surg. 2007;193:96–9.

Part II

Program Optimization

Resident Duty Hours in Surgical Education

9

David J. Rea and Matthew Smith

The topic of duty hours in surgical education is one that stirs a great deal of emotion in all surgeons. As surgeons, we are products of our own training environments and inherently biased about how the time spent in patient care and educational endeavors has shaped our current abilities and surgical careers. It is not uncommon for a group of surgeons to wax poetic about our training programs, the "surgical giants" who influenced us in both a positive and negative manner, and the tragicomic events that have taught us important lessons about patients and surgical disease that we find fundamental to our personal approach to surgical problems. The rigors of the surgical education process have made an indelible imprint on our lives as "physicians who operate."

The heart of the many debates of the role of duty hours in surgical education has been the question of how much "time" is needed to educate a knowledgeable and technically competent surgeon who can independently take care of surgical patients. The research of psychologist K. Anders Ericsson has extensively evaluated high performing individuals, and his findings have suggested that it takes about 10,000 hours of deliberate practice to attain expert performance [1]. This 10,000 hours has been studied across varied disciplines including music, sports, and medicine [2]. A similar thesis has been argued by Colvin in his book *Talent is Overrated* [3]. Whatever natural aptitude we have can be supplanted by deliberate practice with highly skilled coaching to guide our activities. How does this apply to what surgeons do? Is it valid to compare practicing a musical instrument or a golf swing to the breadth of knowledge that surgical residents must master to adequately

D.J. Rea, MD, FACS (✉) • M. Smith, DO
Division of General Surgery, Department of Surgery, Southern Illinois University School of Medicine, 701 N First Street, PO Box 19638, Springfield, IL 62794-9638, USA
e-mail: drea@siumed.edu

T.S. Köhler, B. Schwartz (eds.), *Surgeons as Educators*,
https://doi.org/10.1007/978-3-319-64728-9_9

diagnose, manage, and treat patients with surgical problems? Many professionals involved in teaching learners would argue that surgical residents learn at different rates depending on the task and the characteristics of the learner, and so a one size fits all, time-based approach is too narrow.

As surgeons we have all been exposed to the aphorisms of our elders, which usually sound something like this. "The problem with being on call only every other night is that you miss half of the good cases!" In this staid witticism is the assumption that spending more time in the care of patients results in a greater breadth and depth of knowledge that will ultimately make one a better surgeon. The other unfortunate assumption is that unless you spend extraordinary hours in the care of patients, you will not be as prepared as you could be (or *should* be) for the challenges of a surgical career. As stated in a commentary written in the Journal of the American Medical Association, "Extensive duty hours are a *necessary* component of resident education and a public symbol of a profession that requires hard work and dedication." [4].

It was common knowledge that the work hours for residents often exceeded 80 hours per week, and this was especially true of surgical training programs. In the historical past, residents often lived in the hospitals where they trained (hence the origin of the name "residents") taking call every other night. While in the more modern era, the situation is not that extreme, for all intents and purposes there was only incremental change. In a cross-sectional study conducted by the ACGME of weekly work hours by a postgraduate year PGY-1 and PGY-2 residents across multiple specialties, it was found that general surgery residents worked on average 102–105 hours per week. Eighty-nine percent of residents exceeded the "80-hour" workweek [5]. Similar violations of the 80-h workweek were seen in neurologic surgery (110 h per week), orthopedic surgery (93 h per week), urology (98 h per week), and obstetrics-gynecology (91 h per week). Resident physicians more likely to have higher than average work hours included those who were male, single, childless, and at the PGY-1 level. Conversely, those with lower than average work hours included PGY-2 level, married residents, those with children, and female residents. Other studies corroborate this data [6].

There are certainly detrimental effects to spending long hours performing the work required of a resident physician. The realm of cognitive and psychomotor performance, sleep deprivation has been well studied. In 1971, Friedman et al. published a study that demonstrated after sleep deprivation of an actual night on call; interns made significantly more errors interpreting an electrocardiogram than when they were in a rested state [7]. More recent work has shown that sleep deprivation can lead to increased serious medical errors in residents when they are *actually* practicing medicine, as opposed to in simulated medical scenarios. In the study by Landrigan et al., they observed the incidence of medical errors made by internal medicine interns who worked in the medical intensive care unit and cardiac intensive care unit [8]. In the traditional model of resident work hours, interns worked 77–81 h per week with up to 34 h of continuous duty; in contrast, the intervention group worked 60–63 h per week with up to 16 h of continuous duty. Interns that worked a traditional schedule made 36% more serious medical errors than interns who were in the intervention group, despite no significant difference in patient acuity. The majority of these errors were medication related, but the rate of diagnostic errors was 5.6 times that of the intervention group. Interestingly, the rate of procedural errors was low and similar between the two groups.

Other studies confirm that sleep deprivation does have a measurable effect on psychomotor ability of surgical residents. Grantcharov et al. demonstrated that a typical night on call (with little to no sleep) resulted in a significantly longer time to complete laparoscopic tasks, more task errors, and unnecessary movements than in a rested state [9]. Similar results have been reported by other authors using laparoscopic simulators and other modalities. Studies also suggest that one night of sleep deprivation (less than 3 hours of sleep in a 24-hour shift) creates a psychomotor impairment that equivalents to being legally intoxicated [10]. Various studies have both corroborated and refuted the assertion that sleep deprivation impairs surgical ability [11–13]. To quote Dr. Thomas McCall's perspective on resident fatigue, "Common sense suggest resident's abilities are impaired by fatigue. Few would choose to ride in a car driven by a resident coming off a 36-hour shift" [14].

The effects of fatigue on resident well-being have been extensively studied. In the early work by Friedman et al., interns scored significantly less in areas of surgency (exhibiting high levels of positive affect), vigor, elation, egotism, and social affection when fatigued as opposed to rested. Not surprisingly, fatigue left them feeling more sadness [6]. In a review of studies that examined the effects of sleep deprivation and fatigue on resident physicians, Samkoff and Jaques outlined the findings from numerous studies that included manual dexterity, vigilance, and mood [15]. It has been noted that sleep deprivation can lead to more sadness and less social affection in resident physicians. Additionally, sleep deprivation led to psychological problems such as memory defects, depersonalization, irritability, difficulty in thinking, depression, etc. Other studies have noted that resident physicians have high rates of major depression and episodes of clinical depression. Even after only 6 months of residency, interns have worse moods as manifested by increased rates of anger, tension, confusion, depression, and fatigue. Even a single night of sleep loss has been shown to increase mood issues, depression, anxiety, and demotivation in residents. Extended work hours can also have deleterious physical consequences for resident physicians as well. It has been shown that fatigued residents are more likely to sustain needle stick injuries and significantly more likely to be involved in motor vehicle accidents [16, 17].

To thoroughly explore the issues of how duty hours have impacted surgical education, we aim to discuss the historical events that have catalyzed the changes in resident physician work hours in the United States and how that event led to policy changes that affected resident education. Then we aim explore attitudes of training programs outside of the United States for purposes of comparison. We will then review some contemporary data that supports a more flexible approach to the issue of duty hours in the surgery and how this impacts patient care and resident satisfaction.

Historical Perspective

The case that brought to public attention of the issue of resident physician work hours is that of Libby Zion. The story is well-known to those in the medical community and impeccably outlined by Brensilver and Asch [18, 19]. In March of 1984, a young woman Libby Zion presented to a major New York teaching hospital with fever and agitation. The patient's care was provided by a team that included a resident and an intern. The patient's clinical course was marked by increasing fever and agitation, which ultimately ended up in cardiopulmonary arrest and death. Although the actual cause of death was never determined, issues that became apparent during the investigation was the lack of supervision of the resident team by the attending physician, the delays in the patient being seen by the house staff, the use of physical restraints, and the use of meperidine in a patient who is taking a monoamine oxidase inhibitor (a drug-drug interaction that can cause serotonin syndrome, a likely contributor to her death). Ms. Zion's father, Sydney Zion, was a well-known New York City attorney, former federal prosecutor, and newspaper magnate. Perhaps through the influence of Mr. Zion, the case went to a grand jury approximately 3 years later on criminal charges, but none were filed. There was criticism by the grand jury, however, about the level of supervision of house staff. Following this, the New York Department of Health initiated an investigation, but the findings were inconclusive and only recommended censure of the involved medical providers. Subsequently, the New York State Board of Regents again reviewed the case, and in this instance the intern and resident were found guilty of gross negligence. The disciplinary action imposed by the board included censure and reprimand of the residents, however.

Following this board review, the New York City Health Commissioner formed a commission whose task was to develop rules that would prevent similar occurrences in the future. This committee was chaired by Dr. Bertrand Bell and was informally known as the "Bell Commission." Following its investigation, the Bell Commission concluded that the Libby Zion case was marked by inadequate attending supervision and impaired house staff judgment *due to fatigue,* both of which contributed in some fashion to the patient's death. Recommendations were made for increasing attending supervision and improved ancillary support for residents. The Bell Commission also recommended work-hour limitations for house staff and emergency room physicians. Trainees' total weekly work schedule should be limited to 80 hours. Single shifts in the hospital should not exceed 24 hours, and emergency room shifts should not exceed 12 hours.

These recommendations were incorporated into the New York State Health Code by then Governor Mario Cuomo in October of 1988 and became effective in July of 1989. Unfortunately, the legislation laid down by the State of New York did not result in timely compliance by many of the training programs that were affected. For many years programs were not compliant, and because of lax enforcement by the New York State Department of Health, these violations went unaddressed. The impact of these regulations on resident training in New York did not go unnoticed. In response to the potential economic impact of these regulations, it was calculated that the requirements for additional personnel and ancillary services in New York State would require hiring over 5000 full-time personnel, which would cost state in excess of $358 million dollars [20].

Changes in Duty-Hour Restrictions in the US Training Programs

The changes proposed by the Bell Commission and its application by the New York State Board of Health catalyzed action by many groups to address the issue of resident work hours across the United States [5]. In April 2001, the Occupational Safety and Health Administration (OSHA) was petitioned by multiple groups including Public Citizen, the American Medical Student Association, The Committee of Interns and Residents, and Drs. Bell and Strohl to create national regulations regarding duty hours for all medical residents and fellows in the United States. Legislation was also introduced in the House of Representative and in the Senate to make into law the regulations that were being requested from OSHA. In late October of 2002, the Occupational Safety and Health Administration denied this petition stating that, "other knowledgeable groups are taking action on this problem." It was clear that government regulation of resident work hours was impending. Impressed to perhaps exert control over the future of its own trainees, the American Association Medical Colleges recommended an 80-hour workweek and published its policy shortly thereafter. Similarly, the House of Delegates of the American Medical Association also recommended an 80-hour workweek averaged over 2 weeks for US medical residents and fellows, with a possible increase of up to 5% for some select programs. Finally, in February 2003, the Accreditation Council for Graduate Medical Education (ACGME) whose mandate, "sets standards for US graduate medical education (residency and fellowship) programs and the institutions that sponsors them, and renders accreditation decisions based on compliance with these standards," approved its final version of its recommendations [21]. The work standards took effect on July 1, 2003 and applied to all programs in all specialties. It set a limit of an 80-hour workweek averaged over a 4-week period, every third night on call as a maximum, and 1 day out of each 7 free from patient care responsibilities. Programs also are required to give residents a minimum of 10-hour rest between duty periods. Additionally, all "on call" activities were limited 24 hour plus an additional 6 h of time for transfer of care, continuity of care, education, and didactic activities. It was prohibited for new patient interactions to occur during this time. Up to 10% variance in specific cases was allowed for sound educational reasons. The ACGME guidelines for 2003 are found in Table 9.1.

In response to duty-hour regulations, studies documented both a positive and negative impact on the surgical residency experience. In a survey of general surgery programs in New York State, Whang et al. examined resident attitudes to the changes mandated by the "405 Regulations" (i.e., the Bell Commission recommendations) [22]. The majority of residents felt "more rested" and had "a better quality of life outside of the hospital" after implementing the regulations. Many residents felt that there was a decrease in the quality of their work, the quality of their training, and the

Table 9.1 Summary of existing and new ACGME rules for supervision and duty hours for residency and fellowship programs

Rule	2003 ACGME standards	2010 ACGME standards (Effective July 2011)
Supervision		
Supervision	Adequate supervision is required for all residents	PGY-1 residents must have direct supervision from an upper-level resident or attending physician who is on site and immediately available to provide assistance at all times
Duty hours		
Maximum hours of work per week	Work is limited to 80 h per week, averaged over 4 weeks; internal moonlighting is included	Work is limited to 80 h per week, averaged over 4 weeks; all moonlighting (internal or external) must be included
Mandatory time free of duty	Residents must have 1 day free from educational and clinical responsibilities in 7 days, averaged over 4 weeks	Residents must have 1 day free of duty every 7 days, averaged over 4 weeks; at-home call cannot be assigned during these days
Maximum length of duty period	No new patients may be accepted after 24 h on duty. Residents may remain on duty for an additional 6 h to participate in didactic activities, transfer care of patients, conduct outpatient clinics, and maintain continuity of medical and surgical care	Duty periods of PGY-1 residents must not exceed 16 h in duration. Duty periods of PGY-2 residents and above may be scheduled to a maximum of 24 h with an additional 4 h to complete work; no clinic or admissions after 24 h
Minimum time off between scheduled duty periods	There should be a 10-h period between all daily duty periods and after in-house call	Residents must have 8 h between duty periods and should have 10 h between duty periods. Residents must have at least 14 h free of duty after 24 h of in-house duty
Call		
Maximum in-house on-call frequency	In-house call can occur no more frequently than every third night, averaged over 4 weeks	PGY-2 residents and above must be scheduled for in-house call no more frequently than every third night
At-home call	Hours spent in the hospital while on at-home call must count toward the 80-h workweek limit	Time spent in the hospital by residents on at-home call must count toward the 80-h workweek
Maximum frequency of in-house night float	NA	Residents must not be scheduled for more than 6 consecutive nights of night float

NA denotes not applicable, *PGY* postgraduate year

quality of patient care and a decrease in the continuity of care of their patients. They also felt there was a decline in the case volume and a shifting of responsibility from the junior residents to the senior residents.

A second study surveying residents on the cusp of the ACGME-mandated change in resident duty hours also highlighted the potential positive and negative impacts of the changes [23]. In a sampling of resident from programs in New England, the majority of respondents to the survey were "happy" and "would choose surgery again" if in medical school (81% and 78%, respectively). The majority felt that the ACGME restrictions would have a positive or very positive effect on their personal lives (82%) and work life (62%), while nearly 30% said that there would be a negative or very negative effect on patient care. Seventy-five percent of the junior-level residents felt that "work hour limits would have a positive impact on resident work life," as compared to only 26% of the senior-level residents. Fifty-eight percent of the junior-level residents felt that "work hour limits would have a positive impact on patient care," as compared to only 26% of the senior-level residents. When asked to describe their "ideal" schedule, these residents thought that every fourth night on call and 85–86 hours per week was preferred.

More detailed data was provided by Barden et al. from Weill Medical College in New York City, as they reported on the outcomes of complying with the Bell Commission recommendations as applied to their surgical residents before and after the limitations [24]. As work hours decreased, they saw a statistically significant increase in the ABSITE (American Board of Surgery In-Training Exam) score for the junior residents, but this did not translate to a similar increase in performance for the senior residents. Contrary to the data from the survey by Whang et al., the number of cases for the graduating senior residents actually increased after implementing the 80-hour workweek. Additionally, it was felt that while there was an improvement in resident quality of life, they felt that the continuity of care suffered as a result. There was also a feeling by the residents and faculty that the limitation of work hours did not improve basic science knowledge or clinical decision-making. Sadly, the conclusion of this study was "that both residents and faculty have serious concerns about the impact of work hour reductions on the quality of surgical training and patient care," suggesting that coming duty-hour reforms would be viewed poorly by surgery educators and trainees.

Duty Hours in Non-US Training Programs

The issue of duty hours for resident physicians is not only an issue that became important to trainees in the United States. The public concern over the details of the Libby Zion case did have a ripple effect for other training programs in Western European countries. Not all countries changed their practice policies quickly, however. Most of the changes in work hours in Canada, Europe, and elsewhere outside of the United States are driven by issues surrounding resident well-being and fatigue more than purely a patient safety issue. The resident training system in Canada is managed in a provincial fashion, and as of recently, there were no nationalized standards for resident work hours. In most provinces, there was a 24-hour maximum of consecutive work hours with a time set aside for "handover" of patients. In Canada, in-house call and home call are treated differently so that residents can work up to and over 80 hours in a 7-day period depending on the breakdown of their call schedule. In 2011, however, a Quebecois labor arbitrator successfully argued that a consecutive 24-hour shift was dangerous to the resident's health and violated provincial and national charters. This eventually resulted in a maximum work shift of 16 consecutive hours in Quebec. Currently, a task force is underway in formulating a universal consensus from national stakeholders [25].

Major changes in resident duty hours occurred shortly after the Libby Zion case in Europe. Work hours are governed by the European Working Time Directive (EWTD), whose focus is to protect the health and welfare of all workers in the European Union (EU) nations. This directive has several elements, including a 48-hour workweek, 11 hours of rest between 24-hour duty periods, a minimum of one 24-hour period off every 7 days, and a maximum shift of 8 hours for "stressful" positions. These guidelines have been in place for all workers but started to apply to resident physicians in 2008 [26]. The compliance of the EU nations is highly variable. Denmark has been compliant and, in fact, has an even lower 37-hour workweek. Sweden and Norway also have a 40 hours workweek for resident physicians that has been in place since prior to EWTD [27, 28]. Finland and Germany are felt to be compliant although hard data is lacking. The United Kingdom fully adopted the EWTD in 2009, but some reports suggest that a significant proportion of junior doctors are exceeding the maximum work hours [29]. It is unknown whether the other EU member nations are compliant as no data exists. It is felt by authorities that they are probably not, but some member nations recently became part of EU and may not have been able to adopt the EWTD quickly. With the impending withdrawal of the United Kingdom (and perhaps other nations) from the EU, it will be interesting to see if EWTD restrictions are preserved or discarded in favor of new regulations. In Australia and New Zealand, the training scheme has begun to fall into line with the framework of the EWTD.

The severely limited work hours for non-US resident physicians have been viewed with derision by medical educators in the United States as it seems that the hours spent training seem impossibly limited. Many of these changes have occurred in the recent past, and it may be too early to determine if these training paradigms will continue to be successful in producing high-quality physicians in the surgical specialties. It is perhaps sobering to remember that some of the working time limitations also apply to the attending (consultant) physicians in these countries, and therefore other physicians cannot compensate for diminished working hours. If these countries can continue to produce competent and knowledgeable surgeons under greater time constraints, perhaps we in the United States could adopt some of the methods to increase the efficiency of our training programs.

Repercussions of the 80-Hour Era

Following the implementation of the 2003 ACGME work-hour restrictions, numerous studies were published on the theme of duty-hour restrictions. Compliance with the new duty-hour requirement was found to be lacking. With the restriction of resident work hours, it was felt by some that surgical residents were graduating with less surgical experience and familiarity with specific surgical procedures. Fonseca and coworkers reported that graduating chief residents lacked appropriate confidence in elements of vascular surgery and flexible endoscopy [30–32]. The level of confidence seemed to relate to program size, case volume, and geography, among other things. Additional work from the same group also suggested that a laparoscopic intensive training program also diminished confidence in open surgical procedures. Other studies have disputed this finding and noted that the majority of chief residents were comfortable to go directly into practice, especially if they graduated with more than 950 cases during their residency [33]. Additionally, 80% felt comfortable being on call at a level I trauma center. Procedures that engendered the most discomfort included bile duct explorations, pancreaticoduodenectomies, hepatic lobectomies, and esophagectomies. The later finding is not surprising as the volume of these cases tend to be clustered at higher volume centers with a strong presence of surgery fellows, which means most residents in training have a limited exposure to these cases.

In a similar vein, the readiness of residents for surgical practice became a vital issue as residents began to graduate wholly trained under the ACGME guidelines that began in 2003. Napolitano et al. surveyed "young surgeons" and "older surgeons" about their readiness for surgical practice after graduation and found significantly differing views [34]. The surveyed young surgeons were Fellows of the American College of Surgeons (ACS) less than age 45, while the older surgeons were also ACS Fellows over the age of 45. The response rate in this survey was 10% in both groups; 94% of young surgeons agreed or strongly agreed they were ready for practice after graduation, whereas 59% of older surgeons agreed or strongly agreed with that statement. A similar disparity was evident when asked if they were ready for a surgery attending role. The older surgeons' comments were directed mainly at issues with residency training and limited work hours, while younger surgeons' comments were centered on unfamiliarity with the business side of surgery.

Other literature has been published that examined the effects of duty-hour reforms on graduating surgical resident case volumes before and after the change. Ferguson et al. reported that at Harvard Medical School, case volume in general and vascular surgery did not change during this period [35]. It was noted that graduating chief residents (PGY-5) performed more cases *after* the duty-hour reforms went into effect, mainly due to increased cases on their private practice general surgery service. The case volumes of the PGY-1 through PGY-4 residents did not change during the transition period. Other single institution reports painted a bleaker picture of resident operative volume as a result of the duty-hour changes. In a report from

Carlin et al. from Henry Ford Hospital, there was a significant decrease in operative volume that occurred after July 2003 [36]. Their analysis found a significant decrease in operative case volume in the PGY-1, PGY-2, and PGY-4 residents. The PGY-3 and PGY-5 years appeared unaffected as noted in the article by Ferguson. This decline in volume was noted for their role as primary surgeon, first assistant, or teaching assistant roles. These two manuscripts suggested that the work hour's restrictions caused a shift of operative cases to the more senior resident years from the junior resident years. This is worrisome as the burden of operative teaching would then be spread over fewer years, with less time to work on basic operative skills prior to needing to master more complicated material.

A larger review of operative case logs submitted to the ACGME as mandated for graduating chief residents in general surgery demonstrated overall stability in chief resident case numbers [37]. The number of total cases performed by resident in the year prior to duty-hour reforms (2002–2003, mean = 938) was no different than after (2003–2004, mean = 932). The number of cases performed as a chief resident was also the same across these years as well (2002–2003, mean = 249 vs. 2003–2004, mean = 246). This number of cases also was in line with the average number of chief cases for the prior 5 academic years studied and was well above the established minimum of 150 cases set by the American Board of Surgery. Programs who opted for the variance of an extra 8 hours per week of duty hours (15 programs at that time) as offered by the ACGME did have more cases performed by their graduating chief residents, but no change was noted before or after July 2003.

A second large study that looked operative case volume reported there was a significant change in surgical resident operative volume after the initiation of duty-hour change in 2003 [38]. Despite the significant drop in total case numbers, since the 2003–2004 academic year, there has been an annual *increase* of 8.8 total major cases for graduating chief residents. When examining only the chief resident cases, no significant change was noted after work-hour restrictions went into effect, despite a prior trend of annual decline of 1.9 cases per year. This study also highlighted the change in case types over time for graduating chief residents. For example, 47.1% of the total chief resident case volume was alimentary/intra-abdominal for the earliest cohort (1989–1993), compared to 65.2% in the most recent cohort (2007–2010). In a similar fashion, there has been a decline in the percentage of vascular cases performed as chief resident from 21.8% to 11.7% and in trauma surgery from 8.6% to 3.4%. Some of these changes may reflect changes a shift away from rotations that do not provided defined category (e.g., cardiac surgery) for the RRC, the inability of fellows and chief residents to both log a case (thereby shifting such cases to earlier years in training), and the rise of integrated programs in areas like vascular surgery. A separate analysis looking specifically at trauma operations found that there was no significant change in trauma operations after July 2003 [39]. There has been a steady decline in the ACGME-designated operative trauma cases since 1989, when chief residents graduated with a mean of 72.5 trauma cases, compared to a mean of 39.3 since 1999. Clearly, this trend is based on advances in the management of solid organ injury and the shift to non-operative/endovascular management [40, 41].

In December of 2008, the Institute of Medicine (IOM) released a publication entitled "Resident Duty Hours: Enhancing Sleep, Supervision, and Safety" [42]. This body was asked by Congress to evaluate the most recent evidence on the topic of resident work hours and provide recommendations for schedules and patient handoffs. The IOM cited the ACGME duty-hour changes from 2003 but felt that current evidence that work-hour limits outlined in that recommendation were not restrictive enough. Additionally, they highlighted the need for better resident supervision, appropriate workloads for residents, and accurate handoffs of patients. They also recognized that different specialties have different types of patient complexities and degree of intervention required, which would suggest that a "one size fits all" approach to duty hours is inappropriate. Based on their findings and those of Landrigan (noted previously) and Czeisler et al., the IOM recommended changes to resident duty hours as noted in Table 9.1 [8, 43]. The surgical community was not particularly pleased with further reductions in duty hours [44]. The ACGME reviewed the IOM report and published its own revision to the duty-hour standards entitled, "The ACGME 2011 Duty Hour Standard - Enhancing Quality of Care, Supervision and Resident Professional Development" [45]. Fundamentally, this increased the intensity for resident supervision and curtailed work hours for interns to 16 hours of continuous duty per shift.

Recent Developments in Duty-Hour Reforms

Out of concerns that further restrictions in resident duty hours may have serious consequences for the breadth and depth of surgical resident training, the question was asked whether we had been too conservative with our duty-hour restrictions and if we could safely increase the hours worked by residents in a thoughtful manner without a compromise in patient outcomes. With duty-hour changes now the "law of the land," no sweeping changes were likely to be made to reverse these changes without carefully performed studies that occurred prospectively. To design a study without reproach, it was now necessary to petition the ACGME to waive specific duty-hour requirements for a large group of residents in order to randomize them to the standard duty-hour arm (the current ACGME restrictions) or a more flexible arm. Two separate studies were proposed, one to examine this question in general surgery residents and in internal medicine residents. The Flexibility in Duty Hour Requirement for Surgical Trainees (FIRST) trail was designed by relevant stakeholders in surgical resident education [46, 47].

One hundred and seventeen general surgery programs were randomly assigned to the current ACGME duty-hour policy group (59 programs; the standard-policy group) or the more flexible policies (58 programs; the flexible-policy group). The data obtained on patient-level outcomes came from reporting to the American College of Surgeons National Quality Improvement Program (ACS NSQIP) by hospitals affiliated with the surgical training programs that participated. The NSQIP program has been well described elsewhere and includes data abstracted from the patient medical record by trained abstractors; in this case they were not informed to which study arm the residents at their hospital were assigned [48–51]. The study was of noninferiority design. The ACGME duty-hour restrictions that were waived are shown in Table 9.2. Most of the programs chose to be flexible in the areas of maximum shift length for interns and higher level residents, the minimum time off between shifts, and 24-h call periods. The maximum work, week, and mandatory time free of duty and on-call frequency were immutable.

Table 9.2 Duty-hour requirements and adherence rates according to study group

Requirement category	Standard-policy group		Flexible-policy group	
	Standard ACGME policies	Adherent programs[a] *no. (%)*	Policies[b]	Adherent programs[a] no. *(%)*
Maximum shift length	PGY 1 (interns): duty periods may not exceed 16 h	59 (100)	PGY 1 (interns): duty periods can exceed 16 h	58 (100)
	PGY 2-5 (residents): duty periods may not exceed 28 h (24 h plus 4 h for transition)	59 (100)	PGY 2–5 (residents): duty periods can exceed 28 h (24 hr plus 4 h for transition)	49 (84)
Minimum time off between shifts	Residents must have ≥8 h off between shifts but should have 10 h off between shifts	59 (100)	Residents are not required to have ≥8-10 h off between shifts	47 (81)
	Residents must have ≥14 h off after 24 h of continuous duty	57 (97)	Residents are not required to have ≥14 h off after 24 h of continuous duty	51 (88)
Maximum work h/wk	Residents must not work >80 h/ week, averaged over 4 weeks[c]	—	Residents must not work >80 h/week, averaged over 4 weeks[c]	—
Mandatory time free of duty	Residents must have 1 in every 7 days off from all educational and clinical duties, averaged over 4 weeks[c]	—	Residents must have 1 in every 7 days off from all educational and clinical duties, averaged over 4 weeksl	—
Frequency of on-call duty	Residents must not be on call more frequently than every third night[c]	—	Residents must not be on call more frequently than every third night	—

ACGME denotes Accreditation Council for Graduate Medical Education, and PGY postgraduate year

[a]Program adherence was defined by residency program directors regarding which policies were followed at their institution during the trial period (100% response rate)

[b]Residency programs assigned to the flexible-policy group were allowed to waive four ACGME duty-hour requirements concerning maximum shift length and minimum time off between shifts

[c]These ACGME duty-hour requirements remained the same in both study groups

The study was conducted over a single academic year from July 1, 2014 to June 30, 2015. The randomized design created two well-balanced groups in regard to residents, hospital metrics, residency program types, and patient populations under study. The NSQIP database provided outcomes on 138,691 patients during the study period. As shown in Fig. 9.1, the rate of primary outcomes (e.g., death or serious complications) did not differ between the groups and met criteria for noninferiority. In a similar fashion, the rate of the secondary outcomes was the same in each group and also noninferior. The only exception was renal failure and failure to rescue, which in the adjusted model did not meet criteria for noninferiority. Subgroup analysis of the type of surgery, risk of death, and surgical setting also showed no difference between the two study arms.

The resident-related outcomes in this study were obtained by a questionnaire administered to participating residents (2220 in the standard-policy group and 2110 in the flexible-policy group) during the January 2015 ABSITE exam. Those results are shown in Table 9.3. Importantly, there was no difference between resident dissatisfaction with education quality, overall well-being, patient safety, and work hours between the standard-policy group and the flexible-policy group. The flexible-policy group was significantly less likely to perceive a negative effect of

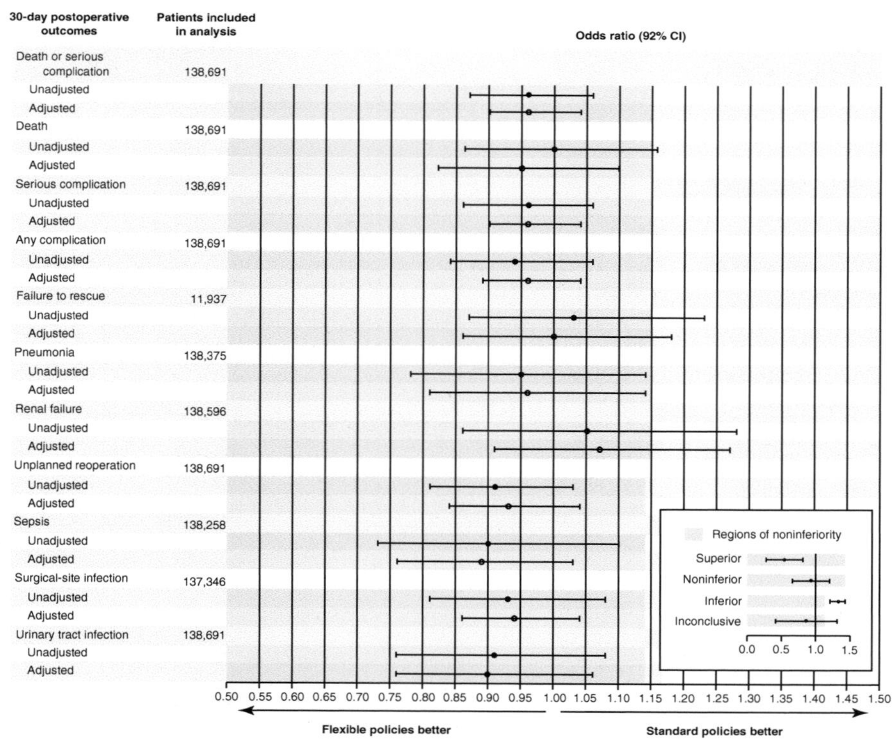

Fig. 9.1 Patient related outcomes from the FIRST trial

Table 9.3 Resident-reported satisfaction and perceptions of well-being, education, and patient safety

Outcome	Standard-policy group	Flexible-policy group	P value[a]	Odds ratio for flexible-policy group (95% Cl)[b]	P value
	no./total no.(%)				
Primary outcomes					
Dissatisfaction with overall quality of resident education[c]	200/1874 (10.7)	194/1768 (11.0)	0.86	1.08 (0.77–1.52)	0.64
Dissatisfaction with overall well-being[c]	226/1876 (12.0)	263/1769 (14.9)	0.10	1.31 (0.99–1.74)	0.06
Secondary outcomes					
Dissatisfaction[c]					
With patient safety	77/1875 (4.1)	62/1770 (3.5)	0.48	0.85 (0.55–1.31)	0.46
With continuity of care	188/1876 (10.0)	83/1769 (4.7)	<0.001	0.44 (0.32–0.60)	<0.001
With quality and ease of handoffs and transitions in care	190/1873 (10.1)	124/1766 (7.0)	0.009	0.69 (0.52–0.92)	0.01
With duty-hour regulations of the program	161/1876 (8.6)	144/1768 (8.1)	0.74	0.99 (0.71–1.40)	0.97
With work hours and scheduling	236/1874 (12.6)	214/1767 (12.1)	0.76	0.95 (0.71–1.27)	0.72
With time for rest	280/1875 (14.9)	329/1768 (18.6)	0.08	1.41 (1.06–1.89)	0.02
Perception of negative effect of institutional duty hours[d]					
On patient safety	491/1891 (26.0)	223/1782 (12.5)	<0.001	0.40 (0.32–0.51)	<0.001
On continuity of care	1053/1892 (55.7)	339/1786 (19.0)	<0.001	0.16 (0.12–0.21)	<0.001
On clinical-skills acquisition	688/1888 (36.4)	232/1777 (13.1)	<0.001	0.24 (0.19–0.31)	<0.001
On operative-skills acquisition	928/1885 (49.2)	337/1781 (18.9)	<0.001	0.22 (0.17–0.27)	<0.001
On resident autonomy	663/1888 (35.1)	232/1782 (13.0)	<0.001	0.26 (0.20–0.34)	<0.001
On operative volume	915/1887 (48.5)	330/1778 (18.6)	<0.001	0.22 (0.17–0.28)	<0.001
On availability for urgent cases	845/1890 (44.7)	266/1783 (14.9)	<0.001	0.20 (0.16–0.25)	<0.001

Table 9.3 (continued)

Outcome	Standard-policy group	Flexible-policy group	P value[a]	Odds ratio for flexible-policy group (95% CI)[b]	P value
	no./total no.(%)				
On availability for elective cases	651/1889 (34.5)	264/1781 (14.8)	<0.001	0.30 (0.24–0.39)	<0.001
On attendance at educational conferences	431/1886 (22.9)	218/1780 (12.2)	<0.001	0.47 (0.36–0.62)	<0.001
On relationship between interns and residents	488/1892 (25.8)	199/1782 (11.2)	<0.001	0.38 (0.29–0.49)	<0.001
On time for teaching medical students	523/1888 (27.7)	262/1781 (14.7)	<0.001	0.45 (0.37–0.56)	<0.001
On case preparation away from hospital	176/1887 (9.3)	427/1781 (24.0)	<0.001	3.37 (2.54–4.47)	<0.001
On participation in research	172/1888 (9.1)	373/1780 (21.0)	<0.001	2.81 (2.12–3.73)	<0.001
On professionalism	240/1891 (12.7)	148/1780 (8.3)	0.002	0.65 (0.49–0.87)	0.003
On job satisfaction	262/1888 (13.9)	226/1782 (12.7)	0.43	0.94 (0.73–1.23)	0.67
On satisfaction with career choice	172/1887 (9.1)	164/1777 (9.2)	0.92	1.03 (0.79–1.33)	0.84
On morale	301/1892 (15.9)	294/1782 (16.5)	0.73	1.09 (0.85–1.40)	0.51
On time with family and friends	168/1888 (8.9)	441/1779 (24.8)	<0.001	3.66 (2.70–4.97)	<0.001
On time for extracurricular activities	172/1886 (9.1)	458/1779 (25.7)	<0.001	3.81 (2.84–5.11)	<0.001
On rest	178/1887 (9.4)	470/1781 (26.4)	<0.001	3.85 (2.88–5.15)	<0.001
On health	128/1883 (6.8)	326/1778 (18.3)	<0.001	3.22 (2.37–4.36)	<0.001
Fatigue always or often affects personal safety[e]	175/1878 (9.3)	188/1774 (10.6)	0.26	1.15 (0.91–1.47)	0.25
Fatigue always or often affects patient safety[e]	118/1878 (6.3)	133/1774 (7.5)	0.17	1.18 (0.91–1.53)	0.21

(continued)

Table 9.3 (continued)

Outcome	Standard-policy group	Flexible-policy group	P value[a]	Odds ratio for flexible-policy group (95% CI)[b]	P value
	no./total no.(%)				
Occurrence during past month owing to duty-hour regulations[f]					
Left during an operation	256/1944 (13.2)	128/1821 (7.0)	<0.001	0.46 (0.32–0.65)	<0.001
Missed an operation	817/1944 (42.0)	544/1821 (29.9)	<0.001	0.56 (0.45–0.69)	<0.001
Handed off an active patient issue	901/1944 (46.3)	583/1821 (32.0)	<0.001	0.53 (0.45–0.63)	<0.001

Denominators represent the number of respondents per survey item in the trial sample of residents. Response rates varied across survey items, ranging from 84 to 87%. When the Bonferroni correction was applied to the 34 resident outcomes assessed, the level of significance was adjusted from 0.05 to 0.0015, and the differences between the study groups were no longer significant for three outcomes: time for rest, quality and ease of handoffs and transitions in care, and professionalism

[a]Cluster-corrected P values were calculated by means of a chi-square test of association between study-group assignment and dichotomized resident outcome

[b]Odds ratios and 95% confidence intervals (Cl) and two-tailed P values were calculated by means of two-level hierarchical logistic regression with program-level random intercepts. Models assessed the association between outcomes and study-group assignment, with adjustment for program-level strata based on 30-day rates of postoperative death or serious complications in 2013 (stratifying variable for randomization). Significant odds ratios of less than 1.00 favor flexible policies over standard policies. Significant odds ratios of more than 1.00 favor standard policies over flexible policies

[c]The numerator represents the number of residents who reported being “very dissatisfied” or “dissatisfied” versus “neutral,” “satisfied,” or “very satisfied”

[d]The numerator represents the number of residents who perceived a “negative effect” of 2014–2015 institutional duty hours versus “no effect” or a “positive effect”

[e]The numerator represents the number of residents who reported that fatigue “always” or “often” affects personal safety or patient safety versus “sometimes,” “rarely,” or “never”

[f]The numerator represents the number of residents who reported one or more occurrences in the past month versus no occurrence

their duty hours on realms of patient safety, patient care, operative experience, and education. Conversely, the flexible-policy group was more likely to perceive a negative effect of their duty hours on realms related to time outside of the hospital (i.e., time with family and friends, extracurricular activities, rest, health, etc.). While the flexible-policy group perceived their duty hours to have less of a negative impact on their sense of professionalism, there was no difference in terms of job satisfaction, career choice decision, or morale. Fatigue as it relates to patient personal safety was similar between both groups. The standard-policy group was significantly more likely have left during an operation and missed an operation or handed off a patient with active issues in the past month than their cohort in the flexible-policy group.

These results demonstrate that more flexible duty hours do not result in inferior patient outcomes, and resident satisfaction was maintained. Other single-center retrospective studies have shown that patient outcomes in other specialties are inferior when resident exceed 80 hours per week [52]. Some limitations of the study exist and are lucidly outlined by Billmoria et al. in their companion article [46]. The intervention period for the study was short, and perhaps running the trial over a longer period time (i.e., 5 years, a full period of residency training) would result in increased job dissatisfaction for the resident working longer hours. The markers of patient safety are important ones (e.g., patient death or serious complication) but perhaps not granular enough to capture errors as a result of resident fatigue.

The landmark FIRST trial demonstrated noninferior outcomes for patients and high levels of resident satisfaction with when duty hours were made more flexible for surgical residents. Another randomized trial has been constructed to examine the effect of more flexible duty-hour policies as it applies to internal medicine trainees. The iCOMPARE trial is led by physicians from the University of Pennsylvania, Johns Hopkins University, and the Brigham and Women's Hospital/Harvard Medical School [53]. As with the FIRST trial, the standard group complies with current ACGME standards including a 16-hour maximum work period for PGY-1 residents. The flexible arm has an 80-hour maximum workweek, 1 day off in every 7, and in-house call no more frequent than every third night (all averaged over 4 weeks). The main outcome will be the measurement of patient safety data and educational outcomes for the internal medicine trainees. The trial began in July of 2015 and has ended in June of 2016. A total of 63 programs enrolled, 31 in the standard policy arm, and 32 in the flexible duty-hour policy arm. As of the writing of this chapter, no data is available about the primary trial endpoints. The results of this trial, if consistent with those of the FIRST trial, will certainly help to justify some relaxation of the standards set for by the ACGME by ensuring patient safety is not compromised. If differences are noted between these studies, this may give way to specialty specific duty-hour restrictions [54].

Several follow-up publications have addressed the residents' perceptions on patient outcomes in the standard duty-hour group compared to those in the flexible duty-hour group. In a recent survey of residents who participated in the FIRST trial, residents in the standard duty-hour group perceived a negative effect on patient safety and continuity of care [55]. Also, PGY-1 residents in the standard duty hours arm were much more likely to have to leave the operating room during a case to abide by the duty-hour rules as compared to the flexible duty-hour group. This did not appear as evident in the PGY-2 or higher group in the standard duty-hour group; the rate of leaving the operating room in the flexible duty-hour group was significantly lower, however. With respect to education and duty hours, there did not appear to be a significant interaction between the duty-hour policy and the degree of dissatisfaction with resident education quality in this study. In terms of the residents' self-perceived domain of well-being as measured by their own health, rest, extracurricular time, and time with family and friends, the flexible policy residents felt more often that their work hours had a negative effect compared to the standard policy arm. This was most prominent at the PGY-1 level, but the effect was significant across all PGY years. This is not unexpected as the length of their time on duty could be considerably longer in the flexible policy arm. However, when asked whether they were "dissatisfied" or "very dissatisfied" with their well-being, there was no difference between the standard and flexible policy arms. Importantly, junior-level residents in the flexible-policy group perceived that the duty hours had

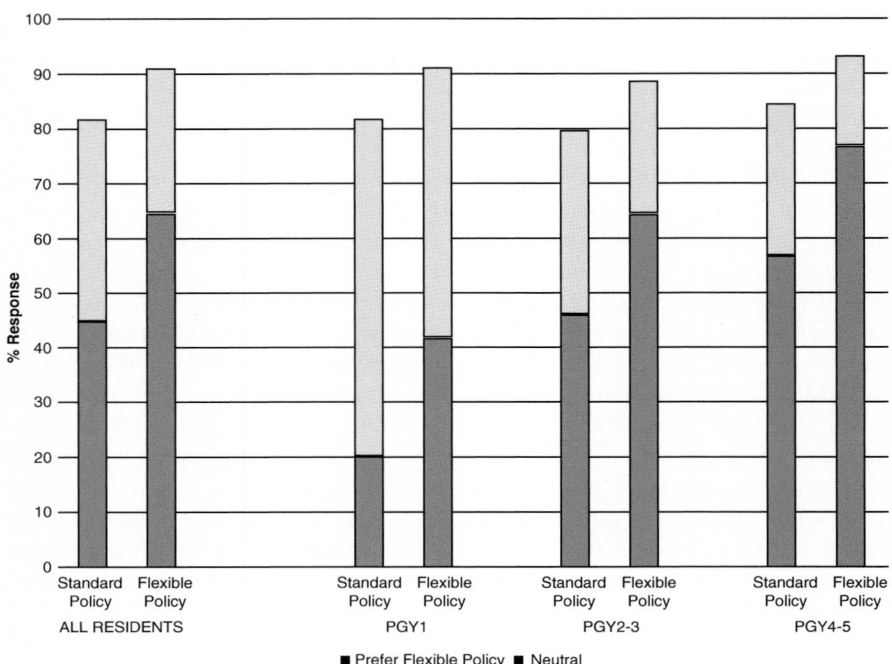

Fig. 9.2 Resident perceptions of flexible duty hours

more of a negative effect on their morale, job satisfaction, career satisfaction, and professionalism when compared to those in the standard policy duty-hour cohort. This effect decreased as the PGY year increased so that senior-level residents in the flexible-policy group perceived that the duty hours had *less* of a negative effect on their morale, job satisfaction, career satisfaction, and professionalism when compared the standard policy arm.

As shown in Fig. 9.2, the majority of residents in the flexible policy arm preferred a flexible duty-hour policy compared to only a minority of residents in the standard policy arm. As the PGY level increased, the proportion of residents who preferred a flexible policy increased dramatically. This was especially evident in the group already assigned to the flexible duty-hour policy (increasing from 41% of interns to 77% of senior residents). It seems that residents themselves overwhelmingly want to train under a flexible duty-hour system, despite their own perceptions that the flexible duty hours have had a negative effect on specific aspects of their out-of-hospital well-being (e.g., rest, health, etc.). As discussed in this article, it would appear that the benefits of this type of training – increased patient safety, better continuity of care, and time in the operating room – would outweigh the negative.

The FIRST trial has caused controversy among those in surgical education as it calls for broad changes in the way duty-hour restrictions are applied and enforced.

Some have called into question the validity of the conclusions drawn by the FIRST trial due to the possibility that surgical residents are underreporting their duty hours. Prior to the conduct of the FIRST trial, several publications noted that falsification of duty hours and noncompliance with ACGME duty hours are common. Drolet et al. published the results of an informal survey in which 62% of surveyed surgical residents falsely report their duty hours, and 67% were noncompliant with ACGME standards [56]. For comparison, duty-hour falsification and ACGME noncompliance occur in 43% and 53% of all residents that were surveyed across all specialties. This behavior was also most prevalent in the PGY-1 year and decreased with increasing PGY level. Other studies have noted similar findings, but perhaps this issue can be viewed as an example of professionalism and a means to identify systemic work-hour issues that need to be addressed on a programmatic level [57].

Billmoria et al. recently reported their own survey of residents who participated in the FIRST trial and the frequency of violating the prescribed duty-hour limitations [58]. In the month prior to the administration of this survey, the group assigned to the standard duty-hour policy, 24% of PGY-1 residents worked more than 16 hours continuously 1–2 times, and 6% did this more than five times. In a similar manner, 25% of PGY-2 through PGY-5 residents worked more than 28 hours continuously on 1–2 occasions, while 4% did this more than five times in the preceding month. Additionally, approximately 20% of residents surveyed had less than 8 hours off between shifts, and 15% had less than 14 hours off after being on call 1–2 times in the preceding month. This occurred more than five times in the preceding month in 4% and 4%, respectively, of residents in the standard duty-hour group. Importantly, 33% of residents worked more than 80 hours per week 1–2 times in the prior month and 16% exceed 80 hours per week 3–5 times in the prior month. This demonstrates that even in highly scrutinized surgery residency programs, violations frequently occur. Clearly, the flexible duty-hour arm of the FIRST trial violated ACGME duty-hour requirements by design. Therefore, it is no surprise that the residents in this group more frequently worked more than 16 hours (at the PGY-1 level), more than 28 hours continuously at the PGY-2 level and above, and more often had fewer than 8 h off between shifts when compared to the standard group. Despite these differences, there was no difference in the percentage of residents who violated the 14-hour off after call rule. When both groups of residents were asked about the reasons that they chose to violate their duty-hour limits, most cited the desire to facilitate care transitions, stabilize a critically ill patient, or operate on a patient they know well. This was certainly more frequent as the PGY level increased. Additionally, many used the extra time to perform "routine" tasks, complete documentation, or round with the team. The minority cited using the extra work hours to attend educational conferences or activities.

Another long-standing argument for limitations of resident duty hours was to allow residents time away from patient care duties to codify the information they learn from patient care with independent and self-directed study of the medical literature. Additionally, some topics with which residents are expected to be familiar are not commonly seen in routine practice, so can only be learned about through diligent study. This knowledge is tested annually as surgical residents take the American Board of Surgery In-Training Exam (ABSITE) and after completion of their final year as they take the American Board of Surgery (ABS) Qualifying Exam (written) and Certifying Exam (oral). In the flexible policy arm, there might be the unintended consequence that the increased time in the care of patients might result in poorer performance on these exams. Although only 2 years of residents and exam data were available, Blay et al. studied exam results in the FIRST trial participants [59]. When comparing the flexible-policy group to the standard-policy group, there were no significant differences in ABSITE score. This finding was consistent over all PGY levels. Additionally, there was no statistical difference in first time pass rates of the ABS Qualifying Exam (Flexible: 90.4% and Standard: 90.5%) or the ABS Certifying Exam (Flexible: 86.3% and Standard: 88.6%). This did not change even when adjusted for the characteristics of the program. This data is limited in that only 2 years of testing is available for review and differences may arise with a larger cohort. Interestingly, the pass rate for the ABS Qualifying Exam over the past 5 years has been fairly steady at 80% [60]. Clearly, the FIRST trial participants are performing well on the Qualifying Exam suggesting they may not have been as impacted by the increase in hours worked which may not be generalizable to all surgical trainees. A similar observation may be made about the recent results from the last 5 years of the Certifying Exam, which have seen pass rates fluctuate between 72% and 80%.

What has been made clear from the FIRST trial is that allowing some flexibility in the duty hours and providing fewer restrictions for residents do not seem to cause harm to patients and provide more satisfaction to surgical residents. This paradigm shift has now been incorporated into recent changes by the ACGME in resident duty hours. As on July 1, 2017, PGY-1 residents will start to have more flexibility in duty hours by allowing them to work 24-hour shifts with an extra 4 h for documentation or education, as opposed to the 16 hour of continuous duty previously allowed [61]. The aim is that this will allow for fewer handoffs and allow for increased educational time for PGY-1 trainees. Also, it will allow more time for PGY-1 resident to acclimate to the resident physician lifestyle and feel more engaged in the care of patients. Additionally, it will certainly ease the now difficult transition between the PGY-1 year and the PGY-2 year. The other limitations on resident duty hours will remain in place (e.g., no more than 80 hours per week averaged over 4 weeks, 8 hours off between shifts, etc.). Importantly, the language of the Common Program Requirements gives resident autonomy and voluntariness to be flexible in how they apply these duty hours in the best interest of caring for patients. Such examples include "to provide care to a single severely ill or unstable patient," "humanistic attention to the needs of a patient of family," or "to attend unique educational events."

As we move forward in the evaluation of the research that has been done in recent years on duty hours and the correlation between needing to provide adequate surgical education and not compromising patient care, it is important that we continue to analyze more long-term data shrewdly. Pendulum shifts will inevitably continue as there have been in the past in the amount of hours worked by residents, with the goal to provide adequate surgical education without compromising patient care or the well-being of the resident population. Some have pleaded that broad-sweeping changes not be made based solely on this data as it stands to avoid shifts that could negatively affect patient care and the wellness of residents. It would seem that the current policy of the ACGME is to look for high-quality data and make incremental adjustments in reforming the duty-hours.

In order to combat the perceived uneasiness of some surgical chief resident to directly enter practice, the American College of Surgeons has proposed the use of a "transition to practice" fellowship [62–65]. These are fellowships that allow a "pseudo-autonomy" of the fellow to operate under the mentorship of a more senior surgeon. Some of these fellowships include performing cases in other surgical disciplines such as urology, neurosurgery, plastic surgery, and orthopedics. Ironically, for many general surgery programs, these rotations were once components of training but have been diminished or removed due to the work-hour restrictions. Some have argued for the advantages of this type of program, but is this really different than an extra year of residency? We can foresee the utility of these types of programs for residents who later in their training decide they would like to work in an environment where they would be a "proceduralist" who needs basic skills in these other surgical disciplines (e.g., a rural surgery practice or as a medical missionary). Perhaps we need to consider the types of residents or programs whose graduates feel they need this type of extra attention and more closely examine why their previous system did not meet their needs. Perhaps this also would suggest that PGY-5 level residents should be given considerably *more* autonomy and even less regulations on their hours to facilitate a smooth transition to practice. These programs are currently not widespread, but we should watch carefully how these are used. Certainly, the fellows in these programs could be seen as cheap (but skilled) labor as opposed to continuing learners.

The long-term effects of residents having trained in the current duty-hour restrictions are something that will not be known for several years to decades. Certainly several scenarios come to mind. Will limitations of duty hours now cause increased job dissatisfaction and burnout among future surgeons when their jobs demand work hours that exceed 80 hours per week? If more senior surgeons have a distrust of the abilities of their newly graduated colleagues, how will that manifest as for the employability of the future generations of surgeons. The issue of burnout has become front and center in the medical community. Although probably not a new phenomenon, burnout has been invoked as a major contributor to physicians leaving medicine. Current data suggest that general surgery and surgical subspecialties are affected by burnout at a high rate than many other specialties [66–70]. Can the current duty-hour restrictions contribute to even high rates of burnout in the future? One could argue that training in an 80 hours per week system and then graduating to a surgical practice where one is expected to work greater than 80 hours per week would create added stress and job dissatisfaction, thereby leading to burnout. This situation could certainly be magnified by choosing to practice in a smaller community where there is less support, and the local surgeon is expected to provide care ceaselessly. If we are also training surgeons with less clinical experience during their residency, we could also imagine that our recent graduates may be less well equipped to handle difficult surgical cases, thereby increasing their personal dissatisfaction with their job, leading to increased rates of burnout as well. The cumulative pressure of these two scenarios may then change the demographics of surgical practice for recent graduates, choosing to practice in larger groups with a larger patient base to insulate them from working beyond 80 hours and from having to tackle cases for which they feel unequipped. This may then further the shortage of surgical providers in small communities in the United States. With all this in mind, it will always be the goal of residency programs across the nation to train and educate future surgeons to be competent surgeons that enjoy their career and provide high-quality care for coming generations.

The issue of duty hours in surgical education has been evolving for the last 40 years. We have seen the extremes of the past, where work hours were excessive and detrimental to residents' physical and emotional health. Unfortunately, the surgical community maintained the status quo for many years – fueled by pride and egotism – to the detriment of many trainees. Spurred on by the very public and tragic death of Libby Zion, the issue of excessive duty hours and resident fatigue was placed squarely in the crosshairs of public opinion; no longer could the medical community sit silently by while this status quo was maintained. Pressures from those inside and outside of the field of medicine led to restricted work hours mandated by the ACGME in 2003. This change then engendered a backlash of concern that the surgical community might be sacrificing surgical competency for resident well-being. Much of the data seemed to suggest that resident experience was unchanged during this tumultuous time, however.

Further restrictions were put in place in 2011 based on data showing negative patient-related consequences of even the 2003 ACGME restrictions. The continued erosion of resident work hours prompted the design of randomized trial to determine if increasing flexibility of resident hours (without increasing the total hours worked) would impact patient care. The landmark FIRST trial showed that when resident work hours were liberalized, no difference in patient outcomes was noted. Importantly, the residents themselves, though with less time for extracurricular activities, felt more of a sense of patient engagement and greater satisfaction with the educational process. This randomized data has now caused the ACGME to reconsider some of the restrictions enacted in 2011. Where the future of duty-hour restrictions is heading is unclear. Are we satisfied that the current system provides that balance of producing highly skilled and competent surgeons who are also emotionally and physically intact at the end of the process? Only careful study and time will tell. As the surgical community goes forward in the future, the new standard of high-quality randomized data will be our best guide at balancing patient and resident outcomes.

References

1. Ericsson KA. Deliberate practice and acquisition of expert performance: a general overview. Acad Emerg Med. 2008;15(11):988–94.
2. Ericsson KA. Deliberate practice and the acquisition and maintenance of expert performance in medicine and related domains. Acad Med. 2004;79(10 Suppl):S70–81.
3. Colvin G. Talent is overrated : what really separates world-class performers from everybody else. New York: Portfolio; 2008.

4. Philibert I, Friedmann P. Williams WT; ACGME work group on resident duty hours. Accreditation Council for Graduate Medical Education. New requirements for resident duty hours. JAMA. 2002;288(9):1112–4.
5. Baldwin DC Jr, Daugherty SR, Tsai R, Scotti MJ Jr. A national survey of residents' self-reported work hours: thinking beyond specialty. Acad Med. 2003;78(11):1154–63.
6. Scher KS, Peoples JB. A study of the on-duty hours of surgical residents. Surgery. 1990;108(2):393–7; discussion 397–9
7. Friedman RC, Bigger JT, Kornfeld DS. The intern and sleep loss. N Engl J Med. 1971;285(4):201–3.
8. Landrigan CP, Rothschild JM, Cronin JW, Kaushal R, Burdick E, Katz JT, Lilly CM, Stone PH, Lockley SW, Bates DW, Czeisler CA. Effect of reducing interns' work hours on serious medical errors in intensive care units. N Engl J Med. 2004;351(18):1838–48.
9. Grantcharov TP, Bardram L, Funch-Jensen P, Rosenberg J. Laparoscopic performance after one night on call in a surgical department: prospective study. BMJ. 2001;323(7323): 1222–3.
10. Mohtashami F, Thiele A, Karreman E, Thiel J. Comparing technical dexterity of sleep-deprived versus intoxicated surgeons. JSLS. 2014;18(4):e2014.00142.
11. Tsafrir Z, Korianski J, Almog B, Many A, Wiesel O, Levin I. Effects of fatigue on residents' performance in laparoscopy. J Am Coll Surg. 2015;221(2):564–70.
12. Olasky J, Chellali A, Sankaranarayanan G, Zhang L, Miller A, De S, Jones DB, Schwaitzberg SD, Schneider BE, Cao CG. Effects of sleep hours and fatigue on performance in laparoscopic surgery simulators. Surg Endosc. 2014;28(9):2564–8.
13. Lehmann KS, Martus P, Little-Elk S, Maass H, Holmer C, Zurbuchen U, Bretthauer G, Buhr HJ, Ritz JP. Impact of sleep deprivation on medium-term psychomotor and cognitive performance of surgeons: prospective cross-over study with a virtual surgery simulator and psychometric tests. Surgery. 2010;147(2):246–54.
14. McCall TB. The impact of long working hours on resident physicians. N Engl J Med. 1988;318(12):775–8.
15. Samkoff JS, Jacques CH. A review of studies concerning effects of sleep deprivation and fatigue on residents' performance. Acad Med. 1991;66(11):687–93.
16. Ayas NT, Barger LK, Cade BE, Hashimoto DM, Rosner B, Cronin JW, Speizer FE, Czeisler CA. Extended work duration and the risk of self-reported percutaneous injuries in interns. JAMA. 2006;296(9):1055–62.
17. Barger LK, Cade BE, Ayas NT, Cronin JW, Rosner B, Speizer FE, Czeisler CA, Harvard Work Hours, Health, and Safety Group. Extended work shifts and the risk of motor vehicle crashes among interns. N Engl J Med. 2005;352(2):125–34.
18. Brensilver JM, Smith L, Lyttle CS. Impact of the Libby Zion case on graduate medical education in internal medicine. Mt Sinai J Med. 1998;65(4):296–300.
19. Asch DA, Parker RM. The Libby Zion case. One step forward or two steps backward? N Engl J Med. 1988;318(12):771–5.
20. Thorpe KE. House staff supervision and working hours. Implications of regulatory change in New York state. JAMA. 1990;263(23):3177–81.
21. http://www.acgme.org/What-We-Do/Accreditation.
22. Whang EE, Mello MM, Ashley SW, Zinner MJ. Implementing resident work hour limitations: lessons from the New York state experience. Ann Surg. 2003;237(4):449–55.
23. Whang EE, Perez A, Ito H, Mello MM, Ashley SW, Zinner MJ. Work hours reform: perceptions and desires of contemporary surgical residents. J Am Coll Surg. 2003;197(4):624–30.
24. Barden CB, Specht MC, McCarter MD, Daly JM, Fahey TJ 3rd. Effects of limited work hours on surgical training. J Am Coll Surg. 2002;195(4):531–8.
25. Temple J. Resident duty hours around the globe: where are we now? BMC Med Educ. 2014;14(Suppl 1):S8.
26. Imrie KR, Frank JR, Parshuram CS. Resident duty hours: past, present, and future. BMC Med Educ. 2014;14(Suppl 1):S1.
27. Søreide K, Glomsaker T, Søreide JA. Surgery in Norway: beyond the scalpel in the 21st century. Arch Surg. 2008;143(10):1011–6.

28. Sundberg K, Frydén H, Kihlström L, Nordquist J. The Swedish duty hour enigma. BMC Med Educ. 2014;14(Suppl 1):S6.
29. Moonesinghe SR, Lowery J, Shahi N, Millen A, Beard JD. Impact of reduction in working hours for doctors in training on postgraduate medical education and patients' outcomes: systematic review. BMJ. 2011;342:d1580.
30. Fonseca AL, Reddy V, Longo WE, Gusberg RJ. Graduating general surgery resident operative confidence: perspective from a national survey. J Surg Res. 2014;190(2):419–28.
31. Fonseca AL, Reddy V, Longo WE, Gusberg RJ. Are graduating surgical residents confident in performing open vascular surgery? Results of a national survey. J Surg Educ. 2015;72(4):577–84.
32. Fonseca AL, Reddy V, Yoo PS, Gusberg RJ, Longo WE. Senior surgical resident confidence in performing flexible endoscopy: what can we do differently? J Surg Educ. 2016;73(2):311–6.
33. Friedell ML, TJ VM, Cheatham ML, Fuhrman GM, Schenarts PJ, Mellinger JD, Morris JB. Perceptions of graduating general surgery chief residents: are they confident in their training? J Am Coll Surg. 2014;218(4):695–703.
34. Napolitano LM, Savarise M, Paramo JC, Soot LC, Todd SR, Gregory J, Timmerman GL, Cioffi WG, Davis E, Sachdeva AK. Are general surgery residents ready to practice? A survey of the American College of Surgeons Board of Governors and Young Fellows Association. J Am Coll Surg. 2014;218(5):1063–72.
35. Ferguson CM, Kellogg KC, Hutter MM, Warshaw AL. Effect of work-hour reforms on operative case volume of surgical residents. Curr Surg. 2005;62(5):535–8.
36. Carlin AM, Gasevic E, Shepard AD. Effect of the 80-hour work week on resident operative experience in general surgery. Am J Surg. 2007;193(3):326–9; discussion 329–30
37. Bland KI, Stoll DA, Richardson JD, Britt LD, Members of the Residency Review Committee-Surgery. Brief communication of the Residency Review Committee-Surgery (RRC-S) on residents' surgical volume in general surgery. Am J Surg. 2005;190(3):345–50.
38. Drake FT, Horvath KD, Goldin AB, Gow KW. The general surgery chief resident operative experience: 23 years of national ACGME case logs. JAMA Surg. 2013;148(9):841–7.
39. Drake FT, Van Eaton EG, Huntington CR, Jurkovich GJ, Aarabi S, Gow KW. ACGME case logs: surgery resident experience in operative trauma for two decades. J Trauma Acute Care Surg. 2012;73(6):1500–6.
40. Hawkins ML, Wynn JJ, Schmacht DC, Medeiros RS, Gadacz TR. Nonoperative management of liver and/or splenic injuries: effect on resident surgical experience. Am Surg. 1998;64(6):552–6. discussion 556-7
41. Bittner JG 4th, Hawkins ML, Medeiros RS, Beatty JS, Atteberry LR, Ferdinand CH. Mellinger JD. Nonoperative management of solid organ injury diminishes surgical resident operative experience: is it time for simulation training? J Surg Res. 2010;163(2):179–85.
42. Institute of Medicine (US) Committee on Optimizing Graduate Medical Trainee (Resident) Hours and Work Schedule to Improve Patient Safety. Ulmer C, Miller Wolman D, MME J, editors. Resident duty hours: enhancing sleep, supervision, and safety. Washington, DC: National Academies Press (US); 2009.
43. Lockley SW, Cronin JW, Evans EE, Cade BE, Lee CJ, Landrigan CP, Rothschild JM, Katz JT, Lilly CM, Stone PH, Aeschbach D. Czeisler CA; Harvard work hours, health and safety group. Effect of reducing interns' weekly work hours on sleep and attentional failures. N Engl J Med. 2004;351(18):1829–37.
44. Fischer JE, Healy GB, Britt LD. Surgery is different: a response to the IOM report. Am J Surg. 2009;197(2):135–6.
45. https://www.acgme.org/Portals/0/PDFs/jgme-monograph[1].pdf.
46. Bilimoria KY, Chung JW, Hedges LV, Dahlke AR, Love R, Cohen ME, Tarpley J, Mellinger J, Mahvi DM, Kelz RR, Ko CY, Hoyt DB, Lewis FH. Development of the flexibility in duty hour requirements for surgical trainees (FIRST) trial protocol: a national cluster-randomized trial of resident duty hour policies. JAMA Surg. 2016;151(3):273–81.
47. Bilimoria KY, Chung JW, Hedges LV, Dahlke AR, Love R, Cohen ME, Hoyt DB, Yang AD, Tarpley JL, Mellinger JD, Mahvi DM, Kelz RR, Ko CY, Odell DD, Stulberg JJ, Lewis FR. National Cluster-Randomized Trial of duty-hour flexibility in surgical training. N Engl J Med. 2016;374(8):713–27.

48. Bilimoria KY, et al. Use and underlying reasons for duty hour flexibility in the Flexibility in Duty Hour Requirements for Surgical Trainees (FIRST) Trial. J Am Coll Surg. 2017;224(4):118–25.
49. http://site.acsnsqip.org
50. ACS NSQIP operations manual. Chicago: American College of Surgeons. 2013.
51. Cohen ME, Ko CY, Bilimoria KY, Zhou L, Huffman K, Wang X, Liu Y, Kraemer K, Meng X, Merkow R, Chow W, Matel B, Richards K, Hart AJ, Dimick JB, Hall BL. Optimizing ACS NSQIP modeling for evaluation of surgical quality and risk: patient risk adjustment, procedure mix adjustment, shrinkage adjustment, and surgical focus. J Am Coll Surg. 2013;217(2):336–46.
52. Ouyang D, Chen JH, Krishnan G, Hom J, Witteles R, Chi J. Patient outcomes when Housestaff exceed 80 hours per week. Am J Med. 2016;129(9):993–9.
53. http://www.jhcct.org/icompare/default.asp.
54. Philibert I, Nasca T, Brigham T, Shapiro J. Duty-hour limits and patient care and resident outcomes: can high-quality studies offer insight into complex relationships? Annu Rev Med. 2013;64:467–83.
55. Yang AD, Chung JW, Dahlke AR, Biester T, Quinn CM, Matulewicz RS, Odell DD, Kelz RR, Shea JA, Lewis F, Bilimoria KY. Differences in resident perceptions by postgraduate year of duty hour policies: an analysis from the flexibility in duty hour requirements for surgical trainees (FIRST) trial. J Am Coll Surg. 2017;224(2):103–12.
56. Drolet BC, Schwede M, Bishop KD, Fischer SA. Compliance and falsification of duty hours: reports from residents and program directors. J Grad Med Educ. 2013;5(3):368–73.
57. Byrne JM, Loo LK, Giang DW. Duty hour reporting: conflicting values in professionalism. J Grad Med Educ. 2015;7(3):395–400.
58. Bilimoria KY, Quinn CM, Dahlke AR, Kelz RR, Shea JA, Rajaram R, Love R, Kreutzer L, Biester T, Yang AD, Hoyt DB, Lewis FR. Use and underlying reasons for duty hour flexibility in the flexibility in duty hour requirements for surgical trainees (FIRST) trial. J Am Coll Surg. 2017;224(2):118–25.
59. Blay E Jr, Hewitt DB, Chung JW, Biester T, Fiore JF, Dahlke AR, Quinn CM, Lewis FR, Bilimoria KY. Association between flexible duty hour policies and general surgery resident examination performance: a flexibility in duty hour requirements for surgical trainees (FIRST) trial analysis. J Am Coll Surg. 2017;224(2):137–42.
60. http://www.absurgery.org/default.jsp?statgeneral.
61. https://www.acgmecommon.org/2017_requirements.
62. Hoyt DB. Looking forward. The American College of Surgeons' transition to practice program. Bull Am Coll Surg. 2014;99(4):8–9.
63. Cogbill TH, Shapiro SB. Transition from training to surgical practice. Surg Clin North Am. 2016;96(1):25–33.
64. Richardson JD. ACS transition to practice program offers residents additional opportunities to hone skills. Bull Am Coll Surg. 2013;98(9):23–7.
65. Sachdeva AK, Flynn TC, Brigham TP, Dacey RG Jr, Napolitano LM, Bass BL, Philibert I, Blair PG, Lupi LK, American College of Surgeons (ACS) Division of Education.; Accreditation Council for Graduate Medical Education (ACGME). Interventions to address challenges associated with the transition from residency training to independent surgical practice. Surgery. 2014;155(5):867–82.
66. Pulcrano M, Evans SR, Sosin M. Quality of life and burnout rates across surgical specialties: a systematic review. JAMA Surg. 2016;151(10):970–8.
67. Jesse MT, Abouljoud M, Eshelman A. Determinants of burnout among transplant surgeons: a national survey in the United States. Am J Transplant. 2015;15(3):772–8.
68. Campbell DA Jr, Sonnad SS, Eckhauser FE, Campbell KK, Greenfield LJ. Burnout among American surgeons. Surgery. 2001;130(4):696–702. discussion 702-5
69. Drolet BC. General surgery resident burnout. J Am Coll Surg. 2017;224(2):217.
70. Elmore LC, Jeffe DB, Jin L, Awad MM, Turnbull IR. National survey of burnout among US general surgery residents. J Am Coll Surg. 2016;223(3):440–51.

Generational Differences and Resident Selection

10

Alison C. Keenan, Thomas G. Leffler,
and Patrick H. McKenna

Generational Differences and Resident Selection

Rapid changes in the demographic characteristics of people entering the workforce have been noted outside of medicine for decades. Generational differences became a popular talking point among leaders across multiple professions when Generation X began to enter the workforce in the 1980s and 1990s. The stark contrast in values and style led to friction with their baby boomer predecessors. While a number of sociologists and demographers study these generational differences and the impact on workforce in depth [18, 28], the medical profession has been late to incorporate the available knowledge into current practice. Recognizing and understanding differences in learning style, personal values, and expectations among different generations is crucial to facilitating success for the current class of young residents and students. This can be challenging in medicine, particularly in surgical fields where dedication is historically measured by long hours and one's career is prioritized over work-life balance. However, failure to properly understand and appreciate the differences between our predecessors, ourselves, and our incoming trainees and applicants will negatively impact our ability to recruit future physicians [1]. The purpose of this chapter is to explore what is known about the three generations currently in the workforce and how we can apply our understanding of the youngest generation to the resident interview and selection process.

A.C. Keenan (✉) • T.G. Leffler (✉) • P.H. McKenna
Department of Urology, University of Wisconsin-Madison, Madison, WI, USA
e-mail: keenan@urology.wisc.edu; leffler@urology.wisc.edu; mckenna@urology.wisc.edu

T.S. Köhler, B. Schwartz (eds.), *Surgeons as Educators*,
https://doi.org/10.1007/978-3-319-64728-9_10

Generational Definitions

Baby Boomers

The baby boomer generation is typically defined as those born from 1943 to 1962 and comprises faculty over the age of 55. The onset of this large generation is defined by a momentous historical event, the end of World War II. As this group approaches retirement, the American Urological Association (AUA) census predicts an impending shortage of urologists, particularly in rural locations (2015 AUA census). Baby boomers have been labeled as loyal and dedicated workers. They have a tendency to respect authority and will work hard out of loyalty to their leaders. They see self-sacrifice as a virtue and believe in the concept of "paying dues" [1]. It is easy to see these characteristics translate into the dedicated and ambitious faculty we know over the age of 55. This generation was the first to be raised in the era of television and saw significant value placed on personal prosperity and growth. This drive for prosperity as well as the value they place on self-sacrifice and loyalty can make them appear inflexible and intolerant when faced with the different attitudes and styles of their younger colleagues. Baby boomers have criticized Generation Xers as lacking work ethic, lacking commitment to their jobs, and overall lacking commitment to their careers [9, 22]. We are no longer seeking to recruit this generation into our residencies, but understanding their position is important when considering how to facilitate their recruitment and selection of residents.

Generation X

Generation X is defined as those born between 1963 and 1982. They comprise faculty over the age of 35 and are the group of physicians that began to see significant changes in duty hour restrictions and training expectations. This generation was defined socially by Watergate, the fall of the Berlin Wall, and the rise of MTV. They have been described by some as pragmatic and value global thinking and diversity. However, pop culture has labeled them as cynical and naïve, lacking respect for authority, and valuing nothing [6]. They are derogatorily referred to as the "Me" generation. The literature reviewing Generation X physicians often cites their desire for autonomy and flexible schedules, their emphasis on personal growth and personal relationships over material success, a preference for the latest technology, and flexible attitudes toward diversity [36, 40, 41]. This is also the generation that saw the introduction of significant numbers of women into the workforce (and medicine), leading to a heightened awareness of the compounded generational and gender differences in current mid-career workers. When this group of physicians first entered the workforce, many in the boomer generation assumed they would work less and be more transient than their elder colleagues. A 2006 survey of internal medicine physicians and departmental staff in Canada explored this notion in depth. They discovered that boomers qualitatively viewed the Gen Xers as less committed to their careers; however, when comparing actual working hours, there was no difference among the groups. In fact, on average, Generation X female physicians worked the most hours per week [22]. It is suggested that the most concrete difference between the baby boomers and Generation X physician is the role that work plays in their life [25]. But in fact, there may be differences in the type of person attracted to medicine from each generation. When assessing the Myers-Briggs personality profiles of surgeons of the boomer generation when compared to Gen X trainees, a statistically significant difference was found in the personality type [37]. Historically, surgeon Myers-Briggs Type Indicator (MBTI) testing had shown a predominance of ESTJ personality type (extraversion, sensing, thinking, judging), while Gen X trainees showed tendency toward ISTJ (introvert), $p = 0.0009$ [37]. While the driver of this difference is unclear, what is important to understand is that there is a fundamental personality difference between many baby boomer and Generation X surgeons. This is important to consider when educating a group of faculty about resident recruitment and selection. What resonates with a boomer may be very different than what resonates with a Gen X faculty member.

Generation Y

Generation Y, also known as millennials, comprises people born between 1982 and 2005. They are the children of the baby boomer generation and are the largest, most educated generation yet. These are our current medical students and residents. Millennials are the resident applicants we seek to properly select and recruit. We are just beginning to examine this generation in a prospective fashion, but they are a topic of much discussion and debate across a number of professions. They deserve extra consideration in our efforts to better understand surgical training and resident selection as this cohort of applicants will be the ones entering the workforce for the next two decades.

Although not marked by a specific historic event that would define the onset of Generation Y, the early years were defined by uncertainty, which has shaped the characteristics of the cohort. The oil bust in the 1980s, threats of global warming, school violence (i.e., the Columbine High School massacre in 1999, among others), the terrorist attacks of September 11, 2001, and a severe economic recession were all significant events that affected this generation in its youth [38]. They are technologically perceptive, and most grew up with easy access to computers and the Internet and expect to have global information available nearly 24/7. A 2007 survey of more than 7000 college students reported that 97% of students owned a computer, and 94% owned a cell phone [23]. Millennials were raised by baby boomers, who had parental guilt about time devoted to work. This drove an intense focus on reinvestment in their children's lives and daily activities, leading to an over-scheduled, overprotected generation of offspring [7]. Parental involvement for this generation is so predominant that many corporations are beginning to include parents in candidate recruitment [34]. Merrill Lynch hosts a "parent day" as a recruitment tool where parents are given a tour of facilities and a presentation on family support in the workplace. Home Depot has a reassuring message to parents on its website. Even the US Army has modified it's recruitment slogan to include parents. While the slogan "An Army of One" appealed to the Me generation (Generation X), the new slogan is aimed at parents directly, "You made them strong. We'll make them Army strong." As inconceivable as it may sound, factoring millennial's parents into the equation when recruiting them for residency positions is something to consider. In fact, in the previously mentioned 2007 study of college students investigating technology access, the authors discovered that the students surveyed talked to their parents 1.5 times a day on average.

Understanding the depth of parental involvement makes it apparent why Generation Y has also been called the "Trophy Generation." They may have been sheltered from failures as the idea that every participant deserved an award took hold [16, 29]. Despite these somewhat negative connotations, the millennials are actually predicted to emerge as the next "Greatest Generation" and are highly competent, high-achieving individuals, even if they are misunderstood by their predecessors [17].

The social fears and uncertainty that colored their formative years have led millennials to value personal connections, community, collaboration, and teamwork more highly than previous generations [19]. Their technological prowess makes them experts at efficiently gathering digital information, file sharing, and video streaming and gives them a willingness to readily adopt new technology. While their history as overprotected children may be seen in a negative light, in fact that may make Generation Y better at responding to authority than their Generation X faculty [31]. This is a particularly relevant aspect of their collective traits when considering resident selection. Generation Y values close relationships with authority figures and mentors, such as they had with their parents. They are likely to value personal connections made during the residency interview process, and these connections may have an important impact on residency selection trends.

The millennial's roots in highly structured childhoods may at times seem to be at odds with their desires for flexibility and learning autonomy; however, the two concepts can blend well. Millennial learners often want clearly outlined expectations and goals, with regular feedback [5, 32]. This can be a more structured approach to surgical teaching than we have historically been used to, but is appealing to Generation Y. Meanwhile, their ability to access information digitally makes them less likely to value scheduled lectures and traditional reading. Finding a way to connect with this generation as well as giving them a structured framework for learning while simultaneously respecting their need for flexibility may be the key to successfully recruit and mentor this group of applicants.

Resident Selection

As anyone who has the privilege of working with residents knows, good residents make our jobs easy and fun. Periodically, an applicant with all the hallmarks of a future chairperson during the resident selection process will struggle to achieve competency or, worse yet, become a problem resident. A problem-free, high-quality residency is every program directors' goal. Careful examination of the data available on resident selection is an important step in putting together an excellent residency program with high-achieving and competent future surgeons. The sheer volume of information and statistics available through the ERAS application, as well as what was gleaned over the course of an interview process, can be overwhelming. Understanding which components of the resident application have the highest value in predicting resident success, and which are less meaningful, is critical to compiling a strong rank list. Self-evaluation of a program's strengths and weaknesses is important in determining the best resident fit for a specific program.

USMLE Performance

A 2014 survey of urology residency program directors ranked USMLE performance and letters of recommendation as the two most important factors when evaluating candidates for a residency position [42]. A 2006 multispecialty study found USMLE step 1 scores and clerkship grades to be the most important selection criteria for urology residency positions [12]. When reviewing the literature available for orthopedic surgical training, similar emphasis is placed on USMLE scores [8]. While considerable debate centers around the validity of using USMLE performance to predict residency success, it remains the only standardized, universal objective method of applicant evaluation [42].

USMLE scores do correlate with in-training examination scores across multiple medical specialties, including urology (24–30). In 2012, Grewal et al. published a retrospective review of 29 urology resident files in an attempt to better understand predictors of success. These authors found that "good" test takers in medical school continued to test well as urology residents and were more likely to be rated as "excellent" urology residents when compared to "below-average" test takers [14]. It is clear that high USMLE scores will predict higher in-training examination scores; however, this study is one of the few to associate USMLE score with overall resident performance. Although USMLE has some predictive value in test scores, it is not predictive of non-cognitive performance. There is evidence that USMLE step 2 (CK) scores are better predictors of resident clinical skill, but these scores are often unavailable for the early urology match process. Overemphasizing USMLE scores in resident selection negatively affects diversity. Given the limited evidence to correlate USMLE scores with actual resident quality, it is important to consider multiple other factors when assessing applications for residency positions.

Letters of Recommendation

As the 2014 survey of urology PDs demonstrated, surgical letters of recommendation (LOR) are highly important in the resident selection process, falling just behind USMLE score. This is facilitated by urology being a relatively small field, allowing most applicants to have contact with, and a letter from, a widely known urologist.

A good letter of recommendation includes comments on technical ability, comparison to previous students, a ranking of current students from the same program, a comment on likability, and whether the home program wishes to retain the applicant [13, 39]. An additionally alluring comment describes an applicant as functioning at the level of an intern [13]. When all of this information is included, these letters are invaluable in giving an overall assessment of an applicant's quality. Unfortunately, LOR are not standardized and often do not include all of the relevant talking points. They are nearly uniformly positive. Additionally, a personal knowledge of the writer may alter the way a letter is interpreted. For example, if a certain writer is known by a program director to give glowing recommendations to all their students, that letter may carry less weight than if read by someone naïve to that writer. This fallacy has led some specialties to move toward standardization of letters of recommendation.

In 1996, the Council of Emergency Medicine Residency Directors pioneered this concept with the adoption of a standardized LOR (SLOR) [24]. The SLOR limits hyperbole and ambiguity and is shown to have superior interrater reliability, independent of the level of experience of the interpreter [10, 33]. SLOR are also faster to interpret than a typical narrative-type LOR. The bottom-line superlative response in the emergency medicine SLOR is "Guaranteed Match." It is the least frequently used superlative phrase [15]. This infrequent but meaningful statement attempts to address the fundamental question of "How should we rank this applicant?" [11]. In 2013, a survey was circulated to all emergency medicine program directors to assess their perspective on the utility of the SLOR. Impressively, 94.3% of programs responded, and 99.3% of responders agreed that the SLOR is an important evaluation tool, which should continue to be used. When they were asked to rank the top three factors in deciding who should receive an interview, 92.7% of responders ranked the SLOR first [30]. Emergency medicine is a larger and less competitive field, and adoption of a true standardized LOR may not be practical in urology. However, standardization of the superlative summary of an applicant would be a useful improvement to our current narrative LOR.

Clerkship Grades

Clerkship grades, particularly receiving honors in surgery and urology clerkships, are a popular method of stratifying residency applicants. There is data to suggest that assessing all clerkship grades has even more value than just looking at the urology and surgery rotation grades. Kenny et al. showed in a [26] meta-analysis that both USMLE scores and medical school clerkship grades correlated with overall resident performance [26]. We may consider surgical clerkships to be the most important when assessing an applicant's affinity and value as a urology resident, but special attention should be paid to applicants who demonstrate consistently poor grades in nonsurgical clerkships. This may be a red flag for arrogance or apathy in candidates who make no effort on clerkships they deem unimportant. Basic science course grades have no correlation with residency performance, in-training examination scores, or board scores and thus should not be heavily weighed.

AOA, Class Rank, and Dean's Letters

AOA status is often cited as in important factor when considering a residency applicant; however, not all schools have an AOA chapter, and AOA status appears to have no correlation with in-training examination scores or residency success. The same can be said of class rank, as well as dean's letters. An attempt to improve the quality and utility of dean's letters was made in 1989 when the Association of American Medical Colleges published specific guidelines on letter creation. Interestingly, in 1998, dean's letter writers at all 124 US medical schools were surveyed about the characteristics of their letters. That year, over 300,000 letters were written, comprising over 1 million pages and costing each medical school an average of $26,000 [21]. Nevertheless, only 65% of schools were determined to produce an adequate dean's letter. They are an expensive, time-consuming, and relatively low-yield component of the resident application package. They can become more meaningful when an applicant has had a negative event occur during medical school, or in explaining any extenuating circumstances experienced by an applicant.

Residency Selection Interview

The residency selection interview process remains a highly program-specific process with wide variability in what individual programs value. For example, in the editorial comment on a 2015 article in urology, the Cleveland Clinic stated that their program places a strong emphasis on applicant research endeavors [2]. Meanwhile, other programs are known to place special importance on former collegiate athletes, assuming they will have good work ethic, technical skills, or team player attitudes. This variability in program-specific preferences ensures that candidates across a broad spectrum of personalities and backgrounds will have an opportunity to match. Understanding what traits are valued at your own institution is critical when considering an applicant rank order.

There is significant research in the business sector on interview best practices. Incorporation of these practices into the residency selection process has been somewhat limited. For example, blinded interviews, in which the interviewer has limited access to data on the applicant, improve interview utility and accuracy [20]. The same can be said for structured interviews with standardized questions [3, 4]. Open-ended, goal-directed questions can maximize information gleaned from the interview. A scripted interview, in which all candidates are asked the same questions, can level the playing field somewhat when assessing applicants post-interview. Sample questions for a semi-structured interview are provided in Table 10.1.

Utilization of known interview best practices appears to be poor. A 2016 survey of general surgery program directors in the USA and Canada revealed only 20% of programs used some form of blinding and a mere 5% used standardized interview questions. Meanwhile, 90% of programs reported basing at least 25% of their final ranking on interview score [27]. The interview is critically important for our ability to assess residency applicants, but there is room for improvement in the way we conduct interviews.

Table 10.1 Sample interview questions for a structured interview

No.	Question
1.	What is the most important thing to you, at this point in your life, other than getting into a urology residency?
2.	What are you looking for in a program?
3.	Do you have any personal connections to this area or this program?
4.	Can you describe a situation in which you were in conflict with another person or group and how you dealt with the situation?
5.	What was your most difficult clinical experience so far and how did you deal with it?
6.	What do you know about this program and why would it be a good fit for you?
7.	What have you liked about other programs, and why?
8.	Tell me about a time you were treated unfairly, and how did you handle it?

Some programs have reported increased applicant and faculty satisfaction with a "candidate-centered" interview format [35]. This interview style seeks to integrate the candidate into a typical workday, matching them with a clinical team to spend time in the OR, on rounds, and in clinic. When considering the increasing number of applicants for urology residency positions, this may be an appealing and successful way to limit the number of working days faculty need to set aside to conduct residency interviews.

Uniformity of the resident selection interview should not be a goal. However, incorporating interview best practices and remembering the generational characteristics of our current applicant pool may be a key to successful resident selection and recruitment. Recall that millennials value and remember personal connections made during the interview process. Therefore, focusing on life issues and common interests in addition to the usual urology specifics may aid in recruiting an especially sought-after applicant.

Conclusions

Generational differences have a profound impact on resident surgical education as well as resident selection. The impact of fundamental differences between generations is always felt most strongly when a new generation enters the workforce, and we are seeing evidence of this currently as millennials come of age. As surgical educators, it is critically important that we understand how to motivate and teach the newest generation of residents. An exploration of the differences between ourselves, our predecessors, and our residents is the first step in improving our ability to be good educators. Understanding our variable priorities and work-related behaviors can also improve our ability to teach other faculty how to best educate the millennial generation.

Selecting the best resident for your program is the next important step after understanding the new generation of applicants. While often maligned, USMLE performance remains the only universal objective measure of applicant stratification. Given its inherent inability to assess the intangibles such as likability, work ethic, and technical ability, the other components of the applicant package remain important. Letters of recommendation could be improved with standardization of the superlative statement, but overall are still a valuable tool in determining a prospective resident's chances of success. Incorporation of interview best practices and exploring new interview formats may increase the utility and accuracy of the residency selection interview. Future efforts should focus on identifying an objective measure of resident competency and success.

References

1. Bickel J, Brown A. Generation X: implications for faculty recruitment and development in academic health center. Acad Med. 2005;80:205–10.
2. Campbell SC, Mishra K. Editorial comment. Program directors' criteria for selection into urology residency. J Urol. 2014;85:735–6.
3. Campion MA, Palmer DK, Campion JE. A review of structure in the selection interview. Pers Psychol. 1997;50:655–702.
4. Campion MA, Pursell ED, Brown BK. Structured interviewing: raising the psychometric properties of the employment interview. Pers Psychol. 1988;41:25–42.
5. Coomes MD, DeBard R. A generational approach to understanding students. In: Coomes MD, DeBard R, editors. Serving the Millenial generation: new directions for student services, number 106. San Francisco: Jossey-Bass; 2004. p. 5–16.
6. Coupland D. Generation X: Tales for an accelerated culture. New York: St Martins; 1991.
7. Eckleberry-Hunt J, Tucciarone J. The challenges and opportunities of teaching "generation Y". J Grad Med Ed. 2011;3(4):458–61.
8. Egol KA, Collins J, Zuckerman JD. Success in orthopaedic training: resident selection and predictors of quality performance. J Am Acad Orthop Surg. 2011;19:72–80.
9. Flynn G. Xers vs. boomers: teamwork or trouble? Pers J. 1996;75:86–9.
10. Girzadas DV Jr, Harwood RC, Dearie J, Garrett S. A comparison of standardized and narrative letters of recommendation. Acad Emerg Med. 1998;5:1101–4.
11. Girzadas DV Jr, Harwood RC, Delis SN, Stevison K, Keng G, Cipparrone N, Carlson A, Tsonis GD. Emergency medicine standardized letter of recommendation: predictors of guaranteed match. Acad Emerg Med. 2001;8:648–53.
12. Green M, Jones P, Thomas JX Jr. Selection criteria for residency: results of a National Program Directors Survey. Acad Med. 2009;84:362–7.
13. Greenburg AG, Doyle J, McClure DK. Letters of recommendation for surgical residencies: what they say and what they mean. J Surg Res. 1994;2:192–8.
14. Grewal SC, Yeung LS, Brandes SB. Predicators of Success in a Urology Residency Program. J Surg Ed. 2012;70(1):138–143.
15. Harwood RC, Girzadas DV Jr, Carlson A, et al. Characteristics of the emergency medicine standardized letter of recommendation. Acad Emerg Med. 2000;7:409–10.
16. Hira NA. What winning means to generation Y. Weblog entry. Available at: http://www.cnbc.com/id/2501105?__source=RSS8blog*&par=RSS. Accessed 1 Nov 2009.
17. Howe N, Strauss B, editors. Millennials rising: the next great generation. New York: Vintage Books; 2002.
18. Howe N, Strauss W. Generations. New York: Random House; 1998.
19. Howell LP, Joad JP, Callahan E, Servis G, Bonham AC. Generational forecasting in academic medicine: a unique method of planning for success in the next two decades. Acad Med. 2009;84:985–93.
20. Huffcutt A. From science to practice: seven principles for conducting employment interviews. Appl H R M Res. 2010;12:121–36.
21. Hunt DD, MacLaren C, Scott C, Marshall SG, Braddock CH, Sarfaty S. A follow-up study of the characteristics of Dean's letters. Acad Med. 2001;76:727–33.
22. Jovic E, Wallace J, Lemaire J. The generation and gender shifts in medicine: an exploratory survey of internal medicine physicians. BMC Health Serv Res. 2006;6:55.

23. Junco R, Mastrodicasa JM. Connecting to the net. Generation: what higher education professionals need to know about Today's students. Washington, DC: Network and Systems Professionals Associations; 2007.
24. Keim SM, Rein JA, Chisholm C, Dyne P. A standardized letter of recommendation for residency application. Acad Emerg Med. 1999;6:1141–6.
25. Kennedy M. Managing different generations requires new skills, insightful leadership. Physician Exec. 2003;29:20–3.
26. Kenny S, McInnes M, Sing V. Associations between residency selection strategies and doctor performance: a meta-analysis. Med Educ. 2013;47:790–800.
27. Kim RH, Gilbert T, Suh S, Miller JK, Eggerstedt JM. General surgery residency interviews: are we following best practices? Am J Surg. 2016;211:476–81.
28. Lancaster L, Stillman D. When generations collide. New York: HarperCollins; 2002.
29. Lipkin NA, Perrymore AJ. Yin the workplace. Franklin Lakes: Career Press; 2009.
30. Love JN, Smith J, Weizberg M, Doty CI, Garra G, Avegno J, Howell JM. Council of Emergency Medicine Residency Directors' standardized letter of recommendation: the program Director's perspective. Acad Emerg Med. 2014;21:680–7.
31. Pew Research Center. Millenials: a portrait of generation next. Washington, DC: Pew Research Center; 2010.
32. Rowse PG, Ruparel RJ, Aljamal YN, Abdelsattar JM, Heller SF, Farley DR. Catering to Millennial learners: assessing and improving fine-needle aspiration performance. J Surg Ed. 2014;71(6):e53–8.
33. Schaider JJ, Rydman RJ, Greene CS. Predictive value of letters of recommendation vs. questionnaires for emergency medicine resident performance. Acad Emerg Med. 1997;4:801–5.
34. Schlitzkus L, Schenarts K, Schenarts P. Is your residency program ready for generation Y? J Surg Ed. 2010;67:108–11.
35. Seabott H, Smith RK, Alseidi A, Thirlby RC. The surgical residency interview: a candidate-centered, working approach. J Surg Educ. 2012;69:802–6.
36. Shields M, Shields M. Working with generation X physicians. Physician Exec. 2003;29:14–8.
37. Swanson J, Antonoff M, D'Cunha J, Maddaus M. Personality profiling of the modern surgical trainee: insights into generation X. J Surg Ed. 2010;67:417–20.
38. Tulgan B. Not everyone gets a trophy. San Francisco: Jossey-Bass; 2009.
39. Wagoner NE, Suriano JR, Stoner JA. Factors used by program directors to select residents. J Med Educ. 1986;61:10–21.
40. Wah L. Managing gen Xers strategically. Manag Review. 2000;89:47.
41. Wasburn E. Are you ready for generation X? Physician Exec. 2000;26:51–7.
42. Weissbart SJ, Stock JA, Wein AJ. Program directors' criteria for selection into urology residency. J Urol. 2015;85(4):731–6.

The Role of Educators in Quality Improvement

11

Sevann Helo and Charles Welliver

Introduction

As healthcare delivery systems struggle to meet the increasing demand of services and resources, they are also under increased pressure to provide high-value care, which is defined as the best healthcare outcomes at the lowest cost [17]. Surmounting pressure from payment reforms such as the Value-Based Purchasing Program of 2012 and the Medicare Access and Children's Health Insurance Program Reauthorization Act of 2015 has forced healthcare organizations to identify areas of improvement. Quality improvement in the healthcare industry strives to improve outcomes, prevent medical errors, and reduce costs.

Medical Errors

In 2016, researchers from Johns Hopkins published a study, which estimated that more than 250,000 medical errors occur each year, making medical errors the third leading cause of death after heart disease and cancer [47, 55]. In addition to the morbidity of medical errors, they are also costly to the US healthcare system. The rising cost of healthcare in the United States presents a major economic burden that totaled $3.0 trillion in 2014, comprising 17.5% of the gross domestic product [40].

S. Helo, MD (✉)
Surgery, Division of Urology, Southern Illinois University School of Medicine, 301 N. 8th St., Springfield, IL 62794, USA
e-mail: Sevannhelo@gmail.com

C. Welliver, MD
Surgery, Division of Urology,
Albany Medical College, 23 Hackett Blvd,
Albany, NY 12208, USA

T.S. Köhler, B. Schwartz (eds.), *Surgeons as Educators*,
https://doi.org/10.1007/978-3-319-64728-9_11

If healthcare spending continues to grow at a rate projected to be 5.8% from 2014 to 2024, this will lead to $5.4 trillion in expenditures by 2024 and represent 19.6% of the gross domestic product [39]. Several studies have documented the association of perioperative complications with increased hospital costs, increased length of stay, and decreased hospital profit margins [10, 19, 20, 33, 56, 78].

In addition to hospital costs, healthcare expenditures may also be reduced by savings in malpractice claims. According to the most recent data available from the Centers for Disease Control and Prevention published in 2007, an estimated 100 million surgical procedures are performed each year in the United States, including 53.3 million ambulatory and 45.0 million inpatient surgical procedures [16, 32]. Surgical *never events* are defined as errors in surgical care that experts agree are always avoidable; these events include retained foreign body, wrong-site, wrong-patient, and wrong-procedure events [15, 27, 31, 46, 52, 64, 67]. A study published in 2013 by Mehtsun et al. [51] utilized the National Practitioner Data Bank to identify malpractice settlements and judgments of surgical never events. The authors identified 9733 paid malpractice settlements and judgments for surgical never events over a period of 20 years, with malpractice payments totaling $1.3 billion. Based on their findings, the authors estimated that more than 4000 surgical never events likely occur each year in the United States and acknowledged that the actual number of surgical never events is likely higher, as many events likely go unreported. Furthermore, the malpractice payments do not take into account the additional financial burden of legal fees, disability care, lost work days, or harm to provider and hospital reputation.

ACGME Core Curriculum

In 1999, the Accreditation Council for Graduate Medical Education (ACGME) and the American Board of Medical Specialties partnered to approve six general competencies that they deemed relevant to all medical specialties [4] as follows: patient care, medical knowledge, professionalism, interpersonal and communication skills, practice-based learning and improvement, and system-based practice. This was later followed by the official launch of the Outcomes Project in 2001, which empowered training programs to transition to an outcome-based (i.e., competency-based) medical education. Recognizing that implementation of the core competencies was difficult for programs that lacked models to teach, implement, and assess this new curriculum, the ACGME moved the accreditation system to focus on a continuous quality improvement philosophy [54]. Beginning in 2007, the specialties of internal medicine, pediatrics, and surgery created developmental milestones to provide a more detailed framework to assess the six competencies [30, 62, 69], which were gradually expanded to include all specialties by 2014.

According to the ACGME, the purpose of the milestones is to guide curriculum development, to provide well-defined learning objectives, and to identify underperforming learners early to support timely intervention. For residents and fellows, ACGME milestones are intended to increase transparency of performance requirements, to encourage self-assessment and self-directed learning, and to facilitate better feedback from the program and faculty [34]. This is a departure from the traditional training method that revolves around the diagnosis and management of disease. The current generation of physicians must be able to objectively evaluate their performance while providing comprehensive care, optimizing communication, defining the goals of the medical care organization, and demonstrating a high level of professionalism. While medical care organizations are adjusting to the shifting healthcare landscape by implementing continuous QI, the role of residents in this process is not well defined. There is a growing body of research regarding different implementation strategies in residency programs across specialties, but these are largely limited to isolated case reports. The remainder of this chapter will focus on different implementation strategies, barriers to implementation, and future direction of quality improvement in graduate medical education.

Quality Improvement

Physician Avedis Donabedian is considered by many to be the father of modern healthcare quality assurance. In his 1966 article "Evaluating the quality of medical care" published in the *Milbank Memorial Fund Quarterly* [22], he divided healthcare quality measures into structure, process, and outcome. In his publication, he described the seven pillars of quality: efficacy, efficiency, optimality, acceptability, legitimacy, equity, and cost [23–25]. Donabedian's influence on healthcare system awareness and design remains an important framework for healthcare quality improvement (QI) to this day.

Key to any QI initiative is the systematic measurement of significant metrics. Performance should be measured over time by using a control and identifying events that deviate from the average range or control limits. The upper and lower control limits define the acceptable range for which a process is assumed to be in control (see Fig. 11.1). Events that fall outside the control limits should be assessed for factors that led to a change in processes.

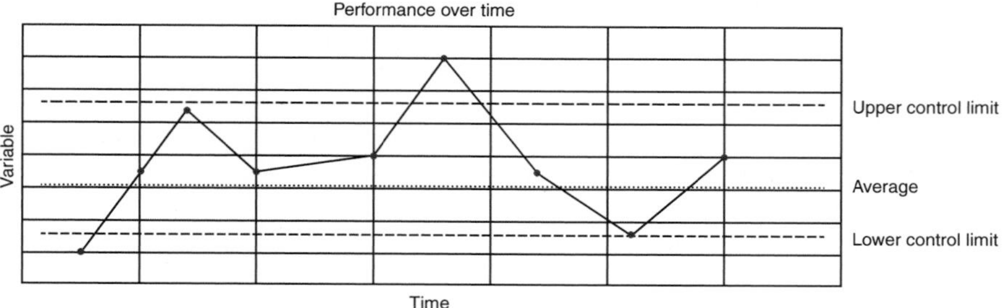

Fig. 11.1 Performance measured over time

Strategies of Quality Improvement Curriculum

Continuous Quality Improvement

Institutions dedicated to preemptive, rather than reactionary, QI generally subscribe to continuous QI, which is founded in the belief that every process presents an opportunity for improvement [7]. It requires that an organization view the processes and operations as a product of the healthcare delivery system on a macroscale rather than an individual patient basis when considering opportunities for improvement. Organizations committed to quality improvement generally approach it from a combination of continuous QI and one of the approaches detailed below.

Plan-Do-Study-Act

The plan-do-study-act (PDSA) cycle is an iterative four-step QI method popularized by Dr. W. Edwards Deming, who was an engineer and management consultant who many consider to be the father of modern quality control [8]. The PDSA cycle is not meant to replace QI methods that an organization already has in place but rather to provide a powerful framework to accelerate improvement. It is a refined take on the traditional trial and error process with the addition of steps for iterative improvement. The PDSA cycle is composed of four logical and sequential steps that with each cycle leads to exponential improvements. The steps in the PDSA cycle are summarized in Table 11.1 and Fig. 11.2.

Advantages of the PDSA cycle include its ability to adapt to the local context, respond to unforeseen obstacles, and deliver effective interventions for complex problems [70]. The PDSA cycle also lends itself to teamwork with well-defined roles that can be performed over the long term. While short-term goals may be achieved, the PDSA cycle enhances an organizations' continuous improvement strategy and can be transitioned from one team to another if the members of the team change over time.

Canal et al. applied the PDSA cycle to surgical residents during an outpatient ambulatory surgery rotation [12]. Residents received a didactic lecture on the application of the PDSA cycle for QI from a faculty member for 1 h a week over the course of 6 weeks. During this time, residents presented their project ideas to one another, voted on which project they wanted to implement, and then worked on their

Table 11.1 Plan-do-study-act cycle

Plan	Identify the change that you would like to implement Select team members who will be involved Evaluate what resources will be needed Determine what data will be collected
Do	Test the feasibility of your plan on a small scale Be prepared to restructure the plan based on preliminary results
Study	Analyze the data to evaluate whether the previous step achieved the desired outcome Summarize lessons learned, unintended consequences, successes, and failures
Act	Decide whether to adapt, adopt, or abandon the approach selected during the "plan" stage

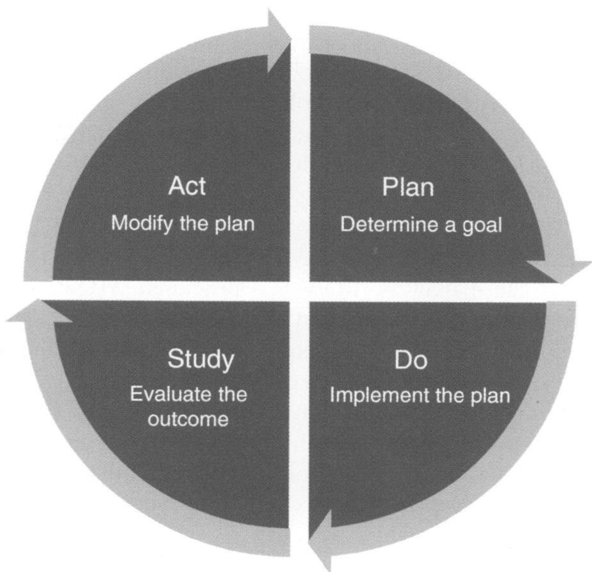

Fig. 11.2 Plan-do-study-act cycle

projects as a group. Examples of projects included developing an ultrasound curriculum for the residents, standardizing discharge forms, developing a research curriculum for research residents, creating a mentoring system between research residents and surgery interns, and improving resident attendance at the chairman's conference. Authors noted that barriers to successful project implementation included getting the residents to follow through on projects, which was most easy to do during the residents' research year when they didn't have as many competing clinical demands. The advantage of the approach, however, was that because the residents were involved in every step of the process, they were invested in the project's success.

Tess et al. described their creation of a QI curriculum, which was supplemented with online modules [71]. Internal medicine residents at Beth Israel Deaconess Medical Center (Boston, Massachusetts) were asked to complete a QI project during their second year. Residents were grouped into teams of three and asked to use the PDSA cycle. Their projects targeted quality measures, patient satisfaction, workflow redesign, and handoff issues. The authors highlighted that implementation of this QI curriculum improved resident attitudes about the culture of safety and their perception about the teaching quality of their rotation.

Authors at the University of Wisconsin (Madison, Wisconsin) reported their experience with the implementation of a practice-based learning and improvement curriculum in PGY-2 general surgery residents. Residents were asked to select a QI project and then discuss their ideas with two hospital quality improvement staff and the residency program manager to discuss feasibility. The residents were instructed to use the PDSA model, read several assigned readings, and attend meetings with the Surgical Quality Improvement Committee, institutional review board, and the faculty National Surgical Quality Improvement Project director. Progress reports and results were then presented at a departmental conference. The authors noted that this *bottom-up* approach gave the residents greater ownership over problems that they identified and areas that were of interest to them. They also noted that this kind of approach to implementation of a QI program requires institutional buy-in and initially may be difficult to engage administrators.

Root Cause Analysis

Root cause analysis (RCA) is a structured systematic approach used to investigate the various factors that led to a patient safety incident or adverse event [2]. The origins of the RCA technique stem from its use in the engineering industry as a method of identifying systems-problems that result in underperformance, variations in production processes, and design failures [1]. Its use in healthcare began in the 1990s as a method to establish the "what, how, and why" of patient safety incidents. An RCA is generally performed by a multidisciplinary team using one of the following problem-solving techniques: Five Whys analysis, Pareto analysis, or fault tree analysis, among others [65, 77, 81]. It is best utilized to retrospectively review an adverse event to determine the sequence of events and the systemic factors that led to the undesired event and can be integrated with other QI tools. Several institutions have reported using RCA in their morbidity and mortality conferences [5, 66, 71], as it lends itself to retrospectively review adverse events. The Veterans Affairs National Center for Patient Safety has a detailed step-by-step guide on how to perform an RCA that may be found online [76].

Five Whys Analysis

The *Five Whys* approach is a method intended to progressively delve deeper into why an adverse event occurred with each subsequent *why*, until the root of a problem is identified [66]. Once the initial problem is specified, a consecutive series of *why* questions are asked, with each answer becoming the subject of the next question. Each subsequent response should generate a more profound investigation, and potential improvement strategies are identified. See Fig. 11.3 for an example of the application of the *Five Whys* in a situation where a patient who should have been ordered for venous thromboembolism (VTE) prophylaxis is diagnosed with a pulmonary embolism.

This example identifies several errors in the system including the lack of inclusion of VTE chemoprophylaxis in standard order sets. While exclusion of VTE chemoprophylaxis in the patient's orders was due to a human error by the resident who forgot to include it, if the standard of care is for all postoperative patients at risk for a VTE to be administered with VTE chemoprophylaxis, then it should be included in all order sets. Additionally, the healthcare organization may consider adding an automated alert to all providers caring for postoperative patients to confirm whether or not their patient should be on VTE chemoprophylaxis.

"Five Whys" Approach

A post-operative patient who did not receive VTE chemoprophylaxis is diagnosed with a pulmonary embolism.

1. **Why** did the patient not receive VTE chemoprophylaxis post-operatively?
   - *The patient was not ordered for VTE chemoprophylaxis.*
2. **Why** was VTE chemoprophylaxis not ordered for the patient?
   - *The resident entering the patient's orders forgot to order VTE chemoprophylaxis.*
3. **Why** did the resident who entered the patient's orders forget to order VTE chemoprophylaxis?
   - VTE chemoprophylaxis was not a part of the order set that the resident used.
4. **Why** is VTE chemoprophylaxis not a part of the order set?
   - Not all surgeons want their patients on VTE chemoprophylaxis post-operatively.
5. **Why** do not all surgeons want their patients on VTE chemoprophylaxis post-operatively?
   - The risk of post-operative bleeding varies depending on surgical procedure, technique, and individual patient characteristics.

Fig. 11.3 Stepwise Five Whys approach as applied to an example of a postoperative patient who did not receive VTE chemoprophylaxis and is diagnosed with a pulmonary embolism

Pareto Analysis

Vilfredo Pareto was an Italian economist born in 1848 who was known for the *Pareto principle*, or *80-20 rule*, in which he recognized that 80% of the property was owned by only 20% of the inhabitants [63]. This principle was later popularized in the 1950s by business management consultant Joseph M. Juran [37], who sought to increase financial returns through increased efficiency by focusing company resources on the sectors that generated the highest revenue [60]. While it has largely been studied in business management, it can be applied to healthcare QI and resident education [28, 42, 53]. It can be applied to healthcare delivery as illustrated by the following example:

> A surgical department is allotted a set amount of block time to schedule their operative cases, but the department's surgical wait times are becoming increasingly longer as the practice expands. Using the Pareto principle to reduce wait times while working within the confines of the allotted block time, the department may review case times for their 10 most commonly performed procedures to identify which cases take the longest to perform on average. After identifying which cases dominate the utilization of the department's block time, members of the team can work together to increase efficiency in the operating room by standardizing instruments sets or equipment needed, defining clearer roles for all personnel in the room, and improving surgical technique.

Fault Tree Analysis

Fault tree analysis is a tool used to understand how the interaction of several individual faults leads to a negative outcome [48, 82]. It is a technique particularly useful in risk and safety analysis. At the top of the fault tree, the undesired event is listed. A hierarchy tree is then constructed starting from the undesired event until all potential causes are identified. Figure 11.4 depicts an illustration of a fault tree

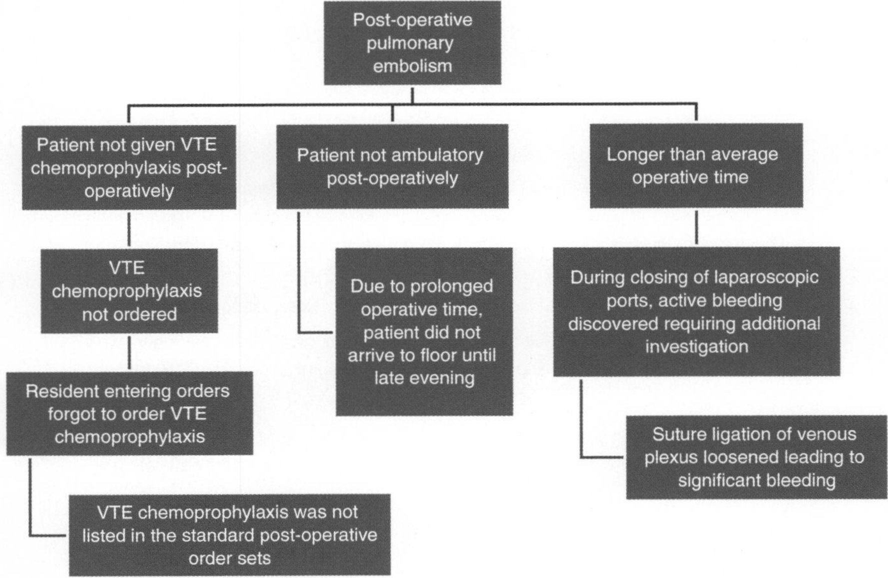

Fig. 11.4 Example of Five Whys analysis applied to postoperative pulmonary embolism

analysis using the example of a patient who experiences a postoperative pulmonary embolism, which was used in the *Five Whys* section.

In this fault tree analysis example, several errors contributed to the patient having a pulmonary embolism. The patient was not on VTE chemoprophylaxis, which was due to a human error in entering the order, but there should have been safety checks in place including an alert to the physician that no VTE chemoprophylaxis was ordered for the patient, and it should be listed in the standard order set for postoperative patients if the standard of care is to put patients on VTE chemoprophylaxis. An additional risk factor for the patient developing a pulmonary embolism was his immobility immediately postoperatively. While patients may typically ambulate postoperatively, this patient was not transferred to the floor until the late evening when the standard practice on the floor was to allow patients to rest, rather than to encourage them to ambulate. Knowing that this patient was at increased risk for a VTE event, the physician caring for the patient might have specifically asked the patient and the nurse caring for him to ambulate several times before going to bed. Lastly, this patient experienced an intraoperative complication of acute blood loss that was due to an incorrectly placed suture on the venous plexus that later became dislodged and led to significant bleeding. This led to an operative time that was longer than average, conferring additional risk to the patient. Although this was due to a technical error, further assessment may reveal that a different kind of suture or technique may prevent this from happening in the future.

In 2012, Smith et al. reported their experience with a departmental initiative to implement a QI program in the Internal Medicine Residency Program at Mount

Sinai Hospital (New York City, New York) by using RCA to address a patient care issue [66]. Residents attended a QI conference every 4 weeks during which a preselected teaching case was presented. A resident on an elective or outpatient block was chosen to investigate the case and gather relevant details in the weeks prior to the session. During the session, chief residents and faculty members facilitated a group discussion with a focus on identifying system-wide failures and solutions. Over the course of 22 months, 46 interventions were suggested, 25 of which were initiated and 18 of which were determined to be successful. The authors noted that "empowering residents to take a more active role in performance improvement yields significant change and does more than simply educate about basic QI methodology." They also aptly pointed out that residents are key frontline providers who spend the most time working within clinical care systems and can therefore provide important insight into areas that need improvement. An important observation the authors also made was that suggestions were more likely to advance if administrators with decision-making authority were present.

For institutions that are limited on time or resources to individualize a QI project, authors from Vanderbilt University Medical Center (Nashville, Tennessee) advocate using the traditional morbidity and mortality conference as a means of establishing a culture of safety while teaching the ACGME general competencies. In their publication, they described retrospectively reviewing morbidity and mortality cases that had been presented [38]. They identified seven categories that were then evaluated to see which of the six ACGME general competencies were addressed. During a 21-month period, 11 cases were discussed, which generated 23 QI initiatives. The initiatives were classified as procedure related, process related, patient related, communication error, medication error, ethics related, and device related. Several other authors have reported similar success with the application of an RCA to morbidity and mortality conferences [5, 58, 59].

Six Sigma and Lean Methodology

Six Sigma is a QI strategy invented by Motorola, Inc. (Schaumburg, Il) in the 1980s, named after the statistical measure of variation, *sigma*, which is the standard deviation of a normal distribution [14]. The concept of Six Sigma reflects the number of standard deviations that it takes to achieve an error-free rate of 99.9996%. In manufacturing, a level of Six Sigma is equivalent to less than 3.4 defects per million units produced, a concept referred to as defects per million opportunities (DPMO). A defect rate can be defined by any measure that is relevant to the process being improved. Setting the goal to achieve a Six Sigma strategy does not guarantee achievement of that goal but does lay the groundwork for improvement. The field of surgical anesthesia serves as a good example of the application of this principle. In the 1970s–1980s, the risk of death related to anesthesia was 1 in 10,000–20,000 – or 25 to 50 per million [29] – but through the advent of several QI measures, that risk has decreased to 1.1 per million [45].

Lean methodology stems from the Toyota Production System created by Toyota Motor Corporation engineer Taiichi Ohno in the 1950s [84]. He revolutionized the automotive production system by focusing on eliminating inefficiency and waste,

Table 11.2 Lean Six Sigma five-step process

*D*efine	The team should determine the following: What is the goal of the project? How will success be defined? Who will be involved? What is the timeline of the project?
*M*easure	Data is collected from several sources to determine the depth of the errors in the system
*A*nalysis	Deviations from the norm are identified to look for sources of process variation
*I*mprove	The team should brainstorm solutions and develop strategies for project completion
*C*ontrol	Based on the previous steps, the team should develop policies, guidelines, and safety checks to enforce the use of the new policy

hence the term *lean*. Since then, lean methodology has been applied to many industries, including healthcare. For a lean approach to take hold within an organization, management must yield the role of micromanaging problem-solving to the employees who are on the ground floor of daily operations. A *lean* system seeks to maximize steps that add value in the most logical sequence to deliver an unobstructed workflow to deliver the services that the customer needs. This is often referred to as a value stream, which is the entire series of steps necessary to produce a product or service. A value stream approach attempts to improve the entire process, not just to optimize the individual parts. Examples of waste in the healthcare system include time spent in the waiting room, wasted inventory, inefficient work area ergonomics, and time transporting patients between departments for multispecialty care.

Six Sigma and lean methodology have been utilized within healthcare quality improvement since 1998 [18, 75]. They are complementary processes that can be combined to create *Lean Six Sigma*, which is a five-step process referred to as the DMAIC cycle – *define*, *measure*, *analyze*, *improve*, *and control*, which is summarized in Table 11.2.

Educators at the University of Michigan (Ann Arbor, Michigan) reported on their implementation of a QI curriculum for internal medicine residents [41]. A team of residents, led by a faculty familiar with the lean thinking approach, piloted a project to evaluate the response to an inhospital cardiopulmonary arrest. They participated in interactive didactic sessions led by their faculty mentor. A hypothetical cardiopulmonary arrest case with patient safety and quality implications was then developed. The team used this example to identify areas of waste and then, using their experiences, developed a current state value stream map of a cardiopulmonary arrest response that was supplemented with data to better understand the process. Through a literature review and reflection on previous experience, the team was able to develop a plan of how an ideal cardiopulmonary arrest response could be performed. This led to changes in the training modules and exercises used to train the cardiopulmonary arrest response teams.

Internal medicine residents at Columbia University (New York City, New York) [83] applied the use of Lean Six Sigma methodology to standardize supply rooms on general medicine units. Through this simple intervention, they were able to reduce mean search times by greater than 90 s, with 92% of participants reporting that they found supplies more rapidly and 86% reporting less frustration after the intervention. Educators have reported similar success using Six Sigma and lean methodology to speed the delivery of hospital discharge documents to primary care physicians [3], decrease the time that residents spend rounding while increasing patient contact time [13], and develop a more efficient postoperative pathway [35].

Challenges of Implementing a Quality Improvement Curriculum

While residents, faculty, and healthcare organizations can benefit from implementing QI projects within their institutions, there are several challenges to the implementation process.

Time

Finding the time to juggle a busy clinical schedule with the demands of an academic program and work-hour restrictions may leave little room for residents and faculty members to participate in a QI program. Residents may take advantage of a research year or elective rotation to complete a QI project, circumstances permitting. A larger project may require a long-term time commitment that exceeds the time allotted to a resident during a research rotation or elective or even surpass a resident or faculty member's time at the institution. This should be taken into account when selecting an intervention and the team members to carry out the project.

Education

The first step toward developing a QI project involves educating the team on the principles and methods of QI. Practice-based learning and improvement teaching may be delivered during resident teaching conferences, morning report, clinical case conferences, grand rounds lectures, or integrated into morbidity and mortality conferences [26, 38, 43, 44, 59, 68]. For institutions that lack the resources or time to deliver didactic lectures, self-guided online modules may be beneficial [11, 71, 74]. This allows a centralized educational curriculum that can be used to train residents and faculty across departments and geographic locations to accommodate their demanding schedules. The Institute for Healthcare Improvement, US Health and Human Services Department, and Centers for Disease Control and Prevention offer several ideas and online resources for institutions interested in QI [36, 72, 73].

Resident Involvement

Resident directly involved in QI reports greater competence in designing and conducting interventions and proficiency in practice-based learning skills [9, 21, 80, 85]. The level of resident involvement in part depends on whether an institution employs a *top-down* or *bottom-up* approach. A *top-down* approach is institution driven; interventions are chosen at the institutional level, and professionals within the organization are selected from a range of positions. Residents typically play a more passive role in this strategy. In contrast, *bottom-up* approach begins with a resident in the trenches who identifies a patient safety or quality issue. This approach allows residents to identify issues that otherwise might be missed by the management, permits residents to see the benefits of their efforts, and ensures that residents are personally invested in the success of their project [57, 61].

Faculty Participation

While residents are good at identifying patient safety and quality issues, faculty participation is critical to make a complex, sustained intervention [79]. The role of faculty members is to contribute their knowledge and mentorship, which may be challenging if they lack formal training in QI. In this situation, faculty members devoted to assess and improve their own clinical outcomes may serve as good role models to help residents identify and carry out an intervention. Given the increased pressure to deliver high-value care, many organizations are hiring QI professionals and support staff. In the academic setting, this presents an opportunity for faculty members devoted to QI to negotiate this responsibility into their workload so that they may be compensated for their involvement [5, 66, 71]. Institutions have also reported success by offering faculty credit for Maintenance of Certification as a valuable incentive for their participation [6].

Institutional Buy-In

Perhaps the most challenging barrier to implement a QI program is institutional buy-in; success is dependent on interdisciplinary communication and compromise. Effective implementation of almost any QI intervention requires the support from the administrative staff and senior officials within the organization at both the institutional and Graduate Medical Education office level [50]. Educators from Kansas City University (Kansas City, Missouri) [49] reported the value in linking practice-based learning and improvement to program and institutional accreditation, noting that it increased the perceived value of involvement in a QI curriculum.

Conclusion

QI efforts benefit the institution implementing them, the employees in the organization, and the patients they are designed to serve. The application of practice-based learning and improvement in conjunction with a QI curriculum permits resident and faculty members to directly apply the ACGME core curriculum competencies. Depending on the level of involvement within an institution, a QI project may be implemented in a *top-down* or *bottom-up* approach. An effort should be made to include faculty members who can serve as mentors, as well as multidisciplinary staff within the hospital to deliver a comprehensive solution.

References

1. Amo MF. Root cause analysis. A tool for understanding why accidents occur. Balance (Alexandria, Va). 1998;2(5):12–5.
2. Bagian JP, Gosbee J, Lee CZ, Williams L, McKnight SD, Mannos DM. The veterans affairs root cause analysis system in action. Jt Comm J Qual Improv. 2002;28(10):531–45.

3. Basta YL, Zwetsloot IM, Klinkenbijl JH, Rohof T, Monster MM, Fockens P, et al. Decreasing the dispatch time of medical reports sent from hospital to primary care with lean six sigma. J Eval Clin Pract. 2016;22(5):690–8. https://doi.org/10.1111/jep.12518.
4. Batalden P, Leach D, Swing S, Dreyfus H, Dreyfus S. General competencies and accreditation in graduate medical education. Health Aff (Project Hope). 2002;21(5):103–11.
5. Bechtold ML, Scott S, Dellsperger KC, Hall LW, Nelson K, Cox KR. Educational quality improvement report: outcomes from a revised morbidity and mortality format that emphasised patient safety. Postgrad Med J. 2008;84(990):211–6. https://doi.org/10.1136/qshc.2006.021139.
6. Bernabeo E, Hood S, Iobst W, Holmboe E, Caverzagie K. Optimizing the implementation of practice improvement modules in training: lessons from educators. J Grad Med Educ. 2013;5(1):74–80. https://doi.org/10.4300/jgme-d-11-00281.1.
7. Berwick DM. Continuous improvement as an ideal in health care. N Engl J Med. 1989;320(1):53–6. https://doi.org/10.1056/NEJM198901053200110.
8. Berwick DM. A primer on leading the improvement of systems. BMJ (Clin Res ed). 1996;312(7031):619–22.
9. Berwick DM, Hackbarth AD, McCannon CJ. IHI replies to the 100,000 lives campaign: a scientific and policy review. Jt Comm J Qual Patient Saf. 2006;32(11):628–30. dsicussion 31–3
10. Birkmeyer JD, Gust C, Dimick JB, Birkmeyer NJ, Skinner JS. Hospital quality and the cost of inpatient surgery in the United States. Ann Surg. 2012;255(1):1–5. https://doi.org/10.1097/SLA.0b013e3182402c17.
11. Bonnes SL, Ratelle JT, Halvorsen AJ, Carter KJ, Hafdahl LT, Wang AT, et al. Flipping the quality improvement classroom in residency education. Acad Med (J Assoc Am Med Colleges). 2017;92(1):101–7. https://doi.org/10.1097/ACM.0000000000001412.
12. Canal DF, Torbeck L, Djuricich AM. Practice-based learning and improvement: a curriculum in continuous quality improvement for surgery residents. Arch Surg. 2007;142(5):479–482.; discussion 82-3. https://doi.org/10.1001/archsurg.142.5.479.
13. Chand DV. Observational study using the tools of lean six sigma to improve the efficiency of the resident rounding process. J Grad Med Educ. 2011;3(2):144–50. https://doi.org/10.4300/jgme-d-10-00116.1.
14. Chassin MR. Is health care ready for six sigma quality? Milbank Q. 1998;76(4):565–91. 10
15. Cima RR, Kollengode A, Garnatz J, Storsveen A, Weisbrod C, Deschamps C. Incidence and characteristics of potential and actual retained foreign object events in surgical patients. J Am Coll Surg. 2008;207(1):80–7. https://doi.org/10.1016/j.jamcollsurg.2007.12.047.
16. Cullen KA, Hall MJ, Golosinskiy A. Ambulatory surgery in the United States, 2006. Natl Health Stat Rep. 2009;11:1–25.
17. Curfman GD, Morrissey S, Drazen JM. High-value health care — a sustainable proposition. N Engl J Med. 2013;369(12):1163–4. https://doi.org/10.1056/NEJMe1310884.
18. DelliFraine JL, Langabeer JR 2nd, Nembhard IM. Assessing the evidence of six sigma and lean in the health care industry. Qual Manag Health Care. 2010;19(3):211–25. https://doi.org/10.1097/QMH.0b013e3181eb140e.
19. Dimick JB, Pronovost PJ, Cowan JA, Lipsett PA. Complications and costs after high-risk surgery: where should we focus quality improvement initiatives? J Am Coll Surg. 2003;196(5):671–8. https://doi.org/10.1016/S1072-7515(03)00122-4.
20. Dimick JB, Chen SL, Taheri PA, Henderson WG, Khuri SF, Campbell DA Jr. Hospital costs associated with surgical complications: a report from the private-sector National Surgical Quality Improvement Program. J Am Coll Surg. 2004;199(4):531–7. https://doi.org/10.1016/j.jamcollsurg.2004.05.276.
21. Djuricich AM, Ciccarelli M, Swigonski NL. A continuous quality improvement curriculum for residents: addressing core competency, improving systems. Acad Med (J Assoc Am Med Colleges). 2004;79(10 Suppl):S65–7.
22. Donabedian A. Evaluating the quality of medical care. Milbank Mem Fund Q. 1966;44(3):166–206.
23. Donabedian A. Explorations in quality assessment and monitoring. Ann Arbor: Health Administration Press; 1980.

24. Donabedian A. The criteria and standards of quality. Explorations in quality assessment and monitoring, vol. 2. Ann Arbor: Health Administration Press; 1982.
25. Donabedian A. Explorations in quality assessment and monitoring, The methods and findings of quality assessment and monitoring: an illustrated analysis, vol. 3. Ann Arbor: Health Administration Press; 1985.
26. Folcik MA, Kirton OC, Ivy ME. A two-tiered quality management program: morbidity and mortality conference data applied to resident education. Conn Med. 2007;71(8):471–8.
27. Gawande AA, Studdert DM, Orav EJ, Brennan TA, Zinner MJ. Risk factors for retained instruments and sponges after surgery. N Engl J Med. 2003;348(3):229–35. https://doi.org/10.1056/NEJMsa021721.
28. Gibbard A. Health care and the prospective Pareto principle. Ethics. 1984;94(2):261–82.
29. Goldstein A Jr, Keats AS. The risk of anesthesia. Anesthesiology. 1970;33(2):130–43.
30. Green ML, Aagaard EM, Caverzagie KJ, Chick DA, Holmboe E, Kane G, et al. Charting the road to competence: developmental milestones for internal medicine residency training. J Grad Med Educ. 2009;1(1):5–20. https://doi.org/10.4300/01.01.0003.
31. Greenberg CC, Gawande AA. Retained foreign bodies. Adv Surg. 2008;42:183–91.
32. Hall MJ, DeFrances CJ, Williams SN, Golosinskiy A, Schwartzman A. National Hospital Discharge Survey: 2007 summary. Natl Health Stat Rep. 2010;(29):1–20. 4.
33. Healy MA, Mullard AJ, Campbell DA Jr, Dimick JB. Hospital and payer costs associated with surgical complications. JAMA Surg. 2016;151(9):823–30. https://doi.org/10.1001/jamasurg.2016.0773.
34. Holmboe ES, Yamazaki K, Edgar L, Conforti L, Yaghmour N, Miller RS, et al. Reflections on the first 2 years of milestone implementation. J Grad Med Educ. 2015;7(3):506–11. https://doi.org/10.4300/jgme-07-03-43.
35. Improta G, Balato G, Romano M, Carpentieri F, Bifulco P, Alessandro Russo M, et al. Lean six sigma: a new approach to the management of patients undergoing prosthetic hip replacement surgery. J Eval Clin Pract. 2015;21(4):662–72. https://doi.org/10.1111/jep.12361.
36. Institute for Healthcare Improvement. Audio and video programs. 2017. http://www.ihi.org/education/audiovideo/Pages/default.aspx. Accessed 25 Feb 2017.
37. Juran JM, Godfrey AB. Juran's quality handbook. 5th ed. New York: McGraw Hill; 1999.
38. Kauffmann RM, Landman MP, Shelton J, Dmochowski RR, Bledsoe SH, Hickson GB, et al. The use of a multidisciplinary morbidity and mortality conference to incorporate ACGME general competencies. J Surg Educ. 2011;68(4):303–8. https://doi.org/10.1016/j.jsurg.2011.02.002.
39. Keehan SP, Cuckler GA, Sisko AM, Madison AJ, Smith SD, Stone DA, et al. National health expenditure projections, 2014-24: spending growth faster than recent trends. Health Aff (Project Hope). 2015;34(8):1407–17. https://doi.org/10.1377/hlthaff.2015.0600.
40. Keehan SP, Stone DA, Poisal JA, Cuckler GA, Sisko AM, Smith SD et al. National Health Expenditure Projections, 2016-25: price increases, aging push sector to 20 percent of economy. Health Aff (Project Hope). 2017. doi:https://doi.org/10.1377/hlthaff.2016.1627.
41. Kim CS, Lukela MP, Parekh VI, Mangrulkar RS, Del Valle J, Spahlinger DA, et al. Teaching internal medicine residents quality improvement and patient safety: a lean thinking approach. Am J Med Qual. 2010;25(3):211–7. https://doi.org/10.1177/1062860609357466.
42. Kramp KH, van Det MJ, Veeger NJ, Pierie JP. The Pareto analysis for establishing content criteria in surgical training. J Surg Educ. 2016;73(5):892–901. https://doi.org/10.1016/j.jsurg.2016.04.010.
43. Kravet SJ, Howell E, Wright SM. Morbidity and mortality conference, grand rounds, and the ACGME's core competencies. J Gen Intern Med. 2006;21(11):1192–4. https://doi.org/10.1111/j.1525-1497.2006.00523.x.
44. Lecoanet A, Vidal-Trecan G, Prate F, Quaranta JF, Sellier E, Guyomard A, et al. Assessment of the contribution of morbidity and mortality conferences to quality and safety improvement: a survey of participants' perceptions. BMC Health Serv Res. 2016;16:176. https://doi.org/10.1186/s12913-016-1431-5.
45. Li G, Warner M, Lang BH, Huang L, Sun LS. Epidemiology of anesthesia-related mortality in the United States, 1999-2005. Anesthesiology. 2009;110(4):759–65.

46. Lincourt AE, Harrell A, Cristiano J, Sechrist C, Kercher K, Heniford BT. Retained foreign bodies after surgery. J Surg Res. 2007;138(2):170–4. https://doi.org/10.1016/j.jss.2006.08.001.
47. Makary MA, Daniel M. Medical error-the third leading cause of death in the US. BMJ (Clin Res ed). 2016;353:i2139. https://doi.org/10.1136/bmj.i2139.
48. Marx DA, Slonim AD. Assessing patient safety risk before the injury occurs: an introduction to sociotechnical probabilistic risk modelling in health care. Qual Saf Health Care. 2003;12(Suppl 2):ii33–8.
49. McClain EK, Babbott SF, Tsue TT, Girod DA, Clements D, Gilmer L, et al. Use of a structured template to facilitate practice-based learning and improvement projects. J Grad Med Educ. 2012;4(2):215–9. https://doi.org/10.4300/jgme-d-11-00195.1.
50. Medio FJ, Arana GW, McCurdy L. Implementation of a college-wide GME core curriculum. Acad Med (J Assoc Am Med Colleges). 2001;76(4):331–6.
51. Mehtsun WT, Ibrahim AM, Diener-West M, Pronovost PJ, Makary MA. Surgical never events in the United States. Surgery. 2013;153(4):465–72. https://doi.org/10.1016/j.surg.2012.10.005.
52. Michaels RK, Makary MA, Dahab Y, Frassica FJ, Heitmiller E, Rowen LC, et al. Achieving the National Quality Forum's "never events": prevention of wrong site, wrong procedure, and wrong patient operations. Ann Surg. 2007;245(4):526–32. https://doi.org/10.1097/01.sla.0000251573.52463.d2.
53. Muller F, Dormann H, Pfistermeister B, Sonst A, Patapovas A, Vogler R, et al. Application of the Pareto principle to identify and address drug-therapy safety issues. Eur J Clin Pharmacol. 2014;70(6):727–36. https://doi.org/10.1007/s00228-014-1665-2.
54. Nasca TJ, Philibert I, Brigham T, Flynn TC. The next GME accreditation system--rationale and benefits. N Engl J Med. 2012;366(11):1051–6. https://doi.org/10.1056/NEJMsr1200117.
55. National Center for Health Statistics. Health, United States. Health, United States, 2015: with special feature on racial and ethnic health disparities. Hyattsville: National Center for Health Statistics (US); 2016.
56. Patel AS, Bergman A, Moore BW, Haglund U. The economic burden of complications occurring in major surgical procedures: a systematic review. Appl Health Econ Health Policy. 2013;11(6):577–92. https://doi.org/10.1007/s40258-013-0060-y.
57. Philibert I. Accreditation Council for Graduate Medical Education and Institute for Healthcare Improvement 90-day project: Involving residents in quality improvement: contrasting "top-down" and "bottom-up" approaches August 2008.
58. Ramanathan R, Duane TM, Kaplan BJ, Farquhar D, Kasirajan V, Ferrada P. Using a root cause analysis curriculum for practice-based learning and improvement in general surgery residency. J Surg Educ. 2015;72(6):e286–93. https://doi.org/10.1016/j.jsurg.2015.05.005.
59. Rosenfeld JC. Using the morbidity and mortality conference to teach and assess the ACGME general competencies. Curr Surg. 2005;62(6):664–9. https://doi.org/10.1016/j.cursur.2005.06.009.
60. Ryan TP. Statistical methods for quality improvement. 3rd ed. Wiley series in probability and statistics. Hoboken: Wiley; 2011.
61. Schumacher DJ, Frohna JG. Patient safety and quality improvement: a 'CLER' time to move beyond peripheral participation. Med Educ Online. 2016;21(1):31993. https://doi.org/10.3402/meo.v21.31993.
62. Schumacher DJ, Lewis KO, Burke AE, Smith ML, Schumacher JB, Pitman MA, et al. The pediatrics milestones: initial evidence for their use as learning road maps for residents. Acad Pediatr. 2013;13(1):40–7. https://doi.org/10.1016/j.acap.2012.09.003.
63. Schumpeter JA. Vilfredo Pareto (1848–1923). Q J Econ. 1949;63(2):147–73. https://doi.org/10.2307/1883096.
64. Seiden SC, Barach P. Wrong-side/wrong-site, wrong-procedure, and wrong-patient adverse events: are they preventable? Arch Surg. 2006;141(9):931–9. https://doi.org/10.1001/archsurg.141.9.931.
65. Shojania KG, Duncan BW, McDonald KM, Wachter RM, Markowitz AJ. Making health care safer: a critical analysis of patient safety practices. Evid Rep Technol Assess (Summ). 2001;(43):i-x, 1–668.

66. Smith KL, Ashburn S, Rule E, Jervis R. Residents contributing to inpatient quality: blending learning and improvement. J Hosp Med. 2012;7(2):148–53. https://doi.org/10.1002/jhm.945.
67. Stahel PF, Sabel AL, Victoroff MS, Varnell J, Lembitz A, Boyle DJ, et al. Wrong-site and wrong-patient procedures in the universal protocol era: analysis of a prospective database of physician self-reported occurrences. Arch Surg. 2010;145(10):978–84. https://doi.org/10.1001/archsurg.2010.185.
68. Stiles BM, Reece TB, Hedrick TL, Garwood RA, Hughes MG, Dubose JJ, et al. General surgery morning report: a competency-based conference that enhances patient care and resident education. Curr Surg. 2006;63(6):385–90. https://doi.org/10.1016/j.cursur.2006.06.005.
69. Swing SR, Beeson MS, Carraccio C, Coburn M, Iobst W, Selden NR, et al. Educational milestone development in the first 7 specialties to enter the next accreditation system. J Grad Med Educ. 2013;5(1):98–106. https://doi.org/10.4300/jgme-05-01-33.
70. Taylor MJ, McNicholas C, Nicolay C, Darzi A, Bell D, Reed JE. Systematic review of the application of the plan-do-study-act method to improve quality in healthcare. BMJ Qual Saf. 2014;23(4):290–8. https://doi.org/10.1136/bmjqs-2013-001862.
71. Tess AV, Yang JJ, Smith CC, Fawcett CM, Bates CK, Reynolds EE. Combining clinical microsystems and an experiential quality improvement curriculum to improve residency education in internal medicine. Acad Med (J Assoc Am Med Colleges). 2009;84(3):326–34. https://doi.org/10.1097/ACM.0b013e31819731bf.
72. United States Department of Health and Human Services HRaSA. Quality improvement tools and resources. 2017. https://www.hrsa.gov/quality/toolsresources.html.
73. United States Health and Human Services Department CfDC. Performance management and quality improvement. 2017. https://www.cdc.gov/stltpublichealth/performance/resources.html. Accessed 25 Feb 2017.
74. Varkey P, Karlapudi S, Rose S, Nelson R, Warner M. A systems approach for implementing practice-based learning and improvement and systems-based practice in graduate medical education. Acad Med (J Assoc Am Med Colleges). 2009;84(3):335–9. https://doi.org/10.1097/ACM.0b013e31819731fb.
75. Vest JR, Gamm LD. A critical review of the research literature on six sigma, lean and StuderGroup's hardwiring excellence in the United States: the need to demonstrate and communicate the effectiveness of transformation strategies in healthcare. Implement Sci. 2009;4:35. https://doi.org/10.1186/1748-5908-4-35.
76. Veterans Affairs Do. VA National Center for Patient Safety. In: Washington (DC): The Department. 2016. http://www.patientsafety.va.gov/professionals/onthejob/rca.asp. Accessed 13 Feb 2017.
77. Vincent CA. Analysis of clinical incidents: a window on the system not a search for root causes. Qual Saf Health Care. 2004;13(4):242–3. https://doi.org/10.1136/qhc.13.4.242.
78. Vonlanthen R, Slankamenac K, Breitenstein S, Puhan MA, Muller MK, Hahnloser D, et al. The impact of complications on costs of major surgical procedures: a cost analysis of 1200 patients. Ann Surg. 2011;254(6):907–13. https://doi.org/10.1097/SLA.0b013e31821d4a43.
79. Weingart SN. A house officer-sponsored quality improvement initiative: leadership lessons and liabilities. Jt Comm J Qual Improv. 1998;24(7):371–8.
80. Weingart SN, Tess A, Driver J, Aronson MD, Sands K. Creating a quality improvement elective for medical house officers. J Gen Intern Med. 2004;19(8):861–7. https://doi.org/10.1111/j.1525-1497.2004.30127.x.
81. Woloshynowych M, Rogers S, Taylor-Adams S, Vincent C. The investigation and analysis of critical incidents and adverse events in healthcare. Health Technol Assess (Winchester, England). 2005;9(19):1–143. iii
82. Wreathall J, Nemeth C. Assessing risk: the role of probabilistic risk assessment (PRA) in patient safety improvement. Qual Saf Health Care. 2004;13(3):206–12. https://doi.org/10.1136/qhc.13.3.206.
83. Yang JX, Hunt TD, Ting HH, Henderson D, Finkelstein J, Davidson KW. Improving value-add work and satisfaction in medical residents training: a resident-led quality improvement

project employing the lean method to improve hospital supply usage. Postgrad Med J. 2016. doi:https://doi.org/10.1136/postgradmedj-2016-134163.
84. Young D. Pittsburgh hospitals band together to reduce medication errors. Am J Health Syst Pharm AJHP (Off J Am Soc Health-Syst Pharmacists). 2002;59(11):1014. 6, 26
85. Ziegelstein RC, Fiebach NH. "The mirror" and "the village": a new method for teaching practice-based learning and improvement and systems-based practice. Acad Med (J Assoc Am Med Colleges). 2004;79(1):83–8.

Role of the Surgeon Educator in Leading Surgical Skills Center Development

12

Michael R. Romanelli, Jennifer Bartlett, Janet Ketchum, and Bradley Schwartz

History of the Program

Surgery has historically been at the forefront of the assessment and integration of surgical skills and simulation into medical curriculum [1]. In the late 1990s, educational leaders of the Southern Illinois University School of Medicine Department of Surgery recognized a need for progression in the development of their resident's skill set outside the traditional environments of the operating room, on the wards, and in the classroom [2]. Thanks to the efforts of key leaders in the Department of Surgery in partnership with one of their teaching hospitals, the SIU Surgical Skills Lab opened in May of 2000. At that time, the SIU Surgical Skills Lab was one of only a handful of centers across the country designed solely to train residents and medical students using surgical skills lab modules; as of 2008, the Residency Review Committee for General Surgery has mandated all of their US postgraduate training programs must have surgical skills laboratories as part of their training facilities [3].

Increased demands in Graduate Medical Education (GME) have influenced shift from the traditional apprenticeship model to integrate additional directed skills

M.R. Romanelli, MA (✉)
Southern Illinois University School of Medicine, J Roland Folse MD Surgical Skills Center, 228 W Miller Street, Springfield, IL 62794-9601, USA
e-mail: mromanelli81@siumed.edu

J. Bartlett, ST • J. Ketchum, CST
J Roland Folse MD Surgical Skills Center at Southern Illinois University School of Medicine, Springfield, IL, USA
e-mail: jbartlett2@siumed.edu; jketchum@siumed.edu

B. Schwartz, DO, FACS
Department of Urology at Southern Illinois University School of Medicine, Springfield, IL, USA
e-mail: bschwartz@siumed.edu

T.S. Köhler, B. Schwartz (eds.), *Surgeons as Educators*,
https://doi.org/10.1007/978-3-319-64728-9_12

training [4]. Reasoning behind this train of thought dates back to 1987, when Barnes highlighted reasons for surgical skills and simulation training including fiscal use of resources in training, increasing complexity of procedures, limitations of available patients, and legal pressures for providers' optimal skills [5]. When the Surgical Skills Lab first opened, the Department of Surgery was accepting 12 surgical residents a year and was responsible for the education of 54 residents across subspecialties including general surgery, orthopedic surgery, otolaryngology, plastic surgery, and urology. Last year, the Surgical Skills Lab provided the environment for and assisted in the training of 160 surgical residents and additional resident subspecialties including internal medicine, family medicine, obstetrics and gynecology, and emergency medicine. In addition to foundational residency skills training, each subspecialty has their own respective curriculum detailed and focused on procedures within their scope of practice. Each year, 176 modules are completed annually. Every day, opportunities for new curriculum and corresponding lab modules are requested and accordingly developed and implemented to meet the needs of learners.

With this extensive growth, the Surgical Skills Lab has outgrown its initial 1600 square foot location and has been established in 2015 as the J Roland Folse Surgical Skills Center named after the founder of the Southern Illinois University Department of Surgery. The Surgical Skills Center relocated to a new 3700 square foot facility in the Memorial Center for Learning and Innovation, a state-of-the-art multimillion-dollar establishment dedicated to the pursuit of advancement and innovation in medical education and care. This move provided the additional space to foster continued aggressive expansion of the center and dramatically advanced the high-fidelity technological capabilities to meet and serve the educational needs of the School of Medicine.

While the Surgical Skills Center has been very fortunate in their move to the new location, the leadership active in this development asserts that surgeons as educators can establish and foster this culture of learning wherever the location might be, from a classroom to a closet or from an empty hospital room to an operating room not in use [6]. Two schools of thought are prevalent in regard to what is the optimal directed training: utilizing low-fidelity task models to train necessary basic operative skills, compared to high-fidelity simulators focused on mimicking the contextual experience of operating [7]. For the Surgical Skills Center, initially mechanical models such as laparoscopic box trainers in consideration of associated costs were determined to be of greatest value for skills improvement, as for many other institutions [8]. As buy-in from medical community leaders has grown, high-fidelity simulators have been integrated into practice to maximize all opportunities of learning.

Residency Boot Camp Curriculum

Surgeons as educators in the School of Medicine were led to recognize the need for a general surgery educational skills practicum determined by incoming interns' variable fund of knowledge and technical skills [9]. Further informed by student and faculty questionnaires supplemented by focus groups, a curriculum affectionately referred to as "boot camp" was developed in 2000 for interns beginning July of their PGY-1 year. This program set out to establish learners' proficiency in training and offer a foundational baseline to track their progress moving forward. These learning modules would later become the foundation of the American College of Surgeons (ACS) and Association of Program Directors in Surgery (APDS) National Surgical Skills Curriculum [3].

For each module, a formal overview is provided to the learner in advance that communicates relevant information including rationale, objectives, a detailed description along with step-by-step walk-through of the module, and criteria for proficiency. Weekly curriculum covers basic surgical skills such as tissue handling, dissection, and wound closure. Learning issues which all PGY-1 surgery residents are required to complete are covered by modules on knot tying, basic suturing, central venous access, chest tube placement, and emergency surgical airway. Attendance and participation in modules are coordinated with the resident call schedule. Modules are planned and scheduled utilizing a block system, which arranges for a learner to experience different modules on days spread over multiple weeks in intervals as opposed to mass practice [10]. Additional times for open skills practice were scheduled to better accommodate the demanding responsibilities of an intern.

Learning modules are led by two faculty members assisted by a skills coach to both lead and assist with discussion of how the skill is integrated into surgery. For select basic surgical skills training, there was determined to be no difference in improvement of a student's performance whether facilitated by a nonphysician skills coach or faculty surgeon [11]. By sharing the responsibilities of teaching, a consistent commitment to a high student/faculty ratio of 4:1 is maintained while avoiding faculty burnout, which has been paramount to the success of the program. By informing learners of common critical errors prior to the learning module, acquisition of skills and performance was enhanced during instruction about correct performance of basic surgical skills [12].

The curriculum culminates in verification of proficiency (VOP) evaluations developed from previous performance-based assessments of technical skills including objective structured assessment of technical skills evaluation methods [13, 14]. Residents are required to demonstrate proficiency on each of the VOP modules by means of the video assessment prior to performing any of the required procedures on the floor or in the operating room. If a learner didn't meet the necessary requirements of their assessment, additional remediation curricula were scheduled until a student met the requirements of the module. The VOP evaluations as shown in Fig. 12.1 empowered educators to swiftly and acutely learn where improvement was necessary on a learner's road to proficiency across a broad spectrum of procedures and practices [13].

We found that faculty volunteerism improved employing an automated video capturing system. This Internet-based program has proved more flexible in that it allows faculty to watch a de-identified learner from the comfort of their home or office. Simultaneously, evaluators are able to fill out their VOP evaluation on a split screen to objectively assess surgical skills performance. Educators have the ability

Bowel Anastomosis Evaluation **Resident:** ____________________ **Date:** __________

Global Characteristics	Satisfactory		Comments
Align the two bowel ends parallel to each other using bowel clamps	Y	N	
Corner sutures left long and clamped (stay sutures)	Y	N	
Appropriate placement of back wall sutures (Lembert .5 cm apart)	Y	N	
Appropriate tension and knots while tying back wall sutures	Y	N	
Appropriate placement of back wall inner layer (running)	Y	N	
Appropriate transition from back to front wall (Connell on inner layer)	Y	N	
Ties inner layer, front wall sutures with appropriate tension	Y	N	
Remove bowel clamps	Y	N	
Appropriate placement of front wall outer layer sutures (Lembert)	Y	N	
Appropriate tension and knots while tying front wall sutures	Y	N	

Economy of Time and Motion

1	Many unnecessary / disorganized movements
2	
3	Organized time / motion, some unnecessary movements
4	
5	Maximum economy of movement and efficiency

Final Rating
Demonstrates Proficiency

☐ Yes
☐ No

Other Summative Comments

Evaluator ____________________

SIU Dept of Surgery, General Surgery Residency Program

Fig. 12.1 Bowel anastomosis verification of proficiency

to annotate the video recording, noting when and what a learner might do to improve their technique. Beard [15] and Driscoll [16] were able to establish construct validity for video assessment of basic surgical trainee's operative skills with strong correlation and evidence.

Surgery Subspecialty Curriculum

Progression of resident's foundational curriculum quickly advanced within subspecialties to incorporate and train residents and fellows for more challenging cases. Often more advanced subspecialty procedural skill modules are coordinated together as team training with various levels of resident learners present. The presence of senior residents to facilitate their juniors' active participation through a procedure has furthered both parties' knowledge foundation in an immersive, student-centered experience [17] in accord with Halsted's concept of "see one, do one, teach one." Additionally, the rationale for certain aspects of each procedure was clarified as different techniques were debated at greater length in feedback discussions than traditionally covered during everyday cases in the operating room.

For general surgery residents as in other subspecialties, advanced laparoscopic skill modules were developed in a stepwise manner based on learner skill level. For the classic laparoscopic cholecystectomy procedure, phase 1 establishes an intern's technical abilities for the procedure utilizing low-fidelity inorganic laparoscopic box trainers in accord with the ACS/APDS Surgery Resident Skills Curriculum. Following demonstration of this proficiency, a learner will progress to a higher-fidelity organic procedure operating on an ex vivo porcine liver with gallbladder. The curriculum culminates in an annual lab in which the entire laparoscopic cholecystectomy procedure is performed from start to finish on a cadaver. This aspect of the learning process enables a resident to focus additionally on nontechnical skills, including communication and teamwork. At our institution, surgery residents work together with students from a local certified surgical technologist community college program to better simulate and integrate interdisciplinary training objectives. This level of learning is paramount for the surgery resident as deficits in nontechnical skills can often result in errors committed in surgery; poor communication has been identified as a causal factor in 43% of surgical errors [18].

Resident Readiness Curriculum

Following the success of the boot camp curriculum, the Surgical Skills Center endeavored to develop a "resident readiness" program to better prepare medical students in the spring of their fourth year for the responsibilities of their resident intern year [19]. Utilizing the American College of Surgeons Graduate Medical Education (ACGME) Committee prerequisites for graduate surgical education, the curriculum was organized around common intern experiences. Learning modules were designed utilizing intensive application of accumulated knowledge and skills for the care of the surgical patient; exercises included mock pages, writing orders, and surgical skills [20]. Leaders at our institution would eventually work with other medical schools to integrate this curriculum into what is now an essential aspect of the American College of Surgery (ACS) and Association of Program Directors in Surgery (APDS) entering surgery resident preparatory curriculum. This coursework has been studied extensively in support of the improved confidence and abilities of fourth year medical students preparing to enter surgical residencies, and we have found the same to be true [21, 22].

Program Support

During the development of the Surgical Skills Center, leaders recognized the importance of gaining buy-in and integration with the School of Medicine and other departments [23–25]. Accordingly, a steering committee was developed to act as a sounding board for discussion of potential opportunities to meet the needs of their learners and determine the best interests and action plans of the Surgical Skills Center. While the steering committee guided the initial direction of the Surgical Skills Center by assembling the personnel, facility, and administrative structure to support the development of its curriculum and continues to meet annually, champions from within the School of Medicine (specifically surgeons as educators) have proceeded to arise to lead endeavors driven to improve learners' skill set [26].

Paramount to the Surgical Skills Center's success has been its steadfast commitment to fostering a culture of continuous improvement. Pursuant of this progression, the Surgical Skills Center has focused on increasing the frequency of direct observation and effective feedback learners receive in a realistic environment to enhance surgical skill in the operating room [27]. By establishing specific performance metrics within an educational framework similar to what is taught perioperatively, a student first talks through critical steps of the procedure during a briefing of the learning module, subsequently receives "intraoperative" coaching if necessary, and undergoes a debriefing following to review performance and identify opportunities for improvement [28]. Unique to the Surgical Skills Center relative to the operating room, performance targets enable a student to safely struggle through critical growth experiences void of any concern for patient safety risk. This approach works to virtually eliminate the amount of guiding often seen in the operating room as it uses autonomy to empower a learner and their facilitator to identify potential gaps in their skill set [29].

The directive of the Surgical Skills Center has been to work closely in conjunction with attending physicians to foster a continuum between the operating room and the surgical skills lab for students, residents, and fellows as yet another learning environment in which faculty-learner collaborations are increased. By minimizing the minutiae of a learning module, the Skills Center empowers the surgeon as educator to focus on coaching skills such as economy of motion, counter-traction, and safe tissue handling, among others. The Surgical Skills Lab better informs assessment of its learners by routinely performing video-based coaching, well supported in the literature to enhance the surgical skills performance of its learners [30]. Based on prior studies of performance, reliable operative assessment for residents should have 20 ratings per year from at least 10 different raters [31]. By acquiring additional data to monitor resident's progress in the Surgical Skills Center, tracking performance and using standardized benchmarks have enabled surgeons as educators to identify those in need of focused remediation. This assessment is essential in identifying and correcting technical deficiencies before they become engrained in a learner's skill set [32].

By supporting faculty development in this dyad model between the Surgical Skills Center and its faculty, surgeons as educators have more time to devote to not only the performance evaluation of their learners but also for themselves [33]. Preparing faculty for learning modules in anticipation of logistics, educational objectives, and potential challenges of a skills lab ensures faculty maintain learners' engagement within the scope of the learning module [34]. By supporting this aspect of the learning module development, additional time has been allotted for faculty to focus on instructional improvement. Consistent evaluations of training and educators as shown below in Fig. 12.2 have led to significant initiatives for improvement in education and evaluation in the Surgical Skills Center. Meeting with program directors routinely to review these assessments has proved pivotal in improving coaching for the better learning of residents.

Vital to providing this curriculum and continuing to meet the learning needs of the Department of Surgery and School of Medicine is the Surgical Skills Center team members' extensive experience in previous surgical environments and ability to think outside of the box in terms of creativity. Porterfield et al. purport in their article on *Simulation and Faculty Development* that "leading a simulation effort requires vision, creativity in management, and team leadership skills" [35]. Experienced surgical scrub technicians empowered and led by surgeons as

SIU SURGICAL SKILL CENTER
RESIDENT EVALUATION FORM

COURSE: ______________________ **DATE:** __________

SYLLABUS	0 – not applicable – did not read it				
Content & Clarity:	1 *session not described adequately*	2	3 *parts of the syllabus were clearly laid out and had relevant content*	4	5 *session described perfectly – syllabus needs no improvement*
Effectiveness:	1 *I did not use any information from the syllabus to prepare for this session*	2	3 *parts of the syllabus prepared me for the session, but it needs improvement*	4	5 *the syllabus was a great source of information – I was completely prepared for the session*
SESSION					
Teaching Expectations:	1 *taught me nothing new about this procedure*	2	3 *Taught me about what I expected*	4	5 *Taught me everything I need to know about this procedure*
Technical Demonstration:	1 *instructor failed to clearly demonstrate even the basic principles*	2	3 *basic principles were demonstrated, but details were lacking*	4	5 *principles and details were demonstrated thoroughly*
Practice:	1 *received no hands-on practice*	2	3 *I could perform this procedure with supervision*	4	5 *received exactly the right amount of practice*
Confidence:	1 *I would not be able to perform this procedure except as an assistant*	2	3 *I could perform this procedure with supervision*	4	5 *I feel I could perform the procedure on a human with no supervision*
BENCH MODEL					
Fidelity of the Model:	1 *was not like human in anyway*	2	3 *was adequate, but needs work*	4	5 *was like operating on a human*

COMMENTS:

PLEASE COMPLETE REVERSE SIDE →

Fig. 12.2 Skills lab evaluation

FACULTY I					
Feedback:	1 instructor did not interact with me	2	3 feedback provided will allow me to address specific deficiencies	4	5 instructor listened attentively, provided clear, effective feedback so that I now exactly what to do to improve
Level of Instruction:	1 instructor disregarded students' prior level of training and knowledge	2	3 instructor appeared to be somewhat sensitive to prior level of training	4	5 instructor was sensitive to the level of training of students and taught accordingly
Stimulates Enthusiasm:	1 the instructor appeared to be going through the procedure to get it over with	2	3 instructor was able to generate some enthusiasm about this procedure	4	5 I became excited about learning the procedure because of the instructor
Instructor's Knowledge:	1 instructor's knowledge of this procedure was barely more than mine	2	3 instructor was able to teach at a satisfactory level	4	5 instructor's knowledge of this procedure is complete – a master

FACULTY II					
Feedback:	1 instructor did not interact with me	2	3 feedback provided will allow me to address specific deficiencies	4	5 instructor listened attentively, provided clear, effective feedback so that I now exactly what to do to improve
Level of Instruction:	1 instructor disregarded students' prior level of training and knowledge	2	3 instructor appeared to be somewhat sensitive to prior level of training	4	5 instructor was sensitive to the level of training of students and taught accordingly
Stimulates Enthusiasm:	1 the instructor appeared to be going through the procedure to get it over with	2	3 instructor was able to generate some enthusiasm about this procedure	4	5 I became excited about learning the procedure because of the instructor
Instructor's Knowledge:	1 instructor's knowledge of this procedure was barely more than mine	2	3 instructor was able to teach at a satisfactory level	4	5 instructor's knowledge of this procedure is complete – a master

COMMENTS:

Return ASAP to Janet Ketchum, Surgical Skills Lab Director, Surgical Skills Lab, MMC, Lower Level Room G36

Fig. 12.2 (continued)

educators have been the backbone of the Surgical Skills Center since it was first established. Not only do personnel work on developing new methods of learning for residents and students, they stay up to date on the latest trends and techniques by consistently working at least 1 day a week in the operating room to anticipate and foresee potential for new innovation and improvement in surgical skills. These labs and module development would be nowhere without their commitment and hard work coupled with their creativity utilizing everyday materials to simulate real-life operative experiences. Embracing and encouraging this culture of creativity among educators and learners have been vital to the progression and innovation of the Surgical Skills Center that has set it at the forefront of skills labs nationally.

Developing the Models for Your Surgical Skills Center

Since the establishment of the Surgical Skills Center, Director and Skills Coach Janet Ketchum CST, CSFA, and Coordinator Jenny Bartlett ST have fostered a commitment to resourceful and novel applications of everyday items as opportunities for realistic simulation of surgical skills training. By integrating everyday experiences witnessing residents and others learn in the operating room with everyday materials, realistic and cost-conscious surgical skills simulators have been developed. Examples range from using pork ribs acquired from a local butcher covered in foam fabric headliner to simulate an easily replicable chest tube model to arranging hamster tubing into the shape of a colon using pegboard for a cost-conscious lower endoscopy insertion model. These novel examples are only a few creative innovations; for a more detailed step-by-step description of do-it-yourself models, we invite you to read *Best Practices in Surgical Education: Innovations in Skills Training* [36] or visit the Surgical Skills Center website [37] as the Surgical Skills Center recognizes collaborative efforts across educational institutions and has dramatically improved the learner's experience. Recently at the Surgical Skills Center, pouring quality plastic molds has been a priority to improve reproducibility and fidelity in light of cost-saving efforts.

Focus on utility and practicality of models has deterred excess use of anatomically precise expensive cadaveric models for routine learning modules; however, as more advanced learning modules require commitment to anatomical acuity, the Surgical Skills Center has risen to meet learning needs, often acquiring cadavers when necessary. Additionally, more resources have since been devoted to the acquisition of high-fidelity surgical skills trainers such as laparoscopic skills trainers, colonoscopy/esophagogastroduodenoscopy trainers, and arthroscopy trainers. During the move to the new location, significant resources were allocated to develop a space dedicated to improving ease of use for learners and diversity in maximizing interdisciplinary learning opportunities.

External Support

By teaming with a supportive local hospital, relationships with scrub technicians and nursing staff have empowered significant cost-saving initiatives through instrumentation loaning programs, and the acquisition of functional expired surgical items including sutures and other instruments has fueled the resource-intensive environment of learning. By maintaining positive relationships with surgical manufacturing companies, box trainers and laparoscopic instruments were donated for students to train on and improve their skills by task challenges such as moving rubber items in between poles, picking up nuts and beans, and cutting mesh in a variety of shapes. Additionally, many surgical companies provide educational research grants that are attainable given the nature of a Surgical Skills Center's directives [38]. It is important to note that when trying to find solutions to meet the learning needs of one's programs, an institution doesn't have to spend exorbitant amounts of money to achieve its goals.

Looking to the Future, Both Ours and Yours

Reflecting on our growth over the years, both in success and in failure, select priorities have kept our focus aligned and enabled us to continue to progress. While the size of a program, location of the skills lab, and available support at your institution may change over time as ours have, what makes a Surgical Skills Center program successful are continual learning needs assessments, a supportive culture of learning and leading, and most importantly the physical environment for learners and teachers to interact, practice, and discuss the details of their craft outside of the pressures of the live medical environment. While the needs of our institution have changed throughout the years, continual reassessment has been paramount to the development of our program and, most importantly, the learning of our students.

Now more than ever, the SIU School of Medicine J. Roland Folse, M.D. Surgical Skills Center is recognizing the value in the learning needs assessments and corresponding curriculum we set forth 16 years ago. Prioritizing the learner's needs and embracing a pursuant culture of learning are the primary reason behind why we believe the initial residency boot camp curriculum at our institution expanded so quickly. Attending surgeons were pivotal in leading the development of curriculum. As the Surgical Skills Center maintains its commitment to continuous innovation, it has overcome new challenges of learning in ways we didn't think were possible; it is the supportive culture of embracing change in learning that sets a program apart.

Recently, orthopedic surgeons in the community endeavored to provide continued medical education opportunities for their learning community. By utilizing technological advances provided by the Surgical Skills Center in conjunction with the Memorial Center for Learning and Innovation, surgeons were able to live stream arthroscopy procedures on a cadaver model to improve the education of their residents, peers, therapists (both physical and occupational), and all care providers along the orthopedic service line in pursuit of improved coordinated care. Moving forward, we anticipate the Surgical Skills Center's further integration into the medical and local community while fostering a commitment to interdisciplinary teamwork among care providers [39].

References

1. Gallagher AG, Ritter M, Champion H, Higgins G, Fried MP, Moses G, Smith D, Satava RM. Virtual reality simulation for the operating room. Ann Surg. 2005;241(2):364–72.
2. Scott DJ, Dunnington GL. The new ACS/APDS skills curriculum: moving the learning curve out of the operating room. J Gastrointest Surg. 2008;12:213–21.
3. Britt LD, Richardson JD. Residency review committee for surgery: an update. Arch Surg. 2007;142:573–55.
4. Aucar JA.The History of Simulation. In: Tsuda ST, Scott DJ, Jones DB (eds), Textbook of simulation. Woodbury, CT: Cine-Med, Inc; 2012. p. 3–14.
5. Barnes RW. Surgical handicraft: teaching and learning surgical skills. Am J Surg. 1987;153(5):422–7.
6. Gould JC. Building a laparoscopic surgical skills training laboratory: resources and support. JSLS. 2006;10(3):293–6.

7. Maran NJ, Glavin RJ. Low- to high fidelity simulation: a continuum of medical education? Med Educ. 2003;37:22–8.
8. Berg DA, Milner RE, Fischer CA, et al. A cost-effective approach to establishing a surgical skills laboratory. Surgery. 2007;143(5):712–21.
9. Sanfey H, Dunnington G. Verification of proficiency: a prerequisite for clinical experience. Surg Clin North Am. 2010;90(3):559–67.
10. Catania A. Learning. 2nd ed. Englewood Cliffs: Prentice Hall; 1984.
11. Kim MJ, Boehler ML, Ketchum JK, Bueno R Jr, Williams RG, Dunnington GL. Skills coaches as part of the educational team: a randomized controlled trial of teaching of a basic surgical skill in the laboratory setting. Am J Surg. 2010;199(1):94–8.
12. Rogers DA, Regehr G, MacDonald J. A role for error training in surgical technical skill instruction and evaluation. Am J Surg. 2002;183(3):242–5.
13. Sanfey H, Ketchum J, Bartlett J, Markwell S, Meier AH, Williams R, Dunnington G. Verification of proficiency in basic skills for postgraduate year 1 residents. Surgery. 2010;148(4):759–66.
14. Martin JA, Regehr G, Reznick R, et al. Objective structured assessment of technical skill (OSATS) for surgical residents. Br J Surg. 1997;84(2):273–8.
15. Beard JD. Setting standards for the assessment of operative competence. Eur J Vasc Endovasc Surg. 2005;30:215–8.
16. Driscoll PJ, Paisley AM, Patterson-Brown S. Video assessment of basic surgical trainees' operative skills. Am J Surg. 2008;196:265–72.
17. Hertel J, Millis B. Using simulations to promote learning in higher education: an introduction. Sterling: Stylus Publishing; 2002.
18. Gawande AA, Zinner MJ, Studdert DM, et al. Analysis of errors reported by surgeons at three teaching hospitals. Surgery. 2003;133:614–21.
19. Lyss-Lerman P, Teherani A, Aagaard E, et al. What training is needed in the fourth year of medical school? Views of residency program directors. Acad Med. 2009;84:823–9.
20. Willis RE, Peterson RM, Dent DL. Usefulness of the American College of Surgeons' fundamentals of surgery curriculum as a knowledge preparatory tool for incoming surgery interns. Am J Surg. 2013;205:131–6.
21. Zeng W, Woodhouse J, Brunt M. Do preclinical background and clerkship experiences impact skills performance in an accelerated internship preparation course for senior medical students? Surgery. 2010;148:768–77.
22. Okusanya OT, Kornfield ZN, Reinke CE, et al. The effect and durability of a pregraduation boot camp on the confidence of senior medical student entering surgical residencies. J Surg Educ. 2012;69:536–43.
23. Seropian MA. General concepts in full scale simulation: getting started. Anesth Analg. 2003;97:1695–705.
24. Haluck RS, Satava RM, Fried G, et al. Establishing a simulation center for surgical skills: what to do and how to do it. Surg Endosc. 2007;21:1223–32.
25. Alinier G, Hunt B, Harwood C. Development of a new multi-professional clinical simulation centre at the University of Hertfordshire. Simul Healthc. 2006;1:198.
26. Strachan A. What shall we do with our simulation centre? Simul Healthc. 2006;1:188.
27. Bonrath EM, Dedy NK, Gordon LE, Grantcharov TP. Comprehensive surgical coaching enhances surgical skill in the operating room. A randomized controlled trial. Ann Surg. 2015;262:205–12.
28. Roberts NK, Williams RG, Kim MJ, Dunnington GL. The briefing, intraoperative teaching, debriefing model for teaching in the operating room. J Am Coll Surg. 2009;208:299–303.
29. Sandhu G, Teman NR, Minter RM. Training autonomous surgeons: more time or faculty development? Ann Surg. 2015;261:843–5.
30. Singh P, Aggarwal R, Tahir M, Pucher PH, Darzi A. A randomized controlled study to evaluate the role of video-based coaching in training laparoscopic skills. Ann Surg. 2015;261:862–9.
31. Williams RG, Verhulst S, Colliver JA, et al. A template for reliable assessment of resident operative performance: assessment intervals, numbers of observations and raters. Surgery. 2012;152:517–27.

32. Sanfey H, Williams R, Dunnington G. Recognizing residents with a deficiency in operative performance as a step closer to effective remediation. J Am Coll Surg. 2012;216:114–22.
33. Chen XP, Williams RG, Sanfey HA, Dunnington GL. How do supervising surgeons evaluate guidance provided in the operating room? Am J Surg. 2012;203:44–8.
34. Krueger PM, Neutens J, Bienstock J, et al. To the point: reviews in medical education teaching techniques. Am J Obstet Gynecol. 2004;191:408–11.
35. Rogers DA, Peterson DT, Ponce BA, White ML, Porterfield JR. Simulation and faculty development. Surg Clin N Am. 2015;95(4):729–37.
36. Saltzman, PD. Best Practices in Surgical Education: Innovations in Skills Training. Somerville, NJ: Ethicon Endo-Surgery, Inc; 2010.
37. Surgical Skills Model Assembly. 2013. Accessed Jan 2016. http://www.siumed.edu/surgery/surgical_skills/model_assembly.html
38. Park AE, Moses GR. Funding for simulation centers and simulation research. In: Tsuda ST, Scott DJ, Jones DB (eds), Textbook of simulation. Woodbury, CT: Cine-Med, Inc; 2012. p. 517–24.
39. Jones A. The changing face of a medical simulation centre. Simul Healthc. 2006;1:196.

Modern Theory for Development of Simulators for Surgical Education

13

Yasser A. Noureldin and Robert M. Sweet

Introduction

Over the past few decades, different types of simulators have been introduced and assessed for validity evidence for surgical training and assessment [1–3]. However, the lack of a standardized process for simulator design and development has led to a mismatch between the needs of surgeons and the products available. While technological gaps in anatomic, physiologic, and tissue fidelity were obvious, there lacked a systematic way of addressing these issues. Each simulation laboratory or company used its own process in isolation. This was reflected in the heterogeneity of the usability, robustness, effectiveness, and applicability of available simulation systems for medical/surgical education. In parallel, the American College of Surgeons-Accredited Education Institutes (ACS-AEI) were rapidly spreading all over the world, and simulators were becoming an integral part of the medical and surgical training curricula. This expanded upon the demand for effective, usable simulation systems to be developed.

In this chapter, a modern theory for a standardized process for design and development of simulators used for medical/surgical education is presented and discussed. This theory depends on the concept of "backward design" as part of the Understanding by Design® Framework (UbD™) which was introduced by Wiggins,

Y.A. Noureldin, MD, MSc, PhD
WWAMI Institute for Simulation in Healthcare (WISH), University of Washington, Seattle, WA, USA

Urology Department, Benha University, Benha, Egypt
e-mail: dryasser.noor@fmed.bu.ed.eg

R.M. Sweet, MD, FACS (✉)
UW Medicine, Department of Urology, University of Washington, Seattle, WA, USA

WWAMI Institute for Simulation in Healthcare (WISH), University of Washington, Seattle, WA, USA
e-mail: rsweet@uw.edu

T.S. Köhler, B. Schwartz (eds.), *Surgeons as Educators*,
https://doi.org/10.1007/978-3-319-64728-9_13

G. and McTighe, J. [4, 5] and the current "Standards for Educational and Psychological Testing" which was produced by collaborative efforts of a committee from the Educational Research Association, the National Council on Measurement in Education, and the American Psychological Association [6], as well as the Guidelines for Simulation Development which was developed by the Technology and Simulation Committee of the Accredited Education Institutes Consortium [7].

Theory of Simulators Design and Development

According to the Standards for Educational and Psychological Testing 2014, test/simulator development is defined as "the process of producing a measure of some aspects of individual's knowledge, skills, abilities, attitudes, or other characteristics by developing tasks and combining them to form a test/simulator, according to a specific plan". A simulator-specific design/development plan should include all steps and considerations in this process. The design/development plan is guided by the expected interpretation of simulator scores for an intended use(s). Simulator development is a multidisciplinary and interprofessional process that occurs through collaboration of physicians, engineers, and industry. This process has four phases: first involves assessment of the requirements from the physicians' perspective, second is translating physicians' requirements to engineers' requirements, third involves the development of a prototype(s), and fourth is a validation process. The transition to a manufactural product is an additional critical step but is beyond the scope of this chapter.

Phase I: Assessing the Requirements from the Physicians' Perspective Identifying a training gap or unmet training need is considered an "opportunity" whereby simulators can fill or satisfy. According to "backward design" principles, the desired training objectives and outcomes should be firstly identified to guide the development process. Training objectives and desired outcomes should be delineated in collaboration with authoritative societies. During the needs assessment process, the following questions must be considered: What will the desired simulator replace (e.g., live patient, expensive teaching technology, or animals)? What are the curricular needs? What are the educational objectives to address? Will this simulator be the most effective educational tool from a cost perspective? Is a demonstration of proficiency necessary and/or required for credentialing or certification? Will the data derived from a simulation-based curriculum improve the quality of care and patient safety? What is the required level of fidelity broken down into anatomic, physiologic, tissue and affective aspects of fidelity. and what learning objective domains are predominant (cognitive, psychomotor, communication, or affective)?

Given the fact that the design and development of simulators are usually led by engineers, it is the responsibility of the physicians to give a clear and detailed answers about all aspects of the surgical procedure such as the indications, purpose, how is it performed, and what is considered success and what is considered failure. This is considered an excellent opportunity for engineers (developers) to interact with physicians and learn about terminology, anatomy, disease, surgical instruments, and surgical procedure. A process called "cognitive task analysis" was found to be optimal for this kind of interaction between developers and physicians. First, gross task or "procedure" deconstruction into a number of steps is performed, and cognitive task analysis (CTA) is then performed for each step of the procedure to clearly describe the specifications and necessity of each step, delineate the visible and hidden anatomic structures, explain the important cues which lead to correct or wrong decision, describe the interactions and behaviors of tissues, and enumerate the errors (*commission, omission, or execution*) which could be made during each step. Watching a video of a faculty instructing a trainee would be an appropriate method for demonstrating critical clinical aspects and the important outcome measures of the procedure [8].

Phase II: Translating Physicians' Requirements to Engineers' Requirements Clinicians' perspectives, obtained from the CTA, are then translated into engineering and art design requirements. During this phase, the characteristics of the task or the procedure to be simulated should be fully understood. If anatomic fidelity is a requirement, carefully edited anatomic datasets need to be imported and edited accordingly. If physiologic fidelity is a requirement, verification of the function of the system as it relates to other organs critical for a given learning objective is important. If tissue fidelity is a requirement, tissue behaviors that need to be observed are identified by collecting tissues and studying its physical and biomechanical properties. This will lead to creation of more realistic "high-fidelity" tissue samples which could be later used to obtain the desired organs. Anatomic data are obtained from DICOM images from computed tomography (CT) and magnetic resonance imaging (MRI) scans. The CTA also serves to identify and weigh each task, decisions based on each task, and what needs to be assessed. Furthermore, performance metrics are delineated and, whenever possible these should be used to give tutoring and feedback in the form of an exportable performance reports. These performance reports have pronounced importance with the increasing role of simulators in objective assessment of technical skills to avoid the "halo effect" of subjective evaluation. If there is a requirement to reproduce the feelings of interacting with the likeness of a real human (affective domain), then verbal and nonverbal cues need to be carefully thought out, and presented to elicit this response in the learner [9].

The development process is guided by a set of specifications which vary according to the nature of the simulator and the intended use of the interpretation of simulator scores. These specifications are created by the developers and include a statement of purpose(s), target users or populations, content frameworks, construct to be measured, tasks, and scoring. Specifications concerning the intended use should mention whether the simulator score(s) interpretation will be primarily criterion-referenced, where absolute interpretations are always used, or norm-referenced, where relative interpretations are always used. Content specifications should delineate what is to be included to represent all aspects of the construct to be measured, and this could be guided by theory or by analyzing the content domain. For example, delineating the requirements to be credentialed as urologist is an important content specification for developing a simulator used for credentialing urologists [6]. These content specifications will be used as a guide for subsequent evaluation during the validation process. Following delineation of specifications concerning the content and the intended use of simulator scores, specifications regarding tasks and scoring which eventually lead to performance assessment should be delineated. Task specifications should cover all aspects of the construct in a way that the domain of activities and the vital dimensions of performance covered by each task should be described. In addition, the number of tasks, duration of each task, and how the user interacts with each task should be detailed. Scoring specifications describe how each item or task is being scored and how the overall items are combined to give one overall score. The scoring process is either *analytic* or *holistic*, and both are based on clear performance criteria. The holistic scoring procedure generates only one overall score based on the performance criteria. The analytic scoring procedure generates an independent score for each item of the performance criteria in addition to the overall score. While the analytic scoring procedure could provide an idea about the points of weaknesses and strengths of trainees, the holistic scoring procedure could be used whenever the skills being assessed are highly interrelated, and overall judgment is only required. The scoring process could be performed by either human judges (e.g., physical simulators) or computer algorithms (e.g., virtual reality simulators). In the case of human judges, scoring specifications should include qualifications of judges, how they were trained, and how scoring discrepancies and bias among judges be checked and resolved. In case of computer algorithms, scoring specifications should include how scores are reproduced using algorithms. The degree to which the performance assessment, guided by both the tasks and scoring specifications, reflects the domain or the construct to be measured should be supported by both theoretical and empirical evidence. This is particularly important for the validation process [6].

By the end of this step, a formal "requirements document" is generated, a "technology budget" is identified, and price sensitivity is assessed using the Simulator Value Index (SVI) [10]. The SVI includes 17 parameters into an Excel® spreadsheet, and it could be used to assess the simulator purchase process across stakeholders, institutions, and countries. This step is important for market reassessment as simulation development is expensive and the return on investment is slow.

Phase III: Development of Prototype(s) Following development and evaluation of simulator specifications, development and verification of the items/tasks start where simulator developers start creating items/tasks pool which consists of all proposed items/tasks that are needed to be incorporated in the simulator to train/assess what it is intended to train/assess. Thereafter, a set of items/tasks which meet the simulator specifications are chosen and pretested or reviewed for accuracy, durability, clarity, content, quality, and presence of any construct irrelevance prior to be assigned task-specific description and scoring rubrics. The pretest or review process is performed by reviewers who are aware of the content specifications and target learner population who will be trained/assessed using this simulator. Simulator developers should perform early verification and usability studies using the target population. The analysis of data helps to identify some of the important aspects of the task such as task difficulty and the ability to distinguish among subgroups of target population. This ensures the appropriateness and quality of items/tasks prior to actual use. Thereafter, assembly and evaluation of items/tasks occur where the selected items/tasks are assembled and one or more scenarios satisfying the requirements of simulator specifications are chosen to undergo multistage testing or adaptive testing. Prior to operational or actual use, a field test of these scenarios should be conducted using the intended target populations to assess the appropriateness of these scenarios and robustness of the model in real educational environments. Internal structure including generalizability of the population to use the model and reliability of scores can also be tested.

During this phase, the interdisciplinary team of developers perform a high-level of breakdown to delineate the choice of models, scenarios, what it has to be measured, the method of reporting back, the method of providing feedback, the learning management platform, and connectivity to other platforms. The resulting information is used to make a timeline for the development process and is matched with the "technology budget," and readjustments are done when it seems necessary making sure that the development process will be successful, timely, and within budget. A preproduction prototype that demonstrates the design is then developed prior to heading to pilot production where optimization of the manufacturing process and component selection occurs to optimize the cost with the potential needs. The preproduction prototype is used for verifying the degree to which it satisfies the technical and customer's requirements, and refinement is performed to fill in the identified gaps prior to starting the business process where launching the new simulator occurs [8].

By the end of this step, it is important to document verification standards and create user manuals and/or user guides. These should provide information about the simulator administration in terms of user agreement, instructions to users and administrators, and sustainability and scalability and configurability of the simulator and also describe the environmental and safety considerations. Whenever possible, it is highly recommended to encourage compatibility and interoperability of the simulator in terms of connecting with other part task trainers and transfer of data. Instructions to simulator users and administrators have to be pretested alongside the item/test review prior to operational use to ensure fairness for all target population. For instance, instructions for starting a task and the task language should be the same in case of physical simulators. On the other hand, the same hardware specifications (e.g., memory, speed, monitor size, display resolution) and software specifications should be consistent in the virtual reality. There has been a recent trend of federal funding for simulation systems focused on the creation of systems with open source and open standards. An open source/open standards physiology engine has been created and continues to be developed [11], and an Advanced Modular Manikin platform is also under development [12]. These promise to rapidly accelerate the applications of simulation systems for surgery and other health-care fields.

Phase IV: Validation It should be noted that this phase is not separate and it is integrated through the other three phases as validation is an "ongoing" process and extends the content to the consequences. Therefore, it starts from the early beginning of the simulator development process to look at the alignment of the content, including skills, knowledge, and scenarios with the construct or domain intended to measure and extends to assessment of the impact of training or assessment of the target simulator. According to the current Standards for Educational and Psychological Testing, validity is "unitary," and validity evidences are collected to either support or refute the interpretation of simulator scores for certain use not for validating the simulator itself. The current standards described five sources for validity evidence: content evidence, internal structure evidence, response processes evidence, relations with other variables evidence, and consequences evidence [6, 13]. The required level of validity evidence for a simulation-based curriculum intended solely to train residents would require a different amount of evidence then a curriculum intended to credential or certify an individual (high-stakes exam) [14].

References

1. Noureldin YA, Stoica A, Kassouf W, Tanguay S, Bladou F, Andonian S. Incorporation of the da Vinci surgical skills simulator at urology objective structured clinical examinations (OSCEs): a pilot study. Can J Urol. 2016;23(1):8160–6.
2. Noureldin YA, Fahmy N, Anidjar M, Andonian S. Is there a place for virtual reality simulators in assessment of competency in percutaneous renal access? World J Urol. 2016;34(5):733–9.
3. Noureldin YA, Elkoushy MA, Fahmy N, Carrier S, Elhilali MM, Andonian S. Assessment of photoselective vaporization of prostate skills during urology objective structured clinical examinations (OSCE). Can Urol Assoc J. 2015;9(1–2):e61–6.
4. Wiggins G, McTighe J. Understanding by design. Alexandria: Association for Supervision and Curriculum Development (ASCD); 2005.
5. McTighe J, Wiggins G. Understanding by design® framework. Alexandria: Association for Supervision and Curriculum Development (ASCD); 2012. Accessed online on June 1st 2017 from the website http://www.ascd.org/ASCD/pdf/siteASCD/publications/UbD_WhitePaper0312.pdf.
6. American Educational Research Association, American Psychological Association, and National Council on Measurement in Education. Standards for educational and psychological testing. Washington, DC: American Educational Research Association; 2014.
7. Millo Y, George I, Seymour N, Smith R, Petinaux O. Guidelines for simulation development: a set of recommendations for preferred characteristics of surgical simulation; developed by the technology and simulation committee of the accredited education institutes consortium; 2014. Accessed online on June 1st 2017 from the website https://www.facs.org/~/media/files/education/aei/guidelines%20for%20simulation%20interactive.ashx.
8. Hananel D, Sweet RM, Stubbs J. Simulator development – from idea to prototype to product. In: Aggarwal R, Korndorfer J, Cannon-Bowers J, editors. ACS principles and practice for simulation and surgical education research. 1st ed. Chicago: American College of Surgeons; 2015. p. 138–52.
9. Hananel, D. Sweet, R. Deconstructing fidelity for simulation in healthcare. Submitted to Simulation in Healthcare.
10. Rooney D, Cooke J, Hananel D. The creation of a simulator value index tool by connected consensus. Simul Healthc. 2014;9(6):427. DOI 10.1097/01.SIH.0000459322.91351.95.
11. BioGears Human Physiology Engine. Accessed online on May 30th from the website https://www.ara.com/projects/biogears-human-physiology-engine.
12. Sweet RM. The CREST simulation development process: training the next generation. J Endourol. 2017;31(S1):S69–75. DOI 10.1089/end.2016.0613. Epub 2016 Dec 22.
13. Sweet RM, Hananel D, Lawrenz F. A unified approach to validation, reliability, and education study design for surgical technical skills training. Arch Surg. 2010;145(2):197–201.
14. Korndorffer JR, Kasten SJ, Downing SM. Validity and reliability. In: Tsuda ST, Scott DJ, Jones DB, editors. Textbook of simulation: skills and team training. 1st ed. Woodbury: Ciné-Med Publishing; 2012. p. 81–4.

The Surgical Workplace Learning Environment: Integrating Coaching and Mentoring

14

Jeanne L. Koehler and Emily Sturm

Aesop's Fable: The Two Crabs [1] *"My dear," called out an old Crab to her daughter one day, "why do you sidle along in that awkward manner?" "Why don't you go forward like other people?" "Well mother," answered the young Crab, "it seems to me that I go exactly like you do. Go first and show me how, and I will gladly follow."*

Moral: Example is the best precept.

Introduction

Preparing surgeons who excel across a number of domains is a priority for medical schools and residency programs, and this preparation is certainly an expectation of patients. The Accreditation Council for Graduate Medical Education (ACGME) has developed a number of milestones with the focus on developing "highly competent physicians to meet the 21st century health and health care needs of the public" [2] (p. 13). The Milestones Guidebook includes six competencies: patient care, medical knowledge, professionalism, interpersonal and communication skills, practice-based learning and improvement, and systems-based practice.

Given the life-and-death reality of the surgical environment and the surgeon's tremendous level of responsibility, it is hard to argue against expecting excellence across a number of competencies; however, the complex surgical learning environment may not be ideal for fostering student and resident growth across all

J.L. Koehler, PhD (✉)
Department of Medical Education, Southern Illinois University School of Medicine, Springfield, IL, USA
e-mail: jkoehler53@siumed.edu

E. Sturm, MD
Department of Surgery, Southern Illinois University School of Medicine, Springfield, IL, USA

T.S. Köhler, B. Schwartz (eds.), *Surgeons as Educators*,
https://doi.org/10.1007/978-3-319-64728-9_14

competencies. Gofton and Regehr [3] summarize characteristics of this taxing learning environment:

> *The context of surgical practice is not generally an easy environment in which to function. It is marked by stress, responsibility, and pressure. It requires the management of multiple inputs and demands during critically emergent situations. It is often performed under suboptimal psychomotor conditions of sleep deprivation or after previous tiring surgeries.* [3] *(p. 4)*

Not only is surgical practice a taxing learning environment, but also learners come into the environment performing at markedly different levels across the different targeted competencies. And certainly no one arrives to the surgical setting operating at peak performance in all areas. If our goal within surgical education is to ensure learners grow and develop the knowledge, skills, and attitudes needed to be effective surgeons, then education must be seen as a continuous process with learning as a social endeavor within the practice environment. Taking a process, continuous learning approach recognizes learners' differing performance levels, provides flexibility for the complexity of the surgical learning environment, and promotes the importance of ongoing, tailored, specific feedback across the competencies. Although this seems to be an insurmountable task within the busy surgical setting, creating a learning culture of mentoring and coaching within a workplace learning environment may help demonstrate that meaningful professional relationships are central for long-term growth and development in both life and work [3].

This chapter provides a brief overview of workplace learning, explores the roles of coaches and mentors within these environments, provides a brief overview of research around coaching and mentoring within surgical work environments, and offers pathways for building stronger cultures for coaching and mentoring. The chapter integrates a modern tale of a surgical resident to provide an example of how coaching and mentoring provide help within a very hectic workplace learning environment.

A Modern Tale of Surgical Mentoring and Coaching

Recently, a surgical resident experiencing a performance issue came into our medical education office. He explained, "I need help with my communication skills. I don't know what that means." Interestingly, this resident knew basic aspects of communication: speaking clearly, body language, and active listening. He also fully accepted communication was an area for improvement. However, prior feedback had been relatively vague, his awareness of his communication style within the fast-paced surgical environment was limited, and he was uncertain how to improve his performance. As the saying goes, we can't fix what we don't know is broken. Given his limited awareness of the specific performance gap, he was seeking an outside perspective to help. This resident's story is not unique, as many students and residents find themselves grappling with varying performance issues within the clinical learning environment. While not unique, this story does provide a practical example of how the role of mentors and coaches may enhance performance in the busy world of surgical education.

Workplace Learning

As medical students and residents become immersed in the clinical years, they transition from school-based learning environments into live, workplace learning environments. Traditionally, the basic science years align closely with school-based educational settings: classrooms, labs, self-directed/online learning time, and, for some, problem-based learning in teams and small groups. The learning structure in the basic science years is clearly defined (schedules, teacher directed), the knowledge is broken down into smaller chunks (units, classes), professors and/or tutors direct the learning process, and assessments are formal (tests, quizzes). The curriculum is carefully crafted, objectives are clearly defined, and evaluations of performance are standardized. When entering the clinical years, learning moves away from the clearly defined structures of school-based learning and into a more dynamic, less structured workplace learning environment. Some students and residents may have little prior experience learning "on the job." Workplace learning tends to be more process oriented, socially constructed, and ambiguous, and when learners enter the particularly demanding surgical context, they may need guides to help adjust to a more hands-on, relational approach to growth and development [3].

Researchers have explored the nature of workplace learning through a variety of lenses (e.g., workplace learning, action learning, situated learning, and learning organizations) [4–13]. While the lenses differ, the underlying arguments have similarities: people within work environments are constantly learning in both formal and informal ways [14]. The history of surgical education supports the idea that learning through the practice of work is central to developing the necessary knowledge, skills, and attitudes to become a surgeon. As a result, surgical education has heavily relied on an apprenticeship model. The student/resident is proximally close to an experienced surgeon who models, provides opportunities for practice, and, in time, oversees the growth from novice to competent to proficient [15]. The apprenticeship model might be questioned, and other models may have been offered, but what continues within surgical education is a commitment to learning in the workplace.

This chapter scratches the surface of workplace learning; however, other chapters may provide a more robust exploration. For this chapter, Billett [6] provides four premises in connection with learning in the healthcare workplace:

- Learning occurs all the time.
- Workers engage in work activities they also remake and potentially transform.
- As clinical knowledge is a product of history, culture, and situational requirements, it has to be accessed and engaged with to be secured by workers.
- Learning and development are two separate but interdependent processes.

Operating within the above premises, we argue, is the social and cultural nature of working with others. In the surgical workplace, rounding, sharing experiences, communicating with patients and families, making mistakes, and conducting team-based procedures are done with high levels of social interaction. For brevity, we will focus on Billet's final premise that aligns with Vygotsky's social development theory [16]. Learning is not necessarily development. For example, a student might learn a piece of knowledge, a skill, and even demonstrate he/she has learned it; however, he/she may not have developed proficiency or enhanced his/her skills as a result of that learning. To explore the separate but interdependent nature of learning and development, let's return to the resident who recognized a need to improve his communication skills.

A Modern Tale of Surgical Mentoring and Coaching (Cont.)

Through the ongoing performance review process, the resident found out his communication skills were an area of concern. Recognizing communication was an issue, he began to read articles and books about effective communication. When meeting with him, he demonstrated he knew the elements of effective communication. He explained that in the few weeks prior to reaching out, he tried implementing the strategies. With frustration, he shared he was continuing to struggle in the surgical setting and, in particular, when attending physicians were present. Learning about communication skills had provided knowledge; however, defining the skills was not sufficient for ***developing*** *communication skills within the context of the surgical workplace.*

Given the dynamics of the work environment, learning new concepts or trying to address competency gaps outside the application environment is not necessarily sufficient for improving performance. To learn and develop, individual engagement in the workplace setting must be part of the learning process. Billett [7] reviewed five different workplaces focusing on individual engagement at work. He found guided learning strategies including *modeling*, *mentoring*, *coaching*, *questioning*, *analogies*, and *diagrams* enhance learning and workplace performance.

If we accept guided learning strategies are important to improving performance, then better integrating them within surgical education is important. Coaches and mentors would play an important role in offering modeling, questioning, sharing analogies, and helping learners to diagram their progress. In the surgical workplace learning environment, residency program directors, attending surgeons, residents, students, nurses, and other key members of surgical teams are able to serve as coaches and mentors but would also receive benefits of being coached and mentored. To help medical learners with continuous learning and performance, an important step is to recognize and adopt guided learning strategies. Creating a culture of coaching and mentoring within surgical workplace learning environments embeds guided learning strategies in the natural flow of the workplace. When these professional learning relationships are closely connected to the needs of the learner (to grow, improve, address a shortcoming) and the emphasis is on continuous growth, problem solving, and ongoing development, an action learning environment is created [17]. Changing the learning cultural to actively include coaches and mentors may be difficult. Prior to moving forward, it is useful to define coaches and mentors and explore whether or not coaching and mentoring positively impacts performance.

Coaching and Mentoring: Definitions and Impacts

If asked, many of us would be able to identify someone who has coached us in our careers, and some of us would be able to identify someone who has served or is serving as a mentor. When discussing what exactly is a coach or mentor, it is easy to find a number of attributes that cross both mentors and coaches. As social beings, we come to rely on one another for friendship, safety, support, laughter, wisdom, and survival. This natural state of supportive interaction makes clearly delineating the lines between friend, teacher, guide, mentor, and coach difficult. Each of us may operate in any of those roles given the particular situation and time. Although difficult to distinguish between a coach and mentor within the surgical education environment, definitions, characteristics, and attributes help frame the purpose and nature of the different relationships [18–23].

	Coaching [18–20]	Mentoring [21–23]
Definition	A relationship "designed to improve existing skills, competence and performance, and to enhance their personal effectiveness or personal development or personal growth" [18]	"Is a dynamic, reciprocal relationship in a work environment between an advanced career incumbent (mentor) and a beginner (protege) aimed at promoting the career development of both" [23]
Typical characteristics of the relationship	Short term Task oriented Performance focused Strategist (may not have expertise in specific field) Promotes problem solving Focus is on skill development	Ongoing, long term Career and life focused Development focused Expert, respected in field Provides vision and advice Emphasis on a reciprocal relationship
Attributes of coach/mentor	Works to identify goals and needs of learner Engages in direct observation Provides specific performance feedback Collaborates with learner to create an action plan (verbal or written) Provides follow-up and ongoing assessment	Is committed and trustworthy Offers a vision and guidance Shares resources and wisdom Provides a network of support Encourages mentee's ideas and work Engages in constructive feedback Challenges mentees Acknowledges contributions Shares in success and benefits

With a clearer definition in place, the question becomes: Do coaches and mentors impact performance in the workplace and even more specifically in surgical education and academic medicine?

Benefits of Coaching and Mentoring

Recognizing that learning and development is situated in the workplace and is fostered through authentic relationships gives credence to the roles of coaching and mentoring. Having a mentor and/or coach impacts not only performance but also has positive impacts on other aspects of individual development. A meta-analysis of coaching scholarship indicates coaching has positive effects on individual-level outcomes that include performance/skills, well-being, coping, work attitudes, and goal-directed self-regulation [24]. Coaching, based on this analysis, is an important interventional strategy from a number of vantage points. In addition, coaching has a strong effect on changing behaviors [25]. It is no surprise that formalized coaching programs are being integrated in surgical programs to promote individual performance improvement [26]. And the concept of coaching has expanded beyond face-to-face coaching to include video-based coaching with the aim of improving surgical technical skills [27, 28]. Coaching is being implemented in varying ways and is proving to be useful in performance improvement.

Mentoring shares some similarities with coaching; however, it is more career and long-term focused. Within academic medicine and in surgical education, the importance of mentoring is emphasized, "Mentoring is essential to the complex professional and personal development of contemporary surgeons" [29] (p.717). In similar ways to coaching, mentoring has positive impacts within workplace learning. Mentoring can be split into two types, career and psychosocial, with career mentoring consisting of organizational, job specific, exposure, challenges, and protection. Psychosocial mentoring consists of role modeling, acceptance and confirmation, counseling, and friendship [30]. It is possible that a mentor offers both career and psychosocial mentoring at the same time. Or learner may seek out a psychosocial mentor from another department. For example, a surgical resident may seek out an attending in internal medicine because they have a similar background (cultural, ethnic, gender, family, religion, language), and their partnership provides a sense of comfort and friendship. Mentors may come within and beyond the surgical education setting. Based on a meta-analysis of both types of mentoring scholarship, mentoring research indicates: [31]

- Career mentoring has a correlation to compensation and promotion.
- Mentees involved with more psychosocial mentoring were more satisfied with the mentoring experience.
- Both forms of mentoring were connected with higher career and job satisfaction.
- Mentored versus nonmentored results revealed strong effects for career-specific variables such as career commitment, expectations for advancement, and career satisfaction.

In addition, mentoring, particularly in academic medical settings, appears to offer additional benefits. Impacts have included increasing organizational stability (sharing of institutional memory), assisting medical schools in recruiting and retaining new faculty members, addressing gender and cultural inequities, building scholarly productivity, and increasing medical students, residents, and faculty members with more personal development and career guidance [30–37]. In addition, surgical trainees who have participated in mentoring relationships have found them to be useful in the learning process [38]. A return to the story of the resident helps illustrate how both coaching and mentoring provide relationships that can help surgical residents and students improve their performance and develop competencies.

A Modern Tale of Mentoring and Coaching (Cont.)

During a meeting with his mentor, the surgical resident had shared his ongoing struggles around communication. The mentor recognized this resident would benefit from targeted coaching, and the mentor recommended visiting a coach (called a performance and learning strategist to help alleviate the stigma that sometimes comes with being coached). The surgical resident sought out the help of our learning and performance strategist, and the strategist began to serve as the resident's communication coach. The resident selected a day and asked the strategist to shadow him within the clinical setting. During the shadowing, the strategist took detailed field notes focusing on the resident's communication with nurses, peer residents, attending physicians, and patients. During the shadowing, the strategist served not as an evaluator but rather as an observer carefully watching and documenting interactions. During transition times, the strategist and resident talked about the resident's successes, frustrations, and background. After the visit, the resident and strategist went through the field notes. As the resident reviewed the notes with the strategist, he noticed areas of concern:

- *I walk away from people before finishing my sentences.*
- *I use a lot of qualifiers when attending physicians are present, and this reflects uncertainty even when I am certain.*
- *I didn't answer the intern's question and instead went on to a new topic.*

The resident also identified areas of strength:

- *I take my time when answering patient's questions.*
- *I am confident when explaining tough concepts to my peers.*
- *I value when peers raise different points of view.*

As the resident and strategist debrief continued, the two discussed approaches to addressing those areas the residents saw as areas of concern. He decided he would be mindful when speaking with others and ensure he kept eye contact until the end of the conversation. He planned to focus on using clear and concise language when talking with attending physicians, and he planned to get rid of statements of uncertainty in times of certainty such as, "I am not sure, maybe the issue might be, I can't be certain but." He would ask his peers to hold him accountable for not answering questions or going on without addressing a key issue.

The resident created a performance plan with the help of the coach and sat down with his mentor to review his plan of action. The mentor was able to offer additional guidance on strategies, and the mentor also shared stories of how he too continued to work on his communication. By the next performance cycle, the attending physicians had confidence the resident had gained proficiency in communication skills, and they commented on his marked improvement. At that point, the resident and the mentor continued to explore career progression as well as the resident's scholarship.

Embedding Coaching and Mentoring Within Surgical Education

If we accept that coaching and mentoring are vital to learning and developing within the complex surgical workplace, then we must identify ways in which to build coaching and mentoring experiences. At this time, a culture of mentoring and coaching is not yet a common practice in academic medicine. A systematic review of mentoring studies in academic medicine indicates that fewer than 50% of medical students and 20% of faculty members have mentors [34]. If access to coaches and mentors within surgical education aligns with the prior research in academic medicine and coaching and mentoring seems to positively impact performance across different competencies, then it is easy to see why surgical education faculty and leaders may want to implement strategies to develop coaching and mentoring relationships in surgical education.

Before rushing to establish formal coaching and mentoring programs, it is important to recognize that ideal coaching and mentoring relationships are *organic*, *purposeful*, and *reciprocal*. Creating a program in which mentors or coaches are assigned externally tends to be less successful than programs in which the coaches, mentors, and learners are actively involved in establishing the partnerships. When mentors, coaches, and learners have few shared interests with each other, they are placed in awkward situations, and the connection suffers from an artificial arrangement. Mandatory assignments make it difficult to find a topic, purpose, or shared connection to discuss. Assigning mentors mandatorily is attractive as this approach ensures every learner is matched with a coach or mentor, but that is often where the benefits of mandatory assignments end.

Building formal coaching/mentoring programs often starts with reflecting on the current organizational structure and culture. When integrating coaching/mentoring, having a deep understanding of the organizational environment is imperative. This includes but is not limited to the culture, work flows, system design, and reward structures [39, 40]. A few questions to consider are as follows:

- Is mentoring and coaching already happening? Where is it happening? How is it working?
- Who is taking an active role as a coach and/or mentor? What qualities do they possess? What do learners say about being coached and mentored?
- What resources do students, residents, and faculty members access when they need help or assistance? Who is providing help when students, residents, and faculty members face difficulty?
- What perception do our students, residents, and faculty members have about coaching and mentoring? Is it seen as continuous learning or remediation?
- Are those who serve as coaches and mentors rewarded? If so, how? If mentoring and coaching is currently limited or missing, how would coaches and mentors be rewarded?

While specific frameworks and models of mentoring and coaching programs have been offered, it is important to develop mentoring/coaching strategies that closely align within one's department and organization [26, 39, 40, 41]. Having varying mentoring/coaching models makes it difficult to research mentoring and coaching organizations; however, ensuring mentoring and coaching relationships are embedded with the surgical workplace learning environment is the greater priority.

In order for mentoring and coaching to work well, a supportive culture needs to be in place. In a supportive culture, learners inherently have opportunities to connect with mentors and coaches. Given the depth of competencies required of future surgeons, surgical learners need access to a wide range of coaches and mentors with varying skill sets. By having wide range of access to coaches and mentors, learners will be able to align their experiences with their goals as well as build both formal and informal relationships focused on development. Depending on the current culture of the surgical setting, the process for building a mentoring and coaching program may range from a relatively natural transition to a more difficult, cumbersome process. There are a few strategies that can help create and/or bolster a mentoring and coaching program.

Find Advocates and Leaders for Coaching and Mentoring Most leaders are motivated to ensure their students, residents, and faculty members are performing at their best. Deans, department chairs, program directors, and teaching faculty members serve as the leadership backbone of surgical education. In order to create a successful mentoring and coaching culture, generating their buy-in for coaching and mentoring is a must. To build a case for the power of mentoring and coaching, the existing research around the impacts of coaching and mentoring is a good place to start. Some of this research has been briefly referred to within this chapter, but the chapter does not provide an exhaustive literature review. Exploring and sharing the literature around coaching and mentoring often generates interest. In addition, most people have stories in which a coach and/or mentor served a pivotal role in their personal and professional development. When people recognize the role coaching and mentoring played in their own success, they often want to create the same kind of learning opportunities for others. Facilitating conversations around coaching and mentoring in existing committee meetings, during casual hallway conversations, and through formal one-to-one appointments is a good way to find those who will advocate and lead coaching and mentoring initiatives. In addition, these conversations generate interest and provide insight into people who are interested in being a coach and/or mentor. For mentoring/coaching programs to last, there needs to be a champion who will move through the next steps. Identifying who (person, committee, department) will be responsible for having an ongoing commitment to mentoring and coaching is a priority.

Provide Training and Development Around Coaching, Mentoring, and Coachability The research on mentoring and coaching has led to the creation of a wide range of training programs that help prepare people to coach and mentor others. Prior to integrating coaching and mentoring in a formal sense, a wise strategy is to offer training for students, residents, and faculty members. It is important for the organization to pick the coaching/mentoring training program that fits best or to design a training program that matches the organizational needs. Regardless, coaching and mentoring training should:

- Set shared expectations of the different roles.
- Clarify responsibilities and desired outcomes.
- Provide strategies and tips for fostering successful relationships.
- Create a learning environment in which coaching and mentoring is central.
- Identify questions and concerns so program can be modified and adapted to fit organizational needs.
- Communicate approaches to use if the partnership is not working.

Plan for Difficulties and Be Prepared to Handle Mentoring and coaching are built around people building working relationships with one another. Conflict, communication breakdown, and discomfort with the partnership do happen (as they do with all relationships). Mentors, coaches, and learners all need to know how to handle when partnerships are not working well. With any coaching/mentoring program, there needs to be steps for how to discontinue a partnership in a professional, safe way. Thinking through how this can be handled ahead of time and communicating that thoroughly can mitigate the negative effects of a failed partnership.

Create Mentor and Coach Profiles and Share Those Broadly Once coaches and mentors are trained, the next step is to make students, residents, and faculty members aware of who is willing to serve as a coach and mentor. Some organizations create profiles that are specifically focused on how a person can serve as a coach and/or mentor. Profiles may include interests, specific skill sets, and career aspirations. The profile allows for students to identify people within the greater organization that align with their goals, interests, and learning needs. In addition, these profiles help departmental mentors and leaders identify potential connections for coaching. The sharing of these profiles broadly allows for those newer to the organization to find resources and form connections more quickly.

Model an Inquiry Mindset That Integrates Coaching and Mentoring at All Levels With this step, we return to our beginning fable. We tend to follow the habits of our role models. If our role models are not focused on continuous development through coaching and mentoring, then the chances are their learners will not perceive coaching and mentoring as an important aspect of ongoing development and improved performance. The idea that we may need a coach or mentor may be perceived as having a weakness that needs remediated. This negative perception can ruin mentoring and coaching before these relationships ever get going. If those in positions of leadership (residents, attending, directors, department chairs) model the importance of continuous improvement through engaging with coaches and mentors, then those at the other levels of the organization will follow suit. While it might be difficult for leaders to model individual coaching/mentoring, they can do so through a group approach to adopting a coach or mentor. Let's say a surgical team faces a problem within the clinical setting (teamwork, workflow, communication, and performance). The attending decides to use an inquiry mindset to explore the problem and seeks out the help of a coach/mentor at the group level. The team could collectively work with the coach/mentor to demonstrate how coaching and mentoring can help impact performance. Incorporating the process of coaching and mentoring within the workplace learning environment helps to solidify a coaching and mentoring culture.

Assess Mentoring and Coaching and Modify as Needed As with any aspect of surgical education, it is important to assess and measure the impact coaching and mentoring is having within the learning environment. This may not mean creating a completely separate assessment. If an organization does yearly evaluations (student/resident evaluations, employee satisfaction surveys), then adding additional questions around coaching and mentoring is a simple step. In addition to asking survey questions about coaching and mentoring, continuing to have conversations about coaching and mentoring at the individual, departmental, and organizational level can provide insight and ideas on how to continue to improve coaching and mentoring.

Summary

In a property insurance workplace learning environment, a much different setting than surgical education, the education department had a motto to encourage educational innovation, "Go ahead and give it a try, we aren't flying planes around here." This statement reflects the learners were in a workplace environment where they could try a number of different educational strategies and no one would be hurt. *This is not the case in surgical education.* Surgeons, surgical residents, and surgical students have patient lives in their hands. To correct this saying for surgical education, "We are flying planes around here." With such important stakes in the workplace learning environment, the educational strategies and innovations need to be closely connected to the workplace environment, based on evidence of positive impact on performance, and situated in a supportive culture of learning. Mentoring and coaching can provide authentic relationships that are closely aligned with the performance needs and goals of our learners. Creating a robust coaching and mentoring program means learners have access to a wide range of coaches and mentors that can connect with the competencies and milestones of becoming a high performing surgeon: patient care, medical knowledge, professionalism, interpersonal and communication skills, practice-based learning and improvement, and systems-based practice. The surgical workplace learning environment is rigorous, demanding, and stressful. A culture of mentoring and coaching provides a social support system for those experiencing one of the most challenging learning environments. In addition, mentoring and coaching models learning as a lifelong endeavor in which social, workplace relationships help us not only learn but also develop.

References

1. Aesop, Griset E. Aesop's fables. New York: Fall River Press; 2010.
2. Holmboe ES, Edgar L, Hamstra CS. The milestones guidebook. American Council of Graduate Medical Education; 2016.
3. Gofton W, Regehr G. Factors in optimizing the learning environment for surgical training. Clin Orthop Relat Res. 2006;449:100–7.
4. Billett S. Towards a model of workplace learning: the learning curriculum. Stud Contin. 1996;18(1):43–58.
5. Billett S. Constituting the workplace curriculum. J Curric Stud. 2006;38(1):31–48.
6. Billett S. Learning through health care work: premises, contributions and practices. Med Educ. 2016;50(1):124–31.
7. Billett S. Learning through work: workplace affordances and individual engagement. J Work Learn. 2001;13(5):209–14.
8. Hager P. Current theories of workplace learning: a critical assessment. Int handb Educ Policy. 2005;1:829–46.
9. Lave J, Wenger E. Situated learning: legitimate peripheral participation. Cambridge: Cambridge university press; 1991.
10. Revans RW. What is action learning? J Manag Dev. 1982;1(3):64–75.
11. Marsick VJ, O'Neil J. The many faces of action learning. Manag Learn. 1999;30(2):159–76.
12. Marsick VJ, Watkins KE. Demonstrating the value of an organization's learning culture: the dimensions of the learning organization questionnaire. Adv Dev Hum Resour. 2003;5(2):132–51.
13. Yang B, Watkins KE, Marsick VJ. The construct of the learning organization: dimensions, measurement, and validation. Hum Resour Dev Q. 2004;15(1):31–55.
14. Marsick VJ, Watkins KE. Informal and incidental learning. NewDir Adult Contin Educ. 2001;2001(89):25–34.
15. Dunphy BC, Williamson SL. In pursuit of expertise. Toward an educational model for expertise development. Adv Health Sci Educ. 2004;9(2):107–27.
16. Vygotsky L. Interaction between learning and development. Readings Dev Children. 1978;23(3):34–41.
17. Pedler M. Action learning in practice. Surrey: Gower Publishing Ltd; 2011.
18. Hamlin RG, Ellinger AD, Beattie RS. The emergent 'coaching industry': a wake-up call for HRD professionals. Hum Resour Dev Int. 2008;11(3):287–305.
19. Marsick VJ, Watkins K. Informal and incidental learning in the workplace (Routledge revivals). New York: Routledge; 2015.
20. Eraut M. Learning from other people in the workplace. Oxf Rev Educ. 2007;33(4):403–22.
21. Healy CC, Welchert AJ. Mentoring relations: a definition to advance research and practice. Educ Res. 1990;19(9):17–21.
22. Daloz LA. Mentor: guiding the journey of adult learners (with new foreword, introduction, and afterword). San Francisco: Wiley; 2012.
23. Berk RA, Berg J, Mortimer R, Walton-Moss B, Yeo TP. Measuring the effectiveness of faculty mentoring relationships. Acad Med. 2005;80(1):66–71.
24. Theeboom T, Beersma B, van Vianen AE. Does coaching work? A meta-analysis on the effects of coaching on individual level outcomes in an organizational context. J Posit Psychol. 2014;9(1):1–8.
25. Sonesh SC, Coultas CW, Lacerenza CN, Marlow SL, Benishek LE, Salas E. The power of coaching: a meta-analytic investigation. Coaching: An Int J Theory, Res Pract. 2015;8(2):73–95.
26. Greenberg CC, Ghousseini HN, Quamme SR, Beasley HL, Wiegmann DA. Surgical coaching for individual performance improvement. Ann Surg. 2015;261(1):32–4.
27. Hu YY, Peyre SE, Arriaga AF, Osteen RT, Corso KA, Weiser TG, Swanson RS, Ashley SW, Raut CP, Zinner MJ, Gawande AA. Postgame analysis: using video-based coaching for continuous professional development. J Am Coll Surg. 2012;214(1):115–24.

28. Singh P, Aggarwal R, Tahir M, Pucher PH, Darzi A. A randomized controlled study to evaluate the role of video-based coaching in training laparoscopic skills. Ann Surg. 2015;261(5):862–9.
29. Sanfey H, Hollands C, Gantt NL. Strategies for building an effective mentoring relationship. Am J Surg. 2013;206(5):714–8.
30. Zellers DF, Howard VM, Barcic MA. Faculty mentoring programs: reenvisioning rather than reinventing the wheel. Rev Educ Res. 2008;78(3):552–88.
31. Allen TD, Eby LT, Poteet ML, Lentz E, Lima L. Career benefits associated with mentoring for protégés: a meta-analysis. J Appl Psychol. 2004;89(1):127–36.
32. Mark S, Link H, Morahan PS, Pololi L, Reznik V, Tropez-Sims S. Innovative mentoring programs to promote gender equity in academic medicine. Acad Med. 2001;76(1):39–42.
33. Sambunjak D, Straus SE, Marusic A. A systematic review of qualitative research on the meaning and characteristics of mentoring in academic medicine. J Gen Intern Med. 2010;25(1):72–8.
34. Sambunjak D, Straus SE, Marušić A. Mentoring in academic medicine: a systematic review. JAMA. 2006;296(9):1103–15.
35. Straus SE, Chatur F, Taylor M. Issues in the mentor–mentee relationship in academic medicine: a qualitative study. Acad Med. 2009;84(1):135–9.
36. Straus SE, Johnson MO, Marquez C, Feldman MD. Characteristics of successful and failed mentoring relationships: a qualitative study across two academic health centers. Acad Med: J Assoc Am Med Coll. 2013;88(1):82.
37. Straus SE, Graham ID, Taylor M, Lockyer J. Development of a mentorship strategy: a knowledge translation case study. J Contin Educ Heal Prof. 2008;28(3):117–22.
38. Hauer KE, Teherani A, Dechet A, Aagaard EM. Medical students' perceptions of mentoring: a focus-group analysis. Med Teach. 2005;27(8):732–4.
39. Sambunjak D. Understanding wider environmental influences on mentoring: towards an ecological model of mentoring in academic medicine. Acta medica academica. 2015;44(1):47.
40. Sinclair P, Fitzgerald JE, Hornby ST, Shalhoub J. Mentorship in surgical training: current status and a needs assessment for future mentoring programs in surgery. World J Surg. 2015;39(2):303–13.
41. Klinge CM. A conceptual framework for mentoring in a learning organization. Adult Learn. 2015;26(4):160–6.

Optimizing Research in Surgical Residents and Medical Students

15

Danuta I. Dynda, Bradley Holland, and Tobias S. Köhler

Introduction

Excuse me Doctor, how can I get involved in research?

Residents and medical students pose this question to faculty at medical schools and residency programs across the country. Research is quickly becoming a strongly recommended option for medical students and an outright requirement in medical schools, surgical residencies, and fellowship programs throughout the United States [1]. In the ever-increasing competitive environment for residency, fellowship, and academic positions in general surgery and especially its varying subspecialties, research has become the go-to option for gaining that competitive edge for these highly sought-after positions. The first challenge is to inspire surgical trainees to utilize and amplify their natural curiosity. The next challenge is to find the right research opportunities within their respective departments and institutions while having actual time to commit to these projects without hurting other aspects of their training (i.e., class load and rotations). The final challenge remains on how to go about conducting this research with the appropriate training and oversight so as to produce a timely, quality finished product that is publishable or presentable without violating any rules.

D.I. Dynda, MD (✉) • B. Holland, MD
Division of Urology/Center for Clinical Research,
Southern Illinois University School of Medicine,
301 N. 8th Street, 4th Floor, Springfield, IL 62794-9665, USA
e-mail: ddynda@siumed.edu

T.S. Köhler, MD, MPH
Urology, Mayo Clinic, Rochester, MN, USA

T.S. Köhler, B. Schwartz (eds.), *Surgeons as Educators*,
https://doi.org/10.1007/978-3-319-64728-9_15

Inspiring Research

Whatever you can do, or dream you can, begin it: boldness has genius, power and magic in it. W.H. Murray

The earth used to be flat and was located at the center of the universe, and smoking used to be good for you. Without curiosity, questioning of the status quo, and the scientific method, we still might believe the previous lists were true. Anyone who has children knows they are naturally curious, often asking *why*? a bewildering amount of times consecutively. What happens to this natural curiosity as we age and become capable of answering some of these questions for ourselves? Surgical trainees are some of the most hardworking and intelligent humans on the planet. How can we help (re)foster their natural curiosity and inspire them to try to answer questions they are passionate about?

Other chapters in this textbook demonstrate the power of culture in an organization. Is the culture in your department one of intellectual curiosity? Does the faculty lead by example and attempt and accomplish noteworthy research? Surgical trainees should be taught to question what they are taught. A flattened hierarchy where this type of questioning is allowed improves patient care and stimulates the intellectual curiosity from everyone. What are the scholarly requirements for your department? Our division currently requires one prepared manuscript submitted for publication per resident per year along with mandatory abstract submissions and presentations in our local and regional meetings. There is a rich history of surgical education culture at Southern Illinois University School of Medicine (SIUSOM) – starting with its founders declaring it as a core value. SIUSOM holds annual internal surgical research days where research is acknowledged and celebrated. Competitions and awards for best research are given to faculty (junior and senior), residents and fellows, and medical students. Does your department create the means and opportunity to do research for faculty and surgical trainees? How is research production rewarded or compensated? SIUSOM was determined to try to balance academic accomplishments in research and teaching with clinical productivity To accomplish this, the Academic Incentive Program (AIP) was created [2]. In brief, this system utilized a list of teaching, research, and academic service activities with which full-time faculty used to report activities. Clinical faculty members received incentive income based on credits earned based on 5% of practice plan receipts. Similar successful systems have been developed at other institutions.

Dr. Donald Coffey, Professor of Urology, Oncology, and Pharmacology at Johns Hopkins University School of Medicine, poses his “real final exam” to any student, resident, or fellow that has come through his laboratory or classroom with the hope that it will provoke their scientific thought process and serve as a guide in research and in life [3]. He states:

I have no more insight into science than many others; I was just naïve enough to list the obvious to which most of us are blinded because of measurements by false yardstick and examples which are always in vogue. I know that with time you can expand and improve your own list. In my weakness, I give students so many sheets or handouts of useless data to memorize that I thought a few important concepts might be worth sharing with you.

It consists of the following questions and statements upon which he elaborates (we highly recommend you read the entire original version which elaborates upon all of the bulleted points and contains inspirational wisdom).

- *If this is true, what does it imply?*
- *Generate more than one concept to explain your data and then give all possibilities equal attention and effort.*
- *You don't have to assume anything that you can prove.*
- *The experiment that didn't come out the way you thought it would is the only experiment that is really going to teach you something new.*
- *Every datum is screaming to tell you something, but you must do the listening and thinking.*
- *What you are thinking about while you are coming to work determines your real interest and will direct your accomplishments for the day.*
- *A complex experiment is usually the least productive.*
- *It is time to do some experiments; others must wait.*
- *You are going to be surprised at the simplicity and beauty of the real answer.*
- *All new ideas are resisted by you, authorities, the editors, study sections, department chairmen, peers, and friends. If this discourages you, you should retire early. However, most criticism can be constructive if you listen with an open mind.*
- *A good paper is simple, clear, and to the point.*
- *If two good investigators disagree and a paradox seems to exist, both of their data are probably correct, and we just need a new explanation to encompass both observations.*
- *Give everyone credit.*
- *Do not be fooled by the authority of the printed page.*
- *Many bright people are paralyzed by negative thinking.*
- *The most important ingredients are honesty, desire, clear thinking, confidence, and hardwork.*

Dr. Coffey concludes his article with:

> *If you are lucky, the world will be paying you a modest salary for what you consider your hobby, and you, in turn, will be contributing to some important answers for our present and future society. As you teach and lead, you will amplify your efforts and those of others, and if appropriate, the influence will continue after you cease. What you learn from courses, lectures and books that are reflected in your course grades will be a very small faction of your FINAL EXAM. Good luck in your careers.*

Finding the Right Research Project

> *Try to learn something about everything and everything about something. Thomas Henry Huxley*

Residents

The Accreditation Council for Graduate Medical Education (ACGME) has outlined requirements for scholarly activity and changed the focus from structure and process to tangible scholarly outcomes in 2013 [4]. The requirements differ between specialties based on the ACGME specialty-specific references for Designated Institutional Officials (DIO), but there are three consistent requirements across all specialties and subspecialties [1]:

- *The curriculum must advance residents' knowledge of the basic principles of research, including how research is conducted, evaluated, explained to patients, and applied to patient care.*
- *Residents should participate in scholarly activity.*
- *The sponsoring institution and program should allocate adequate educational resources to facilitate resident involvement in scholarly activity.*

These ACGME requirements have forced institutions to implement policies requiring that all residents complete at least one research project in some kind of capacity during the tenure of their training [1]. Some program requirements may go beyond the basic minimum. In order to help facilitate this requirement, some of these programs provide designated or protected research time which can range from a 1 month research-only rotation, a full research year, to just protected time incorporated into each week [5, 6].

Residents seek to do research for three primary reasons. First, they do it to fulfill their ACGME and institutional requirements for their postgraduate training, usually resulting in a one-and-done project. Second, they want to further specialize and will apply to fellowship programs or to an academic position and know that the more research they do the greater likelihood of being accepted to their top institutions. Finally, they have a genuine interest in research and answering questions that are posed to them or they see as being recurrent in their training and want to strive to seek out those answers.

Medical Students

The Association of American Medical Colleges (AAMC) conducted a survey in 2012–2013 asking all medical schools whether or not they have a research requirement for students. Of the 136 schools that responded, 49 medical schools confirmed a research requirement [7]. The types of research allowed to fulfill the requirement included basic science, biology/chemistry/physics, bioengineering/informatics, clinical, translational, public health/health services, or ethics/humanities/social sciences. The survey showed an even distribution among students on when they conducted the research throughout the 4 years, including a fifth category designated for the time frame between the first and second year.

As medical students pass through their 4 years of schooling, they must decide which specialty they want to go into. If they choose to go into general surgery, or some of its subspecialties like orthopedics, urology, and ophthalmology, the level of competitiveness intensifies with each level of subspecialty. Through the years students have sought out varying ways to differentiate themselves from the pack with ever-increasing USMLE scores, high-honoring courses, doing volunteer work, and taking on research. The USMLE scores average above 230 (out of a 192 pass) if not into the 250s and beyond in order to increase ones chances to obtain a surgical specialty residency [8, 9]. The 2016 National Resident Matching Program (NRMP) charting outcomes report verified that those allopathic seniors matching into the surgical specialties had two to three times as many abstracts, presentations, and publications than nonsurgical with specialties with up to 13 recorded research activities on average [9]. Those students who matched into surgical specialties also produced more research than those who did not match into the same specialty [9]. With only 49 medical schools requiring research programs and with NRMP reports, students are often left to fend for themselves in finding research opportunities at their perspective schools in order to enhance their residency applications to obtain a residency position in their desired field of medicine.

It is often used as a means of gaining a competitive edge for medical students hoping to obtain residency positions in the surgical disciplines, surgical residents planning further fellowship training, or fellows and residents seeking academic positions upon completion of training.

Types of Research

Research is difficult to define because it is in itself a broad topic and can be conducted in a myriad of ways. When focused within the realm of medicine, there is still a plethora of options that fellows, residents, and students can choose to get involved in. As the AAMC reported in their 2012–2013 survey, students conducted research in a variety of fields including the basic sciences, informatics, clinical, translational, and epidemiological. Below we will outline the types of projects that medical students and residents alike could participate in.

Benchtop Research

Depending on the institution, basic science laboratory work may be an option for conducting research. Some surgeons may have their own laboratories, or residents/students can approach faculty in departments like microbiology and immunology, pharmacy, and physics, in order to help in their laboratories. Benchtop research can seem daunting and difficult to initiate from the perspective of a medical student or resident. It comes with its own set of difficulties involving biohazard training, animal handling training, and Institutional Animal Care and Use Committees (IACUCs) submissions. Another difficulty with benchtop research is the inherent cost factor with regard to laboratory space, materials, animals, and their associated costs. Many students and residents often join an already established laboratory to assist in ongoing projects or add to the concepts already being conducted in the laboratories. A simple google search identifies a plethora of research summer programs ranging for 4–6 weeks and even up to 1 year in length that are available for medical students. Residents, when conducting benchtop research, often join the laboratory of a faculty member or use their facilities to conduct their research.

Case Reports

Case reports are easy ways for students and residents to delve into the foray of scholarly activity. We advise our students to offer up their services in writing up a case report any time they hear a physician say "*well I have never seen that before*" or "*that's interesting!*" Case reports are usually simple write-ups of 1–3 cases that do not require institutional review board (IRB) involvement since they do not meet the Common Rule [10] definition of research (a systemic investigation, including research development, testing, and evaluation designed to develop or contribute to generalizable knowledge). Of note, many publications are starting to require some form of letter or acknowledgment from the IRB or the actual patient before publishing the case report. Case reports are a great introduction because they have minimal IRB involvement, still require a thorough literature review, initiate critical thinking in requiring a thorough review of a patient chart in order to parse out the necessary information, and provide exposure to the manuscript writing and submission process.

Retrospective Chart Reviews

Retrospective chart reviews are great research projects for medical students and residents alike. It is a widely used methodology that is applied in many healthcare-based disciplines [11, 12]. They involve critical thinking and planning along with exposure to actual protocol development. Chart reviews most often provide exposure to exempt and expedited IRB submissions and the intricacies of the consent waiver process. They allow for the residents/students to identify their own questions and, through the review process and subsequent analysis, obtain an answer. They are also a great starting point to obtain preliminary data that can result in further studies. Conducting chart reviews also provides exposure to the creation of databases and the application of statistical analysis of the extracted data.

Quality Outcomes

In the late 1990s, quality outcomes studies became a hot topic and have evolved into a necessary part of most medical practices and hospital administrations. The main goal of outcomes studies is to enhance good outcomes and diminish bad ones. Outcomes studies can be further categorized into the following categories: morbidity, mortality, pain, functional status, satisfaction, and costs [13]. Quality outcomes do not require IRB approval because their main goal is not to create generalizable data but to acquire information that will impact and influence local practice. However, a research determination should be submitted to the IRB to verify that the quality outcomes study is indeed not human subject research. These determinations are required by most publications, and most IRBs will not produce such a determination after the fact. The vast majority of quality outcomes studies are performed as retrospective chart reviews of already recorded medical records, although they can be designed to be prospective. Quality outcomes are not only conducted in hospital and academic institutions, but they are also necessary for private practices since the passing of the Affordable Care Act since reimbursement is now also associated with high-quality services [14].

Prospective Randomized

Prospective randomized studies are more complex endeavors that require extensive literature review, detailed protocol development, and, depending on the risk to patients, a potential full IRB review. They also require a greater time commitment during the hours of business to allow for not only screening but also to be able to meet with patients to conduct the consenting process. For residents/students, prospective randomized trials are more feasible if there is an extended frame of time dedicated to research. Multicenter randomized clinical trials (RCTs) fall into this category. Although residents and students have limited exposure as to their involvement in RCTs because of their ever-changing schedules and rotations, they can witness and obtain experience to such studies if they are conducted in any departments through which they rotate or train in. All RCTs also have an added complexity involving confidentiality clauses requiring stringent lists of the associated research personnel allowed access to the study with great regulatory effort needed to add and remove personnel, thus limiting rotating residents and students in the possibilities of fully participating in them.

Population Studies

Population studies are the current "hot" topic in research. These studies are used to measure the impact of an intervention in a particular population (i.e., minorities, women, rural vs. urban). They help to define if disparities exist between different populations and if interventions need to be adjusted in order to bridge these disparities. The National Institutes for Health (NIH) and office of disease prevention has identified six population studies [15] and has over 50 funding opportunities pertaining to a search on disparities alone [16, 17]. Population studies do require IRB involvement, but they, depending on the study design, can fall into exempt, expedite, and full board review categories.

Regulations and Research Training

In order to conduct any research, certifications, orientations, and other trainings are required. They are based on federal, state, local, and often institutional policies put in place to protect both researchers and their subjects whether human or animal. Residents and students must make sure to familiarize themselves with all of these prior to conducting any research.

Regulatory and Administrative Rules

The Office of Human Research Protections (OHRP) is a subsidiary of the US Department of Health and Human Services (HHS). Their main purpose is to provide guidance on ethical and regulatory issues in biomedical and behavioral research and protecting human subjects in research. They offer compliance and reporting with regard to regulatory oversight and reports of incidents. OHRP is also the registering body of IRBs [18].

The Federal Drug Administration (FDA) and HHS define an IRB as an "appropriately constituted group that has been formally designated to review and monitor biomedical research involving human subjects" [19]. Under FDA regulations, IRBs have the authority to approve, modify, monitor, or outright reject research projects if they are deemed dangerous for patients. The IRB is the regulatory body that most residents/students will submit research proposals to before conducting their research. From anecdotal experience, the IRB is also the research organization that may provide them with the most frustrations in the research process. IRBs are often local as part of the medical school or academic institution. One city can have multiple IRBs located at collaborating institutions and hospitals which can either have an agreement that an approval at one is honored at all or each collaborating institution where the research will take place requires a separate IRB review and approval, greatly increasing the work required in the submission process and can delay the start of a research project. At some institutions, especially with regard to multicenter clinical trials, a central IRB can be utilized for research review.

Besides IRB review, some institutions may require additional administration sign-offs from department chairs, associate deans for research, medical student affairs, or other departments prior to starting any research. Depending on the type of research project, these administrative webs can be difficult to navigate without significant time and effort to assure all the necessary parties have been notified. Any animal studies require review by the institutional IACUC committee with extensive detail required by the investigator to identify every detail of research details involving animals.

Formal Research Training and Certifications

Prior to conducting any research, all IRBs and IACUCs require some form of certification and/or training. IACUC certification at the least requires animal handlers' training conducted through the institution where the research will be conducted. IRBs require completion of a certification course on at least human subject research that lasts for a 2–3-year term, after which renewal courses are completed to keep up the certifications. With research becoming more of a requirement than an option, most institutions instruct residents and students to complete or renew (if expiring shortly) their research training at the start of their school and residency programs.

The overwhelming majority of research training is conducted through the Collaborative Institutional Training Initiative (CITI Program) founded in March 2000 [20]. Institutions register with the CITI Program and choose which modules and courses they want made available to their researchers; these courses include but are not limited to animal care and use, biosafety and biosecurity, conflicts of interest, good clinical practice (GCP), good laboratory practice, information privacy and security, responsible conduct of research, and human subject research. The human subject research course is the base requirement needed to able to conduct the majority of clinical research outlined in this chapter. All of these courses are conducted online at www.citiprogram.org and include modules consisting of reading followed by quizzes that require a minimum of 80% passing to achieve certification.

There are several other training opportunities available to help learn about the theoretical concepts on conducting research. Some institutions hold annual clinical research training seminars that they provide instruction and insight for young investigators or new (to the institution) investigators [21]. The NIH office of extramural research offers an online course on protecting human research participants at https://phrp.nihtraining.com as well as providing training courses for their own investigators. The FDA collaborates with the NIH on the training offered online. For students and residents with a burning desire to earn a more formal research education, there are opportunities for the completion of a certificate in clinical research (usually 1 year programs) or masters in research [22, 23].

Even with all of the required training and optional graduate level research training available, as with any discipline and especially medicine, learning and reading are not the same as actually conducting it.

Executing Research

For every complex problem there is a simple answer, and it is wrong. H.L. Mencken

Collecting the information may be the easiest part of any research project. The most difficult aspects are coming up with the question, designing the study, analyzing the data appropriately, and having enough time to do it in. The ultimate goal is to produce a timely, quality finished product that is publishable or presentable without violating any rules.

The Logistics

After research training is completed and a question has been identified, the actual process to set up the study has to begin. After a thorough literature review is conducted to verify that the question posed is novel, a protocol must be written. Case reports aside, a protocol (templates available with most IRBs) should include objectives, background, study design, methods, data analysis, inclusion and exclusion, identified research team (if necessary), and a clear outline of data points to be collected. A carefully crafted research protocol in the beginning produces approximately three quarters of the manuscript required at completion. Care must be taken to review the study methodology so as to not to fall into some common mistakes that are often identified (especially in retrospective chart reviews) in the peer review process [11] listed below:

- *Ill-defined and poorly-articulated research questions*
- *Failure to consider sampling size and strategy*
- *Inadequate operationalization of variables in the study*
- *Failure to clearly train and monitor data abstractors, as well as identifying how many were involved in the project*
- *Not using standard abstraction forms*
- *Not providing adequate instruction for data abstraction*
- *Poorly developed inclusion/exclusion criteria*
- *Not addressing interrater and intra-rater reliability*
- *Not performing a pilot test*
- *Failure to address confidentiality and ethical considerations*

Upon submission to and eventual approval from the IRB, clear communication between the research team needs to become a regular occurrence in order to allow for troubleshooting; even the most brilliantly written protocols may require amendments when actually carrying out the protocol. There needs to be open communication that allows for immediate correction of any issues. Better to ask and correct right away, then not ask, complete the data collection incorrectly, and find out at the end. Regular communications will also allow for progression of the study, preventing the study from limping toward a finish line at a snail's pace.

The Limitations

There are several limitations when conducting research with residents and medical students. As mentioned already, attempting to involve residents/students in randomized clinical trials comes with increased regulatory effort by research coordinators and logistical difficulty with a monthly rotation schedule offering little benefit for all parties involved. When possible, students and residents should be made aware of RCTs taking place and be provided with brief overviews of the studies along with the option to witness the consenting process.

Some study projects may not be feasible because they have costs required to complete the project. Funding is a common issue in carrying out basic science research, which often come with built-in costs to cover, at least materials (i.e., test tubes and pipettes) and, at most, extremely costly reagents, animals with required boarding costs, and either purchased or rented equipment. Funding has become a serious issue in today's political and economic environment. As an example, the NIH budget is a clear indicator as to the chance that research will be funded. Since 2003, the rate of funding has steadily declined from upward of 30% down to 17% in 2013 [24]. What has not decreased, is the number of investigators seeking funding. The decrease in funding opportunities at the NIH has forced all investigators to seek funding from other external sources forcing a highly competitive application process with most external funding opportunities.

Lack of institutional support from administration and/or faculty is another limitation. Few things are more frustrating to a student or resident, than to be given couple sentences of a research concept and left on their own to complete said project only to then be asked months later where the completed manuscript is. Another difficulty with faculty is the potential to delay progression of the study, especially in the manuscript phase, due to a hectic schedule. Residents and medical students also want to see studies come to an end in order to provide the all-important outcome of the research project which will help them to fulfill requirements or become more competitive candidates of residency and fellowship.

The biggest limitation to conducting research with residents and medical students is time. Residents and medical students have already strained schedules filled with classes, clinical rotations, call, and, in the case of surgery, procedures that fill their days, nights, and some weekends. On top of that, residents are limited in the amount of hours they are allowed to work, and both students and residents must continue to study in preparation for USMLE and in-service exams. Some programs offer research electives for students and designated research-only rotations for residents (1–2 months). There are research internships available to medical students, most commonly between their first and second years, which allow for a 4–8-week exposure to research ranging from benchtop research to translational exposure [25, 26]. The problem with the vast majority of research projects is that they cannot be accomplished in a 1–2-month time frame. Even these summer research internship programs acknowledge in their application process that this short time may not be enough to complete a project. Sometimes the IRB process can alone take multiple months to complete before final approval is obtained.

Research Infrastructure

Although the ACGME focus has shifted from structure and process to scholarly activity outcomes (i.e., abstracts, presentations, publications), structure and process have to be in place to facilitate the outcomes as does committed mentorship and consistent oversight. The most productive outcomes will come when a multi-tiered team is in place to help residents and medical students in their research endeavors. This research infrastructure should consist of faculty (both clinical and basic), statisticians (if available), and dedicated research personnel.

Faculty

At most institutions and IRBs, no resident or medical student can conduct research without direct involvement with at least one faculty member. The difficulty lies in identifying highly involved faculty that are not only productive with research but are willing to devote time to guiding medical students and residents throughout the entire process of the research project. Faculty should engage residents and students and make themselves available for meetings and clarifications.

Statistics

If possible and available, statistical support is highly recommended to the research infrastructure. Masters and PhD-level statisticians can provide expert knowledge into the design of any research project. Utilizing their knowledge from the very beginning provides the establishment of a concise data analysis plan, advice on database setup and input, and help in the all-important analyses upon completion of all data collection. Statisticians seem to have this uncanny ability to analyze complete data sets in hours in comparison to "certain" research team members who may take days longer to complete the same analysis. Along with the analysis, the statisticians are also able to provide input for presentations and manuscripts.

Research Personnel

Dedicated research personnel can play a critical role in a successful research team in producing scholarly activity. This person(s) can be a faculty member tasked as the research director akin to a residency director or a medical student director. This person(s) could also be a nurse or research coordinator with no other duties. The main task of this researcher is to facilitate the design, execution, and completion of research projects. The need for such a person in the research infrastructure is based on the fact that all of the other team members have tasks and responsibilities that will usually take priority over a research project (i.e., patient care, rotations, classes, procedures, and tests). They are also needed because many aspects of the logistical side of research must be conducted during business hours when most faculty, students, and residents are otherwise occupied. They can help to assure that all ethics and regulations are followed in accordance with federal, state, and local guidelines. They can also provide input into study design and feasibility from a logistical and institutional perspective. These researchers can provide guidance and oversight with IRB interactions, and they can provide support with grant submission. They should be the facilitators, rarely originators, of all things research related. Of all of the recommendations and commentary in this chapter, the single biggest driver of quality research volume from medical students and residents has been the addition of our research manager. Hiring the correct individual to quarterback the department's research will amplify and improve the current level of research at your institution.

Do's and Don'ts

To have success with robust research output, we suggest a list of do's and don'ts to consider when involving resident and medical students in research and growing the research infrastructure at an institution.

Don'ts

- Force anyone to work on a research topic who has no interest in it; if you do, you all but guarantee that it will either not be finished or it will take much longer than expected.
- Overload residents with projects. Allow the residents to dictate how much they are able to handle. Be cognizant of their hours worked and their need to have somewhat of a work-life balance.

- Take advantage of medical students by overloading them with too much work.
- Judge residents and students too harshly on their writing skills. We have all had pages bleed red. Medical writing is a skill that is attainable with mentorship and practice.
- Expect the dedicated research personnel to write up all protocols, abstracts, presentations, posters, and manuscripts. In most cases, they will not be a trained physician in your specialty and doing so will greatly diminish the scholarly output.
- Ask a resident or medical student to participate in a project and then take an inordinate amount of time to respond or do your part when the time comes. This is the biggest research enthusiasm killer we have seen. Students and residents are very excited to share their work (a type of which they may be doing for the first time) with you. Acknowledge its receipt immediately and find something about it that's great and tell them. Give them a realistic time frame when your thorough response and next steps can be expected.

Do's

- Engage residents from the beginning of their training to help establish and reinforce the research culture in the residency.
- Identify medical students as early as possible (even in their first year) allowing them as much time as possible to get involved and actually complete as many projects as they are willing to take on.
- Assure students that saying no to a project is always an option because they are students first. Ten research projects will not help their residency prospects if their board scores and grades suffer.
- Allow residents and medical students to help in invited scholarly activity that will help increase the tally of scholarly output, provide almost sure-bet publications, and add another aspect to practice medical writing.
- Do advocate for resident and medical student presentations and national, regional, and local conferences.
- Create research teams that include at least one faculty, resident, and student (more if necessary). This allows for coverage and progression of studies during busy times of certain team members.

Summary

Creating a solid research infrastructure that includes willing faculty, residents, students, statisticians, and research personnel creates mutually symbiotic relationship for all parties involved. Faculty are able to take on more scholarly activity knowing that they will have help in completing their commitments. The increased research output will fulfill the ACGME research requirement by residents, but it will also increase scholarly activity for faculty that may lead to grant funding and academic advancement. Residents and students will become more competitive candidates for fellowship and residencies. Studies have shown the importance of research to surgical education. Sabir et al. showed that 63% of residents were satisfied with the research requirement, and the same number felt it should continue; 80% of graduates of the residency program felt that scholarly activity improved their career [27]. Cultivating research helps to cultivate the career of residents guiding many into academia [28] and increasing their publication productivity during residency as well as after graduation [29].

With regard to medical students, as reported in the AAMC, the more students are able to produce with regard to research, the greater their likelihood of matching into their chosen specialty. Studies have shown that supportive programs increase student interest and output even resulting in subsequent research after graduation [30, 31]. Authors of these chapters can attest that when our research program started in 2013, there was only one student involved in research. When word spread about the research support and the department actively seeking out students to work with, the numbers grew, resulting in as many as 12 students at SIU working on projects at any given time and successfully matching four students in the Urology match in 2016.

Most importantly, patients will benefit. Medicine advances when questions are asked and research is conducted to answer those questions. Creating research programs and the research infrastructure needed to facilitate scholarly activity will resonate well past the length of one project; it will awaken a curiosity in new generation of researchers.

References

1. Specialty-specific References for DIOs: Resident/Fellow Scholarly Activity ACGME [Internet]. ACGME; 2017 [cited 2017 Mar 12]. Available from: https://www.acgme.org/Portals/0/PDFs/Specialty-specific%20Requirement%20Topics/DIO-Scholarly_Activity_Faculty.pdf.
2. Williams RG, Dunnington GL, Folse JR. The impact of a program for systematically recognizing and rewarding academic performance. Acad Med. 2003;78(2):156–66.
3. Coffey DS. The real final exam. Prostate. 1999;39(4):323–5.
4. Philibert I, Lieh-Lai M, Miller R, Potts JR, Brigham T, Nasca TJ. Scholarly activity in the next accreditation system: moving from structure and process to outcomes. J Grad Med Educ. 2013;5(4):714–7.
5. Resident Rotations [Internet]. SIU School of Medicine. [cited 2017 Feb 2]. Available from: https://www.siumed.edu/surgery/urology/resident-rotations.html.
6. UCLA Urology Residency Program [Internet]. UCLA Urology Intranet UCLA Urology Residency Program. [cited 2017 Feb 2]. Available from: https://urology.healthsciences.ucla.edu/intranet/education/pages/residency-info.
7. Medical Student Research Requirement [Internet]. Association of American Medical Colleges. [cited 2017 Mar 3]. Available from: https://www.aamc.org/initiatives/cir/427194/26.html.
8. Rinard JR, Mahabir RC. Successfully matching into surgical specialties: an analysis of National Resident Matching Program data. J Grad Med Educ. 2010;2(3):316–21.
9. Charting Outcomes in the Match for U.S. Allopathic Seniors [Internet]. Charting Outcomes in the Match for U.S. Allopathic Seniors. National Resident Matching Program; 2016 Sep. Available from: https://www.nrmp.org/wp-content/uploads/2016/09/Charting-Outcomes-US-Allopathic-Seniors-2016.pdf.
10. Protections Ofor HR. Federal Policy for the Protection of Human Subjects ('Common Rule [Internet]. HHS.gov. US Department of Health and Human Services; 2016 [cited 2017 Apr 4]. Available from: https://www.hhs.gov/ohrp/regulations-and-policy/regulations/common-rule/index.html.

11. Vassar M, Holzmann M. The retrospective chart review: important methodological considerations. J Educ Eval Health Prof. 2013;10:12.
12. Gearing RE, Mian IA, Barber J, Ickowicz A. A methodology for conducting retrospective chart review research in child and adolescent psychiatry. J Can Acad Child Adolesc Psychiatry. 2006;15(3):126–34.
13. Krousel-Wood MA. Practical considerations in the measurement of outcomes in healthcare. Ochsner J. 1999;1(4):187–94.
14. Linking quality to payment [Internet]. Medicare.gov – the Official U.S. Government Site for Medicare. [cited 2017 May 6]. Available from: https://www.medicare.gov/hospitalcompare/linking-quality-to-payment.html.
15. Defined Population Studies - Phases of Prevention Research [Internet]. National Institutes of Health. U.S. Department of Health and Human Services; [cited 2017 May 5]. Available from: https://prevention.nih.gov/prevention-research/phases-prevention-research/defined-population-studies.
16. NIH Fact Sheets - Health Disparities [Internet]. National Institutes of Health. U.S. Department of Health and Human Services; [cited 2017 May 5]. Available from: https://report.nih.gov/NIHfactsheets/ViewFactSheet.aspx?csid=124.
17. Search criteria "disparities."NIH Guide to Grants and Contracts [Internet]. National Institutes of Health. U.S. Department of Health and Human Services; [cited 2017 Jun 11]. Available from: https://grants.nih.gov/funding/searchGuide/nih-guide-to-grants-and-contracts.cfm?searchTerms=disparities&PAsToo=1&Expdate_On_After=&RelDate_On_After=&RFAsToo=1&NoticesToo=0&OrderOn=RelDate&OrderDirection=DESC&Activity_Code=&Activity_Code_Groups=&PrimaryICActive=Any&View=&status=1.
18. U.S. Department of Health and Human Services. Office for Human Research Protections [Internet]. HHS.gov. HHS.gov; [cited 2017 May 5]. Available from: https://www.hhs.gov/ohrp/.
19. Commissioner Oof the. Search for FDA Guidance Documents - Institutional Review Boards Frequently Asked Questions – Information Sheet [Internet]. U S Food and Drug Administration Home Page. Office of the Commissioner; [cited 2017 May 5]. Available from: https://www.fda.gov/RegulatoryInformation/Guidances/ucm126420.htm.
20. Braunschweiger P, Goodman KW. The CITI program: an international online resource for education in human subjects protection and the responsible conduct of research. Acad Med. 2007;82(9):861–4.
21. Education and Training Offerings [Internet]. SIU School of Medicine. [cited 2017 Jun 11]. Available from: http://www.siumed.edu/ccr/education-and-training-offerings.html.
22. Hands-On Preparation for a Rewarding Career [Internet]. Masters Degree in Clinical Research UCSD. [cited 2017 Jun 11]. Available from: https://clre.ucsd.edu/.
23. Harvard T.H. Chan School of Public Health [Internet]. Certificate Program in Clinical Research Methods. [cited 2017 Jun 11]. Available from: https://www.hsph.harvard.edu/clinical-research-methods/.
24. Rock Talk [Internet]. National Institutes of Health. U.S. Department of Health and Human Services; 2015 [cited 2017 Jun 11]. Available from: https://nexus.od.nih.gov/all/2015/06/29/what-are-the-chances-of-getting-funded/.
25. Molnar H. Research Programs and Opportunities [Internet]. Johns Hopkins Medicine, based in Baltimore, Maryland. 2016 [cited 2017 May 5]. Available from: http://www.hopkinsmedicine.org/som/students/research/.
26. Medical School [Internet]. UT Southwestern Medical Center. [cited 2017 May 5]. Available from: http://www.utsouthwestern.edu/education/medical-school/academics/research/electives/.
27. Sabir M, Penney DG, Remine SG, Mittal VK. Scholarly activities—essential to surgical education. Curr Surg. 2003;60(4):459–62.
28. Bhattacharya SD, Williams JB, De La Fuente SG, Kuo PC, Siegler HF. Does protected research time during general surgery training contribute to graduates' career choice? Am Surg. 2011;77(7):907–10.

29. Ozuah PO. Residency research requirement as a predictor of future publication productivity. J Pediatr. 2009;155(1):1–2.
30. Zier K, Friedman E, Smith L. Supportive programs increase medical students' research interest and productivity. J Investig Med. 2006;54(4):201–7.
31. Dyrbye LN, Davidson LW, Cook DA. Publications and presentations resulting from required research by students at Mayo Medical School, 1976–2003. Acad Med. 2008;83(6):604–10.

16 Promoting Professionalism

Hilary Sanfey

Introduction

Unprofessional behavior can be defined in different ways. Such behavior represents a deficiency in one of the Accreditation Council for Graduate Medical Education (ACGME) competencies [1], i.e., the individual *fails to meet the standard of performance in one or more of the ACGME competencies* [2]. Since unprofessional behavior can have a wide impact on colleagues and patients, such behavior meets the American Medical Association (AMA) definition of "disruptive behavior," i.e., *personal conduct whether verbal or physical that negatively affects or that potentially may negatively affect patient care. This includes but is not limited to conduct that interferes with one's ability to work with other members of the healthcare team* [3]. In 2008, the Joint Commission further defined such behavior as "behavior that undermines a culture of safety" [4]. This is appealing because it reminds us that our most important consideration should be the safety of our patients and that institutional leaders are required to have policies in place that address such behaviors regardless of the underlying cause. On the other hand, any reasonable conduct to advocate for patients and recommend improvements in patient care is appropriate [5]. Physicians who criticize the healthcare system in good faith with the aim of improving patient care should not be silenced or reprimanded. Individual whistle-blowers with good ideas, even when well presented, may be falsely labeled disruptive as a tactic to silence them. A good message can be destroyed by a bad delivery, and the focus becomes the objectionable delivery rather than the issues that caused the physician to express anger [6].

H. Sanfey, MB, BCh, MHPE, FACS
SIU School of Medicine, Department of Surgery,
PO Box 19638, Springfield, IL 62794, USA
e-mail: hsanfey@siumed.edu

T.S. Köhler, B. Schwartz (eds.), *Surgeons as Educators*,
https://doi.org/10.1007/978-3-319-64728-9_16

Aggressive behaviors are obvious and include yelling, the use of foul and abusive language, threatening gestures, public criticism of coworkers, insults and shaming others, intimidation, invading one's space, slamming down objects, and physically aggressive or assaultive behavior. Fortunately, most of these are unusual [7]. What are much more common are passive-aggressive behaviors such as hostile avoidance or "cold shoulder" treatment; intentional miscommunication; unavailability for professional matters, e.g., not answering pages or delays in doing so; using a condescending language or tone; expressing impatience with questions; indulging in malicious gossip; adopting a sarcastic tone of voice; and/or resorting to implied threats, especially retribution for making complaints [7].

There is a wealth of literature to demonstrate that these behaviors contribute to medical errors, poor patient satisfaction, and preventable adverse outcomes, as well as increasing the cost of care. They also lower morale to the extent that other healthcare professionals particularly nurses and administrators seek new positions in more professional environments [8–11]. While these studies refer to practicing physicians and not necessarily to residents, physicians in practice who behave in an unprofessional manner frequently exhibited those same unprofessional behaviors during residency and during medical school [12]. One barrier to addressing such behavior is that disruptive physicians are often successful and accomplished practitioners, who profess high standards of patient care and clinical practice. Aside from their interpersonal behavior, they are valuable members of the profession because of their knowledge and technical expertise.

Prevalence

Although disruptive physicians consume considerable attention, 50% of the concerns are associated with only 9–14% of physicians [13], and this minority is responsible for 50% of malpractice claim costs [14]. Leape and Fromson [15] report that 3–5% of physicians present with a problem of disruptive behavior. According to a 2004 survey of physician executives, more than 95% reported regularly encountering disruptive physician behaviors, and 70% reported that such behaviors nearly always involved the same physicians and most commonly involved conflict with a nurse or other allied healthcare staff. Nearly 80% of the respondents said that disruptive physician behavior is underreported because of victim's fear of reprisal or is only reported when a serious violation occurs [16]. Physicians, when evaluating themselves, are less likely to perceive such problems. Sexton et al. found that 75% surgeons, but only 45% of anesthesiologists, and 30% of surgical nurses expressed satisfaction with the relationship they had with colleagues [17].

Anecdotal data suggest that allowing residents to graduate on time without adequate remediation is not unusual, particularly when the deficiency is in interpersonal communication or professionalism [18]. In a single-institution study, 25% of residents, who graduated on time and passed the American Board of Surgery examinations on the first attempt, received marginal performance evaluations [19]. Nationally, the cumulative risks of termination are 3.0–19.5%, respectively, for all surgical residents [20]. Although many "voluntary" resignations may not be entirely voluntary, there is still some discrepancy between the 3% who are terminated and the reported prevalence of unprofessional behavior. Some of these residents might be successfully remediated; however, it is likely that many graduate without correction. Some reasons for this include the lack of assessment standards and unproven remediation options [21–23]. In addition, program directors are often faced with scanty or conflicting documentation. Frequently, there is inadequate oversight of trainee performance at the bedside or in clinic by attendings, so problems that are blatantly obvious to other healthcare professionals are not identified in a timely manner. Sometimes there is a "halo" effect whereby occasional lapses in professionalism are tolerated in the surgical resident who is well liked and has excellent technical skills. Further barriers to accurate evaluation include concern at the anticipated appeal process, loss of popularity or role as resident advocate, and possible retaliation from the resident. Finally, residents are employees who provide an essential service; therefore, the faculty are reluctant to increase the workload on colleagues by removing a resident from clinical duties [24].

Identification

There are some flags that permit identification of at-risk residents. One single-institution study identified a number of variables including age at entry older than 29 years, no participation in team sports, and/or a lack of superlative comments in the dean's letter as predictors of unsatisfactory outcome [19]. In a review of letters of recommendation, Stohl et al. found that comments about excellence in patient care and interpersonal and communication skills were predictive of the more successful residents. On the other hand, applicants at risk were those who were described as loners, who applied late, and who had letters predominantly from specialties other than their chosen field [25]. While these individuals should not be excluded, extra vigilance might be required. In another single-institution study, 82% of the problems in resident behavior were identified in first year of training [18]. In an internal medicine study, Yao and Wright [26] noted that 60% of program directors identified problem residents through critical incident reports, for example, a patient complaint. In addition, 75% of program directors most frequently became aware of problem residents because of verbal complaints from the faculty, and only 31% identified problems from written evaluations by the faculty. Because behavioral problems are frequently identified early in training, the first 6-month review is a time for critical evaluation of new residents; indeed, there is a case for conducting quarterly reviews of new residents. Any problem arising at any time should be brought to the attention of the program director.

Remediation

Gerald Hickson and colleagues at Vanderbilt have a successful four-step program for disruptive physicians [27]. The authors note that most physicians rarely exhibit unprofessional behavior, and a small percentage will exhibit a single unprofessional incident. This could be an isolated event and unlikely to recur or the first observation of a pattern of behavior. The first report of such behavior is the subject of an informal "cup of coffee" conversation and treated as an anomaly unless it recurs [27]. If the behavior is repeated, then the next step is a confidential nonpunitive awareness intervention, followed by an authority intervention if problems continue, and finally there is a disciplinary action by the highest level of administration [27]. About 60% of physicians improve after level 1 interventions, and recidivism is less than 2%. Another 20% require additional authority interventions to improve [27]. At each intervention, the program director or chair should describe the specific problem behavior and the expected behavior and set a timeline for improvement with consequences for failure to improve. The responsibility for improvement rests with the individual resident or other physician. While each intervention is documented if this is a single incident that is not repeated, the supervisor may choose to remove the documentation from the physician's permanent file.

In the course of the intervention, unprofessional behavior should be described in nonjudgmental language that focuses on the behavior and not on personality. For example, if a resident is described as *driving the nurses and other residents crazy to the extent that everyone groans when he or she appears and breathes a sigh of relief when they rotate off service*, then this resident is behaving in a manner that creates divisiveness and is disruptive to team function. This is a deficiency in the ACGME competencies of both interpersonal skills and communication skills as well as systems-based practice because of the impact on team function. Therefore, it should be described as such with specific examples. If the resident *is manipulative*, *gets others to do his/her work*, *shows up late for assigned activities*, *and/or is delinquent in administrative tasks*, then this resident is exhibiting a deficiency in the ACGME competency of professionalism. Finally, if *patient care is impacted by a delay in communications/poor follow through/team dysfunction*, then this is an obvious deficiency in the ACGME competency of patient care. Sometimes supervising physicians are the last to hear about clinical performance problems because the natural response of residents is to fill in these gaps in patient care themselves. Therefore, the nurses and administrative staff are frequently a more reliable source of information.

There are some guiding principles for addressing unprofessional behavior that include setting very clear expectations as to what is meant by professional behavior, modeling such behavior, and holding all accountable. Some specific interventions that are worth suggesting include encouraging self-reflection in order to gain insight, increasing self-awareness through feedback from nurses or others with whom the individual resident works so the message is presented from different sources, and structured mentoring [24].

There is a spectrum of unprofessional behavior that runs from a single unprofessional event at the less serious end of the spectrum to misconduct at the most extreme. Determining whether to call such behaviors unprofessional or misconduct is often at the discretion of the chair or program director. However, the difference is important as the consequences for misconduct are more severe. By definition, misconduct is a behavior that is wrong, that one knows (or should know) is wrong, and therefore will not be cured by remediation. One approach to assigning culpability is to use the reason criteria and ask if the individual intended to cause harm, came to work impaired, knowingly and unreasonably increased risk, and if another person in the same situation would act in a similar manner [28]. All incidents of alleged misconduct should be investigated and a report generated that considers extenuating circumstances. The individual should be given notice of the charge and an opportunity to be heard, but if found culpable they do not have to be given an opportunity to repeat misconduct as long as the final decision is made through a process that is reasonable.

An important component of the interview, particularly where unprofessional behavior is deemed out of character for that individual, is the identification of possible contributing factors. Underlying causes include impairment due to substance abuse or other psychiatric disorders, external life stressors, personality characteristics, lack of training, or system factors. Some of the more common, treatable factors include transition or separation issues, nervousness, and cultural differences about what is considered appropriate behavior. More serious problems include external stressors such as family illness/marital discord and major illness. In a study of medical students, Dyrbye et al. found a relationship between unprofessional behaviors and burnout, in that these behaviors were more common in students with burnout [29]. A small percentage of individuals will have a significant mental health or substance abuse problem. However, a doctor-patient relationship does not and should not exist between a physician and their supervisor; therefore, if there is a need for referral, this should be made as a request for a "fitness to practice" examination to employee health/employee assistance or the Physician Wellness Program and not as a direct patient referral. The Americans with Disabilities Act [30] mandates that educators must make reasonable accommodation to ensure that a resident with a disability can complete the curriculum; however, the resident must ask for accommodation before a performance deficiency occurs. Performance problems should be addressed as a performance or a behavior problem and not as a health issue. For example, stress must be discussed as it relates to poor performance—not mental health. In addition, the Americans with Disabilities Act limits when a psychiatric evaluation can be required and is usually restricted to decisions about fitness to practice. After such evaluations, the supervisor should receive notification that appropriate follow-up is occurring but not medical details.

How an individual responds during the feedback intervention provides insight on their willingness to improve and the extent to which they are prepared to take responsibility for their own learning and improvement. This response is the most useful predictor of successful remediation [31]. The more defensive the recipient becomes and the more he/she argues, the more likely it is that this person has what is termed a fixed mindset, i.e., is deficient in practice-based learning and improvement, and these are the individuals who are a challenge to remediate [32]. Residents with a "growth" mind-set believe their success is based on hard work and learning, while those with a "fixed" mind-set attribute their success to innate ability and their failures to the actions of others. The latter are a challenge to remediate.

If there is no improvement after an intervention, then it is key to follow through with the previously discussed consequences. Failure to do this has a negative impact on the behavior and morale of all in the workplace. Roberts et al. suggest that in making decisions about a resident, consideration should be given to whether the resident's performance can be improved sufficiently to perform effectively as a member of the healthcare team and whether this improvement is likely to be sustained in practice as well as during training [33]. Other considerations are the cost of remediation in time, effort, and resources, as well as the hidden cost of retaining a resident in terms of the increased workload on colleagues due to "work-arounds," double checking, and low morale. The amount of time spent discussing a resident is frequently a measure of the severity of the problem! All complaints about a resident should be taken seriously and fully investigated. Even if the complaint is not made in writing, it should be documented by the supervisor although it will be up to his/her discretion to keep the documentation as part of the individual's permanent file. If the complaint is valid, then a determination needs to be made about future action in terms of remediation/termination or probation. If the decision is to remediate or place the resident on probation, then there has to be a clear action plan and timeline for reevaluation. Finally, judgments about a physician's behavior should be fair and unbiased and not based on personal friendships, dislikes, antagonisms, jurisdictional disagreements, or competitiveness among members of the staff. Invoking discipline with no option for assistance automatically creates an adversarial relationship in which the physician becomes invested in justifying the disruptive behaviors. A program of assistance allows for constructive change to the benefit of the individual physician, patients, and members of the healthcare delivery system and allows a return to normal functioning.

Addressing the Climate

The hidden curriculum refers to the parallel, implicit curriculum by which students acquire the values, norms, and expectations of professional practice. For the most part, it is taught through role modeling. Most professional value training is acquired through resident interaction. Furthermore, we know that student values change during medical school. There is a conflict between the values that students take with them into medical school and observed behaviors. For example, the structure of medical training promotes competitiveness, and the institutional rewards system recognizes individuals not teams or collaboration, and teaching is often undervalued. Furthermore, modern hospital culture is centered outside the patient room. All of this has a somewhat negative impact on students and also on junior residents. Although not intended, medical training by its nature can serve to encourage unprofessional behavior among those who already have personalities that are so inclined. Abusers often have a past history of having been abused themselves. Many medical students and residents experience abuse during their training in the form of "belittling" or "humiliation" by "malignant" and "egotistical" attendings [34–36]. Those who survive their hazing experiences can identify with those in power who previously abused them. Having achieved full status as physicians, some physicians, having paid their dues, feel entitled to reenact abuse on others. As has been stated,

"Today's abused student is tomorrow's source of social control as a resident or attending physician" [37]. Krizek [38] writes that the nature of surgical training and the rigors of practicing surgery are impairing since external stressors can provoke disruptive behaviors in physicians predisposed to such behavior. Functioning as a physician places demands on coping skills that are psychologically draining.

Often the greatest challenges are dealing with a system that enables and rewards unprofessional behaviors which are often goal directed [39, 40]. For example, staff will often work around uncooperative or even abusive residents and will page an off-call pleasant resident to see a patient or complete a task, thus "rewarding" bad behavior by allowing the unprofessional individual to sleep through the night undisturbed. Clearly we cannot hold our residents to a higher standard of professionalism than our faculty colleagues. If the faculty achieve their goals by yelling or abusing the OR/administrative staff, then the residents learn that this is acceptable professional behavior. Recognizing and addressing such behavior through a system-level response will increase the likelihood of successful remediation.

A lack of documentation is often presented as a reason for not dealing more strictly with unprofessional behavior. However, at least with regard to residents and students, the courts have unfailingly confirmed that as long as the individual was provided with "notice and an opportunity to cure and the faculty decision regarding termination or probation or extension of training is conscientious and deliberate," they will not second-guess the academic decision [41]. The best way to ensure that decisions are not arbitrary or capricious is to use a competency or progress committee. A large percentage of deficiencies only become apparent when the faculty meet to discuss performance because this allows patterns of behavior to become apparent and provides evidence that strengthens individuals' preexisting convictions about performance deficiencies leading to a corporate judgment that is more stringent than that of individual raters [42, 43]. The minutes of this meeting will provide more robust documentation than that of the individual attending. Another consideration is that faculty members with only occasional contact with residents tend to be more generous with their ratings; thus, these ratings need to be interpreted with caution. Narratives are often more useful than numeric ratings in identifying issues. The best way to ensure that decisions are not arbitrary or capricious is to use a clinical competency committee. Problems are often identified in committee discussions that are not raised by individuals permitting the identification of patterns of behavior when an individual saw only a single instance [42–44]. Such committees serve as checks and balances, particularly in identifying the marginal resident.

Conclusion

The guiding principles for addressing unprofessional behavior include setting very clear expectations as to what is meant by professional behavior, modeling such behavior, and holding others accountable. All complaints should be taken seriously and fully investigated to get both sides of the story. Program directors should incorporate an assessment of trustworthiness and ability to take responsibility for personal behavior into resident evaluations and note system problems that enable unprofessional behavior by providing secondary gain for such activities. Once a problem has been identified, the individual must be provided with a notice of deficiency and an opportunity to improve, with consequences for failing to address the deficiency. In addition to participation in a remedial program, the opportunity for feedback and reflection and post-intervention assessment are necessary to determine the next steps. Whatever final decision is made, as long as the process is fair and reasonable, that is, the decision was not arbitrary or capricious, the decision will be upheld by the courts. Finally, legal proceedings and grievance hearings are costly and time-consuming, so prevention is better than cure. Therefore, the importance of intervening early is emphasized.

References

1. ACGME. ACGME program requirements for graduate medical education in general surgery. 2017. http://www.acgme.org/Portals/0/PFAssets/ProgramRequirements/440_general_surgery_2016.pdf. Accesses 2.23.17.
2. Lucey CR, Boote R. Working with problem residents: a systematic approach. In: Holmboe ES, Hawkins RE, editors. Practical guide to the evaluation of clinical competence. Philadelphia: Mosby Elsevier; 2008. p. 201–16.
3. American Medical Association. AMA code of medical ethics: opinion 9.045: physicians with disruptive behavior. 2017. http://journalofethics.ama-assn.org/2016/11/coet1-1611.html. Accessed 2.23.17.
4. Joint Commission. Behaviors that undermine a culture of safety. *Sentinel Event Alert*. Issue 40, July 9, 2008. https://www.jointcommission.org/assets/1/18/SEA_40.PDF. Accessed 2 .23.17.
5. Cohen B, et al. Model Medical Staff Code of Conduct. American Medical Association 2009 http://www.ismanet.org/pdf/news/medicalstaffcodeofconduct.pdf. Accessed 2.23.17.
6. Physicians with disruptive behavior. Report of the Council on Ethical & Judicial Affairs AMA Report. 2000; 2-A-00:2.
7. Reynolds NT. Disruptive physician behavior: use and misuse of the label. J Med Regul. 2011;98(1):8–19.
8. Rosenstein AH, O'Daniel M. Disruptive behavior and clinical outcomes: perceptions of nurses and physicians. Am J Nurs. 2005;105(1):54–64.
9. Rosenstein AH, O'Daniel M. A survey of the impact of disruptive behaviors and communication defects on patient safety. Jt Comm J Qual Patient Saf. 2008;34(8):464–71.
10. Hickson GB, et al. Patient complaints and malpractice risk. JAMA. 2002;287:2951–7.
11. Stelfox HT, Ghandi TK, Orav J, Gustafson ML. The relation of patient satisfaction with complaints against physicians, risk management episodes, and malpractice lawsuits. Am J Med. 2005;118(10):1126–33.
12. Papadakis MA, Hodgson CS, Teherani A, et al. Unprofessional behavior in medical school is associated with subsequent disciplinary action by a state medical board. Acad Med. 2004;79:244–9.
13. Hickson GB, Moore IN, Pichert JW, Benegas M. Balancing systems and individual accountability in a safety culture. In: Berman S, editor. From front office to front line: essential issues for health care leaders. 2nd ed. Chicago: Joint Commission Resources International; 2012. p. 1–35.
14. Moore IN, Pichert JW, Hickson GB, Federspiel CF, Blackford JU. Rethinking peer review: detecting and addressing medical malpractice claims risk. Vanderbilt Law Rev. 2006;59:1175–206.
15. Leape LL, Fromson JA. Problem doctors: is there a system-level solution? Ann Intern Med. 2006;144:107–55.

16. Weber DO. Poll results: doctors' disruptive behavior disturbs physician leaders. Physician Exec. 2004;30(5):6–14.
17. Sexton JB, Thomas EJ, Helmreich RL. Error, stress, and teamwork in medicine and aviation: cross sectional surveys. BMJ. 2000;320:745.
18. Williams RG, Roberts NK, Schwind CJ, Dunnington GL. The nature of general surgery resident performance problems. Surgery. 2009;145(6):651–8.
19. Naylor RA, Reisch JS, Valentine RJ. Factors related to attrition in surgery residency based on application data. Arch Surg. 2008;143(7):647–52.
20. Yeo H, Bucholz E, Ann Sosa J, et al. A national study of attrition in general surgery training: which residents leave and where do they go? Ann Surg. 2010;252(3):529–53.
21. Dudek NL, Marks MB, Regehr G. Failure to fail: the perspectives of clinical supervisors. Acad Med. 2005;80(10 Suppl):S84–7.
22. Hauer KE, Ciccone A, Henzel TR, et al. Remediation of the deficiencies of physicians across the continuum from medical school to practice: a thematic review of the literature. Acad Med. 2009;84(12):1822–32.
23. Torbeck L, Canal DF. Remediation practices for surgery residents. Am J Surg. 2009;197(3): 397–402.
24. Sanfey H, DaRosa D, Hickson G, et al. Pursuing professional accountability: an evidence based approach to addressing residents with behavior problems. Arch Surg. 2012;147(7):642–7.
25. Stoll M. In the best medical schools. New York: Princeton Review Publishing; 1999.
26. Yao DC, Wright SM. National survey of internal medicine residency program directors regarding problem residents. JAMA. 2000;284(9):1099–104.
27. Hickson GB, Pichert JW, Webb LE, Gabbe SG. A complementary approach to promoting professionalism: identifying, measuring, and addressing unprofessional behaviors. Acad Med. 2007;82(11):1040–8.
28. Reason JT. Managing the risks of organizational accidents. Aldershot: Ashgate Publishing; 1997.
29. Dyrbye LN, Harper W, Moutier C, et al. A multi-institutional study exploring the impact of positive mental health on medical students professionalism in an era of high burnout. Acad Med. 2012;87(8):1024–31.
30. Americans With Disabilities Act. Updated March 25, 2009. https://www.ada.gov/pubs/ada.htm. Accessed 2.23.17.
31. Kennedy TJ, Regehr G, Baker GR, Lingard L. Point-of-care assessment of medical trainee competence for independent clinical work. Acad Med. 2008;83(10 suppl):S89–92.
32. Dweck CS. Mindset: the new psychology of success. New York: Random House; 2006.
33. Roberts N, Williams R. The hidden costs of failing to fail residents. J Grad Med Educ. 2011;3(2):127–9.
34. McMurray JE, Schwartz MD, Genero NP, et al. The attractiveness of internal medicine: a qualitative analysis of the experiences of female and male medical students. Ann Intern Med. 1993;119:812–8.
35. Daugherty SR, Baldwin DC Jr, Rowley BD. Learning, satisfaction, and mistreatment during medical internship: a national survey of working conditions. JAMA. 1998;279(15):1194–9.
36. Elnicki M, Linger B, Asch E, et al. Patterns of medical student abuse during the internal medicine clerkship: perspective of student at 11 medical schools. Acad Med. 1999;74(10 Suppl):S99–101.
37. Eckenfels EJ, Daugherty SR, Baldwin DC, et al. A sociocultural framework for explaining perceptions of mistreatment and abuse in the professional socialization of future physicians. Ann Behav Sci Med Educ. 1997;4:11–8.
38. Krizek TJ. Ethics and philosophy lecture: surgery… is it an impairing profession? J Am Coll Surg. 2002;194(3):352–66.
39. Williams BW, Williams MV. The disruptive physician: a conceptual organization. J Med Licens Discip. 2008;94(3):12–20.
40. Williams BW. The prevalence and special educational requirements of dyscompetent physicians. J Contin Educ Health Prof. 2006;26(3):173–91.

41. Board of Curators of the University of Michigan v Horowitz, 435 US 78, 98 S Ct 948; 1978.
42. Schwind CJ, Williams RG, Boehler ML, Dunnington GL. Do individual attendings' post-rotation performance ratings detect residents' clinical performance deficiencies? Acad Med. 2004;79(5):453–7.
43. Williams RG, Schwind CJ, Dunnington GL, Fortune J, Rogers D, Boehler M. The effects of group dynamics on resident progress committee deliberations. Teach Learn Med. 2005;17(2):96–100.
44. Wu JS, Siewert B, Boiselle PM. Resident evaluation and remediation: a comprehensive approach. J Grad Med Educ. 2010;2(2):242–5.

Optimizing Success for the Underperforming Resident

17

Karen Broquet and Jamie S. Padmore

Introduction

Residents who fail to meet standards across one or more competencies or demonstrate problem behaviors that are significant enough to require intervention by program leadership are conceptualized variously as "problem residents" [1], or "residents in difficulty" [2, 3]. Approximately 10% of residents across multiple specialties struggle with underperformance at some point [1–5]. Among surgical programs, the prevalence may be closer to 20–30% [6–9]. More than 90% of program directors report having at least one problem resident in the past 1–3 years [1, 4, 5, 10]. Given enough time, it is likely that all program directors will encounter one or more underperforming resident. Proactively addressing underperformance is highly stressful for program directors and faculty. It can take a disproportionate amount of time, be interpersonally uncomfortable, have an impact on faculty and resident morale, and can sometimes lead to the painful decision that a particular resident who may be far advanced in training does not possess the requisite skills to become a competent safe practitioner in the specialty. In addition, underperforming residents often come to a program director's attention via verbal reports with a paucity of corresponding written documentation [11, 12], leading to concerns of fairness, due process, or legal ramifications for taking action. Helping a resident reach his or her potential and succeed in training can be a gratifying experience. Conversely, not addressing underperformance can lead to further problems as the trainee progresses through training, including a threat to patient safety [13]. In this chapter, we will

K. Broquet, MD, MHPE (✉)
Southern Illinois University School of Medicine, PO Box 19656, Springfield, IL 62794, USA
e-mail: kbroquet@siumed.edu

J.S. Padmore, DM, MSc
Georgetown University School of Medicine and MedStar Health,
3900 Reservoir Road, NW, Med-Dent Building, NW-110, Washington, DC 20007, USA

T.S. Köhler, B. Schwartz (eds.), *Surgeons as Educators*,
https://doi.org/10.1007/978-3-319-64728-9_17

review practical steps in recognizing and assessing underperforming residents, making an educational formulation and developing a learner-centered remediation plan. We will also discuss common concerns and practices regarding due process and academic legal issues. Although the work of helping an underperforming resident succeed or exit the program falls to all educators, the information in this chapter is specifically geared toward program directors.

Predicting Performance Problems

A program director, even with the benefit of hindsight, may well review a struggling resident's file only to find no warning signs of the difficulties to come. However, some pre-matriculation predictors have been identified in the literature. The presence of even one negative comment in the Dean's letter, failing one or more courses during medical school, low USMLE scores, transferring in from another program, and time lapse between medical school and residency have all been associated with being placed on warning status or probation [7, 8, 14–16]. Guerrasio et al. [14] retrospectively compared 102 trainees on probation across multiple specialties at one institution. Those on probation were more likely than matched controls to have transferred from another training program, to have taken time off between medical school and residency, and to have scored lower on all three USMLE examinations. They also found that being male, married, older, not Caucasian, or an international medical graduate were all independently associated with being on probation, but not associated with poorer graduation or board certification outcomes. Other studies have found no association with underperformance and gender, age, marital status, or being an international medical graduate [4, 7–9]. Yaghoubian et al. [7] retrospectively analyzed remediation and attrition across six general surgery programs over 11 years. They found a positive association between remediation and lower USMLE Step 1 and 2 scores, as well as (ironically) having received honors in the third-year surgery clerkship.

Post-matriculation, even in the absence of identified deficits on rotation evaluations, low in-training examination performance has been associated with both remediation and low board passage rates [14, 17, 18]. The presence of any complaint or critical incident should also be taken seriously. Resnick et al. [8] retrospectively reviewed all founded complaints against general surgery residents in one institution over a 10-year span. The vast majority (83%) of complaints were for unprofessional conduct toward perceived subordinates, and 80% of the complaints were filed against 15% of the residents. A high number of complaints were associated with the resident leaving the program prior to graduation. Twenty-six percent of all residents received at least one complaint. A resident who received one complaint had a 55% chance of receiving an additional complaint. In other words, a resident with one complaint was twice as likely to receive another as a resident with no complaints.

The presence of one or more of these risk factors may well be balanced by multiple positive factors, and none are robust enough to predetermine lack of success in residency. However, a resident with any of these risk factors may well benefit from added structure or frequency of feedback and assessment during the early part of training. In particular, verbal expressions of concern from supervisors or complaints from staff, nurses, or patients, even in the face of average or above rotation ratings, should be taken very seriously.

Identifying and Assessing Lapse in Performance

Underperforming residents may come to a program director's attention from a variety of sources. Program directors and chief residents are most likely to be the first to identify a problem [1, 10]. Underperformance can be identified by a plethora of methods, but the most common are direct observation of clinical skills by supervising faculty, by standardized cognitive or clinical performance assessments, or via critical incidents or external complaints. Sometimes subtle deficits are identified only after Clinical Competency Committee (CCC) review and discussion [10]. A CCC is required by the Accreditation Council for Graduate Medical Education (ACGME) for all residency programs [19]. The CCC is an advisory body that is appointed by the program director and is comprised of at least three faculty members. Residents are restricted from being members of the CCC. It is critically important to underscore that the CCC is *advisory* to the program director. The program director is the ultimate decision-maker and should consider the recommendations of the CCC regarding resident performance prior to rendering decisions on progress, promotion, remediation, and dismissal. The ACGME CCC Guidebook for Programs [20] provides detailed information for program directors regarding the operation and function of the CCC. The CCC should utilize multiple assessment sources when evaluating resident performance. The discussion that takes place between faculty in the CCC can provide valuable insight to emerging resident performance issues. Schwind et al. [12] and Williams et al. [21] address the topic of group decision-making in clinical evaluation, noting the committee structure provides for a broader base of information used for decision-making, allows for calibration of disparate raters and identification of a presumed "bad day" vs. a pattern of performance issues, and promotes reasoned decision-making. Holmboe et al. [22] emphasizes the "wisdom in the group." Hemmer [24, 25] and Hauer et al. [23] reinforce this concept by adding that group conversations regarding performance are much more likely to uncover deficiencies in knowledge and professionalism and improve feedback that subsequently can positively impact learner performance. It is rare for a resident to self-identify underperformance. Physicians as a rule tend to overestimate their performance, and those functioning in the lower range overestimate their performance even more [1, 26, 27].

Program directors are twice as likely to get faculty input about an underperforming resident verbally as via written evaluations [10]. Consider this scenario:

You receive a call from Dr. A about a PGY2 he is supervising. Dr. A tells you that he is very concerned about Resident B's clinical judgment and patient care skills. You are surprised because Resident B's written evaluations have consistently been in the good or above range, including those by Dr. A. You ask the CCC to review Resident B at their next meeting, after which the CCC chair tells you the CCC has agreed unanimously that Resident B is in need of remediation.

Numeric rotational evaluation ratings often fail to provide accurate feedback regarding resident performance; however, information from the comments section can be more valuable. This underscores the importance of establishing a multifactorial assessment system that solicits performance feedback through multiple sources and evaluators. Even when supervisors recognize underperformance in a resident, they are often reluctant to rate a resident as unsatisfactory or even lower numerically in the performance range [11, 12, 21]. Schwind et al. [12] reviewed all rotation evaluations for surgical residents over a 5-year period at one institution. Less than 1% of the individual evaluations even nominally noted a deficit, while 28% of the residents were identified as having deficits requiring some level of intervention. There are a number of contributors to this. If the supervisor is not consistently directly observing the resident, he or she may not observe performance deficits. Performance in technical/operative skill, which is more likely to be directly observed, is more accurately rated than other competency areas. Subtle deficits or incidents may fade in the supervisor's memory between their occurrence and the time of evaluation. Deficits in knowledge base and clinical judgment may be masked by the compensation of other team members. In other instances, raters feel they lack documentation of the day-to-day observations to support a low or failing rating, lack confidence in the validity of the overall assessment system, lack confidence in the availability or efficacy of remediation options, or may fear repercussions in the event of an appeal or grievance [11, 12, 21, 28]. Williams et al. [21] offer the following suggestions to maximize the accuracy of rotation ratings:

1. Maximize both the number of ratings and raters to increase the situations and tasks observed, and dilute any idiosyncrasies of individual raters. Thirty-eight ratings per resident per year are recommended to assure a reproducible estimate of performance.
2. Include nurses and patients as raters. In general, accurate assessment of interpersonal skills requires a greater number of ratings for reliability. Nurses and patients tend to be more accurate raters in this competency.
3. Use simulations and standardized observed clinical encounters liberally to ensure observation and assessment of all aspects of performance.

4. Make sure all faculty are trained in good feedback skills and encouraged to give frequent real-time feedback to learners. This helps the faculty rater recall observations and reduces the potential for the resident to be surprised in the event deficits are identified.
5. Ensure that rating forms are short and only include items that raters can actually observe and assess.
6. Familiarize all raters with the rating instrument and the expected standards of performance associated with each level on the rating scale.
7. Provide raters with convenient access to evaluation instruments as close to the end of the evaluation period as possible.
8. Do not ask individual faculty members to make pass-fail assessments. Ask them only to provide quality ratings about performance for the CCC and provide written details to support the ratings.
9. Analyze resident ratings in context (i.e., compare with historical average ratings for past residents at the same level of training) and longitudinally (look for trends in ratings over time).
10. Utilize the CCC for all resident progress decisions, reviewing all data. If performance deficits are identified, act on them in a prompt and fair manner.

In addition to being frustrating for the faculty and program director, it is very confusing for a resident to be counseled about underperformance after having received several months or more of satisfactory rotation evaluations. In many programs, residents routinely receive copies of their rotation evaluations, but not all of the other assessment data points, or updates on early CCC concerns. This can create a situation in which the resident enters serious discussions about their performance or even their progress in the program, with the belief that the process is unfair or the decisions are being made on a basis other than clinical performance, such as personality conflict or discrimination. It is never useful to have a conversation about the vagaries of competency-based assessment at this point. While there are no easy solutions to this dilemma, these steps can help residents maintain a more complete picture of their progress:

1. At orientation and frequently thereafter, educate residents about all assessment instruments and processes utilized by the CCC.
2. Ensure that residents are getting frequent and focused feedback, so any discussion about underperformance is not unexpected.
3. Make sure residents have access to all of the assessments in their file, not just rotation evaluations.

Underperforming residents may come to attention either because of specific behaviors or lapses or poorly differentiated concerns on the part of supervisors. The first step is to gather information to more fully define the problem. When a resident is early in training and the concerns are not impacting patient care, it can be tempting to view them as growing pains, hoping the resident improves. However, this is not in the resident's or the program's best interest. Even with a minor lapse, intervention should occur sooner rather than later, as early identification of, and feedback about, underperformance or problem behaviors can help modify behaviors before they become more serious or refractory to change [29]. At a minimum, this fact-finding phase includes assessing the initial report(s) for validity and severity; reviewing other available data such as past evaluations, milestone assessments, CCC discussions, 360-degree evaluations, etc.; and meeting with the resident, to incorporate the resident's perspective of the problem. In meeting with the resident, it is very important to approach the subject with an attitude of concern and assurance that the goal is to help the resident be as successful as possible. Discussion of the areas of concern should be accompanied by clear information on the expected performance outcomes or behaviors. Residents receive this initial news with varying degrees of insight and receptiveness and generally require multiple conversations to process the information. When a resident presents with significant deficits in clinical performance or judgment, a program director will need to decide, after careful review of institutional policies, whether the resident can continue to practice safely under supervision or if the deficits are so severe that they need to be removed from clinical service to preserve patient safety while a clear educational formulation and remediation plan are being developed. In these instances, it is vital to include appropriate GME office leaders, human resources, and/or legal representatives in the discussion. Commonly described performance deficits are listed in Table 17.1.

An underperforming or problem resident is likely to have deficits across multiple competency and performance domains. Although deficits may occur across all

Table 17.1 Common performance deficits

Interactions or relationships with others
Insufficient knowledge/ITE score
Technical skills
Communication skills
Case presentations
Effective handoffs
Clinical judgment
Clinical reasoning
Data interpretation
Ability to put everything together
Decision-making
Ability to manage patients
Dependability
Punctuality
Absences
Medical records delinquency
Bad attitude/lack of apparent interest or motivation
Lack of honesty or trustworthiness
Time management
Slow pace of work
Inappropriate, disruptive, unethical, or illegal behaviors

Adapted from Williams et al. [4] and Tabby [6]

Table 17.2 Cognitive vs. non-cognitive deficits

Cognitive	Non-cognitive	
	Professionalism	Organizational
Knowledge base Clinical reasoning and judgment Clinical decision-making Technical skills	Interpersonal conflicts Dependability Disruptive behaviors Dishonesty Misconduct	Time management Multitasking Level of organization

Adapted from Williams et al. [6], Tabby et al. [4], Audétat et al. [2]

ACGME competencies, residents most commonly exhibit deficits in medical knowledge, patient care, professionalism, and interpersonal skills and communication [1, 2, 4–7, 14, 30]. Because most of our assessment instruments, milestone information, and evaluations are either organized via ACGME competencies or specifically mapped to them, this is a useful starting point for delineating behaviors of concern and targeting assessment. An equally useful framework is to conceptualize deficits as cognitive or non-cognitive, as outlined in Table 17.2. This model is more closely tied to observable behaviors and lends itself more to designing a behavior-based remediation program. More importantly, it draws attention to professionalism issues that may not be remediable.

Contributing Factors

In order to succeed, it is up to the underperforming resident to demonstrate improvement in the behaviors or skills of concern. However, deficits don't arise in a vacuum, and often underlying contributing factors can be identified for the performance problems. If possible, targeting remediation interventions to the underlying cause will maximize the chances of success. Common contributors and possible interventions are listed in Table 17.3.

Consider this scenario:

Resident S received above-average faculty ratings throughout most of his PGY1 year. During PGY2, you are noticing a downward trend of mostly average ratings with a smattering of below average. Your chief resident recently came to you with concerns that Resident S seemed withdrawn and not quite as on top of things. You've just received an incident report that Resident S failed to follow up on a critical lab value for a patient.

Residency training has long been identified as a high-risk time for symptomatic levels of stress, burnout, and depression. Between 22% and 43% of residents experience some level of depression during residency [31–33], and 50–75% suffer from burnout [34–37]. Burnout and depression are not synonymous with performance impairment, and indeed the prevalence of both in residents is much higher than the

Table 17.3 Contributors and potential resources

Underlying contributor	Resources/interventions
Family or relationship stress	Employee Assistance Program Stress management Resident support group Schedule decompression Promotion of self-awareness and self-care
Chronic interpersonal or personality problems	Faculty mentoring Assignment of coach More frequent feedback Liberal use of 360 degree evaluations Discussion with risk manager about relationship between interpersonal skills and malpractice rates
Insufficient fund of knowledge	Assignment of reading/study materials with frequent mini-assessments
Psychiatric illness (disclosed by trainee)	Mental health evaluation and treatment Schedule decompression Leave of absence
Substance misuse	Referral to physician health program
Cultural issues	Mentor/advisor Cultural competence experiences
Poor study habits	Assignment of reading/study materials with frequent mini-assessments Mentor/advisor
Poor organizational skills	Performance and learning strategy evaluation
Poor test-taking skills	Mentor/advisor

Adapted from Reamy and Harman [3], Yao and Wright [10], Tabby et al. [4], Sullivan et al. [29]

prevalence of underperformance, but it is a significant risk factor. Burnout in residents has been associated with lower in-service scores, professionalism issues, lower quality patient care, and greater self-reported medical errors [35, 36, 38–40]. Depression has also been associated with more self-reported medical errors [32]. Mental health issues such as depression, anxiety, and personality disorders have been described as a causative factor in up to 22–38% of problem residents [1, 3, 4] and substance misuse in 5–14% [1, 3]. A resident with suspected or identified psychiatric illness or substance abuse presents unique challenges for the program director, who is in the difficult role of being a physician and a supervisor. Program directors should first and foremost focus on managing performance, describing performance concerns, providing examples, and holding residents to performance standards. Even in the face of concern that there may be underlying medical issues impacting the resident's performance, program directors must be cognizant that they are not the resident's physician and refrain from attempting to diagnose. While the program director must be aware and respectful of laws such as the Americans with Disabilities Act (ADA), which allow employees (residents included) to keep their medical information private, in some instances, it's necessary to make a judgment about the resident's level of safety or risk for suicide and to enlist support from the GME office, human resources, occupational health, or physician wellness services. Most of the time, a resident with significant stress or psychiatric symptoms is open to a program director's expression of concern or recommendation to obtain an evaluation by a mental health professional. Other times, a resident may be resistant to this. Having a carefully constructed discussion with the resident regarding their performance and asking the resident if there are any issues that may be impacting performance is typically the right approach. For example, "I'm very concerned about you. Some of the things I'm seeing make me worry that you are experiencing stress or other issues that are making it hard for you to succeed. I'd like to ask you access some resources that may be helpful to you." When a resident is forthcoming about a medical or psychiatric issue, the program director can offer assistance, including helping the resident to request a medical accommodation. However, if the resident is not forthcoming about a medical or psychiatric issue, then the program director is somewhat limited in what can be done, other than being supportive and managing performance.

If a program suspects that a resident is impaired (unable to practice safely, even under supervision), a fitness for duty evaluation is warranted. By definition, if a resident is sent for a fitness evaluation, it implies a belief that the resident is not fit to work and needs to be removed from the clinical workplace. The resident should be placed on a leave of absence until the fitness evaluation can be completed and the results returned. It is not something that can be put off until after the resident is done with call duty that night or until other residents are back from vacation to cover. If a resident is exhibiting symptoms of impairment, a fitness for duty evaluation that includes a drug screen should be done immediately, while the resident is exhibiting the signs and/or symptoms. If, after consultation with the DIO or other individuals as outlined in your particular institutional protocols, it is determined that a resident is in need of a fitness for duty evaluation, it is important for the program director and resident alike to have a full understanding of what can be gleaned from this. In the case of a mental health fitness evaluation, a psychiatrist or another examiner may be asked to examine the trainee, prepare a report of detailed diagnostic findings and treatment options (if appropriate), and offer an opinion regarding fitness for duty. The report will limit the evaluator's expert opinion to questions of psychiatric impairment, not assessments of unsafe medical practice due to lack of skill, knowledge, or training. Specific questions center on the presence of impairment as a result of psychiatric illness. Illness may refer to psychiatric disorders including substance abuse disorders, as well as physical disease or disability. Behavioral concerns such as boundary violations, unethical or illegal behavior, or interpersonal conflicts may precipitate an evaluation but do not necessarily result from disability or impairment due to a psychiatric illness. A fitness for duty evaluation must address the specific functional tasks of the particular trainee's duties. Therefore, the following information should be provided to the examiner: a criterion-based job description, or a list of resident responsibilities, the specific questions the program would like to address, and any collateral information that can help the evaluator to more fully understand the resident's functional level. Since the purpose of a fitness for duty evaluation is to provide information to an employer or program director, the resident needs to know in advance of the limits of confidentiality and sign appropriate releases for the examiner to provide a report [41].

For residents struggling with problematic non-cognitive learning behaviors unrelated to psychiatric illness, assessment by an educational specialist may be helpful. High-yield non-cognitive behaviors that are most likely to benefit from a performance and learning strategy intervention include organizational skills, time management, cognitive skill development, interpersonal or communication skills, or test-taking difficulty. A resident with a pattern of chronic non-compliance with program policies, expectations, or follow-up on prior educational interventions is not likely to benefit from this type of assessment.

When a resident has extraordinary external stresses or has disclosed a psychiatric illness, both the program director and the faculty must be very careful to keep their compassion and empathy for the resident separate from the expectations for performance standards. Mental health treatment or learning strategy assistance may be an important part of a remedial plan to assist the resident to succeed, but participation in such is not a reasonable performance outcome measure. Residents should be educated to consider requesting a medical accommodation to allow for extra assistance to perform the essential duties of their job.

In assessing for underlying causes, a program director must be open to the possibility that causative factors may lie within the program rather than within the resident. Excessive clinical volumes or call demands may be exceeding the capabilities of residents with more limited reserves. If a resident is exhibiting unprofessional behaviors, being rude to subordinates, or throwing things in the OR, he or she may be emulating behaviors that are being role modeled by faculty. It is not uncommon for an underperforming resident to perceive that they are being held to a different standard than another resident. Academic decisions for individual learners are made based on individual factors and review of the entire academic record.

Developing a Learner-Centered Remediation Plan

Remediation may carry different connotations for different institutions. For some, remediation may imply a formal institutional action, such as letter of deficiency or academic probation. For others it may encompass an informal warning status. Remediation programs may include focused activities that parallel regularly scheduled rotations, repeated rotations or experiences within a standard length of training, or extension of training. In this chapter, we define remediation broadly as "the process of improving or correcting a situation" [42]. As an adult learner with expected competence in practice-based learning and improvement, the resident should be actively involved in developing the plan. As described by Hauer et al. [23] and Sullivan and Arnold [29], a sensible remediation plan requires the articulation of clear goals and expectations for acceptable performance. The goal of any remediation is behavioral change. Therefore, the expected outcome behaviors should be as specific as possible. (See Table 17.4 for examples).

Development of a remediation plan should be guided by sound educational principles as well as program and institutional policies on academic progression and due process. In addition to a clear description of the performance deficits and

Table 17.4 Examples of behavior-based performance outcomes

You are expected to	Your progress will be assessed via
For a resident with dependability issues	
You are expected to	Your progress will be assessed via
Arrive promptly to all clinical and educational activities Complete all duty hour, charting, and other residency administrative requirements in a timely manner Log all procedures within 1 week Respond promptly and courteously to pages and phone calls from clinical and administrative staff	Attendance and punctuality for all clinical and educational activities Timely and satisfactory completion of all rotational requirements, including medical records and procedure logs Prompt and professional response to all emails, pages, etc. Satisfactory performance as assessed by the CCC Absence of patient or staff complaints
For a resident with deficiencies in clinical reasoning and decision-making	
You are expected to	Your progress will be assessed via
Formulate an appropriate and complete differential diagnosis for patients, and present this to supervisors in an organized manner Formulate an appropriate plan of care for patients, and present this to supervisors in an organized manner Manage patient care, including answering nursing questions, responding to patient care concerns, and completing orders as appropriate Proactively contact your chief resident or attending if you are uncertain about how to manage a patient	Successful completion of five observed clinical encounters with reflection and debriefing Successful performance in verification of proficiency exam in the skills lab, to be scheduled in the last week of this plan Improvement in mean rotation ratings for key items Absence of critical incidents or complaints by patients or staff Satisfactory performance as assessed by the CCC

expected performance outcomes, the following should be defined in advance and adhered to scrupulously:

- Time frame for remediation
- Prescribed learning activities
- Adjustments to schedule (decompression, repeat of previous rotation)
- Monitoring and feedback process
- Schedule and criteria for reassessment
- Consequences for not meeting the expected standards

The outlined criteria for reassessment should delineate any assessment activities that are not part of the program's regular performance assessment structure, such as additional standardized objective clinical examinations. Because of limitations in supervisor rotation evaluations described earlier, it is best to avoid using "satisfactory performance on all rotation evaluations" as an expected outcome. A more appropriate approach is "satisfactory performance as adjudged by the CCC." To reinforce accountability, the plan may be signed by the program director and the resident.

An essential component of any remedial program is the provision of prescribed learning activities that are tailored to the problems and the resident's learning needs.

For example, a period of increased direct supervision and standardized objective clinical examination exercises would be useful for a resident with difficulties in clinical reasoning and judgment, but not a deficit in medical knowledge. A resident with deficits in interpersonal relations or emotional self-regulation would be better served by a plan that includes clear behavioral expectations and consequences, coaching or mentoring, and frequent 360 degree feedback than a series of assigned readings. For residents struggling with significant stress management, substance use, or mental health issues, referral for formal treatment or outside resources or support, schedule decompression, or a medical leave of absence may well be part of the plan. However, it is important for the resident to understand that any activities in the remedial plan are being put in place to assist them and it is ultimately their responsibility to demonstrate the expected performance standards. (See Appendix A for sample plans).

Once a plan is initiated, the activities should offer the resident opportunities for focused deliberate practice on the deficiency areas with frequent feedback and encouragement for self-reflection. There should be at least one identified advisor or mentor who is meeting regularly throughout the plan's duration to assist in these. The resident should be updated frequently regarding progress. This approach maximizes the chances of success for the remediation plan and minimizes the chances for a learner to misperceive how he or she is progressing and have a surprise at the end of the reassessment.

The final step is the reassessment at the end of the prescribed period of remediation, utilizing the assessment parameters that were outlined in the plan. If the resident is still not meeting performance standards, and the program feels that the resident has the capabilities to succeed, the plan may be updated and continued. If the resident is successful and is performing adequately at the end of the plan, this should be stated explicitly to the resident and documented in the resident's file as well.

Impact of Learning Climate

The process of identifying and providing intervention for performance deficits is smoother in a program with a safe learning climate. Components of a safe learning climate include shared mission and values, commitment to a common purpose, clear expectations and performance standards, the ability to speak up without fear of intimidation or retaliation, and, most importantly, the perceived accuracy of performance feedback and assessment [43]. Accuracy of evaluations is a concern for both program directors and residents, although program directors worry more about grade inflation or leniency and residents worry more about fairness or unwarranted over-attention to lapses of competence. The motivation of faculty can have profound effects on the accuracy of evaluations. If a program leader sends the strong message that careful observation, accurate assessment, and frequent feedback are important, the faculty is more likely to be assiduous in directly observing residents, rating them honestly, and providing feedback. The level of trust held by faculty raters that the assessment system is fair may account for up to one third of rating variance. Raters with the highest degree of trust provide the most accurate and least lenient ratings [28]. Likewise, the resident's level of trust that the assessment system is fair and just strongly impacts a struggling resident's willingness to accept feedback regarding their performance and progression in the program.

Despite active efforts to increase diversity in surgical training and a steady increase in the number of women residents [44], representation in surgical programs remains low for Asian-Americans (17%) and for African-Americans, Latin Americans, and international medical graduates (about 5% each). The number of minority surgical faculty, particularly in academic programs, remains even lower [45–47]. An underperforming minority resident may experience some unique challenges in processing and navigating remediation. It's not uncommon for minority residents to enter training with a history of discriminatory experiences and may perceive the overall assessment system as less fair as a result. Because of the relative paucity of minority faculty, minority residents may have fewer opportunities for role modeling or mentoring. And, even with the best of intentions, faculty and CCC members may carry some level of stereotypical assumptions about minority trainees. Active steps to maintain and cultivate a positive learning environment that is respectful and as free as possible of implicit bias can go a long way in mitigating some of this. Most academic institutions have an official well versed in diversity who can provide support and consultation to the minority resident, program director, or both. Residents can be encouraged to bring an advocate or support person to formal discussions of their remediation or progress in the program.

The Nonreflective Learner

Every resident wants to succeed, and the majority of residents who receive feedback that their performance is not where it should be actively embrace recommendations on how to improve it. However, learners come to us with varying levels of self-reflection. Occasionally a program director will encounter a resident who lacks insight into the presence, nature, or seriousness of the deficits. This is more common when the deficits lie in domains with a higher level of assessment subjectivity, such as clinical judgment or interpersonal skills, or when deficits are identified later in training. A nonreflective resident will often selectively attend to positive feedback or assessments in areas in which they are performing well and tune out information about deficits. At the completion of training, the program director must certify that the resident is an independent lifelong learner, and a resident who is very resistive to feedback and unable to reflect upon performance does not meet this standard. In an effort to be supportive, kindhearted supervisors may unwittingly reinforce this pattern by giving frequent words of encouragement to the resident but less (or no) ongoing feedback about the performance areas of concern. If supervisors are also less than direct and honest on their written evaluations, it creates a greater dissonance between the resident's and the program director's assessment of performance. This can be mitigated somewhat by following the assessment and feedback guidelines outlined earlier in the chapter. We cannot overemphasize the importance of ensuring that every supervisor provides frequent, honest, and accurate performance feedback to all residents. Learners who are not exposed to feedback early in their training tend to become less receptive to it as they progress. Frequent feedback also reinforces that the assessment system is a just one. If informal feedback is occurring on a regular basis, there should be no surprises for the resident at more formal assessment points [48].

Remediating a resident with significant performance problems is stressful in the best of circumstances. Sometimes, even in the presence of frequent, honest, and accurate feedback, if the resident lacks insight about the deficits or has significant interpersonal difficulties, the process can become adversarial. Organizing and implementing a remediation plan for a willing resident take a significant amount of faculty time and effort. If the resident is angry or repeatedly challenges feedback and performance assessment, it can become emotionally draining as well. Nonreflective residents may want to revisit and parse the details of every incident or complaint instead of reflecting or looking at the larger pattern. It is important to allow the resident a forum to have his or her concerns heard, addressing any that may be reasonable while taking care not to get sidetracked by repeated discussions of incident details that have already been thoroughly evaluated and discussed. Consistently and firmly refocus the discussion to the discrepancy between the expected standards of the program and the resident's performance and behavior. No matter how challenging the resident is, it is wise to not respond with anger and to avoid the temptation to diagnose any personality issues, as that has no bearing on the performance standards. The most important thing for the program director to remember is that resident training is a collective effort. Fellow program directors, departmental chair, faculty members, the DIO, and human resources or legal colleagues can all be valuable sources of support.

How Do You Know if Your Remediation Is Successful?

Knowing if and when a given intervention or remediation for a resident has been successful is a difficult issue for program directors and CCCs. The success rate for an intervention for a discrete medical knowledge deficit, such as in-training exam performance, may be 75–100% [17, 18, 49]. Remediation is generally more successful for deficiencies in medical knowledge and least successful for problems in professionalism, communication, and interpersonal behaviors [1, 6, 17, 18, 49, 50]. Papadakis [51–53] has reported an association between professionalism concerns in medical school and residency and disciplinary action by a medical board but did not include info on whether attempts at remediation had occurred. For many residents, especially those with deficiencies in multiple areas, the deficits may persist over time, and repeated episodes of remediation may be needed [2, 6].

Graduation rates from 52% to 94% have been reported for identified underperforming residents, with lower rates corresponding to those residents on formal academic probation status [3, 4, 6, 7, 9, 14]. The interpretation of graduation rates as a successful outcome measure for underperforming surgery residents is complicated by the high attrition rate of about 20% among general surgery residents, irrespective of in-residency performance [54]. Unfortunately, as measured by board certification and licensure, residents who underperform may experience continued difficulties after graduation [6, 14]. Among the 102 residents on probation across all specialties described by Guerrasio et al. [14], 52% ultimately graduated. These graduates were less likely than their matched peers to be in practice or fellowship (96% versus 100%), and those that were in practice were less likely to be board certified (64% versus 100%) and more likely to have an encumbrance on their medical license (6.9% versus 0%). In a retrospective analysis of categorical general surgery residents in 1 program over 30 years, Williams et al. [6] identified 17 residents with substantial problems. They found the residents often had deficits in multiple areas and continued to have substantial performance problems at the end of the program, even with interventions. Sixteen out of the 17 residents ultimately graduated from the program, although two repeated a year. They continued to underperform after graduation. Compared to matched controls, they were less likely to be board certified (59% versus 100%) and less likely to hold active medical licensure (88% versus 100%).

The Legal Context of the Poorly Performing Resident

Are residents considered employees or students? On November 26, 1999, the National Labor Relations Board (NLRB) rendered a decision holding resident physicians to be "employees" under the National Labor Relations Act (NLRA). This decision reversed two prior decisions (1976, 1977) that residents were not employees (but instead, students) under the NLRA. The impact of the 1999 decision allowed for residents to organize in labor unions and collectively bargain as "employees" with full rights and protections of the NLRA; however, this decision also opened legal pathways for residents to take action against their employers under employment laws. Principles adopted by the ACGME related to the NLRB decision are outlined in Fig. 17.1

1. Residents are first and foremost students, rather than employees, and all accreditation standards and activities reflect this distinction.
2. Residents need to be protected as students with respect to their educational environment and the clinical settings in which they learn.
3. Residency settings vary substantially from place to place throughout the country. Thus, solutions to the resident protection issues which have been articulated should be implemented at local levels rather than by a single national plan. Institutions must be accountable for addressing resident concerns and issues at the local level.

Fig. 17.1 ACGME Principles

The bottom line is that residents are actually both employees and students. Like other employees, they receive an employment agreement/contract, receive a paycheck and benefits, contribute to retirement accounts, and, in many cases, even track their time. But they are also students, applying to accredited academic programs, enrolled in programs with a curriculum they must meet, and seeking to achieve an academic credential at the end of the educational period. This nuance is fundamental to approaching resident problems and issues and for program directors and institutions to be able to take appropriate actions that are defensible in a court of law. Therefore, prior to approaching the "how to" of dealing with problems that arise with residents, it is important for a program director to understand the legal context of both academic *and* employment law.

The ACGME. While there are no laws that require employers to have written policies or for employees to have written contracts, the ACGME requires institutions to provide written agreements for employment and to have policies that govern the many aspects of the resident's working environment [19]. In most institutions, employment-based lawyers with little academic/educational law experience advise GME programs to create policies that are very employment centric. Generally speaking, many policies try to be as detailed as possible, which creates a situation where the more you write, the worse the policy becomes. Good working policies provide a framework and allow for discretion and interpretation based on the framing principles.

Regardless of the employment and academic law principles and subsequent application described in this chapter, if a hospital and/or residency program does not follow their written policies, they will be at risk in any subsequent legal reviews and actions. At the heart of employment law are the requirements that employers do not discriminate (against those in protected statuses), follow their written policies, and comply with their written contracts.

Employment Law Employment laws derive from three primary sources: common law, federal statutes, and state statutes. In addition, many local jurisdictions, such as cities or counties, regulate different aspects of employment. Thus, precise rules governing employment for any particular hospital depends on the location of the hospital. However, common law governs the fundamental nature of the employment relationship. Although residents are almost always hired pursuant to written contracts or agreements, for a definite term, it is important to understand the nature of at-will employment, in order to understand the ways in which resident employment is different from other forms of employment. An at-will employment relationship is one with no specified term. Where no term is specified, either party may terminate the relationship at any time, for any lawful reason, or no reason, with or without notice.

Due process in employment matters follows a fairly simple framework:

1. Notice of the charges (allegations, accusations) against you
2. An opportunity to be *heard*
3. A reasonable decision-making process

Within the structure of employment settings, progressive discipline is a commonly utilized construct to assure due process has been followed. Progressive discipline typically resembles a "stepwise" process such as a verbal warning, written warning, and suspension prior to a termination action. These processes, while effective in many employment settings, generally are not effective in an academic setting like residency training, which is better suited to the principles of assessment, feedback, learning, and performance.

Academic Law and Resident Due Process

Two Supreme Court decisions provide the context and framework for academic due process, including the concept of a CCC.

University of Missouri v. Horowitz (1978) [55] *Case Summary*: Ms. Horowitz excelled in her first 2 years of medical school but received criticism from the faculty as she began her clinical rotations in years 3 and 4. She was provided feedback in her rotational evaluations criticizing her attendance, slovenly appearance, hygiene, and bedside manner. Despite feedback, Ms. Horowitz's behavior did not improve. The school's faculty evaluation committee ultimately recommended her dismissal from medical school. Ms. Horowitz appealed the dismissal decision to the Dean. The Dean allowed Ms. Horowitz the opportunity to be evaluated by seven independent physicians. At the conclusion of the rotations, the faculty provided feedback to the Dean of varied opinion; three physicians said she was fine, three said she was deficient, and one physician was indifferent. Based on the feedback of the independent faculty evaluators, the Dean upheld the dismissal decision. This case and the issue of academic due process were ultimately argued in front of the Supreme Court of the United States. The Court supported the University's decision based on the following:

1. Ms. Horowitz was provided *notice* of her deficiencies through private verbal feedback and her rotational evaluations.
2. Ms. Horowitz was provided an *opportunity to cure* her deficiencies.
3. The *decision was made carefully and deliberately*. The regularly called meeting of the faculty, called for the purpose of evaluating academic performance, was noted as being a reasonable decision-making process consisting of faculty members, expected to evaluate student performance.

Of note, the Court decision noted that the rotations with the seven physicians was *much more process than was due to Ms. Horowitz*, as the rotational evaluations provided her with notice (of her deficiencies) and an opportunity to cure.

University of Michigan vs. *Ewing (1985)* [56] *Case Summary*: Mr. Ewing was enrolled in the 6-year BS/MD program at the University of Michigan. After 4 years, he was eligible to write the NBME Step 1 exam. Mr. Ewing failed the exam and was subsequently dismissed from medical school. He sued, citing at least 11 other students who previously failed the exam and were allowed to stay enrolled in school and retake the test; some were allowed to retake the exam three and four times. In fact, Mr. Ewing was the only student in the history of the school who was dismissed based on failure of Step 1. The decision to dismiss Mr. Ewing was made by the faculty committee charged with reviewing academic performance. This committee reviewed Mr. Ewing's *entire academic record* and determined that based on his overall performance (including several incompletes, required repeats of courses, and the lowest score ever recorded on the NBME exam at this school), he did not have the ability or aptitude required of a physician and had no chance of ever succeeding.

The Court sided with the school noting:

1. "The narrow avenue for judicial review of the substance of academic decisions precludes any conclusion that such decision was a substantial departure from accepted academic norms as to demonstrate the faculty did not exercise professional judgment."
2. The decision-making process was "conscientious and made with careful deliberation," citing the regularly called faculty meeting structure, the "Promotion & Review Board."
3. The faculty rightly reviewed Mr. Ewing's entire academic record, not just a single test, rotation, or incident, to provide context to the decision.

Like due process in employment law, academic due process provides for a similar framework. The decision in the Horowitz case defines academic due process with an important nuance, the opportunity to cure:

1. Notice (of deficiencies)
2. Opportunity to *cure*
3. A careful and deliberate decision-making process

An opportunity to cure an academic deficiency is reasonable in the residency setting, allowing for a resident who is not performing on target to receive feedback of their deficiencies, formulate a plan, and show improvement. An opportunity to cure would not be appropriate for behavioral situations, where the law, or practical management, does not need to allow an individual an opportunity to repeat bad behavior. This premise will be further deconstructed in this chapter as we differentiate between academic and professional misconduct issues in residency.

The "reasonable decision-making process" as we know it in residency education is the CCC, that is, a regularly called meeting of the faculty for the purpose of discussing student (resident/fellow) performance. In both Missouri v. Horowitz ("Horowitz") and Michigan v. Ewing ("Ewing"), the faculty evaluation committee was identified as being a vital component of the "reasonable decision-making process." This structure of a faculty committee is the legal construct supporting the importance of the CCC in today's evaluation systems in medicine and by the ACGME. The Ewing case further supported the idea that a faculty decision-making committee rendering academic performance decisions that are conscientious and made with careful deliberation (i.e., they are not arbitrary or capricious) constitutes reasonable decision-making. When making academic decisions regarding resident/fellow performance, promotion, or dismissal, the CCC provides the structure recognized by the highest court in academic cases.

Due process	
Academic	Misconduct
Notice Opportunity to *cure* Reasonable decision-making	Notice Opportunity to *be heard* Reasonable decision-making

Resident Misconduct

Prior to approaching an issue involving a problem resident, program directors should pause and decide if the challenge is one of pure academic issues or of behavioral misconduct. Issues that are academic in nature can be dealt with most simply and directly by assuring the resident receives feedback (notice of deficiencies) and an opportunity to cure. Earlier in this chapter, we discussed the many ways in which residents can be provided feedback that meet the framework of academic law.

However, behavioral problems can be more difficult to navigate. When a potential behavioral issue arises with a resident, program directors should begin the process by talking with the resident regarding the allegation made and providing the resident with an opportunity to be heard – to hear their side of the story. In most situations, hearing the resident's side of the story provides an unknown perspective to a situation. Once the resident has an opportunity to be heard, then the program must determine the next steps.

- Does the resident not contest the allegation? If they admit to the allegation, then perhaps no further investigation needs to be done. At that point, the program director may be able to determine what the appropriate next step is, including dismissal.
- Does the resident contest the allegation? If the resident provides a different perspective or contradictory information, then it's incumbent on the program director to inquire further. This may mean conducting an investigation to learn additional facts from other people, documents, or records.

Deficiency in Professionalism or Misconduct?
You receive a phone call concerning Dr. Jones, a fifth-year resident who is due to graduate in 1 month. To date, there have not been any serious performance issues with Dr. Jones, but he has "pushed the envelope" a few times with issues related to honesty and integrity. The program administrator is reporting to you that she has collected the resident's procedure logs, and based on the ledger, it appears that Dr. Jones has falsified information in the logs. It is noted that all of the entries for the past 10 months are written with the same pen and in the same format and appears at face value to have been entered all at once. You tell the administrator to bring you the documents; you examine them personally and agree with her assessment. You then look up a couple of the patients listed in the log and confirm that the information is either incorrect or nonexistent in the medical records. You share this with several of the core faculty, and all are in agreement that Dr. Jones must be fired for this serious breach of honesty.

Question to consider: Is this matter an academic issue or misconduct? Since it deals with behavior (conduct), it should be treated as misconduct until more information can be received. In order to treat the matter as misconduct, the program director should meet with the resident, present the allegations, and hear Dr. Jones' side of the story (e.g., notice of charges, an opportunity to be heard, and a reasonable decision-making process). This should happen prior to the program director, or the faculty, assessing judgment.

You meet with Dr. Jones and share the information, allegations, and procedure log. Dr. Jones quickly admits, without shame, that he procrastinated and in fact wrote all 10 months' worth of procedures in 1 day; furthermore, he notes there were several that he couldn't remember exact dates or names. However, he shares with you that the associate program director (a fairly new graduate of your program) told him to do this and said it was common practice and it wasn't a big deal.

Question to consider: How does this information provided by the resident change this situation? Since the resident was acting under the direction of the associate program director, does it change your view of the situation? If you had not received this information, how would your decision-making process have been different in this scenario? What steps should you take now that you have more information?

Conducting an inquiry does not mean trying to be a police detective or basing decisions on irrefutable evidence. In fact, many times, the person conducting the inquiry may receive ambiguous information or nuanced information from many sources. A misconduct inquiry is not a court trial; the program director should gather as many facts as possible in order to make the best possible decision.

In some situations, a program director may determine that the resident in fact did engage in misconduct, but either made an honest mistake or has faith that the resident can learn from the situation and improve. Only after an inquiry can this determination be fairly made. If the program director determines the resident should be given another chance to show they can learn from the misconduct, then remediating under the competency of professionalism is an appropriate next step.

Documentation

When defending a legal case, contemporaneous documentation of events, actions, or conversations is very helpful in determining whether or not something actually happened. While there is no law that requires evaluations or performance feedback to be written, the ACGME requires written rotational evaluations and semiannual evaluations of performance. Of course, it is natural within an academic clinical setting that a faculty member provides a resident/fellow with routine verbal feedback. Although it is not recorded, this verbal feedback constitutes notice and opportunity to cure [55].

While it is always helpful to have written performance documentation, lack thereof should not deter evaluators from doing the right thing and utilizing this information as part of the overall evaluation process. One critical role of the CCC is to elicit feedback from faculty members regarding performance in a variety of settings and situations and for the faculty to discuss performance based on individual experiences and opinions. In many situations, this discussion at the CCC may be the first time that issues emerge and indicate a pattern of performance or behaviors. This discussion is the heart of the CCC and should not be discounted just because there is not a rotational evaluation or other assessment tool or form to support the discussion. Research shows that the discussion among the faculty members in the CCC often provides more accurate and robust information regarding learner performance than the written evaluation alone, which may not represent a complete view of actual performance (see previous section on the CCC).

The Appeals Process

The ACGME requires each Sponsoring Institution to have a policy that provides residents/fellows with due process relating to the following actions regardless of when the action is taken during the appointment period: suspension, nonrenewal, non-promotion, or dismissal [19]. Many institutions have structured "hearings" or multiparty review panels to hear and decide upon resident appeals. However, there is no requirement for a "hearing" or even a panel consisting of multiple people. Due process can be as simple as a meeting, with a single neutral reviewer. Padmore, Richard, and Filak [57] describe review processes in detail, demonstrating that a single reviewer can be more effective and less resource intensive than a hearing or review panel.

The appeals process should be limited to assuring that (a) departmental/hospital/university policies were followed, (b) the resident received notice and opportunity to cure [or be heard], and (c) there was a reasonable decision-making process and (d) determining if there were any extenuating circumstances that have not previously been considered. If all of these items are in compliance, then it is generally inappropriate for a review panel to change or reverse the decision of a department regarding competence or performance.

The Final Summative Evaluation

The ACGME requires the program to prepare a final summative evaluation (FSE) for each resident [58]. The FSE should be competency based, fair, and balanced and provide a narrative assessment of the entirety of the resident's performance in your program. The FSE should be comprehensive enough that it is maintained as the historic document of record describing the performance of the trainee for decades to come. The FSE should be provided upon request to other training programs, licensing boards, and credentialing bodies. It is good practice to provide the resident with a copy of the FSE upon departure from the program. The FSE for an underperforming resident, or a resident who has been dismissed from the program, can be especially important. The FSE should be carefully written and honest. The FSE is very different from a letter of recommendation (LOR). The FSE is comprehensive and balanced. Letters of recommendation are intended to be positive and written to persuade another decision-maker and generally do not include both strengths and weaknesses. Departments should have a policy on who can write letters of recommendation and under what circumstances. The institution can have substantial risk when dismissing a resident, if conflicting messages in the form of the FSE and LOR are communicated to others.

Summary

In this chapter, we have reviewed steps in identifying, clarifying, and addressing deficiencies in resident performance. Performance issues are most commonly identified via direct observation of clinical skills by faculty, standardized cognitive or clinical assessments, and critical incidents or complaints. Faculty may be reluctant to document concerns about underperformance on written evaluations. Verbal expressions of concern or complaints, even in the face of average rotation evaluations, should be taken seriously. Residents often have deficiencies in multiple domains, although the competencies of medical knowledge, patient care, professionalism and interpersonal skills, and communication are the most common. Remediation efforts are felt to be more successful in medical knowledge and less so with deficits in clinical reasoning or professionalism. When underperformance is identified, the nature and extent of the deficiencies should be elucidated as clearly as possible. This educational formulation should include assessment for any underlying or contributing factors such as resident stress or burnout, time management or organizational problems, unreasonable service expectations, or inadequate medical school preparation. A remediation plan should be targeted to the deficits and formulated with active input by the learner and CCC. It should clearly outline the expected performance outcomes, as well as the prescribed learning activities and any adjustments to the resident's regular schedule, the process for monitoring and feedback, timetable and criteria for reassessment, and consequences for not achieving the expected standards. We also reviewed the parameters of a good learning climate which include clear expectations and performance standards, consistent feedback, and the perceived accuracy and fairness of performance feedback and assessment. We discussed some of the challenges of the nonreflective learner and reinforced the vital importance of consistent, focused, direct, and accurate feedback.

We reviewed the legal context of underperformance, in that residents are both employees and students. In instances of academic or remediable professionalism deficiencies, a resident must be afforded notice of the deficiency and an opportunity to correct it. In instances of misconduct, a resident must be afforded a notice of the deficiency and an opportunity to be heard. In both cases, any decisions made regarding progress in the program must be made thoughtfully and deliberately, with active CCC involvement. In the case of serious deficiencies, or if the resident is unable to progress in the program, scrupulous adherence to program and institutional policies is paramount, as is involvement of other appropriate administrators, which generally include at a minimum the DIO, and representatives from legal and human resources.

Appendix A
Remediation Plan: Sample 1

This is an initial remediation for a PGY1 resident with a discrete deficit in medical knowledge and good insight. This is a program-level remediation. The resident is not being placed on official academic deficiency or probation status.

Dear Merle,

As we discussed last week in your semiannual review meeting, it is the consensus of the faculty that you have a deficiency in the ACGME competency domain of medical knowledge. As you know from our discussion, we are concerned that you are not learning to your ability. You identified time management and lack of reading as your primary challenge. You and I discussed the options and activities that you thought would be useful. These were very helpful as I worked with the Clinical Competency Committee to outline a sensible remediation plan for you.

This letter is to formally outline your remediation plan to improve your level of medical knowledge.

We encourage you to take the following steps:

- Schedule a short time for focused reading and reflection every day.
- Take a self-assessment examination at least monthly. Let these guide your focused reading.
- At the beginning of each rotation, review the goals and objectives for medical knowledge. Talk with your attending at the beginning of each rotation to get input on the most appropriate learning resources for those objectives.
- Every patient is an opportunity for specific reading. If your knowledge is pegged to patient, you will never forget.

It is ultimately your responsibility to take the steps necessary to your improve your level of knowledge. To assist you, the following help will be organized:

- Dr. Nelson has agreed to be your advisor. We recommend you meet with her at least monthly.
- You have access to our Specialty Question Bank and Self-Assessment Program.
- Dr. Cash and Dr. Owens are trained Board Examiners – they have agreed to give you periodic mini-oral exams upon request.

This remediation plan will be in place until next February. Your regular semiannual review will occur midway through this plan, and Dr. Nelson will review individual evaluations with you as they come in. The parameters the CCC will use to assess your progress will include:

- Faculty ratings and comments regarding medical knowledge on your evaluations, with emphasis on the final few months.
- Oral examination assessment cards from the final 3 months of this plan.
- Your in-service exam score. (This exam is just one piece of information, but scores are predictive of eventual success in board certification exam for our specialty. Improvement up to at least the 35th percentile for your PGY group should be a goal).

You will be promoted to your PGY2 year. Despite the knowledge deficits, your clinical skills are very good, and we trust you to assume PGY2 clinical and supervisory responsibilities. We do not plan any alterations to your regular schedule, but if at any point you feel like you need that, we can revisit. If you meet your learning goals in February, we will consider the remediation completed. If you have not met your learning goals by then despite active participation in the plan, we will either continue or modify it. In most instances, a plan that requires extension includes a more formal letter of deficiency.

We are all aware that the birth of your twins created some significant time management challenges for you. I'm pleased to hear that they are now sleeping through the night! Every faculty member is invested in your success and is devoted to helping you become the great doctor we know you can be.

Sincerely,

Signed by Program Director and Resident

Remediation Plan: Sample 2

This is a PGY2 resident with significant, ongoing deficits in multiple domains, with limited insight. Deficits have persisted despite several months of a program level remediation plan. This Sponsoring Institution uses a "letter of deficiency" process in lieu of a traditional probation process.

Dear Jamie,

I. Notice of Deficiency

This letter is to notify you that you are being given a letter of deficiency due to insufficient progress in the competency areas of medical knowledge, patient care, professionalism and practice-based learning, and improvement. Your faculty recognizes that you have been working very hard to improve your performance. However, your performance remains significantly below your level of training. These concerns have been discussed with you on numerous occasions over the past several months, both in your rotation feedback sessions and in monthly progress meetings with your advisor and myself. To review, the assessment of your progress is based on the following:

- Continued variability and unpredictability in performance.
- Reporting of patient data without processing or interpreting it.
- Continued instances of missing details in patient care or presenting wrong information.
- Continued instances of medication errors.
- Faculty continues to have concerns that you respond to feedback in a defensive manner or with excuses.
- Continued tardiness to conferences, clinical obligations, responding to pages, and completing medical records.
- Marked decrease in your ITE score.

At your level of training, you should be able to:

- Consistently demonstrate a predictable clinical performance on a day-to-day basis.
- Demonstrate an appropriate level of medical knowledge as demonstrated on evaluations and ITE.
- Attend to detail in caring for patients. Information presented should be accurate and correct.
- Be able to accurately order medications in the inpatient and outpatient setting.
- Accept feedback professionally and use self-reflection to analyze your own performance and areas for improvement.
- Respond to pages promptly, and keep current with medical records.

II. Opportunity to Correct Deficiency

It is ultimately your responsibility to take the steps necessary to meet expectations. To assist you in meeting the expectations, the following help will be organized:

Dr. Patel will continue as your advisor. Dr. Johnson will be your preceptor in the clinic.

We have made time available in your schedule for your meetings with our academic coach.

We will continue to limit the number of patients that you care for. The faculty does not believe that you are ready to assume a supervisory role.

You have identified EHR fluency as a time management problem. You now have Dragon access for the terminals both on the ward and in the outpatient clinic.

Jamie, your faculty is very worried about your health and wellness. We are concerned that you may have other issues in your personal life that are interfering with your ability to perform to your full potential. When you appear anxious and overwhelmed, your memory, performance, and organization are all markedly below average. We would once again strongly encourage you to utilize the employee assistance program.

In addition to your monthly evaluation review with Dr. Patel, your performance will be reviewed quarterly by the CCC with updates provided to you. Your progress in this letter of deficiency will be reassessed at the end of April. If you have demonstrated significant improvement at that time, this letter of deficiency may be rescinded or continued. If you are not achieving standards by then, we will have to consider either having you repeat all or part of your PGY2 year or termination.

Your faculty stands ready to help you, and we want to see you reach your potential as a physician. We encourage you to make use of all the resources available to you.

Sincerely,

Signed by Program Director, Resident, and DIO

Remediation Plan: Sample 3

This is an example of a last chance agreement with a resident who had unprofessional behavior related to substance misuse. It is more of a contract than a traditional remediation plan and is therefore between the resident and the employing hospital.

Last Chance Agreement

This agreement is made this day of, 20, by and between [Name of Hospital] Hospital ("Hospital") and, M.D. ("Dr.").

WHEREAS, Dr. __________, who is enrolled in Hospital Graduate Medical Education program and subsequently employed by Hospital, was referred for a full medical assessment and evaluation of fit for duty following documented substance abuse on (date). Dr. __________ was subsequently referred to (Treatment Center) for a professional evaluation. Dr. __________ has been cleared to return to the residency program under the conditions set forth in this Last Chance Agreement.

In addition, Dr. __________ has admitted to several instances of unprofessional conduct that will not be tolerated.

WHEREAS, Dr. __________ desires to enter into this agreement with Hospital, allowing Hospital to provide continued monitoring and oversight, and WHEREAS, Dr. __________ understands and agrees that he would not be allowed to re-enroll in the residency program, but for his agreement to and compliance with these terms, and further understands and agrees that this is his last chance to demonstrate that he is capable of meeting all professional expectations and curricular requirements and completing his residency training program at Hospital.

THEREFORE, IN CONSIDERATION of the mutual covenants and promises contained in this Agreement, the Parties do hereby agree as follows:

1. Professional Conduct. Dr. __________ affirms his understanding that his strict compliance with the terms of this Agreement is necessary as a condition of his enrollment in the residency and his employment at Hospital. He further affirms his understanding that non-compliance with this Agreement and non-compliance with the Hospital GME House Staff Manual Policies, and Hospital Policies, will lead to immediate dismissal from the residency training program and termination of his employment.
2. Conditions of Employment and Training:
   (a) Dr. __________ shall submit to ongoing compliance with therapy as recommended by his provider and the Hospital Physician Health and Wellness Committee.
   (b) Dr. __________ agrees to be monitored by the Hospital Physician Health and Wellness Committee for the remainder of his residency training and will submit to any required activities or treatment as directed by the Committee.
   (c) Dr. __________ agrees to random drug and alcohol monitoring by Hospital Occupational Health for the duration of his employment.
   (d) Dr. __________ agrees to be an active participant in various Hospital programs, as requested by the institution, to share his personal experiences with other residents to assist with their learning and professional development.
   (e) Dr. __________ agrees to meet with faculty mentor, Dr., at least monthly, to discuss and receive direction on his performance.
3. Abstinence from Improper Behavior. Dr. __________ agrees to maintain total abstinence from any outbursts, improper behavior, improper or poor communications, or other behavioral issues that are not supportive of a Just Culture, and Hospital's commitment to clinical quality and patient safety.
4. Job Performance Standards. Dr. __________ agrees and understands that he is expected to comply with all residency and job performance standards and requirements and with Hospital/department policies, practices, and procedures. He is expected to report on time for all work shifts, meetings, appointments, patient procedures/consultations, and other work-related requirements. Dr. __________ acknowledges that he will be subject to the appropriate disciplinary action for his non-compliance with this Paragraph 4, including dismissal from the residency program.

5. Notice to Management and Human Resources. Dr. __________ acknowledges and agrees that Hospital's GME Office has the right to provide his management staff, the Hospital VPMA and Chief Medical Officer, and anyone else with a need to know with notice that he is working under this mandatory Agreement and of his compliance or non-compliance with its terms and conditions.
6. Binding Agreement. The parties acknowledge that the terms of this Agreement are lawful and binding. Dr. __________ further acknowledges and agrees that any violation of the terms of this Agreement will result in his immediate termination from employment and dismissal from his fellowship training program and render him ineligible for employment at any other System Health facility. A violation of this Agreement will be reported to Dr. __________'s immediate supervisor, GME, and the Hospital VPMA/CMO, as well as the State Board of Medicine.
7. Term of Agreement. The parties agree that this Agreement will remain in force during Dr. __________'s employment.

I, __________, MD, acknowledge that I have read and understand the terms and conditions of this Agreement. I agree to abide by all terms of this Agreement without exception. I understand and acknowledge that my employment with Hospital will be terminated due to my non-compliance with this Agreement and/or with the policies and procedures of Hospital. I further acknowledge that I had the opportunity to ask questions and receive appropriate answers to clarify any portion of this Agreement and that I fully understand the terms and implications of the Agreement. I enter into this Agreement voluntarily, willingly, and without duress or coercion.

Signed by Resident and DIO/Hospital Representative

References

1. Dupras DM, Edson RS, Halvorsen AJ, Hopkins RH, McDonald FS. "Problem residents": prevalence, problems and remediation in the era of core competencies. Am J Med. 2012;125(4):421–5.
2. Audétat MC, Voirol C, Béland N, Fernandez N, Sanche G. Remediation plans in family medicine residency. Can Fam Physician. 2015;61(9):e425–34.
3. Reamy BV, Harman JH. Residents in trouble: an in-depth assessment of the 25-year experience of a single family medicine residency. Fam Med. 2006;38(4):252–7.
4. Tabby DS, Majeed MH, Schwartzman RJ. Problem neurology residents: a national survey. Neurology. 2011;76(24):2119–23.
5. Silverberg M, Weizberg M, Murano T, Smith JL, Burkhardt JC, Santen SA. What is the prevalence and success of remediation of emergency medicine residents? West J Emerg Med. 2015;16(6):839–44.
6. Williams RG, Roberts NK, Schwind CJ, Dunnington GL. The nature of general surgery resident performance problems. Surgery. 2009;145(6):651–8.
7. Yaghoubian A, Galante J, Kaji A, Reeves M, Melcher M, Salim A, et al. General surgery resident remediation and attrition: a multi-institutional study. Arch Surg. 2012;147(9):829–33.
8. Resnick AS, Mullen JL, Kaiser LR, Morris JB. Patterns and predictions of resident misbehavior – a 10-year retrospective look. Curr Surg. 2006;63(6):418–25.
9. Bergen PC, Littlefield JH, O'Keefe GE, Rege RV, Anthony TA, Kim LT, Turnage RH. Identification of high-risk residents. J Surg Res. 2000;92(2):239–44.

10. Yao DC, Wright SM. The challenge of problem residents. J Gen Intern Med. 2001;16(7):486–92.
11. Dudek NL, Marks MB, Regehr G. Failure to fail: the perspectives of clinical supervisors. Acad Med. 2005;80(10 Suppl):S84–7.
12. Schwind CJ, Williams RG, Boehler ML, Dunnington GL. Do individual attendings' post-rotation performance ratings detect residents' clinical performance deficiencies? Acad Med. 2004;79(5):453–7.
13. Roberts NK, Williams RG. The hidden costs of failing to fail residents. J Grad Med Educ. 2011;3(2):127–9.
14. Guerrasio J, Brooks E, Rumack CM, Christensen A, Aagaard EM. Association of characteristics, deficits, and outcomes of residents placed on probation at one institution, 2002-2012. Acad Med. 2016;91(3):382–7.
15. Sanfey H, DaRosa DA, Hickson GB, Williams B, Sudan R, Boehler ML, et al. Pursuing professional accountability. Arch Surg. 2012;147(7):642–7.
16. Brenner AM, Mathai S, Jain S, Mohl PC. Can we predict "problem residents"? Acad Med. 2010;85(7):1147–51.
17. Edeiken BS. Remedial program for diagnostic radiology residents. Investig Radiol. 1993;28(3): 269–74.
18. Harthun NL, Schirmer BD, Sanfey H. Remediation of low ABSITE scores. Curr Surg. 2005;62(5):539–42.
19. Accreditation Council for Graduate Medical Education Institutional Requirements. Available at http://acgme.org/Portals/0/PDFs/FAQ/InstitutionalRequirements_07012015.pdf. Accessed 19 Sep 2017.
20. Clinical Competency Committees: a guidebook for programs. http://www.acgme.org/Portals/0/ACGMEClinicalCompetencyCommitteeGuidebook.pdf. Published January 2015. Accessed 28 Apr 2017.
21. Williams RG, Dunnington GL, Klamen DL. Forecasting residents' performance-partly cloudy. Acad Med. 2005;80(5):415–22.
22. Holmboe ES, Sherbino J, Long DM, Swing SR, Frank JR. The role of assessment in competency-based medical education. Med Teach. 2010;32(8):676–82.
23. Hauer KE, Ciccone A, Henzel TR, Katsufrakis P, Miller SH, Norcross WA, et al. Remediation of the deficiencies of physicians across the continuum from medical school to practice: a thematic review of the literature. Acad Med. 2009;84(12):1822–32.
24. Hemmer PA, Pangaro L. The effectiveness of formal evaluation sessions during clinical clerkships in better identifying students with marginal funds of knowledge. Acad Med. 1997;72(7):641–3.
25. Hemmer PA, Grau T, Pangaro LN. Assessing the effectiveness of combining evaluation methods for the early identification of students with inadequate knowledge during a clerkship. Med Teach. 2001;23(6):580–4.
26. Hodges B, Regehr G, Martin D. Difficulties in recognizing one's own incompetence: novice physicians who are unskilled and unaware of it. Acad Med. 2001;76(10 Suppl):S87–9.
27. Davis DA, Mazmanian PE, Fordis M, Harrison RV, Thorpe KE, Perrier L. Accuracy of physician self-assessment compared with observed measures of competence: a systematic review. JAMA. 2006;296(9):1094–1102.
28. Govaerts MJ, van der Vleuten CP, Schuwirth LW, Muijtjens AM. Broadening perspectives on clinical performance assessment: rethinking the nature of in-training assessment. Adv Health Sci Educ Theory Pract. 2007;12(2):239–60.
29. Sullivan C, Arnold L. Assessment and remediation in programs of teaching professionalism. In: Teaching medical professionalism. New York: Cambridge University Press; 2009. p. 124–49.
30. Zbieranowski I, Takahashi SG, Verma S, Spadafora SM. Remediation of residents in difficulty: a retrospective 10-year review of the experience of a postgraduate board of examiners. Acad Med. 2013;88(1):111–6.
31. Collier VU, McCue JD, Markus A, Smith L. Stress in medical residency: status quo after a decade of reform? Ann Intern Med. 2002;136(5):384–90.

32. Sen S, Kranzler HR, Krystal JH, Speller H, Chan G, Gelernter J, Guille C. A prospective cohort study investigating factors associated with depression during medical internship. Arch Gen Psychiatry. 2010;67(6):557–65.
33. Mata DA, Ramos MA, Bansal N, Khan R, Guille C, Angelantonio ED, Sen S. Prevalence of depression and depressive symptoms among resident physicians: a systematic review and meta-analysis. JAMA. 2015;314(22):2373–83.
34. West CP, Shanafelt TD, Kolars JC. Quality of life, burnout, educational debt, and medical knowledge among internal medicine residents. JAMA. 2011;306(9):952–60.
35. Dyrbye LN, Massie FS Jr, Eacker A, Harper W, Power D, Durning SJ, et al. Relationship between burnout and professional conduct and attitudes among US medical students. JAMA. 2010;304(11):1173–80.
36. Shanafelt TD, Bradley KA, Wipf JE, Back AL. Burnout and self-reported patient care in an internal medicine residency program. Ann Intern Med. 2002;136(5):358–67.
37. Holmes EG, Connolly A, Putnam KT, Penaskovic KM, Denniston CR, Clark LH, et al. Taking care of our own: a multispecialty study of resident and program director perspectives on contributors to burnout and potential interventions. Acad Psychiatry. 2017;41(2):159–66.
38. West CP, Huschka MM, Novotny PJ, Sloan JA, Kolars JC, Habermann TM, Shanafelt TD. Association of perceived medical errors with resident distress and empathy: a prospective longitudinal study. JAMA. 2006;296(9):1071–8.
39. West CP, Tan AD, Habermann TM, Sloan JA, Shanafelt TD. Association of resident fatigue and distress with perceived medical errors. JAMA. 2009;302(12):1294–300.
40. Shanafelt TD, Balch CM, Bechamps G, Russell T, Dyrbye L, Satele D, et al. Burnout and medical errors among American surgeons. Ann Surg. 2010;251(6):995–1000.
41. Anfang SA, Faulkner LR, Fromson JA, Gendel MH. The American Psychiatric Association's resource document on guidelines for psychiatric fitness-for-duty evaluations for physicians. J Am Acad Psychiatry Law. 2005;33(1):85–8.
42. Cambridge English Dictionary. Cambridge, UK: Cambridge University Press. 2017. http://dictionary.cambridge.org/us/dictionary/english/remediation. Accessed 23 Jan 2017.
43. Goleman D. Leadership that gets results. Harv Bus Rev. 2000;78(2):78–90.
44. Davis EC, Risucci DA, Blair PG, Sachdeva AK. Women in surgery residency programs: evolving trends from a national perspective. J Am Coll Surg. 2011;212(3):320–6.
45. Daniels EW, French K, Murphy LA, Grant RE. Has diversity increased in orthopaedic residency programs since 1995? Clin Orthop Relat Res. 2012;470(8):2319–24.
46. Butler PD, Longaker MT, Britt LD. Major deficit in the number of underrepresented minority academic surgeons persists. Ann Surg. 2008;248(5):704–11.
47. National Resident Matching Program. Results and data: 2017 main residency match. http://www.nrmp.org/match-data/main-residency-match-data. Published May 2017. Accessed 1 May 2017.
48. Broquet K, Dewan M. Evaluation and feedback. In: International medical graduate physicians: a guide to training. Switzerland: Springer International Publishing; 2016. p. 41–55.
49. Borman KR. Does academic intervention impact ABS qualifying examination results? Curr Surg. 2006;63(6):367–72.
50. Adams KE, Emmons S, Romm J. How resident unprofessional behavior is identified and managed: a program director survey. Am J Obstet Gynecol. 2008;198(6):692.e1–5.
51. Papadakis MA, Hodgson CS, Teherani A, Kohatsu ND. Unprofessional behavior in medical school is associated with subsequent disciplinary action by a state medical board. Acad Med. 2004;79(3):244–9.
52. Papadakis MA, Teherani A, Banach MA, Knettler TR, Rattner SL, Stern DT, et al. Disciplinary action by medical boards and prior behavior in medical school. N Engl J Med. 2005;353(25):2673–82.
53. Papadakis MA, Arnold GK, Blank LL, Holmboe ES, Lipner RS. Performance during internal medicine residency training and subsequent disciplinary action by state licensing boards. Ann Intern Med. 2008;148(11);869–76.Andriole DA, Jeffe DB. Prematriculation variables associ-

ated with suboptimal outcomes for the 1994–1999 cohort of US medical school matriculants. JAMA 2010;304(11):1212–1219.
54. Yeo H, Bucholz E, Sosa JA, Curry L, Lewis FR, Jones AT, et al. A national study of attrition in general surgery training: which residents leave and where do they go? Ann Surg. 2010;252(3):529–36.
55. Board of Curators of Univ. of Mo. v. Horowitz, 435 U.S. 78, 98 S. Ct. 948, 55 L. Ed. 2d 124 (1978).
56. Regents of Univ. of Mich. v. Ewing, 474 U.S. 214, 106 S. Ct. 507, 88 L. Ed. 2d 523 (1985).
57. Padmore JS, Richard KM, Filak AT. Human Resources and Legal Management of Residents Who Fail to Progress. In: Guide to medical education in the teaching hospital. 5th ed. Irwin, PA: Association for Hospital Medical Education; 2016. p. 273–95.
58. Accreditation Council for Graduate Medical Education Common Program Requirements. Available at http://acgme.org/Portals/0/PFAssets/ProgramRequirements/CPRs_2017-07-01.pdf. Accessed 19 Sep 2017.

Part III

Lessons and Insights of Surgical Education

Surgeons' Reactions to Error

18

"First, Do No Harm": Rectifying the Perceived Hypocrisy of the Hippocratic Oath

Melanie Hammond Mobilio and Carol-anne Moulton

I will not be ashamed to say 'I know not,' nor will I fail to call in my colleagues when the skills of another are needed for a patient's recovery. [1].

Introduction

"First, do no harm"—the powerful mandate that springs to mind when we think of the role of the medical professional is thought to be captured succinctly within the Hippocratic Oath. The trouble is, the words themselves are actually not found anywhere within the oath. This vow—one that so many consider to be synonymous with entering the world of medical practice—is in fact a much lengthier and involved pledge to practice medicine in an ethical manner, without offering the impossible promise that mistakes will never be made. Unfortunately, the stereotype of the ideal surgeon (or more broadly, physician) as one who "does no harm" remains very much present in current surgical culture. This stereotype holds widespread implications for patients, families, and surgeons themselves.

More than a decade ago the American Institute of Medicine published *To Err is Human*, the seminal report that led to heightened public awareness of the large number of morbidities and mortalities associated with surgical complications [2].

M.H. Mobilio
Wilson Centre, University Health Network, Toronto, ON, Canada

C.-a. Moulton (✉)
Wilson Centre, University Health Network, Toronto, ON, Canada

Department of Surgery, University of Toronto, Toronto, ON, Canada

Division of General Surgery, University Health Network, Toronto, ON, Canada

Toronto General Hospital, Toronto, ON, Canada
e-mail: carol-anne.Moulton@uhn.ca

T.S. Köhler, B. Schwartz (eds.), *Surgeons as Educators*,
https://doi.org/10.1007/978-3-319-64728-9_18

Increased numbers of allegations of negligence and public expectations for solutions have created a pressure to enforce the prevention of surgical error [3]. The medical profession has responded to these pressures by placing greater emphasis on system-wide analyses of quality assurance and quality improvement strategies [4, 5]. These approaches are similar to those used in engineering and aviation, where advances have been made to reduce human factor contributions to error in the workplace [6, 7]. In surgery, the study of error has largely focused on "systems" causes, with little attention directed toward identifying causes for individual surgeon error or failures of self-regulation.

One NEJM study on adverse events in hospitalized patients notes that "unfortunate decisions and actions" occurring during care were a leading cause of death and disability [8]. Subsequent research showed that many of these decisions and actions were actual errors [9]. Definitions of "medical error" have been highly variable, making it hard to study error in epidemiology [10] with the additional issue that the term carries negative connotations of failure and blame. In recent literature, medical error has been defined as an "act or omission that leads to an unanticipated, undesirable outcome or to substantial potential for such an outcome" [11]. This will be the definition of error used in this review.

Adverse patient events are inevitable and common, yet many surgeons are poorly prepared for the emotional reactions they experience when they occur. To date, these reactions are widely considered "part of the job" of being a surgeon, a consequence of being a member of the profession. Although, if asked, most surgeons would acknowledge they experience a negative emotional reaction following an adverse event, the nature and impact of these events in surgical education are not well articulated. Surgical culture typically does not encourage open acknowledgment of these emotions; thus, surgeons would be unlikely to volunteer such information without direct probing into their experiences. In fact, it is quite possible that surgical culture itself may be a major contributor to the negative reactions we experience. With increased rates of burnout, suicide, divorce, and attrition among surgeons, it is important that we begin to understand what contributes to these reactions. Acknowledging and exploring these questions may better prepare the future generation of surgeons and keep our profession healthy.

How do surgeons react to error or patient complications? What factors affect these reactions, and how do these reactions affect future performance? Perhaps the best phenomenological description of these reactions has been provided by Paget [12]. Actions themselves are not distinctly seen as right or wrong, but instead they become right or wrong, in retrospect, in a process Paget calls "complex sorrow." Her work suggests that reactions to medical error are not as simple as once thought. An example of the ongoing interplay between error and practice was highlighted in one study exploring surgeons' reactions to unexpected outcomes or situations. Results indicate that surgeons' reactions to errors affect subsequent decision-making and judgment, and further research is clearly needed if we are to properly understand the association between the two [13].

This chapter will shed light on recent work that explored surgeons' reactions to adverse events. Several psychological theories are proposed, and ways they might help toward a greater understanding of the surgeon in the midst of an adverse event are suggested. While psychological theories help explain the inner workings of our brain and subsequent emotional reactions as human beings to these events, we are also embedded in a very powerful culture that influences our interpretation and experience of events. Therefore, we will also interrogate the surgical culture and accuse it somewhat of being at the epicenter of these reactions. Recognizing that it is impossible to "do no harm" over the course of a surgical career, we will provide a language to conceptualize, understand, and teach the experience of adverse events in surgery in a new way. We argue that, by reducing the stigma around admitting error and instead framing the unavoidable experience of adverse events as an opportunity for growth and reflection, surgeons and learners may open new avenues in which to harness surgical expertise.

To set the stage for what is to follow, it is necessary to first discuss the different terms used when talking about surgical mishaps. When a patient suffers an adverse event following surgery, it is not always possible to link the event with surgeon error. More often than not, the degree to which the surgeon is responsible for that particular event is difficult to ascertain. Surgical procedures will necessarily result in complications in a percentage of patients, even if the surgery was done "perfectly." Other times surgeon error is recognized as the cause of the mishap. In the latter situation, it is clear there is a direct causal link between surgeon error and adverse patient outcomes. It is worth noting that this clear link is not the norm. To further complicate the relationship between surgeon error and adverse outcomes, a surgical error does not always lead to a bad outcome for the patient. Surgical errors can be safely corrected during or after a procedure without necessarily causing harm to a patient. Therefore, it is necessary to state at the outset that a surgeon's reaction to an adverse event might be the same whether or not an error was recognized and/or acknowledged. Granted, the reaction might be more severe if there is a clear link between the error and event, but the nature of the reaction appears to be similar regardless. For this reason, in the section that follows, we will focus on the phases of the reaction generally and not get hung up on the impossible task of quantifying the specific cause of individual events as they relate to surgeon reaction to error.

Phases of Reactions to Adverse Events

What is the nature of the reaction a surgeon experiences after a patient's adverse event?

In a recent qualitative study, as part of a larger research program on surgeon cognition and culture, we interviewed 20 surgeons about their reactions to adverse events. Our aim in this study was to develop a conceptual framework [13] for understanding these reactions for the purposes of providing a tool for self-reflection, discussion, teaching, and further error-reduction strategies.

Luu et al. identified four phases of progression after an adverse event: the kick, the fall, the recovery, and the long-term impact [13]. The initial stage, *the kick*, was characterized by a visceral response of tachycardia, anxiety, and self-deprecation. In this phase, surgeons described a physiological response upon hearing of the adverse event. Whether it was at the bedside, at the operating table, over the phone, or elsewhere, surgeons described a similar response that included a physiological component. This phase was also associated with a sense of inadequacy and shame. Surgeons described wanting to hide and run away. One surgeon described almost running into four parked cars in the parking lot after he heard the news. Others described a preoccupation after hearing about the adverse event such that they could not focus on any other activity. Following this initial phase, surgeons progressed to the next, categorized as *the fall*. Here, surgeons sought to figure out, "how much of this was my fault?" This phase centered on the surgeon seeking information—answers to questions about their role in the error, looking up journal articles around similar complications, talking to colleagues, and, when relevant, rehearsing the event over and over in their heads. Participants described the presence of a "black cloud" or "pall" that affected their emotional well-being as well as their personal and professional lives. Surgeons acknowledged that the impact was typically greater if a direct link between their actions and the adverse event could be established. The third phase, *the recovery*, focused around communication of the event to colleagues. For many, it was easier to discuss the details of the case rather than the emotional impact it had on them personally. The recovery phase appeared to be marked by a commitment to improve in their practice. Surgeons did not want the patient's suffering to be for nothing. By reframing the adverse event into a learning experience, participants appeared to begin the process of granting themselves permission to "move on." The final phase, *the long-term impact*, left a positive or negative impression on the physician depending on how they viewed the adverse event and in some instances resulted in a change to their scope of practice. While most surgeons saw the long-term impact of each adverse event in a negative light, a few described positive impacts, such as increased humanity or emotional maturity within themselves that came from a connection to the patient and/or the patient's family after these events occurred.

It noteworthy that the authors of this study could not find a surgeon that did not describe experiencing these reactions in their practice. Without exception, participants admitted to being affected by adverse events in similar ways, and many wanted to talk further about their reactions with the researchers after the study was completed. Following publication of the study, numerous surgeons—ranging from local to international—have contacted the senior author to share stories of their own experience. It is critical to highlight this point, as many surgeons continue to feel they are unique or "odd" as they are left to deal with their emotions around adverse events. These feelings can contribute to surgeons feeling isolated at an extremely vulnerable time in their practice and ultimately surgeon burnout. We will return to these vitally important issues later in this chapter.

Awareness, then, is the first step toward a healthier experience around adverse events for surgeons. Naming the phases as individuals experience them is an important step toward understanding and is likely quite helpful for surgeons to see that their experience is shared by so many. Understanding the ubiquitous nature of these reactions among surgeons might help prevent the individual surgeon feeling they are all alone in these experiences or not "cut out" to cope with the consequences of surgical mishaps.

The next step is to begin to understand the causal roots of these damaging reactions. Adverse events happen in surgery. Why do we respond to them this way when they do?

Surgeons Are People

Once thought of as infallible and unemotional, physicians and the public now increasingly recognize that doctors are as human as the patients they care for. The mid-1980s was marked by a series of publications in the medical literature that portrayed personal accounts of physicians conveying feelings of guilt, shame, and inadequacy after a medical error [14–16]. This paved the way for acknowledging the internal struggle physicians face, leading internist Dr. Albert Wu to coin the term "second victim" [17]. In an editorial published in 2000, Scott et al. went on to provide a more detailed definition as follows [18]:

> Second victims are healthcare providers who are involved in an unanticipated adverse patient event, in a medical error and/or a patient related injury and become victimized in the sense that the provider is traumatized by the event. Frequently, these individuals feel personally responsible for the patient outcome. Many feel as though they have failed the patient, second guessing their clinical skills and knowledge base.

As clinicians we feel a sense of duty to our patients and honor to our profession. We have all felt the sinking feeling when we realize that we have made a mistake while caring for a patient. Instinctively we look to see who has noticed because we fear the accompanying shame or punishment. We wrestle with the information, who to tell and what to say. In an effort to make sense of what happened, we may replay the events in our mind, what we could have done differently, and how it may have changed the outcome. The thought of confessing breeds fear of punishment and uncertainty about how the patient will react. These negative feelings may leave us feeling anxious, isolated, and insecure.

In addition to its direct emotional effect, complications can negatively impact a physician's performance. Patel et al. reported that 12.2% of surgeons felt it impaired their ability to perform their job and 2% even avoided certain procedures as a result [19]. Survey participants who were negatively affected by a complication reported difficulty concentrating, declining clinical judgment, loss of confidence, trouble sleeping, and difficulty enjoying leisurely activities and daily life—symptoms that overlap with clinical signs of depression [20]. A review of the literature shows other frequently reported symptoms include frustration, embarrassment, anger, blame, worry about reputation, and reduced job satisfaction [21–27]. Pinto et al. described the association between complications and acute traumatic stress, likening it to post-traumatic stress disorder [28]. They determined that general surgeons were more likely to display symptoms of acute traumatic stress than their vascular surgery counterparts, hypothesizing that general surgeons may be less accustomed to life-threatening complications or a complication in a low-risk patient takes a higher toll than if the patient were high risk [28]. According to survey results from Shanafelt et al., surgeons may be more sensitive to burnout than their nonsurgeon colleagues as they were less likely to report that they would become a surgeon again and less likely to recommend their children pursue a career in surgery [29].

Physician burnout and medical errors appear to be intimately associated, although direct causation is more difficult to establish [30, 31]. Both patients and physicians attribute stress, fatigue, and exhaustion leading to medical errors [32, 33]. Fahrenkopf et al. established a relationship between depression and medical errors in pediatric residents when they determined that residents suffering from depression were six times more likely than their nondepressed colleagues to make a medication error [31]. The relationships between adverse events and surgeon wellness and expertise are clear. Next, we will outline what might be going on in a surgeon's head as they navigate the experience of an adverse event.

Inside the Head of the Surgeon: The Psychology of the Surgeon's Reaction to Error

In this section we consider literature from the field of social psychology as a lens through which we might think about surgeons' reaction to error in a new way. Here we will introduce theories of cognitive dissonance, self, and counterfactual thinking.

First proposed by Festinger, the theory of *cognitive dissonance* refers to the notion that if a person holds two psychologically (not necessarily logically) discrepant thoughts, psychological discomfort will occur [34]. Psychologically, individuals are motivated to reduce dissonance, either by changing one or both of the thoughts or by introducing a new thought. For example, a reputable surgeon who takes pride in her operative skills will develop cognitive dissonance if a technical error is made ("I am a very good surgeon" and "I made a mistake"). In order to resolve the discomfort, she can introduce a new thought—maybe that the patient's case was confounding—and thus the error had nothing to do with her technical skill or judgment. A colorectal surgeon who injures the left ureter in a difficult sigmoid resection, for example, may "know" that the ureter was in its normal position in the retroperitoneum but may "think" (by introduction of a new thought) that an unusual variant, such as peritoneal adhesions, "caused" the error, as she deals with her uncomfortable cognitive dissonance.

The *theory of self* utilizes *self-affirmation* to explain the approaches that individuals take when dealing with cognitive dissonance, understanding that the goal of an individual's *self* is to protect their self-integrity. When the image of self-integrity is threatened, the individual will take steps to restore self-worth [35]. There are a variety of ways to maintain self-integrity but, when possible, individuals will choose to respond to threats using indirect psychological adaptations in which they can adapt affirmations unrelated to the immediate situation. These unrelated affirmations allow the individual to realize that their self-integrity and self-worth are independent of the situation [36]. In the previous example, the surgeon determined that her technical skill and self-esteem were independent of error, thus allowing her to self-affirm. When given the choice, individuals will tend to self-affirm in a domain that is unrelated to the perceived threat [37]. An affirmation that is related to the domain—such as admitting the error was in fact a technical one—would increase cognitive dissonance [38]. Self-affirmation is not the only method of dealing with dissonance. Direct psychological adaptations to the threat are also probable, such as denial or avoidance [39], both of which can occur in a surgeon's response to error.

Cognitive theorists describe *counterfactual thinking* as something that occurs when an individual creates a thought around an outcome that did not happen. Using statements that begin with "if only..." or "what if..." they either use an upward counterfactual thought (better than reality) or a downward counterfactual thought (worse than reality). Kahneman and Miller describe the "simulation heuristic," in which individuals travel forward or backward in subjective time in order to examine how things might have turned out differently [40]. Kahneman and Tversky emphasize that the way individuals make sense of events or outcomes they experience is largely determined by their formation of counterfactual thoughts [41].

Surgeons might use counterfactual thinking in their reflections on error. The hepatobiliary surgeon who resects a colorectal liver metastasis for cure resulting in a positive oncologic margin may employ the upward counterfactual: 'He is probably cured anyway with good chemotherapy, it is good I didn't take too much liver." Alternatively, the surgeon may utilize the following downward counterfactual after the same error: "What if the patient's cancer recurs? I will feel really bad."

Markman and McMullen made an addition to the hypothesis, called the "Reflection and Evaluation Model" of counterfactual thinking [42]. In this model, they distinguished between two modes of thinking: evaluative and reflective. Unlike evaluative thinking as Kahneman and Miller had originally described, when a standard—upward or downward—is used as a reference point to evaluate reality, reflection is more experiential. In this model, the individual will vividly simulate the information and imagine themselves in it. As a result, less attention is paid to what actually happened [42]. In the above example, the surgeon using reflective thinking might say, "I likely got enough for the chemotherapy to help with a cure." However, the surgeon using evaluative thinking might say "I got a positive margin, and failed to get a negative margin." A real-life example we can all likely relate to is the student who declares after receiving his test results, "I almost got an A" using reflective thinking as opposed to another who says, "I got a B and I failed to get an A" using evaluative thinking. Choosing one model of thinking over another will tend to favor either positive or negative emotions, depending on both the situation and whether it was an upward or downward counterfactual [43]. Some researchers have argued that upward counterfactuals are an automatic default in response to negative affect (emotion), whereas downward counterfactuals are an effort and controlled process to override the negative affect [44]. However, there is no consensus, and it is often unpredictable what type of counterfactual an individual will produce. In addition, extrapolating from Kübler-Ross' work on the time-dependent seven stages of grief [45], we can expect that counterfactual production may also be time dependent. As time passes and emotions change, the use of counterfactual thoughts changes. In the stages of surgeons' reactions to error described above, we see surgeons moving through different phases, each of which hold may be related to a different cognitive process. It is possible that counterfactual thinking may be most relevant during the *long-term impact* phase [13].

Organizational theorists have been increasingly interested in counterfactual thinking because of its implications for learning. It has been found that individuals are more likely to draw performance-promoting lessons from ambiguous outcomes, such as in surgical error, after they have responded with a self-focused upward counterfactual comparison [46]. In addition, individuals performing under organizational accountability (accountability to superiors) will be less likely to draw performance-promoting lessons. This is because the use of self-focused upward counterfactuals can imply negligence or culpability [47], a key concern for surgeons who must consider both professional and legal implications when admitting error. The additional threat from the organization evokes a reaction called "defensive bolstering," an information processing strategy that leads to a tendency to avoid complex or self-critical thoughts [48]. Defensive bolstering has been shown in physicians performing under organizational pressure [49].

In conclusion, psychological theories support the notion that surgeons experience surgical complications as a personal affront that must be accommodated into their professional sense of self. Thus, complications function as immediate performance feedback that is "self-oriented," emotionally driven, and based on a strong link between "self" and "performance."

Beyond the Individual: The Impact of Surgical Culture on Surgeons' Reactions to Error

Beyond their "personality" and cognitive processes, surgeons—as people—are imbedded within a powerful surgical culture. Two key features of surgical culture are of particular concern as we consider them in relation to surgeons' reactions to error: surgeons' strive for perfection and concerns around reputation.

As a group, surgeons are trained for rapid and confident decision-making with little room for error [50] and reside in a culture where they are forced to artificially contain emotions for fear that they would otherwise be unable to practice. Surgical residents often experience internal conflict as they are taught about the uncertainty of medicine in parallel with the unacceptability of error [46]. Furthermore, unlike many other professions, counseling or "debriefing" on the individual level after medical errors is not routine [46]. Following the occurrence of an error, surgeons are often reluctant to disclose the error to patients and colleagues for fear of malpractice litigation [51], shame, or self-disappointment [46]. Similar findings occur in studies in other areas of medicine, for example, in-depth interviews with general internists found that error, whether perceived or real, result in diminished self-confidence, fear of stigmatization, and feelings of guilt [21].

Social identity theories outline how individuals adopt shared attitudes and identify with social groups [52]. Current surgical culture holds, among other things, "boldness of action" and "a take-charge machismo" in the operating theater as an expectation [53]. Moments of uncertainty can be thought to reveal an underlying lack of expertise, while surgical error can be viewed as incompetence. Surgeons, broadly, are a competitive group who have each achieved a number of successes during their training and practice. Being a member within surgical culture involves comparing oneself to others and often involves judging other surgeons' competency [54] in areas such as peer-reviewed research, academic promotion, or clinical performance. As surgeons typically do not operate together, informal sources of information, including gossip, may be used to compare surgeon performance [55]. Surgeons may solicit information from other members of the interprofessional team, such as nurses, in an effort to obtain insights about the performance of other surgeons, possibly with the aim to be viewed as "the best" in the eyes of their colleagues. Some surgeons are awarded desired reputations (such as the exemplary surgeon, the "go-to" guy, the "surgeons' surgeon"), while others are labeled negatively (the hesitant surgeon, the hack, the incompetent buffoon) [55]. These types of social labels carry with them a great deal of cultural capital and are powerful motivators in moving individuals toward particular behaviors and away from others.

Recent studies of surgical complications and errors have suggested that individual surgeon improvement would lead to better surgical quality of care and that this might be achieved through surgeon-to-surgeon coaching for technical performance [56–59]. However, if coaching is to be a successful strategy for bettering performance, it will need to be accepted by surgeons. Mutabdzic et al. qualitatively explored surgeons' responses to the idea of having a coach paired with them in the OR [60]. Study results indicate that, while participants did recognize the theoretical benefits that having a coach could bring to their practice, they were more concerned with how having a coach might make them appear to their colleagues. Ultimately, fears around appearing incompetent and losing autonomy (i.e., being paired with a coach that the learner surgeon had not chosen) outweighed the potential of a paired learning experience for the surgeons in the study. These findings align with earlier studies [61, 62], where physicians have been seen to be reluctant to ask for and learn from feedback, due to a perceived pressure to appear "competent" in learning. It may be worth considering that medical culture itself has a significant role to play in the aversion to feedback as such hesitance is not seen in other disciplines. In particular, Watling highlights the discrepancy between the learning culture in music, where the emphasis is on improvement, and medicine, where the focus is on the performance of competence. Mutabdzic et al. come to a similar conclusion in their work, concluding the study by noting, "it might be considered ironic that a surgeon's culturally embedded value of performing competence may be the very thing that prevents further development of competence" [60].

Management of Emotions After Adverse Events

How do healthcare providers manage their own emotions that are linked to their patient's adverse events?

Most healthcare providers believe that talking about the incident with someone else is beneficial, typically a trusted senior colleague or significant other [23, 24, 63, 64].

Physicians may turn to a colleague for solace or advice after a medical error, because a colleague is uniquely positioned to provide personal validation, reassurance, and professional affirmation. Such discussions with colleagues may be beneficial unless the individual attempts to minimize the mistake in an effort to avoid emotional concern [21]. In the study by Luu et al. [13], it took some time for the participant surgeons to speak clearly and deeply about their role in the mishap during the acute phase. In the initial time following an acute event (i.e., first 24–48 h), surgeons spoke quite clinically about the facts of the case, but once into recovery, deeper reflections about the surgeons role in the mishap surfaced. Meeting with the patient who was harmed seems to also combat some of the negative feelings associated with the event [63, 65], although it may not be as effective a coping mechanism as discussing the event with medical colleagues [64]. Physicians may also benefit from seeking professional help to deal with a complication [64], although only a minority of physicians report doing so [19].

In a study by Scott et al., a defining moment is described in which the physician can either drop out, survive, or thrive following adverse events [18]. Similarly, Luu et al.'s study suggests that cumulative reactions over time either had a long-term personal growth effect, where surgeons were able to face errors head on and learn from them, or a long-time negative effect, where surgeons were left feeling depleted and wanting [13]. It is interesting to consider the difference between those that thrive and those that drop out or simply survive in surgery. Will arming providers with effective coping tools, including an awareness of the phases and emotional effects described in this chapter, increase the likelihood of surgeons being able to thrive following error? We suspect this will help, but ultimately a change in culture is needed for providers to feel truly supported and accepted following these events.

Conclusion

Echoing Mutabdzic et al., it might be considered ironic that a surgeon's culturally embedded value of *performing strength and shunning vulnerability* may be the very thing that leads to surgeon burnout and ultimate weakness [60]. Returning to the Hippocratic Oath, it is well past time to move beyond the unachievable myth of the ideal surgeon as one who will "do no harm" and, instead, embrace the surgeon as a highly educated, talented, fallible human being with the potential to improve her practice each day. A culture that strives for and values perfection, and fosters invulnerability, leaves surgeons unable to discuss their mistakes openly and transparently, let alone their own emotions surrounding these events. The modern version of the Hippocratic Oath includes a call to embrace vulnerability, to call for help when needed, and to put the patient before all else [1] . When faced with the implications of our current culture on surgeon improvement, surgeon learning, and surgeon wellness, it is clear that it is time for surgical culture to shift toward these ideals. It is time for a change.

References

1. Tyson, Peter. "The Hippocratic Oath Today" PBS.org. http://www.pbs.org/wgbh/nova/body/hippocratic-oathtoday.html 03/27/01. Accessed February 10, 2017.

2. Kohn L, Corrigan J, Donaldson M. To err is human: building a safer health system. Washington, D.C: National Academy Press; 2000.
3. American Medical Association. Council on Ethical and Judicial Affairs, Code of medical ethics: current opinions with annotations, Southern Illinois University Carbondale. Southern Illinois University School of Medicine, School of Law; 2002–2003 ed.
4. Shiloach M, Frencher SJ, Steeger J, Rowell K, Bartzokis K, Tomeh M, Richards K, Ko C, Hall B. Toward robust information: data quality and inter-rater reliability in the American College of Surgeons National Surgical Quality Improvement Program. J Am Coll Surg. 2010;210(1):6–16.
5. Hamilton B, Ko C, Richards K, Hall B. Missing data in the american college of surgeons national surgical quality improvement program are not missing at random: implications and potential impact on quality assessments. J Am Coll Surg. 2010;210:125–39.e2.
6. Dhillon B. Human errors: a review. Microelectron Reliab. 1989;29:299–304.
7. Wiegmann D, Shappell S. Human error perspectives in aviation. Int J Aviat Psychol. 2001;11:341–57.
8. Brennan T, Leape L, Laird N, Hebert L, Localio R, Lawthers A, Newhouse JWP, Hiatt H. Incidence of adverse events and negligence in hospitalized patients. Results of the Harvard medical practice study. N Engl J Med. 1991;324:370–6.
9. Leape L. Error in medicine. JAMA. 1994;272:1851–7.
10. Hofer T, Kerr E, Hayward R. What is an error? Eff Clin Pract. 2000;3:261–9.
11. Shojania K, Wald H, Gross R. Understanding medical error and improving patient safety in the inpatient setting. Med Clin North Am. 2002;86:847–67.
12. Paget M. The unity of mistakes: a phenomenological interpretation of medical work. Philadelphia: Temple University Press; 1988.
13. Luu S, Patel P, St-Martin L, Leung A, Regehr G, Murnaghan M, Gallinger S, Moulton C. Waking up the next morning: surgeons' emotional reactions to adverse events. Med Educ. 2012;46:1179–88.
14. Hilfiker D. Facing our mistakes. N Engl J Med. 1984;310:118–22.
15. Levinson W, Dunn P. A piece of my mind. Coping with fallibility. JAMA. 1989;261:2252.
16. Hilfiker D. Healing the wounds: a physician looks at his work. 1st ed. New York: Pantheon; 1985.
17. Wu A. Medical error: the second victim. BMJ. 2000;320:726.
18. Scott S, Hirschinger L, Cox K, McCoig M, Brandt J, Hall L. The natural history of recovery for the healthcare provider "second victim" after adverse patient events. Qual Saf Health Care. 2009;18:325–30.
19. Patel A, Ingalls N, Mansour M, Sherman S, Davis A, Chung M. Collateral damage: the effect of patient complications on the surgeon's psyche. Surgery. 2010;148:824–828.; discussion 8–30.
20. American Psychiatric Association, American Psychiatric Association. DSM-5 Task Force. Diagnostic and statistical manual of mental disorders DSM-5, DSM-5 Task Force. Diagnostic and statistical manual of mental disorders DSM-5. 5th ed. Arlington: American Psychiatric Association; 2013.
21. Christensen J, Levinson W, Dunn P. The heart of darkness: the impact of perceived mistakes on physicians. J Gen Intern Med. 1992;7:424–31.
22. Newman M. The emotional impact of mistakes on family physicians. Arch Fam Med. 1996;5:71–5.
23. O'Beirne M, Sterling P, Palacios-Derflingher L, Hohman S, Zwicker K. Emotional impact of patient safety incidents on family physicians and their office staff. J Am Board Fam Med. 2012;25:177–83.
24. Pinto A, Faiz O, Bicknell C, Vincent C. Surgical complications and their implications for surgeons' well-being. Br J Surg. 2013;100:1748–55.
25. Schelbred A, Nord R. Nurses' experiences of drug administration errors. J Adv Nurs. 2007;60:317–24.
26. Waterman A, Garbutt J, Hazel E, Dunagan W, Levinson W, Fraser V, Gallagher T. The emotional impact of medical errors on practicing physicians in the United States and Canada. Jt Comm J Qual Patient Saf. 2007;33:467–76.

27. Gallagher T, Mello M, Levinson W, Wynia M, Sachdeva A, Snyder Sulmasy L, RD T, Conway J, Mazor K, Lembitz A, Bell S, Sokol-Hessner L. Talking with patients about other clinicians' errors. N Engl J Med. 2013;369:1752–7.
28. Pinto A, Faiz O, Bicknell C, Vincent C. Acute traumatic stress among surgeons after major surgical complications. Am J Surg. 2014;208:642–7.
29. Shanafelt T, Balch C, Bechamps G, Russell T, Dyrbye L, Satele D, Collicott P, Novotny P, Sloan J, Freischlag J. Burnout and medical errors among American surgeons. Ann Surg. 2010;251:995–1000.
30. West C, Huschka M, Novotny P, Sloan J, Kolars J, Habermann T, Shanafelt T. Association of perceived medical errors with resident distress and empathy: a prospective longitudinal study. JAMA. 2006;296:1071–8.
31. Fahrenkopf A, Sectish T, Barger L, Sharek P, Lewin D, Chiang V, Edwards S, Wiedermann B, Landrigan CP. Rates of medication errors among depressed and burnt out residents: prospective cohort study. BMJ (Clin Res ed). 2008;336:488–91.
32. Blendon R, DesRoches C, Brodie M, Benson J, Rosen A, Schneider E, Altman D, Zapert K, Herrmann M, Steffenson A. Views of practicing physicians and the public on medical errors. N Engl J Med. 2002;347:1933–40.
33. Firth-Cozens J, Greenhalgh J. Doctors' perceptions of the links between stress and lowered clinical care. Soc Sci Med. 1997;44:1017–22.
34. Festinger L. A theory of cognitive dissonance. Evanston: Row; 1957.
35. Steele C. The Psychology of Self-Affirmation: Sustaining the Integrity of the Self. In: Leonard B, editor. Advances in experimental social psychology, vol. 21. San Diego: Academic; 1988. p. 261–302.
36. Sherman D, Cohen G. The psychology of self-defense: self-affirmation theory. In: Mark PZ, editor. Advances in experimental social psychology. San Diego: Academic; 2006. p. 183–242.
37. Aronson J, Blanton H, Cooper J. From dissonance to disidentification: selectivity in the self-affirmation process. J Pers Soc Psychol. 1995;68:986–96.
38. Blanton H, Cooper J, Slkurnik I, Aronson J. When bad things happen to good feedback: exacerbating the need for self-justification with self-affirmations. Personal Soc Psychol Bull. 1997;23:684–92.
39. Sherman D, Cohen G. Accepting threatening information: self affirmation and the reduction of defensive biases. Curr Dir Psychol Sci. 2002;11:119–23.
40. Kahneman D, Miller D. Norm theory: comparing reality to its alternatives. Psychol Rev. 1986;93:136–53.
41. Kahneman D, Slovic P, Tversky A. Judgment under uncertainty: heuristics and biases. Cambridge: Cambridge University Press; 1982.
42. Markman K, McMullen M. A reflection and evaluation model of comparative thinking. Personal Soc Psychol Rev. 2003;7:244–67.
43. Mandel D. Counterfactuals, emotions, and context. Cognit Emot. 2003;17:139–59.
44. Bandura A. Social foundations of thought and action: a social cognitive theory. Englewood Cliffs: Prentice-Hall; 1986.
45. Kübler-Ross E. On death and dying. London/New York: Routledge; 1973.
46. Rowe M. Doctors' responses to medical errors. Crit Rev Oncol Hematol. 2004;52:147–63.
47. Morris M, Moore P. The lessons we (don't) learn: counterfactual thinking and organizational accountability after a close call. Adm Sci Q. 2000;45:737–65.
48. Tetlock P, Skitka L, Boettger R. Social and cognitive strategies for coping with accountability: conformity, complexity and bolstering. J Pers Soc Psychol. 1989;57(4):632–40.
49. Hendee W. Accountability in the acquisition and use of medical technologies. Int J Technol Manag. 1995;10:38–47.
50. Coombs R, Fawzy F, Daniels M. Surgeons' personalities: the influence of medical school. Med Educ. 1993;27:337–43.
51. May T, Aulisio M. Medical malpractice, mistake prevention, and compensation. Kennedy Inst Ethics J. 2001;11:135–46.

52. Shotter J, Gergen K. Social construction: knowledge, self, others and continuing the conversation. Ann Int Commun Assoc. 1994;17(1):3–33.
53. Katz P. The Scalpel's edge: the culture of surgeons. Boston: Allyn and Bacon; 1999.
54. Pratt M, Rockmann K, Kauffmann J. Constructing professional identity: the role of work and identity learning cycles in the customization of identity among medical residents. Acad Manag. 2006;49:235–62.
55. Cassell J. Expected miracles: surgeons at work. Philadelphia: Temple University Press; 1991.
56. Sargeant J, Bruce D, Campbell C. Practicing physicians' needs for assessment and feedback as part of professional development. J Contin Educ Heal Prof. 2013;33(Suppl 1):S54–62.
57. Greenberg C, Ghousseini H, Pavuluri Quamme S, Beasley H, Wiegmann D. Surgical coaching for individual performance improvement. Ann Surg. 2014;261(1):32–4.
58. Schwellnus H, Carnahan H. Peer-coaching with health care professionals: what is the current status of the literature and what are the key components necessary in peer-coaching? A scoping review. Med Teach. 2014;36(1):38–46.
59. Hu Y, Peyre S, Arriaga A, Osteen R, Corso K, Weiser T, Swanson R, Ashley S, Raut C, Zinner M, Gawande A, Greenberg C. Postgame analysis: using video-based coaching for continuous professional development. J Am Coll Surg. 2012;214(1):115–24.
60. Mutabdzic D, Mylopoulos M, Murnaghan M, Patel P, Zilbert N, Seemann N, Regehr G, Moulton C. Coaching surgeons: is culture limiting our ability to improve? Ann Surg. 2015;262(2):213–6.
61. Watling C, Driessen E, van der Vleuten C, Vanstone M, Lingard L. Music lessons: revealing medicine's learning culture through a comparison with that of music. Med Educ. 2013;47(8):842–50.
62. Mann K, van der Vleuten C, Eva K, Armson H, Chesluk B, Dornan T, Holmboe E, Lockyer J, Loney E, Sargeant J. Tensions in informed self-assessment: how the desire for feedback and reticence to collect and use it can conflict. Acad Med. 2011;86(9):1120–7.
63. Aasland O, Forde R. Impact of feeling responsible for adverse events on doctors' personal and professional lives: the importance of being open to criticism from colleagues. Qual Saf Health Care. 2005;14:13–7.
64. Engel K, Rosenthal M, Sutcliffe K. Residents' responses to medical error: coping, learning, and change. Acad Med. 2006;81:86–93.
65. Berlinger N, Wu A. Subtracting insult from injury: addressing cultural expectations in the disclosure of medical error. J Med Ethics. 2005;31:106–8.

Quality Improvement and Patient Safety 19

Ethan L. Ferguson and Chandru P. Sundaram

Introduction

A hallmark of the modern healthcare system is the pursuit of the highest-quality medical care possible. This requires balancing among the available treatment options, those that are cost-effective and those that will provide the best outcome for patients. This process is ever evolving through research and advances in technology. Despite these advances, treatments should remain patient-centered and emphasize patient safety.

In medical education, there is a duty to pass on knowledge and to train the next generation of physicians to practice safely and independently. Previously, physician knowledge and experiential learning were paramount. Particularly in the field of surgery, surgeons focused on experience and operative volume as trainees. In the current era of medical education, however, patient safety and delivery of high-quality medical care are increasingly important and have become necessary components of undergraduate and graduate medical education. In 1999, the Institute of Medicine drew national attention to the need for improvements in quality and safety reporting with their report *To Err is Human* [1]. More recently, the Association of American Medical Colleges (AAMC) and the Association of Faculties of Medicine of Canada endorsed the introduction of patient safety and QI topics early in medical school training [2]. Beginning in 2012 through a Clinical Learning Environment Review (CLER), the ACGME mandated that quality improvement and patient safety be core competencies in every residency curriculum [3]. This is also true of

E.L. Ferguson
Department of Urology, Indiana University, Indianapolis, IN, USA

C.P. Sundaram, MD (✉)
Department of Urology, Indiana University School of Medicine,
535 N Barnhill Dr., STE 420, Indianapolis, IN 46202, USA
e-mail: sundaram@iupui.edu; csundaram@IUHealth.org

T.S. Köhler, B. Schwartz (eds.), *Surgeons as Educators*,
https://doi.org/10.1007/978-3-319-64728-9_19

the accreditation body of Canada, the Royal College of Physicians and Surgeons of Canada (RCPSC) [4]. Despite this requirement, there is no standard for teaching or incorporating patient safety and quality improvement into a surgical residency curriculum [4, 5]. Currently, the extent of QI education varies greatly across surgical residencies; therefore, there is a clear need to understand logistic and structural factors that contribute to implementing QI improvement for residents [6].

This chapter will attempt to summarize available literature regarding trainee engagement in quality improvement and patient safety initiatives.

Value of Quality Improvement/Patient Safety Programs

Resident engagement in quality improvement initiatives is thought to mutually benefit the organization, the resident's educational experience, and patient outcomes. While some projects are purely designed to streamline operations and improve efficiency, many QI projects are focused primarily on patient care. Benefits may include improvements in patient management outcomes, professional and personal development of residents, and more engagement among faculty and trainees [7].

Establishing a Curriculum

Recently, there has been a focus from program directors, administrators, and other members of training institutions to establish a formal curriculum in QI/PS. While many of these curricula are direct responses to ACGME requirements, there also appears to be a paradigm shift within residency training to focus more on patient outcomes, patient satisfaction, and improved relations between colleagues. Several studies have attempted to focus not only on outlining specific examples of successful projects but also outlining a framework for establishing a sustainable curriculum at any training institution.

Canal et al. (2007) outlines a set of four steps for establishing continuous quality improvement, including (1) identifying areas for improvement, (2) engaging in learning, (3) applying new knowledge and skills to practice, and (4) checking improvement. The study also offers a template for continuous quality improvement projects that assures that projects will remain goal-oriented and be more likely to succeed [8]. Table 19.1 is an example of a template for continuous quality improvement projects for trainees to use when developing quality improvement/patient safety projects.

Some healthcare institutions have looked to the business world for suggestions on how to establish quality improvement measures in hospital and residency training settings. On example of a specific model for quality improvement is the "lean model," which is a set of operating philosophies that maximize value for patients by minimizing waste and waiting [10]. Adapted from the Toyota corporation and Henry Ford System on car manufacturing, the lean model has been used in a variety of healthcare systems to improve patient safety and efficacy, decrease length of stay, and enhance financial responsibility by identifying ways to decrease material and

Table 19.1 Template for continuous quality improvement projects that may be used by trainees for quality improvement or patient safety-related projects

Template for continuous quality improvement	
Identify a problem	What is the problem? Why should it be improved?
Background	Have there been other attempts for improvement? Is there information about the problem (literature review, discussions with stakeholders, etc.)?
Establish a goal	What is the focus or aim of the project?
Project logistics	How can we track progress? Can data points be generated? Does the data generated support the goal of the project? Is the project feasible (taking cost, time, resources into account)? What is a reasonable timeline?
Analyze interventions	Are changes actually improvements? How do we know? Will the results be valid or reliable?
PLAN (who? what? where? when?) ***DO*** (setting the plan into motion) ***STUDY*** (analyze project results) ***ACT*** (build on project results to make further improvements and identify new problems)	

End results of plan-do-study-act cycle should identify problems leading to additional projects, hence continuous quality improvement [8, 9]

time wastes in patient care [11]. Examples of activities within the lean model for continuous quality improvement include rapid improvement event (RIE) workshops and value stream mapping, which attempt to quickly and efficiently reinforce valuable measures and eliminate wasteful measures. Residency programs can use the lean model to identify ways to improve patient care (improve admission time, OR turnover, clinic waiting time, etc.).

Another example of a model for quality improvement that may be applied to healthcare is the Six Sigma management strategy that, like lean, has origins in business. Six Sigma relies on statistical methods to systematically eliminate defects and reduce variability in processes and may be used in a variety of quality improvement initiatives [12]. For example, Six Sigma principles may be applied when streamlining a process for preventing bloodstream infections [13]. A downside of this system is the need for advanced proficiency training and certification, which may result in requiring an outside organization to perform data analysis. Although effective, this makes trainee involvement less feasible.

Johnson Faherty et al. (2016) identified models for engagement in resident training programs based on short-, medium-, and long-term quality improvement initiatives. Short-term projects (typically 1–2 weeks) typically build upon and improve prior efforts instead of completely overhauling system. This may involve improvements to workflow within a specific team that can flexibly alter daily routines without negatively impacting patient care. Medium-term projects (up to 6 months) are typically unit or clinic-based and are thought to be focused on attending physicians, nurse managers, and other staff members who remain in a particular area long term. Long-term projects (months to years) focus issues that impact hospital-wide quality measures or issues that affect the healthcare system as a whole [14].

Many other reviews/studies focus on didactic lectures or lecture series as a focus of quality improvement during residency [5, 7, 15]. Didactics have been identified as one of the easiest and most common ways to incorporate teaching on quality improvement and patient safety into resident education [16]. Didactic lectures may take the form of annual seminars, monthly lectures, or even online modules focused on QI-related topics. Trainees may be involved by identifying research topics and giving lectures, as well as participating in discussions. Lectures may serve as inspiration for initiating a novel idea for a project or continuing a national initiative at a local institution.

Methods for Education in QI

Although no set of guidelines exists for the optimal implementation of a QI/PS curriculum, there are many ways that quality improvement can be integrated into surgical education programs. In reality, there is likely no one perfect strategy, and program directors/clinical educators should rely on a combination of strategies to facilitate QI at their institutions. Some methods to improve quality improvement are below:

Rapid Improvement Events (RIEs)

Rapid improvement events (RIEs) allow for prompt identification of problems and strategies aimed at solutions that may be implemented in days rather than weeks to months. RIEs have been used in businesses and in healthcare to expedite change and usually consist of 2–3-day events. In these events, the following are identified: problems, potential actions/changes, impact of change, time frame, and party responsible for change. Historically, RIEs have been used in nursing management and medical administration but may also apply to resident-led QI initiatives [17].

Didactic Lectures

Didactic lectures have been identified as among the easiest and most effective ways to educate large groups of people efficiently and are likely the most common method of QI/PS integration in surgical residency programs [5, 15, 16, 18]. Lectures may be part of an overall patient safety curriculum in which a variety of topics are discussed each year to meet competency requirements. One downside of didactic lectures is that they are a relatively passive form of information acquisition and may or may not result in actual QI changes.

Local Hospital Projects

Local hospital projects aimed at quality improvement or patients' safety are among the most common types of projects that engage residents at academic teaching institutions. The majority of QI/PS-related projects rely on plan-do-study-act cycle

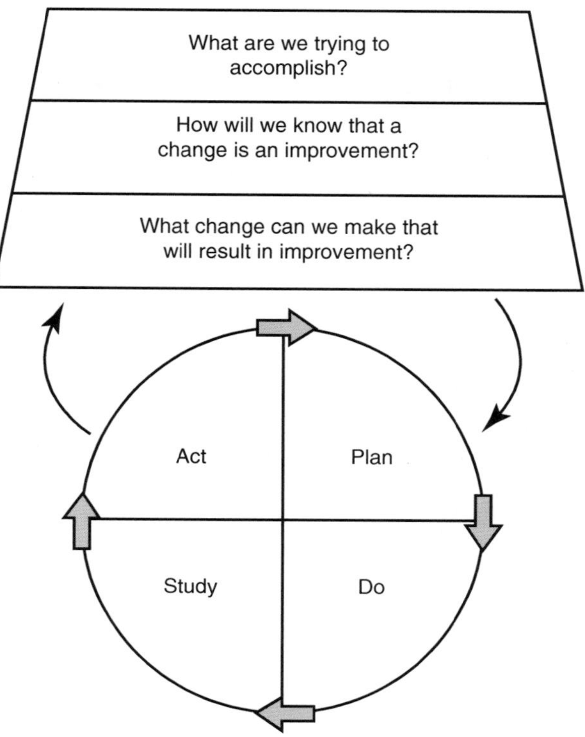

Fig. 19.1 The plan-do-study-act (PDSA) model for continuous quality improvement. After identifying a problem and understanding how changes may result in improvements, the PDSA cycle may be used and outcomes generate ideas for new problems that may benefit from further PDSA cycles, hence continuous quality improvement (Permission requested for use by publisher of Langley et al. (2009))

(Fig. 19.1) in which an idea is generated (plan), a test of that idea is carried out (do), the data are analyzed (study), and appropriate changes are made (act) [9]. Ideally this cycle repeats itself to generate continuous quality improvement. These projects often result in real changes in process improvement that impact patient care directly.

Surgical Simulation and Certification

Surgical simulation is an increasingly important aspect of surgical education in the current era of increasing focus on outcomes and patient safety. Simulation allows trainees to practice safely prior to entering the operating room. It is important to note, however, that simulation should not replace real surgical training opportunities but may be an important adjunct to surgical training. The focus of many simulation programs has been on laparoscopic and endoscopic surgery [19]. Open surgical simulation includes live animals, cadavers, bench models (products from limbs and things, etc.), virtual reality simulators, and computer simulators. These methods have poor data support and are often expensive to initiate but may provide an important long-term adjunct to traditional operative surgical training.

Feedback

Some studies have shown that feedback may improve the quality of care delivered and improve operative skill in surgical residents. Particularly today when trainees are spending less time in the operating room than in previous generations of residents, feedback is important. In a systematic review, Trehan et al. (2015) found that formal feedback was a powerful method to improve performance by reducing total procedure time and improve economy of movement, as well as several improvements in laparoscopic simulator parameters. Feedback may come in a variety of forms including oral or written feedback, self-assessment, video footage review, reviewing outcomes of treatments or surgical procedures, or comparing assessment to peers in the same training program [20]. In the current age of mobile device use, mobile devices may be important in feedback dissemination though there is limited literature regarding this topic.

Journal Club

Evidence-based theory is at the core of quality improvement and patient safety, and intermittent journal clubs (often resident led) are thought to be an effective way to evaluate current literature and to decide whether or not data should be used to impact patient care. Many surgical residencies utilize journal clubs as a component of QI/PS [21]. Generally, a journal article is identified, disseminated for a group to read, presented with an independent interpretation of the methods, results, and conclusions, and finally discussed in a group setting. Although journal clubs have been in existence for many years, formats vary widely even within the same institution, ranging from formal education conferences to informal gatherings. There is no data supporting one type of journal club format over another; however, Al Achkar et al. (2016) offered suggestions for optimizing journal club, including following the same systematic approach for every resident presentation and involvement of a faculty mentor in article selection, as well as article discussion [22].

Promoting Teamwork in Medicine

The scope of medicine has expanded drastically over the last several decades, demanding division of medicine into various specialties that must work together to care for patients. Teamwork and shared expertise lead to better outcomes for patients [23]. Resident participation in interdisciplinary conferences, such as tumor boards, can be beneficial [24]. In addition, resident participation in management huddles with nursing, pharmacists, therapists, and other members of the patient care team helps to ensure the best possible care [11].

Techniques in QI/PS

Surveys

Surveys are instruments used for a wide variety of research initiatives and have been shown to be a useful method for gathering data from a large group of people to assess feelings and attitudes that may otherwise be very challenging to assess. Data may be applied qualitatively or quantitatively to answer research questions. Surveys are extremely valuable in assessing patient satisfaction and quality of care, as evidenced by validated surveys like the SF-36 health outcomes survey and the Hospital Consumer Assessment of Healthcare Providers and Systems (HCAHPS), among others. In addition to research questions, surveys may also assess uptake of information through pre- and post-intervention questionnaires.

An example includes Pringle et al. (2009), which used surveys to examine safety reporting practices and perceptions across a variety of hospitals. Using data from these surveys, they were able to identify which aspects of patient safety needed to be reinforced and at which facility. Information from surveys then helped to guide quality improvement changes across a variety of healthcare campuses [25].

Databases and Data Reporting

Collaborative databases are emerging as an important component of quality improvement and patient safety initiatives. These databases exist in many forms, including some federally supported programs, such as the AHRQ, and specialty-specific organizations, such as the ACS NSQIP (surgery) and the AUA quality registry (American Urological Association's AQUA). Physicians contribute data regarding outcomes and other end points to generate data with statistically impactful numbers of observations, which may otherwise be very difficult or impossible to achieve. The Centers for Medicaid and Medicare Services (CMS) recognizes a number of these databases through the Physician Quality Reporting System (PQRS). Through this system, eligible physicians and/or group practices may be subject to a reduction in payment for inadequate reporting of data for Medicare patients [26].

Large databases and registries including ACS NSQIP and AHRQ may help determine how rates of surgical complications, infections, or other outcomes nationally compare with local rates to identify areas for improvement. These results may drive quality improvement initiatives at the local level [5]. Results may also be analyzed to perform retrospective analyses that can identify healthcare system-wide problems that result in system-wide quality improvement initiatives. Rowell et al. (2007) described how ACS NSQIP data was used to identify problem areas at multiple institutions resulting in QI projects that led to significant improvements in patient outcomes [27].

A statewide initiative known as the Michigan Urological Surgery Improvement Collaborative (MUSIC) is a collaboration among urologists treating prostate cancer in the state of Michigan. The database is designed to share data in order to improve quality and value of care as well as enhance outcomes in prostate cancer treatment. This is an example of a smaller, physician-led quality improvement project that generates useful data that may be used in retrospective analysis and leads to local or national improvements in quality improvement measures [28].

M&M/Safety Reporting

Surgical morbidity and mortality (M&M) conferences have long been utilized quality assurance programs in surgical residency programs with little change in format and structure for nearly 100 years [1]. In these educational conferences, surgical complications are reviewed and discussed in an attempt to learn from mistakes or to be aware of risk factors in patients for certain complications. M&M conferences were made a requirement for all surgical training programs in 1983 by the ACGME. Therefore, resident participation in M&M conferences is generally accepted as a vital aspect of quality improvement and patient safety training in residency training [8]. Although important, a recent study from one institution found that institutional rates of complication reporting are often much lower than national rates or institutional rates reported to ACS NSQIP [1]. Given this result, training programs should accurately review outcomes to ensure their validity.

OR Etiquette and Checklists

An important aspect of patient safety in surgical residencies is ensuring that proper OR etiquette is maintained, including obtaining informed consent, appropriate site marking, time-out before and after all surgical procedures, and appropriate handoff of care. In addition, checklists are an important aspect of modern surgical care and help to reduce otherwise preventable complications. In 2008, the World Health Organization (WHO) published a set of guidelines in a global initiative to improve the safety of surgery. An important component of these guidelines included establishing a surgical safety checklist to ensure that the correct procedure for the correct patient was being performed and that potential life-threatening complications are avoided [29]. This includes separate preanesthesia, pre-incision, and post-procedure time-outs, which have been widely accepted and implemented. Using the WHO surgical safety checklist in the operating room has been shown to be a feasible way to reduce all-cause morbidity regardless of operative site [30].

Role of Trainees

As previously mentioned, the ACGME has mandated QI/PS into all residency curricula, meaning that all trainees should be involved in quality improvement measures of some form. Residents are positioned at the "front lines" of patient care and are therefore in a position to conceptualize real-time solutions to patient problems [11]. While many of these problems will be local or unit-based, others may be generalized to the national healthcare system [14]. In multiple analyses, resident involvement in QI/PS curricular efforts may lead to improvements in clinical processes [31]. There are many examples of resident-led projects that have resulted in real and measurable improvements in quality and safety, some of which may be found in Appendix 1.

Role of Mentors

In order for QI/PS initiatives to succeed, there is a need for effective, longitudinal mentors to facilitate trainee involvement. Mentors have been identified by several authors as vital components of any QI/PS curriculum and are essential to initiating and overseeing projects to ensure their completion [6, 23, 32]. Trainees may have an idea or a plan for initiating a QI/PS project but often lack the resources, connections, or power within their institutions to get ideas off the ground. Mentors help trainees navigate the complex healthcare landscape and facilitate partnerships necessary to start projects and ensure the resources necessary to complete them.

As quality improvement and patient safety become increasingly important aspects of medical education, it is important for faculty members to teach students and residents about QI/PS early in their careers. Faculty members with experience in QI/PS should meet regularly with students and trainees to generate enthusiasm and awareness within their institutions. In addition, when overseeing projects with students or trainees, it is important to meet at regular intervals to ensure completion of ongoing projects. Waits et al. (2014) outlined team action projects in surgery (TAPS) at the University of Michigan, which are multilevel team-based projects led by faculty mentors. Faculty mentors oversee projects led by residents who, in turn, lead and mentor groups of medical students or other groups of student learners. This multitiered system allows residents to gain experience in leadership, while exposing other learners to academic surgery, and to gain research experience. Using this framework, residents at UM successfully instituted projects aimed at enhanced recovery after kidney donation and standardization of VTE ppx and *c. difficile* treatment within their institution [6].

Although designed for program directors and educators within the field of internal medicine, one review outlined the role of clinical educators in implementing sustainable improvements in healthcare [32]. They found that QI initiatives not only improve patient care but also may assist in promotion of faculty mentors through scholarly publication and demonstration of successful leadership. They also discovered that many physicians who took part in efforts to improve resident education or overall quality of care rated their overall professional satisfaction to be improved. Academic surgeons are both responsible for patient care and resident education. Therefore, clinician educators in academic surgical departments are uniquely positioned to address both institutional and system-wide improvements in QI/PS.

Challenges

Resident Factors

A major challenge in implementing meaningful and sustainable quality improvement measures is the natural turnover of trainees in surgical residency programs [4, 14]. The rapid pace and transient nature of residency training, combined with time demands, can result in a lack of ownership over the residency program or patients [4]. Well-established units may be resistant to changes proposed by a trainee who is "passing through" [14]. To address these problems, some residency programs have established team-based approaches in which resident groups take over projects from previous groups to ensure continuity and increase the likelihood of completion [2]. In addition, timing of resident involvement in research in general and let alone long-term QI/PS projects can be challenging. While some residency programs offer dedicated research time, many residencies do not offer protected time or "light rotations" to ensure residents have sufficient time outside of work responsibilities to dedicate to projects [8]. These programs may rely more heavily on didactics to deliver QI/PS-related information to residents.

Work hours have been targeted as a reason for decreased resident effectiveness, although the data supporting this is unclear. Dating back to the Libby Zion case in which a woman died while being treated by a fatigued resident, resident work hours have remained a point of contention [33]. While some suggest that unlimited work hours lead to more errors, others cite that restrictions in work hours result in an overall negative impact because of increased handoffs. The results of the FIRST trial were published in February 2016 and showed no difference in outcomes in residents with less restrictive duty hour policies compared with those with restricted duty hours [34]. In addition, there were no differences in resident dissatisfaction or quality of education. That being said, residents with flexible duty hour policies may have less time available to complete research and/or QI/PS projects.

Some have suggested that there is seasonal variation in the quality of patient care related to the "July effect" when new residents start each year [35]. The literature is somewhat inconsistent on this matter, but some sources suggest that operating room efficiency is decreased and overall mortality may be increased in early training months. Other sources suggest that resident involvement, in general, may have a negative impact on patients no matter what time of year [36, 37]. These results showed that resident involvement increased overall length of stay and decreased OR efficiency but that overall patient care was not affected.

Institutional/Hierarchical Factors

Institutional factors can also limit the success of QI/PS initiatives. This may be related to lack of institutional support or institutional "buy-in" for a given idea [32]. Institutions may vary widely on how much value is placed on QI [4]. Another factor may be related to the hierarchy of medicine and healthcare preventing effective communication. Ginsberg et al. (2013) suggested that there is impaired communication between nurses and physicians related to hierarchy differences at some institutions. Trainee communication may also be impaired [38]. Teamwork must be emphasized to ensure the highest possible quality of care and adequate communication.

Lack of Faculty Mentors

Some sources have suggested that there is an overall lack of qualified mentors available for trainees to support QI/PS projects. This may be related to inadequate knowledge of quality improvement by faculty [4, 14] versus a lack of mentors with interest in quality improvement-related projects.

Limitations in Evaluating QI/PS Curricular Efforts

Many QI/PS attempts at curriculum reform are difficult to assess and analyze because their outcomes are not easily quantifiable and, particularly in local projects, are tailored to specific needs by that institution. As many of these observational studies lack a control group, it is impossible to say definitively whether or not a given intervention was truly successful or not [2]. In this way, it is often difficult for QI-related projects and ideas to gain traction with other training programs.

In addition, it is thought that acquiring meaningful data for QI/PS measures can be challenging. Many database-driven large-scale projects are often retrospective and fail to show any clear benefit on health outcomes [2]. In the Medicare patient population, the CMS has attempted to improve data reporting quality by certifying data registries as qualified clinical data registries (QCDR). Many of these organizations are national data registries mentioned earlier (ACS NSQIP, AQUA, AHRQ, etc.), and other specialty-specific governing bodies are included in this group of data registries [39].

Resources

There are many resources available at the disposal of students, residents, and faculty to utilize for quality improvement projects. One of the most commonly used and largest available resources is the American College of Surgeons National Surgical Quality Improvement Program (ACS NSQIP). ACS NSQIP is a nationally validated risk-adjusted outcomes-based program that is designed to measure and improve surgical care [21]. When creating a curriculum, ACS NSQIP is a useful guide for the development of educational content [36]. Users may evaluate their own institutional outcomes against the national database using observed to expected ratios [1, 5, 27], which rely on confidence intervals to determine if an outcome occurs more or less often than expected. Confidence intervals for O/E ratios with lower limits >1 suggest that patients at an institution experience an adverse event more often than expected. In converse, if the upper limit of the confidence limit for an O/E ratio is <1, this suggests that patients at an institution experience a particular complication less often than expected [27].

When explaining the utility of ACS NSQIP, one author points out that the goal of the database is not to identify and punish underperforming institutions but rather to use reliable data that allows institutions to identify areas of weakness and generate quality improvement measures in response [27]. Analysis of NSQIP data before and after an intervention is implemented helps to determine its effectiveness [27].

The Agency for Healthcare Research and Quality (AHRQ), an agency within the Department of Health and Human Resources, is another resource aimed at producing guidelines improving quality of healthcare through research. The AHRQ produces a variety of literature, and continuing education materials that are widely accessible cover a wide variety of healthcare topics. In addition, the AHRQ website contains data reports that may allow comparison of hospital or practice data to those at the state or national level [40].

The Joint Commission Surgical Care Improvement Project (SCIP) uses large multicenter data sets to power a series of projects aimed at reducing surgical complications. The Joint Commission is an independent, not-for-profit organization that is responsible for accreditation and certification of healthcare organizations in the United States. Measures within SCIP include VTE prophylaxis guidelines and appropriate perioperative antibiotic use. Knowledge of patient safety standards outlined the Joint Commission by residents, and program directors will not only improve patient safety but ensure institutional accreditation [41].

The Institute for Healthcare Improvement (IHI) is an independent, not-for-profit organization that aims to improve healthcare worldwide through an array of educational resources, including the IHI Open School. The IHI Open School is a collection of online modules in QI/PS, including a full curriculum, available to the general public, as well as professional and academic groups. This program is utilized by undergraduates, medical students, residents, and practicing physicians and offers a flexible, organized method to learn about QI/PS. The Open School also offers courses in experiential learning that help learners [42].

Examples of specialty-specific resources are those provided by the American Urological Association (AUA). Some of these include a detailed list of best practice clinical guidelines written and reviewed by leading experts. The AUA offers an AUA Quality Registry (AQUA), which extracts quality metrics from the medical record to generate quality metrics for urologists across the United States. There are also a number of educational resources provided by a department within the AUA focused on patient safety and improved quality of care measures. This department organizes an evolving list of quality improvement guidelines and hosts intermittent quality improvement summits to address important quality-related topics, the most recent of which addressed shared decision making and prostate cancer screening. The AUA is an example of many successful surgical specialty organizations that are not only focused on QI/PS but also provide a number of resources to providers [43].

There are many other available resources available to trainees and clinical educators, many of which are summarized in Table 19.2 [16].

Table 19.2 This table includes a brief summary of available resources related to quality improvement and patient safety education for residents, educators, or program directors

Resource	Description	Webpage
ACS Division of Education	Educational material and online modules for independent study Various topics in QI, patient safety, and error prevention Access to ACS fundamentals of surgery online curriculum and Surgical Education Self-Assessment Program (SESAP)	www.facs.org/education
SCORE (Surgical Council on Resident Education)	Educational videos, online modules for independent study Self-assessment questions available	www.surgicalcore.org
APDS (Association for Program Directors in Surgery)	Organized information and reference material for program directors in surgical training programs Useful for program directors, clerkship directors, surgical educators	www.apds.org
ASE (Association for Surgical Education)	Organized information regarding curricular development Useful for program directors, clerkship directors, surgical educators	www.surgicaleducation.com
SSH (Society for Simulation in Healthcare)	Directory of simulation resources, online courses, and videos Memberships available for purchase	www.ssih.org
IHI (Institute for Healthcare Improvement)	Complete curriculum in healthcare-specific quality improvement and patient safety through Open School online modules and project-based learning	www.ihi.org
AUA (American Urological Association)	Access to guidelines and educational resources related to urology	www.auanet.org

While some resources are surgery specific, others offer general educational materials that may be integrated into surgery training programs [16]. More information is available at respective websites

Conclusions and Future Directions

Quality improvement and patient safety are increasingly important aspects of modern healthcare systems. Local and national initiatives aimed at improved quality of healthcare delivery and patient safety result in real-world benefits to patient morbidity and mortality and help to address the rising costs of healthcare. With well-integrated quality improvement initiatives built into a training curriculum, residents at academic medical centers are poised to learn the tools necessary to become future leaders in QI/PS efforts. Medical schools and residencies are in a position to educate and train the next generation of physicians in QI/PS and to carry on a legacy of high-quality healthcare delivery.

In surgical education, there are many ways that surgical trainees can participate in QI/PS projects and educational initiatives. Some of these are outlined in this chapter and include didactic lectures, local hospital projects, utilizing national database information, participating in morbidity and mortality conferences, utilizing survey data, and many other possibilities. There are also a number of electronic resources at the disposal of residents and program directors, many of which are aimed at QI/PS education.

Although literature review has revealed significant progress from a number of institutions regarding QI/PS in surgical residency, many institutions lack curricular organization. Curricular efforts are, for the most part, focused on didactics and to a lesser extent involve residents in quality improvement projects. In the future, there is a need for more faculty involvement and educators in QI. Currently accreditation standards, such as those through the Joint Commission, require that institutions meet guidelines in order to maintain accreditation. In the future, accreditation standards may target QI/PS assessments to maintain accreditation.

Examples of Successful Resident-Led QI Projects

There are many examples shared in the literature of successful QI- and PS-related projects across a wide array of topics. These projects span topics in surgical and nonsurgical medical specialties. Examples of some topics featured in the literature are shown in the table below:

Project topic	Type	Source
Curriculum development of an ultrasound course for the residents	Surgery	Canal et al. (2007)
Reducing postoperative order errors	Surgery	Canal et al. (2007)
Standardizing discharge forms	Surgery	Canal et al. (2007)
Developing a research curriculum for research residents	Surgery	Canal et al. (2007)
Improve surgical intern satisfaction with the residency by creating a mentoring system between research residents and PGY-1 surgery interns	Surgery	Canal et al. (2007)
Improve resident attendance at the chairman's conference	Surgery	Canal et al. (2007)

Project topic	Type	Source
Improving colorectal cancer screening in a vulnerable adult population seen at SFGH	Medicine	Neeman et al. (2012)
ED door to floor: quality improvement in the admission process	Emergency medicine	Neeman et al. (2012)
Fostering a patient-centered environment: condolence cards in death packets	Medicine	Neeman et al. (2012)
Diabetic patient education on home foot exams	Medicine	Neeman et al. (2012)
Develop an anticoagulation protocol for trauma patients	Surgery	O'connor et al. (2010)
Develop a chest tube protocol for traumatic hemopneumothorax	Surgery	O'connor et al. (2010)
Decrease turnaround time of ORs	Surgery	O'connor et al. (2010)
Improve patient handoffs between residents	Surgery	O'connor et al. (2010)
Study ways to reduce nurse calls to residents on home call	Surgery	O'connor et al. (2010)

References

1. Hutter MM, Rowell KS, Devaney LA, et al. Identification of surgical complications and deaths: an assessment of the traditional surgical morbidity and mortality conference compared with the American College of Surgeons-National Surgical Quality Improvement Program. J Am Coll Surg. 2006;203:618.
2. Wong BM, Levinson W, Shojania KG. Quality improvement in medical education: current state and future directions. Med Educ. 2012;46:107.
3. Accreditation Council for Graduate Medical Education Policies and Procedures, 2/4/2017 ed. http://www.acgme.org: Accreditation Council for Graduate Medical Education (ACGME), 2017.
4. Hall Barber K, Schultz K, Scott A, et al. Teaching quality improvement in graduate medical education: an experiential and team-based approach to the acquisition of quality improvement competencies. Acad Med. 2015;90:1363.
5. Chang DC, Bohnen JD, Mullen JT, et al. Big data and GME: expanding the scope of patient safety and QI training. Bull Am Coll Surg. 2015;100:40.
6. Waits SA, Reames BN, Krell RW, et al. Development of team action projects in surgery (TAPS): a multilevel team-based approach to teaching quality improvement. J Surg Educ. 2014;71:166.
7. O'Connor ES, Mahvi DM, Foley EF, et al. Developing a practice-based learning and improvement curriculum for an academic general surgery residency. J Am Coll Surg. 2010;210:411.
8. Canal DF, Torbeck L, Djuricich AM. Practice-based learning and improvement: a curriculum in continuous quality improvement for surgery residents. Arch Surg. 2007;142:479.
9. Langley GJ, Moen RD, Nolan KM, et al. In: Langley GJ, editor. The improvement guide a practical approach to enhancing organizational performance. 2nd ed. San Francisco: Jossey-Bass; 2009.
10. Lawal AK, Rotter T, Kinsman L, et al. Lean management in health care: definition, concepts, methodology and effects reported (systematic review protocol). Syst Rev. 2014;3:103.
11. Fang DZ, Kantor MA, Helgerson P. Quality improvement in academic medical centres: a resident perspective. BMJ Qual Saf. 2015;24:483.
12. Schweikhart SA, Dembe AE. The applicability of lean and six sigma techniques to clinical and translational research. J Investig Med. 2009;57:748.
13. Frankel HL, Crede WB, Topal JE, et al. Use of corporate six sigma performance-improvement strategies to reduce incidence of catheter-related bloodstream infections in a surgical ICU. J Am Coll Surg. 2005;201:349.

14. Johnson Faherty L, Mate KS, Moses JM. Leveraging trainees to improve quality and safety at the point of care: three models for engagement. Acad Med. 2016;91:503.
15. McKee R, Sussman AL, Nelson MT, et al. Using qualitative and quantitative assessment to develop a patient safety curriculum for surgical residents. J Surg Educ. 2016;73:529.
16. Medbery RL, Sellers MM, Ko CY, et al. The unmet need for a national surgical quality improvement curriculum: a systematic review. J Surg Edu. 2014;71:613.
17. Martin SC, Greenhouse PK, Kowinsky AM, et al. Rapid improvement event: an alternative approach to improving care delivery and the patient experience. J Nurs Care Qual. 2009;24:17.
18. Tess AV, Rosen C, Tibbles C. Mapping quality improvement and safety education to drive change across training programs. J Grad Med Educ. 2015;7:275.
19. Davies J, Khatib M, Bello F. Open surgical simulation – a review. J Surg Educ. 2013;70:618.
20. Trehan A, Barnett-Vanes A, Carty MJ, et al. The impact of feedback of intraoperative technical performance in surgery: a systematic review. BMJ Open. 2015;5:e006759.
21. O'Heron CT, Jarman BT. A strategic approach to quality improvement and patient safety education and resident integration in a general surgery residency. J Surg Educ. 2014;71:18.
22. Al Achkar M. Redesigning journal club in residency. Adv Med Educ Pract. 2016;7:317.
23. Mochan E, Nash DB. Weaving quality improvement and patient safety skills into all levels of medical training: an annotated bibliography. Am J Med Qual. 2015;30:232.
24. Kiersma ME, Plake KS, Darbishire PL. Patient safety instruction in US health professions education. Am J Pharm Educ. 2011;75:162.
25. Pringle J, Weber RJ, Rice K, et al. Examination of how a survey can spur culture changes using a quality improvement approach: a region-wide approach to determining a patient safety culture. Am J Med Qual. 2009;24:374.
26. Physician Quality Reporting System. http://www.cms.gov: Centers for medicare and medicaid services, 2016.
27. Rowell KS, Turrentine FE, Hutter MM, et al. Use of national surgical quality improvement program data as a catalyst for quality improvement. J Am Coll Surg. 2007;204:1293.
28. Program Overview. http://www.musicurology.com: Michigan urological surgery improvement collaborative (MUSIC), 2014.
29. The second global patient safety challenge: safe surgery saves lives. In: World Health Organization World Alliance for Patient Safety. Online: World Health Organization (WHO), p. 28, 2008.
30. Haynes AB, Weiser TG, Berry WR, et al. A surgical safety checklist to reduce morbidity and mortality in a global population. N Engl J Med. 2009;360:491.
31. Wong BM, Etchells EE, Kuper A, et al. Teaching quality improvement and patient safety to trainees: a systematic review. Acad Med. 2010;85:1425.
32. Stevens DP, Kirkland KB. The role for clinician educators in implementing healthcare improvement. J Gen Intern Med. 2010;25(Suppl 4):S639.
33. Lee MJ. On patient safety: have the ACGME resident work hour reforms improved patient safety? Clin Orthop Relat Res. 2015;473:3364.
34. Bilimoria KY, Chung JW, Hedges LV, et al. National cluster-randomized trial of duty-hour flexibility in surgical training. N Engl J Med. 2016;374:713.
35. Englesbe MJ, Pelletier SJ, Magee JC, et al. Seasonal variation in surgical outcomes as measured by the American College of Surgeons-National Surgical Quality Improvement Program (ACS-NSQIP). Ann Surg. 2007;246:456.
36. Hoffman RL, Bartlett EK, Medbery RL, et al. Outcomes registries: an untapped resource for use in surgical education. J Surg Educ. 2015;72:264.
37. Kiran RP, Ahmed Ali U, Coffey JC, et al. Impact of resident participation in surgical operations on postoperative outcomes: National Surgical Quality Improvement Program. Ann Surg. 2012;256:469.
38. Ginsburg LR, Tregunno D, Norton PG. Self-reported patient safety competence among new graduates in medicine, nursing and pharmacy. BMJ Qual Saf. 2013;22:147.
39. 2016 Physician Quality Reporting System Qualified Clinical Data Registries, 6/10/2016 ed. Centers for Medicare and Medicaid Services p. 61, 39.

40. Agency for Healthcare Research and Quality: U.S. Department of Health and Human Services.
41. The Joint Commission: The Joint Commission, 2017.
42. Open School http://www.ihi.org: Institute for Healthcare Improvement (IHI), 2017.
43. Patient Safety and Quality of Care: American Urological Association (AUA), 2017.

Teaching Surgeons How to Lead

20

Jon A. Chilingerian

Where will surgical practice be in 10 years? Uncertainty, pressure, complexity, and novelty confront every health-care organization today. Situations are dynamic as futures unfold. One surgeon, trying to head off a feeling of an impending catastrophe, recently sent me an e-mail with a request for help that said:

> …I am past president of my medical society, and past president of the medical staff at my hospital. Right now, I am struggling to lead our medium sized, single specialty private practice group…We are dealing with falling surgical reimbursements along with crushing practice overhead…while we are struggling with conversion to value-based reimbursement and ICD 10, and meaningful use and crippling physician burnout…

The healthcare environment is turbulent, and surgeons work in an era of patient-driven organizational forms, advances in biomedical science, accelerated technological development, and complex health policy reforms. Medicine is no longer a private relationship between patient and surgeon with a promise of good outcomes [12, 45]. We live in an age of public reporting, online patient communities, and multiple performance requirements [14]. Surgeons not only have to achieve excellent technical outcomes, they must also offer outstanding patient experience and efficient, low-cost care [48]. The ambiguity of how to deliver care that meets those requirements contributes to the uncertainty.

What kinds of solutions exist to solve these problems? Should a struggling surgical group hire outside consultants, restructure, reduce staff, retreat from some insurers and procedures, or partner with a hospital? Reorganizing or restructuring

J.A. Chilingerian, PhD
Brandeis University, Heller School, Waltham, MA, USA

Public Health and Community Medicine at Tufts School of Medicine, Boston, MA, USA

Organizational Behavior and Health Care Management at INSEAD, Fontainebleau, France
e-mail: chilinge@brandeis.edu

T.S. Köhler, B. Schwartz (eds.), *Surgeons as Educators*,
https://doi.org/10.1007/978-3-319-64728-9_20

the surgical group has the appearance of solving the problem, but just as one masters the rules of the game, the environment will change, and instability is destructive to morale.

Another response to an unstable and dynamic environment is to accept the fact that health care will never stop changing. There is no generic management solution to these problems, but the missing ingredient in every health-care organization may be a lack of effective clinical leadership or inadequate depth of clinical leadership inside and throughout the organization. Thus, there is a growing need to train and develop every surgeon to take on a leadership role.[1] Why?

There are at least three reasons why surgeons should be educated and trained to be leaders:

1. There is a new and blossoming science of medicine and management.
2. Complex medical organizations such as hospitals should be led by people trained in the underlying disciplines and applied medical sciences.
3. There is research evidence that managers with clinical backgrounds can run better health-care organizations, and some physician-led multispecialty groups outperform organizations run by lay managers.

First, the merging of the biomedical sciences and the management sciences is occurring through generative emergence. In the same way that biology and chemistry became the powerful new medical science of biochemistry during the nineteenth and twentieth centuries,[2] the new science of medicine and management is emerging. As researchers blend medicine and management science, they are discovering new knowledge, such as the physics of patient flow, the measurement of quality and clinical efficiency, learning from outliers, and the underlying science of improving patient experiences. Through scientific method and rigorous validation, their academic findings are beginning to inform patient care throughout the world.

The clinical research and health services research literature are reporting significant clinical improvements when clinical medicine applies the science of process management. At Intermountain Health Care,[3] *physicians have led more than100 successful patient-centered clinical improvements that reduced practice variations* [32]. For example, when they looked at coronary artery bypass grafts (CABG), there were massive variations in physician practices and twofold variations in cost

[1] When I refer to leadership, I am not referring to head of state, CEO, or chief but the ability to mobilize people to want to struggle for some challenging goal in the front stage for patient care and throughout the organization (see Kouzes and Posner 2016 [34]).

[2] According to Afshar and Han [2], "Advancement of medicine and that of biochemistry are inseparable, and much of modern medicine would not be practiced in the ways, as they are known today, without our understanding of how genetic, pathogenic and environmental factors affect the human body at the biochemical level. Thus, the importance of teaching medical students biochemistry is self-evident" (page 339).

[3] Intermountain Healthcare is a nonprofit health-care delivery system located in Salt Lake City, Utah. It is comprised of 22 hospitals that offer a broad range of clinics and services. They employ approximately 1400 primary care and secondary care physicians.

per case. However, these CABG patients were not sicker; in fact, 80% of the patients had similar severity and complexity. By reducing process variations,[4] CABG outcomes improved and costs were reduced.[5] The new science of medicine and management advances the medical practice such that the lowest-cost care provides the best clinical results.[6]

Second, consider companies in the computer, software, and internet industry, such as Google. Who ought to run a technocratic organization like Google? The answer is, the people trained in the basic underlying science, such as programmers and software engineers (see [24]). Perhaps complex biomedical science organizations, such as academic medical centers, acute general hospitals, or specialty hospitals, should be led by professionals trained in the underlying disciplines and applied medical sciences, i.e., physicians, nurses, and other clinicians trained in the science of medicine.

Third, we have learned from research and from teaching physicians[7] that physician leaders can make a significant difference in health-care delivery outcomes and efficiency in hospitals. Moreover, there is growing evidence that the direct involvement of physicians in health-care management improves overall organizational performance ([6], *AJC*; [18] *Annals of Internal Medicine;* [8, 55]).[8] Historically the most effective health-care organizations are the multispecialty, physician-led groups [56].[9] These organizations nurture and integrate physician leaders who are prepared to bring management science closer to clinical operations and medical decision-making ([16, 32] and [37]).

There is a counterargument however to the assertion that physicians make the best health care leaders. Safe, efficient, accountable, high-quality health care in the twenty-first century demands a broad range of conceptual, technical, analytical, and leadership skills, a range that is nearly impossible for *self-taught* physician leaders to comprehend and manage [7, 19, 47, 59, 60].

---

[4] The science of process management applied to medicine is only one example of the new science of medicine and management.

[5] The new science has been applied to procedures and diagnoses such as prostatectomy, cholecystectomy, pneumonia, and pacemaker implantation [32].

[6] When the science of process management is applied to a surgical care program, every care process will "always" produce parallel clinical cost and patient experiences.

[7] In 1995, Brandeis and Tufts partnered to offer medical students a 4-year, dual MD-MBA degree. Today it is the largest program in the USA. Since 2004, Brandeis offers a 6-day CME leadership program in Advanced Health Policy and Management, in partnership with the American College of Surgeons. Finally, Brandeis launched a 16-month executive MBA for physicians. All of these programs have demonstrated the ability of physicians to take leadership roles and make significant improvements to clinical and managerial services.

[8] Research by Bloom, Homkes, Sadun, and Van Reenen in 2010 on 1200 hospitals found that hospitals with more clinically trained managers outperform all the others. They hypothesized that perhaps clinical managers obtain higher levels of street-level credibility, competence, and authoritative clinical expertise difficult to achieve for nonclinical managers. This is what behavioral scientists call "social proof."

[9] Staller, Goodall, and Baker [56] reported that a matched random sample of employees and employers in the USA and UK found employees reporting to leaders who are experts in the core business had low intentions to change jobs and higher job satisfaction.

Merely promoting well-behaved physicians into "accidental" leadership positions is like allowing a laparoscopic surgeon to do a prostatectomy with a da Vinci robotic device without any advanced training and practice. We need physicians with advanced leadership training, so that they can not only define shared clinical visions, but also build commitment, and implement medical reforms that challenge assumptions, traditional roles, behaviors, and systems of authority (see [55]).

This chapter examines the importance of teaching leadership to surgeons and adding leadership training and development as part of contemporary surgical education. Teaching leadership to medical students, surgical residents, fellows, and other surgeons is a challenge for medical professionalism [38].

There is no end to the many ways we can waste time and distract students with abstract theoretical approaches to leadership or other popular notions. Leaders need to be taught practiced and effective concepts and tools. They also need feedback on their behavior and a safe space in which to reflect with a coach. Leaders who can reflect on their behavior will always be on a steep and asymptotic learning curve: feeling challenged,[10] assessing their own behavior and the outcomes, and learning from small mistakes [1, 7, 20, 30, 50].

Leadership training and development requires activity in the presence of knowledge. It requires an application of knowledge as well as experience and skills and a willingness to commit to the responsibilities of leadership, to understand the importance of a leader as a role model, and to believe in the capability of the team.

It also requires a relentless willingness to:

- Learn from mistakes.
- Take full responsibility for outcomes (never finger-point or excuse yourself from poor results)
- Communicate why the mission and goals are important and meaningful to everyone

Not everyone will agree that every surgeon should be the ascribed or emergent leader. Some surgeons may have notable abilities (knowledge, skills, and experience) to be leaders; they may also have appreciable disabilities. What is certain is that not all leaders are effective in every situation unless they are able to diagnose and analyze the situation and adapt their styles. So, while there may be few "born" leaders, we can train many surgeons to become better leaders. That may be the most important and hopeful lesson for surgical education and the future of health care.

The remainder of this chapter is broken down into six main sections: (1) Leadership Versus Management: Some Definitions; (2) The Surgeon as Leader; (3) Teaching What They Need to Know: Leadership Models Not Leadership Theory; (4) Teaching Leadership to Surgeons Using Cases; (5) Physician-Centered Learning

[10] To deprive leaders of feedback is to cheat them, and yet evolutionary psychologists tell that for most human beings, negative feedback leads to hurt feelings (see [43]).

Techniques: Translating Materials in Classroom Pedagogy with Group Work and Active Learning Techniques; and (6) Key Learning Points and Conclusions.[11] Next we will distinguish leadership from management, and define what leaders do—that is, define how leaders build a group of professionals into willing followers.

Leadership Versus Management: Some Definitions

Imagine we were talking about strategic issues in medical practice 5–10 years ago. Would we be talking about the same things we are talking about today? If we came back 5 years from now, again would we be talking about things that have evolved very differently from what we expected 5 years before?

This runs to the heart of what effective leaders must do. They must understand the evolving situation, all the important variables, and how they are related.[12] As Mary Parker Follett once said, it takes insight to master the current situation and to "…see possible new paths, the courage to try them, the judgment to measure results…" ([23], p. 170). If leaders are effective, they are *creating a future situation* while dealing with the current situation.

Clinical leaders should not be predicting or forecasting but rather anticipating and responding to change—in the surgical sciences, the regulatory environment, the dynamic and highly competitive marketplace, rapidly changing technology, and so on. More than coping with change, clinical leadership is about shaping the upcoming situation.

There is a difference between managers and leaders. To manage an organization literally means to handle many complex activities. Managers plan, recruit people, design and align the organization, establish budgets, coordinate, and report on performance. Managers also decide when people and budgets have to be cut, labs have to be outsourced, service lines have to be "rationalized," and medical suppliers have to be consolidated. As the former CEO of Nissan and Renault, Carols Ghosn once said to a business school audience, "management is about telling people to do things they otherwise don't want to do."

Without *willing followers*, managers lose control of the situation. Managers have a choice. They can rely on authority, rewards, coercion, fear of punishment, or other negative incentives; or use positive leadership strategies to guide and motivate people. Now we can see the challenge of leadership and what leadership means.

The best definition comes from Kouzes and Posner [34]:

> Leadership is the art of mobilizing people to **want to** struggle for shared aspirations.

---

[11] There is an appendix on teaching physicians and mention of several case studies that can be obtained for the author.

[12] The great management prophet, Mary Parker Follett, argued that leadership was all about diagnosing situations. This can be found in a lecture she gave in 1949 entitled "Freedom and Coordination" reprinted in a book published in 2003.

While this entire definition is important, there are two keywords that not only run to the heart of leadership, but can be the measure of one's effectiveness as a leader, i.e., the words "want to." People can be *trained to do* things, *afraid not to do* things, *prepared to do* things, and *paid to do* things, but do they *want to do* them? When they want to, they will not only take on the task, they will work very hard and persist in the face of difficulty.

Leaders turn people resisting change into "willing followers." The tools they use include action plans with clear goals, priorities, timeframes, and targets. They mobilize people to be willing to cut budgets, outsource labs, retreat from some service lines, and consolidate suppliers, because they understand the rationale for making difficult decisions to fix the organization. They persuade key people that the current situation requires difficult and painful changes in order to get to a future situation that fulfills the mission or accomplishes a goal everyone aspires to achieve. Later in the chapter, I will discuss how this happens. Next, I turn my attention to understanding whether surgeons are prepared to be leaders and what it means for a surgeon to lead. I will draw on the sports metaphor of the player-coach.

The Surgeon as Leader[13]

Surgeons are uniquely positioned to be leaders, but are they prepared? Robert Goffee and Gareth Jones once posed the most troubling, look-in-the-mirror, question posed to professionals—"why should anybody be led by you?"[14] They argued that not everyone can be an inspirational leader, and yet authentic leaders are found at every level in an organization. Every surgeon should ask themselves this question, because if you cannot manage yourself, you cannot manage others [22].

Next, to further explore the surgeon as leader, I will raise the following questions:— Is it possible to be both a player and a coach? Is it possible for leaders to continue to practice medicine? I will give an example of one leader trying to play both roles.

A New Imperative: Every Surgeon a Player-Coach?

What does it mean to be a clinical leader? One of the best examples of a clinical leader is Dr. Tomy Mihaljevic, MD, a practicing thoracic surgeon and the former CEO in Cleveland Clinic Abu Dhabi (CCAD).[15]

Being an MD-CEO required being both a team player and a coach, taking on multiple roles—clinical leader, cardiothoracic surgeon, chief strategist, visionary, and figurehead. While being CEO and a physician is daunting, he would not have it any other way. Dr. Mihaljevic explained:

[13] When we try to answer the question, "what is leadership," it is as difficult as answering the question "what is surgical quality?" Like quality, leadership is multidimensional (see [11]).

[14] Goffee and Jones [27].

[15] This section is based on my interviews with Dr. Mihaljevic between 2014 and 2017 and my case study of CCAD.

> If I can borrow a metaphor from the military, I say that medicine ought to be led at the level of the corporal and not the general (as long as each corporal is not only qualified but is also the best soldier). A hospital CEO ensconced in meetings in the C-suite and meetings with VIPS is like a general who is 5 miles away: they can be out-of-touch. So, for me it would be difficult to envision that I could run a hospital effectively without knowing what hospital life is really like...

He went on to say:

> I am a thoracic surgeon and I am a CEO. As a surgeon when I perform a minimally invasive robotic heart surgery, I must be available for that patient 24/7; as the responsible physician working with the most qualified workforce as a team, I can make decisions that put the patient first; in addition, I understand intimately our internal problems...As the hospital CEO, I have morning huddles, administrative meetings and rounds, and other duties. Playing both roles enables me and every other physician leader here at CCAD to understand the clinical, managerial and policy world we deal with every day.

To borrow a player-coach sports analogy, he is developing and executing the medical and operating strategy, holding everyone accountable for patient outcomes, and playing and collaborating on the surgical team, calling signals, managing tactics, and making surprise plays.

To be called a clinical leader, a surgeon needs followers (i.e., other surgeons, residents, anesthesiologists, scrub nurses, circulating nurses, other clinical and administrative staff, etc.). Entrepreneur Derek Sivers, in a 2010 Ted Talk,[16] said that the first follower is "an underappreciated form of leadership." He said, "the first follower transforms a lone nut into a leader." So, the role of the followers is to help keep the leader in control of the situation [23]. This means that leaders need to embrace and value followers who become committed to innovative ideas and important goals. Leaders do not need to push followers; followers are willing participants who see the value of what the team is trying to accomplish.

The surgeon leaders make two primary contributions: first, they heal their patients, and second, they take the lead for the organization. As mentioned, followership is an "underappreciated" form of leadership. My mantra for these leaders is:

> *Every surgeon, a leader; every leader, a collaborative follower and team player.*

If they are prepared to lead, surgeons should be able to engage the best people to diagnose evolving situations—changes in the rules, the competition, and surgical improvements. Through their networks they should be able to ensure a lucid analysis of the future regulatory conditions, technical innovations, changes in population health, reimbursement rules, and the myriad data that affect performance.

They should be able to facilitate an assessment of the strengths and weaknesses of the surgical team, along with future opportunities, risks, and threats in the environment. By engaging the best people, they source new ideas and explore alternatives as well as the full set of consequences.

---

[16] See Derek [51]. Ted Talk. How to start a movement

Beyond assessing the human resources, surgeons have to learn how to adapt the medical strategy as the environment changes. Roles may stay the same, but different people may have to come in to play these roles. Surgical leaders must recruit, train, develop, and interchange people without losing the energy and capabilities of surgical and other teams. Other clinical team members may need help evaluating their style and effectiveness. Leaders must also focus on coaching and developing future clinical leaders and offering continuous leadership education.

For surgeons not prepared to lead, clinical leadership training is essential. Topics for conversation include strategies to:

- Build a group of professionals into a high-performance unit committed to a clear and challenging direction
- Perform an initial team briefing (or huddle)
- Give feedback and have difficult conversations
- Coach a nurse or a resident
- Bring a new technology or surgical procedure into the hospital
- Build commitment to quality and safety goals

In order for leaders to learn these things, we must present the right concepts, tools, and models. I will address which theories or practices to teach next.

Teaching What They Need To Know: Leadership Models Not Leadership Theory[17]

We are interested in teaching surgeons how to understand their own behavior so they can reflect and diagnose the range of leadership situations they will confront. As faculty, we want to introduce usable concepts and tools, and to teach leaders to self-reflect for purposes of training and development. Consequently, the models that we teach should reconstruct realities encountered, and should be grounded in assumptions and behaviors that can be applied.

The theory and practice of leadership has a long and rich history [44]. Reviewing the last 90 years of literature, one can see that just about every method and research technique has been used to study leadership. While progress has been made, one academic, in analyzing the published evidence, found a "bewildering mass of findings" [5]. Other social scientists refer to their own body of leadership research as a "long and frustrating odyssey."

[17] These views are based on over 30 years' experience as a professor working with physician and nonphysician executives in health care as well as executives from other industries. I have conducted observational and ethnographic studies of hospital CEOs with MD and non-MD backgrounds [9]. I conducted quantitative studies of health leaders using multi-rater instruments. I also conducted qualitative leadership studies of surgeons, general managers, symphony conductors, and religious leaders.

Broadly speaking, teaching surgeons about leadership theory may not be relevant to most surgeons' work. These theories have been developed to align with basic social science theories often using standardized measurement and convenient mathematics for purposes of research, publication, or edification. Most of these theories have not been developed to teach people how to lead. However, it will be helpful to begin with a very brief review of the literature, which I will do in the next section.

A Brief Review of Some Leadership Theories

Leadership theory courses often start with ideologues and heroic leaders, such as Moses, Joan of Arc, Genghis Khan, Napoleon, Gandhi, and Mao Tse Tung.[18] All of these are entertaining and interesting as historical leadership studies. From there, the history of leadership follows with a search for "idealized" personality traits of these great leaders. Drawing on psychology, social psychology, sociology, and other social sciences, the literature continues to evolve.

Today, the literature includes descriptive studies of skill sets (technical, interpersonal, and conceptual), contingency approaches, theories of transactional versus transformational or charismatic leadership, path-goal theory, leader-member exchange, and the like.[19] There are no stable theories of leadership. Perhaps studies of clinical and managerial situations reveal far too many variables and insufficient observations to develop a strong theory. Significant variables pop in and out.[20] Every one of these so-called theories of leadership has some strengths, but also some serious criticisms and critiques of their scientific quality.[21] Leaders are left with broad generalizations and platitudes: model the way, challenge the process, enable others, inspire a vision, and encourage the heart, rather than the conditions under which some behaviors will be more effective and more likely to achieve a goal than others.

While leadership theories may be useful for academic research or to explain or describe events and behaviors, teaching surgeons a leadership model that can be applied may be more useful.

[18] All of the leaders mentioned above mobilized people and accomplished some aspiration. They became heroes or villains. It can be said that without Moses, his followers would have remained in Egypt as slaves.

[19] For a more complete description of the rich literature on leadership concepts and theories, see [44], Leadership: Theory and Practice.

[20] A recent example is the review of one of the trendier theories of leadership—charismatic-transformational leadership theory. The review essential closed down this body of work as having, lacking in conceptual clarity, confounding leadership with its effects, suffering from valid measures, and resulting in unstable findings (see [33]).

[21] Some scholars see the leadership as a weak science. There are no "barriers to entry" and no specialty boards examining the knowledge and skills of leadership coaches and leadership gurus. The danger is that some sell what Stanford Business School Professor Jeffry Pfeiffer calls a pseudoscience or "Leadership BS" (see [45]).

Leadership Models Teachable and Useful to Surgeons and Clinicians

Progress has been made in understanding two basic ingredients of leadership behavior: task behavior and relational behavior. Task behavior refers to a leader's words and actions used to accomplish the goals, for example:

- Guiding or teaching people how to perform tasks
- Reviewing roles and responsibilities
- Instructing people about goals
- Offering instruction about how to meet deadlines and performance standards

Task behavior occurs when a leader focuses attention on obtaining goals, overcoming constraints and barriers, and general problem solving.

Relational behavior refers to a leader's words and actions used to make personal connections, for example:

- Expressing appreciation for good work
- Listening to understand people's points of view
- Creating a safe space for people to express opinions
- Listening to people's ideas and concerns
- Maintaining the group's self-esteem
- Treating people fairly and with respect

Relational behavior occurs when a leader focuses attention on listening, praising, recognizing, respecting, and building self-efficacy (or collective efficacy) [3, 4].[22]

If we put these two elements on a horizontal and vertical axis, we get a two-by-two table (see Fig. 20.1). By segmenting the two-by-two table into four quadrants, we can combine these two ingredients and obtain high and low task behavior and high and low relational behavior.

Now we can define a surgeon (or anyone's) leadership style. Style is the pattern of a leader's behavior in terms of the proportion of task versus relational behavior as perceived by the people working with that leader. Leadership styles are malleable and may be altered according to the demands of a situation, resulting in alternative solutions to various situations.

Figure 20.2 is a visualization of these four quadrants, and represents in more detail, the four alternative attention structures and styles of leading:

1. High task/low relational behavior, a very directive style, called the "teacher."
2. High task/high relational behavior, a persuading and clarifying style with two-way communication, called the "hub at the center."

[22] Professionals may be self-confident, but in some situations, they may feel insecure. Self-efficacy is a belief in one's ability to succeed in a specific situation when it involves a task, activity, assignment, or challenging goal. Collective efficacy is also situational; it refers to a group's belief that together they have the resources and capabilities to undertake a challenge and to achieve and perform (Bandura [3]; 2010).

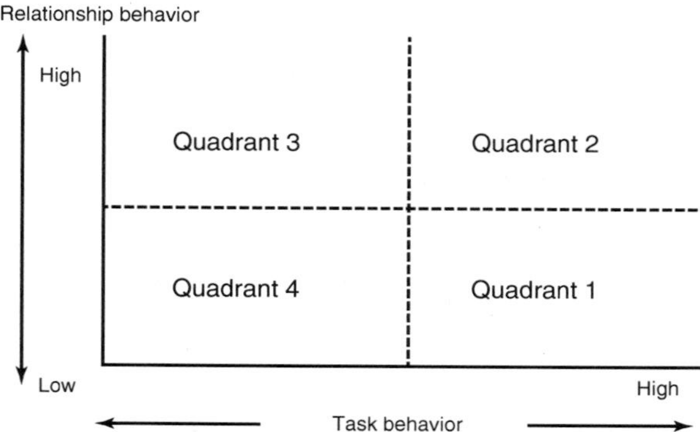

Fig. 20.1 Defining Leadership Style

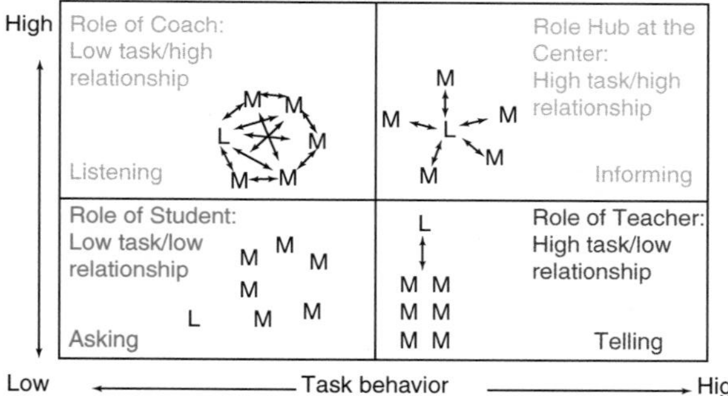

Fig. 20.2 Attention Structure and Leadership Style Alternatives

3. Low task/high relational behavior, a deep listening, facilitating, and following style, called the "coach."
4. Low task/low relational behavior, a delegating and empowering style, called the "student."

The four quadrants shown in Fig. 20.2 also represent the four basic tools of leading:

- Quadrant 4: Asking—using open-ended questions, such as What are the problems, What seems to be working, and What are your ideas?
- Quadrant 3: Listening—gathering important information with no agenda other than to understand feelings and experiences[23]

[23] Here is where training in motivational interviewing can help you to lead by listening, by affirming what people say (in your words), by reflecting in the form of statements that form a hypothesis about what they mean, and by summarizing what transpired during the meeting and the next steps.

- Quadrant 2: Informing—sharing evidence, explaining rationale, clarifying ideas, or giving advice
- Quadrant 1: Telling—teaching how to do a task, setting the goal and the performance standards, and setting expectations (roles, responsibilities)

The idea is that leaders become skillful in using these four tools to get work done through other people. These tools enact both micro- and macroleadership styles. In some situations the "telling" leader is more effective. In other situations, the "asking" leader is more effective. Effective leaders will become adept at knowing which style to use when.

Leaders cannot fixate on one or two styles, but must adapt their style to the people and the evolving situations. Leaders need to know and be able to use all four macrostyles. For any given task, goal, or critical event, leaders will choose among the four styles so that people will better understand the leader and view the leader's behavior as consistent with the situation.

Figure 20.3 is a representation of leadership situations, as matched to the four leadership styles depicted earlier.

- Quadrant 1: a crisis requires more directive and authoritative leader behaviors, i.e., more task behavior than relational behavior.
- Quadrant 2: strategic problem solving requires more clarifying and democratic leader behavior, i.e., a high degree of relational and task behavior, with intense two-way communications.
- Quadrant 3: coordination or interpersonal problems require more participative leader behavior, i.e., lower on task but much higher relational behavior.
- Quadrant 4: a routine situation requires empowering and enabling self-reliance, or delegating leader behaviors, i.e., lower on both task and relational behaviors.

The four attention structures and leader roles in the preceding figure are mapped to the specific leadership behaviors in Fig. 20.4. In each quadrant, the leader has diagnosed the situation, identified the objective, and selected the appropriate leader behavior. Effective leaders must always diagnose and then adapt their style, their attention structure and their role (see Fig. 20.4).

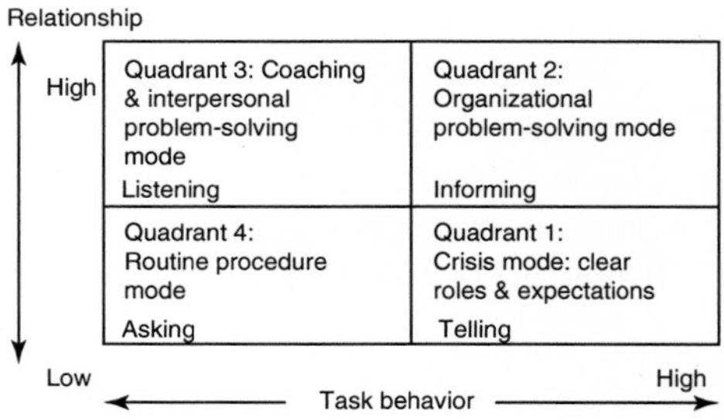

Relationship

High	Quadrant 3: Coaching & interpersonal problem-solving mode Listening	Quadrant 2: Organizational problem-solving mode Informing
Low	Quadrant 4: Routine procedure mode Asking	Quadrant 1: Crisis mode: clear roles & expectations Telling

Low ← Task behavior → High

Fig. 20.3 Leadership Situations Matched to Leadership Style

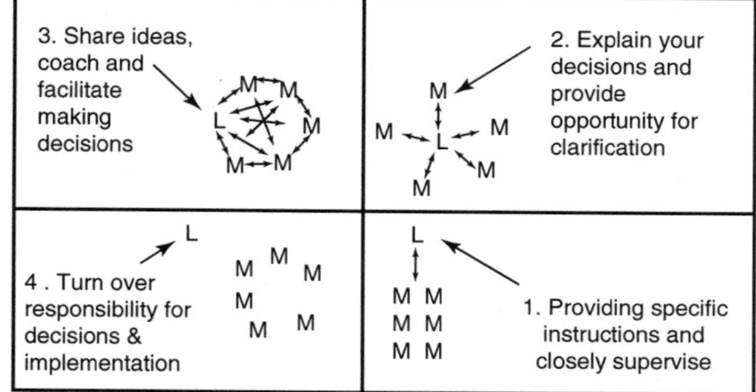

Fig. 20.4 Visualizing the Attention Structure of the Four Leadership Styles

In summary, the work of leadership requires both a relentless diagnosis of the current (or evolving) situation and an ability to adapt style to situation [17, 20, 29, 30, 31]. To do this, leaders must focus their attention so they can understand the situation as a set of important and dominant variables, and then detect the relationships among these variables and the likelihood of their effect on the future. Leadership styles are alternative ways of behaving that can facilitate the results leaders want to achieve [30, 31, 39, 41, 42, 46, 47, 54, 57].

Useful Theories That Underlie Models of Effective Leadership Practices

There are four theories that underlie effective leadership practices and that are particularly relevant to surgical leadership: (1) situational diagnosis, (2) collective intelligence, (3) fair process, and (4) goal theory.[24]

Mary Parker Follett has said of situational diagnosis, that leaders must understand the whole situation in order to effectively diagnose and determine the next steps. In particular, analyzing the situation requires a deep understanding of the interrelations among the environment, people, technology, structures, the work to be done and how all of it is changing [23].

Collective intelligence, the second theory, is the ability of a group to perform a wide variety of tasks. It begins with the following proposition—people are the source of novel ideas and strategic innovations; however, no individual is smart enough to evaluate his or her own ideas. Only through a collaborative process where

[24]There are four underlying theories that help us to explain this—situational diagnosis, collective intelligence, fair process, and goal theory. I do not have time to go into these theories, but I will refer you to the following topics and authors:

1. Diagnosing Situations and the Discipline of Strategic Thinking—[13]
2. Collective Intelligence—[62]
3. Goal Theory—see [40]
4. Fair Process—Kim and Mauborgne 2007 [58] and [13]

challenging discussions take place and the pool of ideas can be enlarged will a group achieve its potential. Collective intelligence occurs when a group can outperform other groups across a multiplex of tasks, e.g., tasks involving superior moral judgment, brainstorming, complex problem solving, conflict resolution, and so on. Groups with collective intelligence (CI) are more diverse; in fact, one study found that *the higher the proportion of women in a group, the greater the collective intelligence* [62]. Groups with CI have superior social sensitivity and equal participation—i.e., no one dominates [62, 63]. Groups displaying CI find the areas of agreement and allow the sources of disagreement to be aired.

The third theory, fair process leadership, has several characteristics [35, 36]. Fair process *engages* key people to analyze the situation, resulting in a framing of the decision. *Fair process also explores* and narrows the list of new ideas, *explains* the rationale for decisions, sets *expectations* about roles and responsibilities, and implements strategy with an eye toward *evaluation* and learning [13, 58].

The fourth important concept that underlies leadership is goal theory [40]. The dirty secret of leadership is that if leaders can get people committed to a goal, these people will adjust their effort level to accommodate the difficulty of the task. If people are able, motivated, and believe the goals are important and possible to achieve, the more challenging the goal, the better the performance. Performance drops if people are not committed to the goal, or the wrong tools or task strategies are used, or if they reach the limits of their abilities.

Here is where we can connect fair process with goal theory. Studies of leadership have found that commitment to strategic goals is directly related to the perception that a process was fair, even if decision makers disagree with the final outcome or alternative selected. Commitment to strategic goals means that the key people are drawn to the strategic goals because they believe the strategy is important; moreover, they will persevere to implement the strategic activity even when there are severe constraints [40].

How to Build Commitment to Goals

The most important lesson to teach surgeons is how to build commitment to goals.[25] Goal theory teaches us that commitment means that people believe that the goal is not only important and attractive, but also possible to attain. If people are committed, they will stick to the goal even in the face of setbacks and disruptive events. My research on effective leaders revealed that there is a clear pattern to overall effective leadership which requires building commitment in critical situations. Some examples of critical situations follow [9, 10].

1. Taking charge of an organization as a new assignment

[25] I am grateful to Dr. Mitch Rabkin, MD; Dr. Michael Jellinek, MD; Reverend Jeffrey Brown; and Maestro Wolfgang Heinzel for allowing me to observe them in situ, to study their leadership styles to learn how they built commitment to goals. I am grateful to my colleague at INSEAD, Dr. Paul Evans, for discussing his framework for building commitment to goals with me.

2. Improving existing programs and processes
3. Attempting simple strategic adaptation (e.g., targeting new patients, new locations, new technologies, new competition, or new regulations)
4. Attempting more complex strategic adaptations (e.g., new markets and industries)
5. Transforming the culture or recreating the organization, for example, reorienting the organization by changing the focus from acute care to population health

When new leaders are settling into their jobs (situation 1) or they must reestablish objectives and strategic plans (situations 2–5), what exactly do they do? To be effective, their goal is to mobilize people to want to find solutions to challenging situations. Research on effective leadership has discovered a pattern of behavior that works quite well to build commitment. Here is a framework and timeline of what effective leaders do over a period of 3 to 4 months[26]:

- During the first 4–6 weeks, leaders plan to spend 100% of their time deep inside the organization talking with the people closest to the customers or the people involved with key processes where the actual work gets done. The Japanese word for this place is called *Gemba*, or place of value.
- Effective leaders start with a hypothesis. There are solutions to all the five leadership situations mentioned above; however, they are buried inside the organization with the people who are closest to these problems. The leader must perform a lucid diagnosis[27] of the root causes of problems and of the opportunities by listening to what people—especially those in the front lines—say when they are asked simple questions, for example:

    1. Why are we in this situation?
    2. What can we do to improve?
    3. What actions should we take?

- The leader merely listens, takes notes, and begins grouping the issues and actions to be done into a few logical categories.
- Often there are open discussions with all internal and external stakeholders—clients, customers, suppliers, bosses, peers, and direct reports. The leader's job again is to ask open-ended questions, to listen, and to take notes on problems and opportunities, as well as the strengths and weaknesses of the organization. Leaders will want to know, What is working in terms of strategy, operations, services, culture, human resources, leadership development, and the like? Alternatively, what is not working in the same areas. Leaders will

[26] To prepare for this 3–4-month period, a leader must activate social networks to answer four questions:

1. Who has "organizational rights" to be involved with this situation?
2. Who has the expertise to help us think about this situation?
3. Who should be consulted prior to or during the dialogue?
4. Who should be informed of the rationale for the decision and the expectations?

[27] For an explanation of how leaders use tools and concepts to improve strategic thinking, see [13].

want to ask stakeholders, e.g., What are your ideas? What is your department's contribution?

- During this 4–6 week period, leaders are assessing the organizational culture while building relationships with subordinates and key stakeholders, and assessing talent and the overall ability and willingness to collaborate.
  - They are beginning to identify the cultural problems, such as "shame and blame," finger-pointing, inability to speak up to authority, weak commitment, low morale, and feelings of underappreciation.
  - They are assessing strategic design and misalignments, such as poor coordination, vague goals and standards, lack of knowledge about costs, inefficiencies, and the need for process improvements.
  - They are discovering customer experiences and the true value proposition, the people proposition, and the value to the organization.
- After 4–6 weeks in the GEMBA, talking with dozens, or for a CEO, hundreds of people, critical issues and hypotheses emerge.
- The next 4–6 weeks are marked by reviewing the diagnoses, separating the facts from assumptions.
  - Groups are formed and are engaged in challenging discussions. They are testing hypotheses, reframing the problems and opportunities, and assessing the full set of consequences, the risks, uncertainties, and tradeoffs.
- The leader's job is to stay out of the content and instead to manage the process—keeping people as rational as possible while ensuring good relationships.
  - The leader also ensures that people use a process of inquiry, not advocacy, allowing challenging discussions, debates, and friendly arguments.
  - The leader asks everyone to explore the uncertainties by exploring the "what ifs" and the contingencies for 2–3 likely scenarios, asking for example, What would happen if we pursued this solution? Or that goal?
  - The discussion allows for more reframing and more argument, building on the ideas of others. Everyone is exploring the alternatives and options.
- The last month of this 3–4 month period is spent communicating the implications of the targets, the rationale, and the plan to get there. Finally, the 3–4 months end with an announcement:

  > Ladies and gentlemen, thank you for the challenging discussions and all your ideas during the last 3–4 months. We have decided that the objective of this group (department, organization, etc.) is X, Y, Z, and this is our strategic action plan to get there. Here are your roles and responsibilities, and now we have to execute the plan.

  Some leaders will make a final commitment:

  > If this plan we developed does not work over the next 12–18 months, and we do not make significant progress towards our goals, I will take responsibility and resign—no excuses. We will do this right or not at all.[28]

[28] Carlos Ghosn, CEO of Nissan and Renault, used reciprocal commitment. Here are our goals and your role and responsibilities. In addition, he publicly promised his resignation if they did not get the expected results in 1 year.

- Most important is the timing and symbolism of this message. The time for debate is over, the time for action is now. What counts now is action in pursuit of the objectives. Here are the goals; here are your roles and responsibilities; these are my expectations, and I will hold you *and myself* accountable to make these goals happen.

Here is a summary of the preceeding explanation of how leaders build commitment to goals. By asking open-ended questions and listening to understand people's points of view, leaders discover two things. First they discover the interests of the people—their hopes, fears, insecurities, concerns, and more. They discover people's perceptions of what they perceive they have to give up and what they perceive is in it for them.

The second discovery is a superordinate goal that all the internal stakeholders[29] strongly agree is the most important goal.[30] The leader puts something in front of people that is significant and that they would be proud to achieve. The solution came from inside, so there is deep engagement and fair process. It allows the leader to align the internal stakeholders, so everyone becomes willing to sacrifice some of their self-interest, and the buy-in is 100%.

This superordinate goal should be perceived as making them better off in one or more of the following: their careers, their compensation, their practice, their learning and mastery, or their feeling of taking responsibility for outcomes. After leaders align stakeholder interests around the more significant goal, implementation begins. This goal should be something so important it creates hope or confident expectation that once through the tough situation, things will be much better.

Figure 20.5 depicts the process and the pattern of leadership behavior toward bulding commitment.

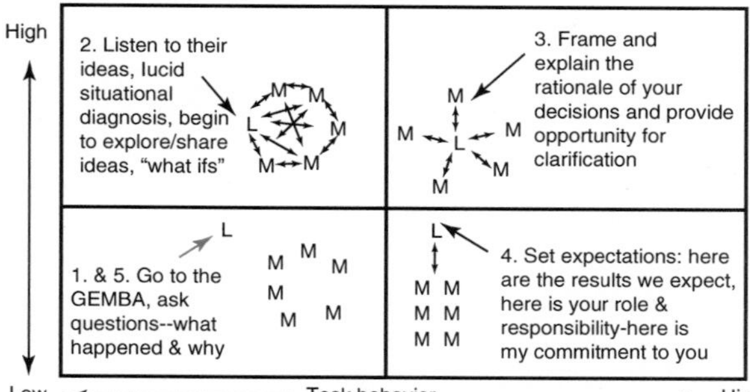

Fig. 20.5 Attention Structure When Building Commitment to Goals

[29] Stakeholders are individuals, groups, institutions, and organizations that can affect your decisions and/or are affected by your decision-making.

[30] How to get "willing followers" is the leadership challenge. It is about giving people a choice and letting them make the decision for themselves without punishment.

Teaching Leadership to Surgeons Using Cases

Some surgeons may believe that leadership is something that comes naturally. They have clocked in so many hours in the operating room; they know how to lead. While that may be true to some extent, there is also a need for self-reflection against some objective criteria.

Perhaps the best way to explore how to teach surgeons about leadership is to ask: How do we combine leadership knowledge with surgical practice? This is fundamental according to Alfred North Whitehead:

> "What the faculty have to cultivate is activity in the presence of knowledge. What the students have to learn is activity in the presence of knowledge…"[31]

Whitehead goes on to say that passive learning that shields the classroom from real-world activities is misplaced. Application is part of knowledge. This seems to align with the basic idea in medical education—see one, do one, teach one. The case method is one way to take real-world problems and translate them into classroom pedagogy.

The Case Method of Instruction

In educating future surgical leaders, the case method has been recognized as a primary pedagogy. Books on teaching medical professionalism advocate case vignettes as a vehicle for bringing real-life situations into the classroom.[32]

Cases are pedagogical tools designed and formulated for classroom learning and post-class discussions. A formal definition of the case comes from one of the true masters of the case method, Professor C. Roland Christianson:

> A case is a partial, historical, clinical study of a situation which has confronted a practicing administrator or managerial group. Presented in narrative form to encourage student involvement, it provides data—substantive and process—essential to an analysis of a specific situation, for the framing of alternative action programs, and for their implementation recognizing the complexity and ambiguity of the practical world.[33]

Cases combine historical, verbal, numerical, visual, and graphical data allowing a fresh process of discovery with each discussion. A case discussion not only teaches people how to think in the situation described in the case but also in diverse situations. Therefore, cases are not about teaching a solution or a way to behave, but cases are about teaching leaders how to think.

In a "good" case, the leaders are facing a complex or novel real-world problem or opportunity. Students are told to prepare the case and make a recommendation. Offering questions in advance such as:

- What are the facts and key issues? What went right? What went wrong?
- Describe the key events. How did the events evolve? What are your assumptions?

[31] Whitehead [61].

[32] Steinert [53].

[33] Christensen and Hansen [15].

- What is your diagnosis of the situation?
- What is your hypothesis or theory about what happened?
- As a surgeon leader, what would you do?
- How would you communicate that idea?

During the case discussion, there is simultaneously too much general information and never enough specific information. There is time pressure and uncertainty in the situation, but the basic question remains: What would you recommend? As a leader you must guide and motivate the group. What is your decision? What would you do?

A student is called upon to answer. When a student gives an answer, the professor then asks, What do the rest of you think? Would that work? Why or why not?

The discussion begins. There are rational and emotional reactions from students. From time to time, there is a covert activation of biases that support the student or argue with the student's thinking. The instructor must weave together the discussion, building on the ideas, summarizing the conditions under which some ideas work and other will not. By enabling a case discussion to become a collaborative experience, it becomes an opportunity for everyone to reevaluate their own ideas and the quality of their thinking and to confront and reflect on their own attitudes, biases, and prior experiences—i.e., an occasion to learn. The responsibility of the instructor is simply to lead the case discussion and, as such, to enact the learning process.

Professionals learn from good stories. Following are several cases I have used when teaching surgeons.

Case 1: Surgical Leadership in the Removal of an Unexploded Ordnance

On March 16, 2006, American soldiers were on a mounted patrol in Afghanistan. As the Americans were coming around a bend in their vehicles, they were ambushed from the left. The Americans were under attack from small arms fire and then heavy arms fire with rocket-propelled grenades (RPGs). One RPG went over the head of the US truck and struck an American soldier, Chaney Moss, in his abdomen piercing his pelvic bone and lodging in his right thigh. As the wounded soldier, Chaney Moss, recalled:

> I felt the cool breeze of the chopper coming and I could see the yellow smoke. I thought about my wife and my girls growing up without me. I had those quiet moments on the helicopter. I thought I was going to die. I didn't think anyone could save me. But if I did survive, I would not be able to function. I felt at peace at one moment. That's if I did die, I died for the right cause and I did the right thing. But you want to fight and you want to live. Your inner feeling is to fight and go on. You can do this. We touched down at OE, and everyone was rushing.

Chaney Moss was brought inside the forward surgical unit. The general surgeon, Captain Oh, took away the dressings and realized that the soldier had live ordnance in him and he told everyone to get out.

The general surgeon recalled the situation and how he reacted as a leader:

> I never saw an RPG before. It looked like some kind of munitions--it had fins on it. The guideline is, you do not bring the soldier in. You leave them outside. I was scared. I was scared "shitless." I have never been so scared in my entire life. You look at the guy and then you think, there is no way I am going to let this guy die.

What this surgical leadership case involves is the essence of what leadership is about.

> *Leadership is a relentless, moment by moment, strategic thinking and communication process that guides and motivates people to want to respond to a given situation.*

Captain Oh, MD, as the responsible surgeon, had to diagnose the situation in the moment, and to mobilize the people to want to deal with this challenging situation. He called in the unexploded ordnance team to radiograph the ordnance, and they discovered that the warhead had broken off, and only the detonator was inside—still enough to kill the patient and wound the surgeon. What should he do?

Although I have written a case study on this, another alternative is to show the video from YouTube.[34] Both typically elicit a great discussion.

Case 2: Developing a Minimally Invasive Esophagectomy (MIE) Program at a Tertiary Hospital—Is the Surgical Team a Real Team?

The leader of the surgical team is Dr. Colon, a thoracic surgeon looking to develop a minimally invasive esophagectomy (MIE) program at the Tertiary Medical Center (TMC). He has done this procedure before at another hospital, but MIE has never been performed at TMC. His surgical assistant will be Dr. Valley, a bariatric surgeon, whom Dr. Colon routinely assists in his laparoscopic bariatric cases. He has never done an MIE before either; however, the abdominal portion is technically similar to his bariatric cases.

The other key players are the anesthesiologists. Their leader is Dr. Kellogg, a thoracic anesthesiologist who is also one of the senior physicians in the anesthesia group. Dr. Kellogg has worked with Dr. Colon before and will be running anesthesia for the MIE. Dr. Arthur is a thoracic anesthesiologist who was recently hired to the practice to assist in the growing number of thoracic cases under Dr. Colon. Dr. Alexis, Dr. Rohit, and Dr. Markus are other anesthesiologists on staff at TMC who are not specialty trained in thoracic cases. Davida and Lucy are the operating room staff that will be assisting in the procedure. Lastly, there is James, the previously healthy 61-year-old with invasive esophageal cancer, who agrees to the first MIE at TMC. There are a series of handoffs after Dr. Kellogg leaves. Here is how this case unfolds.

Dr. Kellogg leaves at 3:00 pm; it is his day to leave early, and he arranges to meet his trainer in the gym. He appears to have made adequate arrangement for handover of the case to another anesthesiologist, Dr. Alexis, but it is not clear whether he handed over details of the complexities—i.e., the fact that it was the first operation of this kind in this hospital or that there had been difficulties with the insertion of the double-lumen tube. It appears that he has made no special arrangements for handover, as he states, "I am going to go check to see who's going to take my room at 3:00 pm."

[34] This is a terrific video case that you can download from YouTube (see https://www.youtube.com/watch?v=KAKaZdFk0eA&spfreload=10).

Ideally the case would be taken over by a specialist thoracic anesthetist. We are told then that he has told the next anesthetist, Dr. Alexis, "all about James' history and signed out on all the things he needs to know." However Dr. Alexis stays for only 1 hour and then hands over to another anesthetist, Dr. Rohit. The surgeon has never worked with Dr. Rohit before. It is not clear if Dr. Kellogg knew that Dr. Alexis was available for only 1 hour, or that there would be yet another handover.

Dr. Rohit arrives at 4:00 p.m., and by 5:30 it seems clear that he is a less experienced anesthetist. He is anxious about "a difficult airway" and because he has been given inaccurate and inadequate information. He calls for another anesthetist to help him. At this time it is late and it may be that Dr. Rohit is a trainee. Certainly managers should be aware that there are difficulties with handovers, with continuity of care, and with poor and inaccurate information, that much care is given by a less qualified workforce, and that is when problems arise.

Following the surgery, there is a rupture of the anastomosis requiring a return to the operating room. It is clear that the clinical outcome is very poor and so in order to save the patient's life, heroic surgery is undertaken, with many further operations, intensive care, and complications with attendant poor quality of life. Despite this, and the direct plea from the patient that Dr. Kellogg stay to see him through, Dr. Kellogg again leaves the operation as soon as his session is completed, handing over on this occasion to another thoracic anesthetist. Once again he has fulfilled his contracted duties and made arrangements for handover but shown no commitment to the surgical team in a time of great difficulty or any empathy for the patient's emotional or medical needs.

It is not possible to be sure that the misplacement of the endotracheal tube into the esophagus caused the anastomosis to rupture. There is always a risk of this complication occurring, and James had been warned that the risk was somewhere around 25–30%. However, it is certainly possible that the tube had disrupted the anastomosis, and if the case were to proceed to litigation, this would be evident to expert advisors. Dr. Colon certainly would be concerned about this and would be likely to favor that explanation over the alternative that it was a direct result of his surgical skills. More important, however, it seems very probable that his working relationship with Dr. Kellogg, one of the few thoracic anesthetists in the department, would be badly, if not permanently, damaged. Dr. Colon is likely to believe that Dr. Kellogg left the team for a trivial social engagement and has contributed to the adverse outcome. As the first case has gone badly, it may be a long time before Dr. Colon has a chance to undertake another.

Both clinicians and managers will be disturbed by Dr. Kellogg's actions and will question his behavior. Did he act unprofessionally? Was he clinically negligent? Should a manager take action in terms of his work commitment or his contract? We make an assumption that he is more financially motivated than focused on the needs of the patients; he doesn't like the extra, stressful work involved in looking after complex, major surgery cases because the insurance doesn't recognize the additional workload. We are told he "made a special effort and was there early," so the operation could start on time at 07:30; we assume that he does not usually come in early, and we might infer that he does not like to stay late. A colleague states that Dr.

Kellogg is the senior partner, he has worked for 18 years, his personal time is his own, and "he doesn't have to give more than is required."

I teach this case by asking "what went right and what went wrong?" Ostensibly, the most important piece of this case was the error itself. The problems began with the handoff that occurred between anesthesiologists and Dr. Rohit stating that James had "a difficult airway" when this was not the case. When time came for the reintubation after the case, Dr. Rohit became apprehensive because James had been mislabeled, and he was unfamiliar with the thoracic case. He brought in another anesthesiologist, Dr. Markus, who passed the tube through the esophageal anastomosis rather than into the trachea. This tore Dr. Colon's anastomosis and led to the complications that ensued. Despite Dr. Colon's high suspicion after the failed intubation, he chose to send James to the ICU rather than to reexamine the anastomosis and possibly order some imaging at that point.

Did Dr. Kellogg, chair of anesthesiology, walk away from the patient? Was he clinically negligent? Did he violate his psychological contract with the team?

And what of the leadership of Dr. Colon? What was the quality of his strategic thinking? Were the "what ifs" developed and understood? Did Dr. Colon build commitment to the goals? Was the team engaged? Why or why not? Is it possible for a surgeon to play both roles i.e., chief technical expert and team leader, planning and implementing this procedure?

Case 3: Flight 1549—Collaborative Leadership in Action

The first responders expected the worst case scenario. An Airbus A320 with 155 passengers crash landed in the middle of the Hudson River. What happened?

On January 15, 2009, US Airways flight 1549 departed New York City's La Guardia Airport at 3:25p.m. Ninety seconds after takeoff, the Airbus 320, headed to North Carolina, hit a flock of Canadian geese. The captain noticed large birds filling the entire windscreen. There was the sound and smell of birds smoldering in the engines. There was a "dramatic loss of thrust" and no sideward motion—conclusion: they lost both engines. What would you do?

In the cockpit, the conversation was as follows:[35]

H1 (Captain): birds
H2 (Copilot): uh oh
H1 (Captain): we got one rol-both of em rolling back
H1 (Captain): ignition start. I'm starting APU.
H1 (Captain): my aircraft
H2 (Copilot): your aircraft
H1 (Captain): get the QRH…lost thrust in both engines
H1 (RDO-1): mayday mayday mayday. Uh this is uh Cactus 1549. We've lost thrust in both engines, we're heading back to La Guardia.

[35] Contact the author for a copy of the case study; however the best way to teach this case is to show the video at https://www.youtube.com/watch?v=pWpSAfF6elI

In this case, the airline captain, Sully Sullenberger, displayed grace under pressure. He took charge by declaring "my aircraft" and made a perfect landing in the Hudson, and all the passengers survived. His leadership during execution had to be flawless.

Upon closer examination, we see that effective leaders like Sullenberger do two things. First, though the entire situation unfolds in less than 5 minutes, the leader must activate and engage the entire team to do their jobs and deal with the situation without panic. Second, leaders must collaborate with key stakeholders by adapting their leadership style moment by moment to respond to the situation.

Though the event was novel and uncertain under severe time constraints, there was amazingly good coordination and "quick-teaming." The team had to be activated quickly, with open lines of communication and shared goals, and able to work together. He said that there was not time to exchange words—but there was mutual observation and listening. This decision-making unit had been strategically designed so that the people and structures supported the critical tasks that had to be accomplished.

Captain Sullenberger said he and the copilot were on the same page—each knew their role and the role the other would play, and so they interacted only when needed. Both had training in crew resource management. Flight attendants sensed panic in the back, so they calmed everyone down, and told passengers, "We lost an engine, so we will circle back." They made sure passengers heads were down, and that there was no pushing and shoving.

Within minutes the first responders arrived—ferries, coast guard, helicopters, boats and divers, hundreds of New York City fire fighters and police. [36]

Alignment of roles, technology, protocols, and the emergency checklists help, but there is also a *clear role* for the leader. As mentioned, Kouzes and Posner define leadership as "the art of mobilizing people to want to struggle for shared aspirations" [34]. This case demonstrates the connection between leadership and strategic thinking. The work of leadership also requires moment-by-moment adjustments, sourcing external knowledge, checking facts, processing information, activating people, all of which was done quickly and efficiently by the leader in this case.

> *Leadership requires a relentless (moment by moment) strategic thinking and communication process that guides and motivates people <u>to want to</u> respond to a given situation.*

Figure 20.6 illustrates how leaders adapt their style based on the demands of the situation. Shifting occurs from very task-orientated behaviors exercising the captain's authority by taking control of the airbus from the copilot (e.g., "my aircraft"). They also ask open-ended questions ("any ideas").

This airline case should be used when teaching case 2 in the OR. It enables the instructor to raise several questions about fast versus slow thinking, quick teaming, activating roles, and adapting styles of leading. It enables the instructor to raise questions about leading the OR team and the various roles and relationships among nurses, surgeons, and anesthesiologists.

---

[36] Luck also plays a role in these situations. It was daytime. If this happened at night, perhaps the outcomes would have changed.

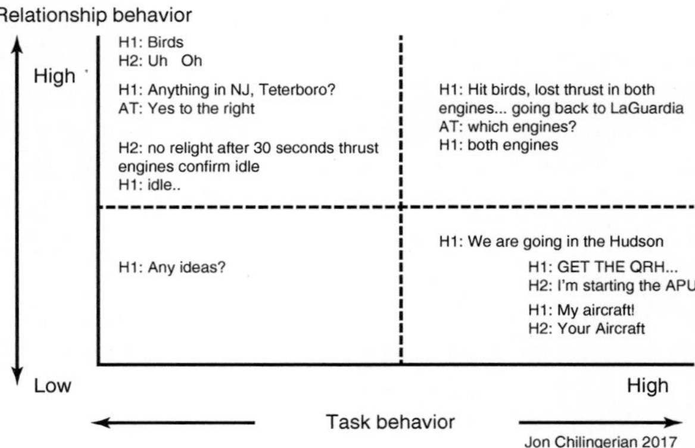

Fig. 20.6 Diagnosing Flight 1549's Situation and Adapting Leadership Style

Leadership Lessons: Diagnose Before You Prescribe and Disagree Respectfully[37]

While leaders are involved in many aspects of organizational life, they are judged based on the effectiveness and quality of decisions made during their tenure as leaders. Research shows that effective leadership practices can promote more effective decision-making [13]. Training physicians to lead requires them to do what they have already been trained to do—diagnose a situation before they seek a solution. This may be an important connection for surgical leaders. People seem to be hardwired to begin strategic thinking by talking about solutions rather than diagnosing the situation.

The job of the leader is to manage the rational decision-making process by avoiding premature discussion of strategic solutions. When people advocate too quickly for one alternative, then opinions, assumptions, and uncertainties become indistingtuishable from known facts. A clinical leader's first obligation is to help the team separate the facts from the assumptions.

Why separate facts from assumptions? The primary source of strategic mistakes is hidden assumptions [21]. Hidden assumptions can lead to two types of ineffective decision processes. If the decision makers have the same assumptions, they will reach closure very fast without considering the full set of consequences; if they have different assumptions, the discussion will be neverending and emotionally charged, at least until the deadlock is broken by abandonment or force (March 1988). In either case, the quality of the decision making will not be very good.

Strategic thinking shifts the group from premature discussion of solutions to an exploration and understanding of the problem, the assumptions and the goals, before deciding on the alternatives. By shifting everyone's focus from solutions to effective strategic thinking, the decision makers have a better understanding of what is at

[37] See [13].

stake and who holds the various points of view. Although strategic thinking slows down the decision process, the pool of information is enlarged as people have more time to think about how the decision may affect the organization in the future.

Effective decision making occurs when groups use both a rational process and a relational process. Physicians, however, may not be trained in how to build relationships via effective group communication. The work of leadership is to ensure that the decision making process is as rational as possible. At the same time, the rational process is used in combination with the relational process as the leader observes how people interact with each other, making certain not to interrupt or be disrespectful.

The leader's job is to coach the group to improve their social sensitivity, their ability to listen, and their capacity to build on each other's ideas. As such, the leader can coach a group to fulfill their potential for collective intelligence. To become a leader is to develop an enhanced understanding of human nature and interaction, and to foster relationships that support the flow of ideas toward effective decision making.

Leadership Lessons from Sports Coaches and Airline Captains

Research has shown that effective leaders increase the likelihood that a team can manage complex, ambiguous, and time-critical situations. Effective leaders adjust the strategy as the situation changes, inspire the team to perform, and enable the team to work together in a highly coordinated way [28].

With this in mind, clinical leaders can learn lessons from sports coaches and airline captains. First, what do good coaches do that clinical leaders can emulate? According to Hackman [28], they build the team during practice sessions. Second, they use pregame warm-ups to keep everyone coordinated. During a game, they check in (at halftime) to make tactical and midcourse corrections. Finally, after the game they review what happened and learn from the experience.

For clinical leaders, team building must happen in a practice field where members of a team can get together with nothing at stake and tinker with ideas aimed at creating a performance unit [26]. For example, the leader can assure that a huddle becomes a forum for dialogue where permission is given to explore complicated and subtle issues allowing each team member to raise conflictual issues essential to the team's work. Leading this type of "practice field" teaches the team to listen to each other's ideas and to suspend one's own views [49].

Research on airline captains who are better leaders finds that they do more team building activities during the first few minutes of a crew's life. These team activities occur in a preflight huddle and informal interactions. They also use low-workload moments during long flights to maintain the crew as a high-performing unit [25].

As I have argued earlier, the surgeon is both coach and player. There are many opportunities in clinic, at meetings, and in the OR when they can guide and motivate other clinicians. In the operating room, every surgeon is leading a team of clinicians: anesthesiologist, scrub and circulating nurses, patient assistants, etc. They should be taught specific skills to build stronger teams.

For example, surgeons could be trained to use the huddles and check lists to get an OR team off to an excellent start. They could be trained to develop "quicker" teams, for when team members have never worked together before. During long surgeries, they can develop practices that rejuvenate their teams. A high percentage of competent, well-trained surgeons experienced in building and leading high-performance teams could become the hospital's most significant resource and capability.

Being a leader is about being a role model. When people think of someone as the leader, everything said, every single word that comes out of that leader's mouth has an impact. And as psychologists teach us:

Whenever you open your mouth you can lose control.

Therefore, surgeons should be in the moment and mindful of the impact they have on the people that they work with day in and day out.

Physician-Centered Learning: Translating Materials in Classroom Pedagogy with Group Work and Active Learning Techniques[38]

Physicians are very capable of independent learning, acquiring the leadership knowledge and applying the concepts and tools to be successful. However, leaders cannot be developed through reading and application alone; to hone their skills, they need to practice in a safe space and obtain feedback. Moreover, physician leadership training programs will have a limited impact if the curriculum is simply taught through didactic lecturing. Active learning helps physicians apply new knowledge to their specific work situation and forces faculty to plan a practical and not just theoretical curriculum. To be more effective and keep physicians engaged throughout the leadership training programs, lecturing needs to be only one aspect of the design.

I recommend that material be presented through a wide variety of modalities. Health care-based case studies, simulations, projects, team-based learning, peer-to-peer learning, breakout group discussions, online tutorials, role-playing, storytelling, interactive exercises, and shadowing are all methods that bring information to life. Multimedia education, in particular, is very effective.

Online and/or blended curriculum design is another successful approach. While some programs have developed online learning components, it is still a small part of current training. Given the time constraints of practicing physicians, however, it is likely that blending residential with online learning will become another important part of successful surgeon training programs.

[38] My colleagues and I have written a white paper developing a leadership curriculum for physicians. Chilingerian, Jon., Ourieff, Sally., Garvin, Lynn., and Harris, Andrea. [14]. *Building a Twenty-first Century Physician Leadership Curriculum.* White Paper: National Physician Foundation.

To maximize engagement, physicians should feel that they are in control of the learning process and not have information simply tossed at them. Leadership content needs to be structured in an integrated learning sequence. Physicians will learn better if they can get direct feedback in an intuitive learning environment. The sessions should allow learners to make direct connections with what they already know and identify the gaps in what they don't know. The faculty can guide them to obtain the knowledge they want to acquire.

I have used a wide range of pedagogical tools, such as lecturing, leading a discussion, case studies, simulations, and role-playing. Lecturing to smart, creative people does not promote the active learning. People begin to feel isolated unless steps are taken to reduce the distance between the "talking head" facilitator and the physicians. It is important that a sense of the learning community is created by personalizing lectures, encouraging participation by asking many open-ended questions, and structuring "icebreaker" sessions for people to get to know each other informally before the formal sessions begin.

Adults learn best when they are participating and actively involved in a face-to-face process and when there is group work involved. Formal learning groups should be established at the beginning of a program and used even in sessions with a lecture format. There are many alternatives to lecturing. Four examples of active learning will be discussed: (1) case method, (2) role-playing, (3) simulations, and (4) multi-rater feedback coaching.

The Case Method

I suggest using the *case method* and *flipped classroom* approach for physician programs. In the flipped classroom, the physicians read a health care case or view a short video case before the session. In-class time is devoted to an introduction of concepts and tools. Group work and plenary discussions are used to discuss the case, and the facilitator avoids lecturing but instead poses questions and probes.[39]

The case method shifts the focus of instruction from the instructor to the physician. A good case brings reality into the classroom by telling a story that provokes discussion. Physicians read the case in advance and try to apply analytic concepts and tools. It encourages participants to take a position on a tough issue, challenging problem, or an intriguing opportunity. It acknowledges the physician's voice as central to the learning experience. Thus, physicians are given more freedom to choose what they will learn, how they will learn, and how they will assess their own learning. In this approach, the faculty takes on the role of facilitator.

[39] In an attempt to get class members to become full partners in the learning process, I encourage the formation of study groups and group work, where students not only present their ideas to fellow students and work collaboratively, but also experience the growing importance of collective intelligence.

Leader Role-Playing

Role-playing starts with a real case situation in which the students must improvise an interaction with real dialogue between two or more characters in the situation. For example, in some case sessions, I select physicians who want to make a yes or no decision. Rather than asking why, I role-play a stakeholder. For example, I might play the role of a boss, a family member, a colleague, or the media in the class during a case study discussion to enliven the focal issue discussion. This method engages the entire class, as they can visualize events, utilize interpersonal communication, and experience conflicting ideas. I do this to illustrate difficult conversations, such as how to say no to your chair, how to negotiate resources, or how to give feedback on a performance gap to a fellow surgeon or an anesthesiologist.

Simulations

Computer- or paper-based simulations are commonly used to teach group problem solving, effective decision making, and techniques for forming teams. They allow students to experience the situation and apply the concepts. Simulations are designed so that the physicians must deal with ambiguity, risks, and assumptions. To do well, physicians have to work together to choose the correct strategy and tactics. I use a 3-hour management simulation on leading change called "Change Pro Business Simulation."[40] The learning goal is to apply some of the theories they have learned, such as diagnosing the technical, political, and sociocultural systems in this organization, identifying resistors and early adopters, building key relationships, mapping and using informal social networks, and leading change.[41] After 3 hours they have a team-based success score based on the number of adopters, and they can see a diffusion curve.

Multi rater Physician Leadership Coaching With Peer Coaching

Along with the use of individual and 360 assessment tools, leadership coaching is a valuable method for educating and training surgeons. While training programs with strong action learning can build physician knowledge, developing new leadership behaviors and skills that build on that knowledge within the complexities of healthcare systems remains a significant challenge for many physicians. Organizations are using executive coaching more and more as a critical tool for developing their physician leaders. Within physician leadership programs, coaching can be integrated

[40] For this simulation, working in groups of five, the students have a clear mission and a time budget of 120 days. They have been sent by headquarters to convince 24 busy managers to adopt a new performance management system. The Change Pro Simulation® is a registered trademark of Learning Ways Pte. Ltd.

[41] Some of the theories include the science of persuasion, diffusion theory, social facilitation and network theory, catastrophe theory, and attitudinal segmentation.

into the curriculum in a variety of ways. Some programs create fully dedicated retreats on interpersonal development using trained coaches to facilitate groups and work with participants. Others use coaches to facilitate the feedback of the assessment tools, to support ongoing team project work, or to deliver content on topics such as conflict resolution and emotional intelligence.

Multi rater Leadership Development Experiences

There are multi rater leadership instruments that are available to quantify the dimensions and styles of a leader's behavior. The participants complete the instrument and select 8–15 anonymous observers (colleagues, boss, direct reports, etc.) to fill out the instrument prior to the training program. Once the self-reported data on leadership behavior is collected and analyzed, there can be a daylong group experience in which physicians share their 360 feedback and support each other in using the report to create specific developmental goals.

The physicians are placed into small diverse learning groups of five physicians. A coach/facilitator works with the group, establishing safety and ground rules with the participants. Each physician then takes 20 min to draw a self-portrait that expresses what is in their head, heart, gut, work, leisure, past and future. Each physician would get an hour during the daylong session to talk about their leadership feedback. When it is their turn, the group shares their observations about the drawing before the physician has explained it. This is followed by the individual's explanation of his or her drawing. Following the sharing of the self-portrait, the person is offered the opportunity to share and discuss their feedback report.

Both experiences promote broad and deep discussion and a strong bond among the group members. The physicians then become peer coaches and learning partners with a focus on supporting the achievement of their chosen development goals.

Key Learning Points and Conclusions

This chapter examined how to teach surgeons to become leaders. I argued that the difference between managers and leaders is a leader's ability to cultivate "willing followers." Effective leaders have mastered the art of mobilizing people to want to take on challenging situations. When surgeons take the lead, they become a player-coach. They must assess the evolving situation moment by moment and the strengths of the clinical team, plugging people into situations that are congruent or complimentary with their skills and experience.

I also introduced a model for determining the right mix of task and relational behaviors, showing how these become ingredients for leadership styles. Leaders learn how to adapt their style to align with different organizational situations, such as developing and implementing new surgical procedures, improving surgical quality and safety, or dealing with crises.

One of the most important lessons for surgeons is learning how to build commitment to goals—not requesting commitment from their colleagues. This process takes 3–4 months, and it begins with deep engagement of all the relevant people in all the technical centers and key care processes in the organization. If leaders build commitment, people believe that the goal and the plan are not only important and attractive, but also attainable. Research shows that people will work hard to achieve the goals even in the face of setbacks and disruptive events.

The leader visits with people inside the organization and asks 2 simple question—(1) Why are we in this situtation? and (2) How can we fix this situation? As the leader listens and aligns the stakeholders, they must put something in front of people that is significant and that they would feel proud to achieve. When solutions come from inside the organization, and not from consultants, there is a perception of fair process. There is deeper engagement, an understanding of the rationale used to make the decision, clearer roles, responsibilities, and expectations. It allows the leader to align the internal stakeholders, so everyone becomes willing to sacrifice some of their self-interest, and the buy-in is 100%. The people become willing followers, who want to go through painful situations in order to fix the organization.

I argue in this chapter that the case method is useful both for teaching leadership and doing research. Good cases not only bring organizational situations, critical events, cultural facets, and "reality models" in the classroom, they require systemic diagnosis that evokes wide-ranging perceptions of cause and effect, sharpening and enlarging debates and discussions. Finally, cases can accomplish deeper learning objectives—e.g., underscoring the importance of having more than one theoretical lens, discovering an emotional response as an intervening variable in decision-making, failing to separate facts from assumptions, or discovering personal biases in the use of heuristics or rules of thumb when making decisions.

Medical professionalism is fundamental to medicine [52]. When surgeons adopt and embrace their role as leaders, medical professionalism can be strengthened and supported. If the purposes of an organization support medical professionalism, surgical leaders have the potential to build commitment to patient-centered care, safety and quality, efficient use of resources, improved access to care, professional competence, better coordination, and scientific knowledge that advances social justice.

When physicians practice good leadership, they can make a significant difference in health-care performance in terms of technical outcomes, patient experience, and decision-making efficiency and costs. As one surgeon leader has said: "In the long run, the best care is always the lowest cost care." Having dozens of surgeons pursuing this idea in hospitals could have a significant effect on performance.

Clinical leadership is an overdue imperative, and yet we remain somewhat ambivalent about whether we should train physicians to take significant leadership roles. In the end, it is up to surgeons to want to take the lead and to commit to becoming a leader capable of managing serious clinical problems such as patient safety, poor quality, clinical inefficiency, poor coordination, incompetence, or the prevalence of disruptive physicians.

Alfred North Whitehead once said:

> The word "education" means, literally, the process of leading out. Thus we are talking of the way in which all your faculties and capacities should be encouraged to expand and unfold themselves. Consider how nature generally sets to work to educate the living organisms which team on this earth. You cannot begin to understand nature's method unless you grasp the fact that the essential spring of all growth is within you. All that you can get from without is some food—material or spiritual—with which to build your own organism, and some stimulus to spur you to some activity. What is really essential in your development you must do for yourselves.

As educators, we can facilitate leadership development, but we cannot really teach surgeons to be effective leaders. What is essential for leadership development, leaders must do for themselves and with the help of their followers.

Appendix: Notes on Teaching Leadership: Approach and Methods

Teaching runs to the heart of what we do as health-care professionals and as leaders. When teaching current or future clinicians about leadership in health-care organizations, we try to understand real problems that clinicians and managers face. We frame those problems into relevant research questions, conduct research and inquiry and write a case or manuscript for publication. Finally, we translate that research into classroom pedagogy.

I have learned by observing masterclass sessions of other professors that many things we do in the classroom have the potential to be important, engaging, and entertaining. However, years of observation and teaching experience do not necessarily ensure effectiveness.

I define my job as guiding and motivating students to learn how to think when they encounter unique managerial or novel research situations. I strive for high levels of involvement in every class, so students can explore real management problems firsthand. Ultimately, I aim for the kind of "self-appropriated" classroom learning that John Dewey and Alfred North Whitehead spoke of—where students wrestle with problems and, in the process of finding their way out, expand and unfold themselves. In an attempt to get class members to become full partners in the learning process, I encourage the formation of study groups and group work where each student not only presents their ideas to fellow students and works collaboratively but also experiences the growing importance of collective intelligence.[42]

I have found that the case method has been useful both for my teaching and my research needs. Good cases not only bring organizational situations, critical events,

[42] Woolley AW, et al. Evidence for a collective intelligence factor in the performance of human groups. Science. 2010;380(6004):686–8.

cultural facets, and “reality models” into the classroom, they require systemic diagnosis that evokes wide-ranging perceptions of cause and effect, sharpening and enlarging debates and discussions. Finally, cases can accomplish deeper learning objectives—e.g., underscoring the importance of having more than one theoretical lens, discovering an emotional response as an intervening variable decision-making, failing to separate facts from assumptions, or discovering personal biases in the use of heuristics or rules of thumb when making decisions.

I believe that professors are obliged to not only *teach* other people’s cases but to research and write original cases to profess their own ideas. Conducting research on organizations and clinical fieldwork on hospital managers and physician efficiency has enabled me to write case studies such as “When the Physician Becomes a Patient,” “Managing a Liver Transplant Decision: Capacity and Medical Strategy,” “Implementing an Advanced Surgery Program at a Tertiary Care Regional Medical Center: Leading Change and the Liabilities of Newness,” “Friederike Bismarck’s Dilemma,” “Baker Medical Center,” or “The Loughbeg Lipitor Factory” (these cases are available from the author). Writing original cases not only provides me with strong links to the practice of management but also exposes students to my current research and thinking, while I learn from their insights.

While the case method is an important part of my teaching, I continue to experiment with a variety of other teaching methods. I am becoming more convinced that multimedia pedagogy, classroom polls, buzz groups, computer simulations, and group work foster effective learning without sacrificing critical thinking, analytical skills, and conceptual skills.

Over the past few years, I have become cognizant of four challenges faced in the classroom. First is the tendency to overload and overburden the students with information, concepts, and knowledge—e.g., too many powerpoint slides and too many final takeaways. The second challenge is knowing when and how to refocus your attention away from the academic content and toward the people and the learning process. The third challenge is avoiding overcontrol of the learning experience, remembering to see what is going on in the moment, and thus allowing the students to create their own learning and even to teach the professor. The fourth challenge is being able to connect with each student as an individual to give every student an equal chance to learn. I will focus on this fourth challenge.

Connecting with each student as an individual turns out to be more complicated than making simple adjustments, such as adding better case studies, finding important and relevant readings, or employing multimedia pedagogy. We have to be clear about each student’s learning goals. We also have to understand students as individual learners and guide them to reach their potential in each and every session. There are auditory, visual, and kinesthetic learning preferences to consider. Some students still enjoy a and lecture; many enjoy active learning; others learn much better in a flipped classroom. I try to employ multiple techniques, and as long as I have been at it, I still have lot to learn.

Here is a case in point. One of my MD-MBA graduate students told me that she needed more time to process ideas discussed in class; when I asked questions in class, she felt unable to participate. She made an appointment and requested more written work to make up for her inability to participate verbally in class. That conversation made me reflect on what I require in the classroom. I realized that it was unfair to require her (or anyone in a similar situation) to make up for being a slower processor by having to do extra work—even by choice. People who are able to acquire and process information faster would not have to do this extra work. This became a serious problem for me, since class participation is very important in my case-based sessions.

I thought about how I teach most sessions. Before class, I instruct students to read, study, and prepare the cases and readings. After most in-class discussions, I ask my students to take 10 min to write down their insights, and I ask them "would anyone like to share their insights?" I generally open the next session with a recap of what we discussed and an opportunity for people to share any additional thoughts.

I reflected on what I was doing and asked myself several questions: Do I give everyone enough time to think and offer a response in class? How much time would slower processors need to respond? Are there better ways to obtain inclusion? Should I offer more group work so people can share ideas? I learned from this student that I have to adapt my teaching style to the wide range of learners in class.

Reflecting on these and other questions is what I love about being a professor. We are continually learning how to connect with every student. We cannot fixate on one style or pedagogy. The teaching challenge requires that we get out of our comfort zones to accommodate our students' needs. We should use blended learning models, with classroom and e-learning, synchronous and asynchronous methods, flipped classrooms, and other innovations in an ever evolving effort to connect with students and enhance the learning process.

References

1. Ackoff R. The art of problem solving. New York: Wiley; 1978.
2. Afshar M, Han Z. Teaching and learning medical biochemistry: perspectives from a student and an educator. Med Sci Educ. 2014;24:339. https://doi.org/10.1007/s40670-014-0004-7.
3. Bandura A. Self-efficacy. In: Craighead EW, Nemeroff CB, editors. Encyclopedia of psychology and neuroscience. 3rd ed. New York: Wiley; 2000. p. 1474–6.
4. Bandura A. Self-efficacy. In: The corsini, editor. Encyclopedia of psychology. 4th ed. Hoboken: Wiley; 2010. p. 1534–6.
5. Bass BM, Bass R. The bass book of leadership: theory, research & managerial application. 4th ed. New York: Simon and Shuster; 2008.
6. Bradley EH, Herrin J, Curry L, Cherlin EJ, Wang Y, Webster TR, et al. Variation in hospital mortality rates for patients with acute myocardial infarction. Am J Cardiol. 2010;106:1108–12. [PMID: 20920648]
7. Bristol Royal Infirmary Inquiry Final Report 2002, The Report of the public inquiry into the children's heart surgery at the Bristol Royal Infirmary, Learning from Bristol (2002). Presented to Parliament by the Secretary of State for Health by command of her Majesty, Crown/London/England.
8. Castro P, Dorgan J, Stephen J, Richardson B. A healthier health care system for the UK. McKinsey Quarterly. McKinsey and Company: 1–5; 2008.
9. Chilingerian J. The strategy of executive influence. Unpublished Ph.D. Dissertation. Massachusetts Institute of Technology (MIT). 1987.

10. Chilingerian JA. Managing strategic issues and stakeholders: how modes of executive attention enact crisis management. In: Thomas H, editor. Building the strategically responsive organization. Sussex: Wiley; 1994. p. 189–213.
11. Chilingerian JA. Who has star quality? In: Herzlinger RE, editor. Consumer-driven health care: implications for providers, payers, and policy-makers. San Francisco: Jossey-Bass; 2004. p. 443–53.
12. Chilingerian J, Savage GT. The emerging field of international health care management. In: Savage GT, editor. International health care management. Amsterdam: Elsevier Press; 2005. p. 3–30.
13. Chilingerian J. The discipline of strategic thinking in health care. In: Jones R, Jenkins F, editors. Management, leadership and development in the allied health professions. Oxford: Radcliffe Publishing, Ltd.; 2006.
14. Chilingerian J, Ourieff S, Garvin L, Harris A. *Building a 21st Century Physician Leadership Curriculum*. White Paper: National Physician Foundation. 2017. Downloaded on 1 Sept 2016: http://www.physiciansfoundation.org/uploads/default/Brandeis_Building_A_21st_Century_Physician_Leadership_Curriculum.pdf.
15. Christensen RC, Hansen A. Teaching and the case method. Boston: Harvard Business School Press; 1987. p. 27.
16. Cosgrove T. The Cleveland way. New York: McGraw Hill Education; 2014.
17. Courtney H, Kirkland J, Vigurie P. Strategy under uncertainty. Harv Bus Rev. 1997;75(6):67–79.
18. Curry LA, et al. What distinguishes top performing hospitals in acute myocardial infarction mortality rates? Ann Intern Med. 2011;154:384–90.
19. Dorgan S, et al. Management in health care: why good practice really matters. *McKinsey Management in Health Care Report*. Center for Economic Performance: LSE. 2009. Downloaded on 24 Feb 2015: http://worldmanagementsurvey.org/wp-content/images/2010/10/Management_in_Healthcare_Report_2010.pdf
20. Dorner D. The logic of failure: recognizing and avoiding error in complex situations. Reading, MA: Perseus Book; 1996.
21. Drucker P. The theory of the business. Boston: Harvard Business Review; 1994.
22. Drucker P. Managing oneself. Harv Bus Rev. 1999;77:64–74.
23. Follett MP. Freedom and control. In: Graham P, editor. Mary Parker Follett. Prophet of management. Washington, DC: Beard Books; 2003.
24. Garvin D. How Google sold its engineers on management. Harv Bus Rev. 2013;91(12):74–82.
25. Ginnett RC. Crews as groups: their formation and their leadership. In: Wiener EL, Kanki BG, Helmreich RL, editors. Cockpit resource management. San Diego: Academic Press; 1993. p. 71–98.
26. Glavin M, Chilingerian JA. Hospital care productions and medical errors: organizational responses to improve care. Curr Top Manag. JAI Press. 1998;3:193–215.
27. Goffee R, Jones G. Why should anyone be led by you? What it takes to be an authentic leader. Boston: Harvard Business School Press; 2006.
28. Hackman JR. Teams, leaders, and organizations: new directions for crew-oriented flight training. In: Wiener EL, Kanki BG, Helmreich RL, editors. Cockpit resource management. San Diego: Academic Press; 1993. p. 47–69.
29. Hammond JS, Keeney RL, Howard R. Smart choices: a practical guide to making better decisions. Boston: Harvard Business School Press; 1999.
30. Janis I, Mann L. Decision making: a psychological analysis of conflict, choice, and commitment. New York: The Free Press; 1977.
31. Janis I. Crucial decisions: leadership in policymaking and crisis management. New York: The Free Press; 1986.
32. James BC, Savitz LA. How intermountain trimmed health care costs through robust quality improvement efforts. Health Affairs (Millwood). 2011;30(6):1185–91. https://doi.org/10.1377/hlthaff.2011.0358. Epub 2011 May 19
33. van Knippenberg D, Sitkin SB. A critical assessment of charismatic-transformational leadership research: back to the drawing board? Acad Manag Ann. 2013;7:1–60.
34. Kouzes JM, Posner BZ. Learning leadership: the five fundamentals of becoming and exemplary leader. New York: Wiley; 2016.
35. Kim WC, Mauborgne R. Fair process: managing in the knowledge economy. Harv Bus Rev. 1997;75:65–75.

36. Kim WC, Mauborgne R. Blue ocean strategy: how to create uncontested market space and make the competition irrelevant. Boston: Harvard Business School Press; 2014.
37. Leonhardt D. Making health care better. *New York Times, Sunday Magazine.* 2009. Downloaded on 3 Jan 2013: http://www.nytimes.com/2009/11/08/magazine/08Healthcare-t.html?rref=collection%2Fbyline%2Fdavid-leonhardt&action=click&contentCollection=undefined®ion=stream&module=stream_unit&version=search&contentPlacement=1&pgtype=collection.
38. Levinson W, Shiphra G, Hafferty FW, Lucey CR. Understanding medical professionalism. New York: McGraw Hill; 2014.
39. Latham GP, Locke EA. Goal setting-a motivational technique that works. Autumn: Organizational Dynamics; 1979.
40. Locke EA, Latham GP. A theory of goal setting and task performance. Englewood Cliffs: Prentice-Hall; 1990.
41. Mintzberg H. The nature of managerial work. New York: Harper and Row; 1973.
42. Mitroff I. Stakeholders of the organizational mind. San Francisco: Jossey-Bass Publishers; 1983.
43. Nicholson N. How hard-wired is human behavior? Harv Bus Rev. 1998;76(4):134–47.
44. Northouse PG. Leadership: theory and practice. 7th ed. Thousand Oaks: SAGE; 2016.
45. Pfeffer J. Leadership BS: fixing workplaces and careers one truth at a time. New York: Harper Collins; 2015.
46. Roberto, MA. Why great leaders don't take know for an answer: managing or conflict and consensus. Philadelphia: Wharton School Publishing; 2005.
47. Roberto MA, Garvin DA. Taking charge of the Beth Isreal Deaconness Medical Center (Multi Media Case) Harvard Business School Press, No. 303–058. 2003.
48. Roth A, Venkataraman S, Tucker A, Jon C. Being on the frontier: identifying high triple performance hospitals. Unpublished Working Paper. 2017.
49. Senge P. The fifth discipline: mastering the five practices of the learning organization. New York: Doubleday; 1990.
50. Schon D. The reflective practitioner. New York: Basic Books, Inc.; 1983.
51. Sivers D. How to start a movement. Ted Talk Downloaded on 20 Sept 2013. 2010. https://www.ted.com/talks/derek_sivers_how_to_start_a_movement
52. Spandorfer J, Pohl CA, Rattner SL, Nasca TJ. Professionalism in Medicine: A Case-Based Guide for Medical Students. NY: Cambridge University Press; 2010.
53. Steinert Y. Educational theory and strategies to support professionalism, and professional identity formation. In: Cruess RL, Cruess SR, Steinert Y, editors. Teaching medical professionalism. 2nd ed. New York: Cambridge University Press; 2016.
54. Stewart RD. Choices and constraints: a model for understanding managerial jobs and behavior. Acad Manag Rev. 1982;7(1):7–13.
55. Stoller J, Berkowitz E, Bailin P, L. Physician management and leadership education at the Cleveland clinic foundation: program impact and experience over 14 years. J Med Pract Manag. 2007;22(4):237–42.
56. Stoller JK, Goodall A, Baker A. Why the best hospitals are managed by doctors. Harvard business review. 2016. Downloaded on 31 Dec 2016 at https://hbr.org/2016/12/why-the-best-hospitals-are-managed-by-doctors.
57. Tichy NM. The cycle of leadership. New York: Harper Collins Publisher; 2002.
58. Van der Heyden L, Blondel C, Carlock RS. Fair process: striving for justice in family business. Fam Bus Rev. 2005;18(1):1–21.
59. Walshe K, Shortell S. When things go wrong: how health care organizations deal with major failures. Health Aff. 2004;23(3):103–11.
60. Weick KE, Sutcliffe KM. Hospitals as cultures of entrapment. *California Management Review.* 2003.
61. Whitehead A,N. Essays in science and philosophy. New York: Philosophical Library, Inc; 1947. p. 218–9.
62. Woolley AW, Chabris CF, Pentland A, Malone TW. Evidence for a collective intelligence factor in the performance of human groups. Science. 2010;330:686–8.
63. Woolley AW, et al. Collective intelligence and group performance. Curr Dir Psychol Sci. 2015;24:420–4.

Teaching Surgical Ethics

21

Sabha Ganai and Karen M. Devon

The Problem

Surgeons deal with ethics in daily practice, whether in the process of obtaining informed consent for a procedure, encountering a sporadic innovation in the operating room, disclosure of errors and complications, or interacting with surrogate decision-makers. Surgeons support patients and their families at the extremes of life and must be comfortable and competent in addressing palliative and end-of-life care. Surgeons must also be able to adequately discuss risk as part of decision-making and should be able to effectively identify and communicate such issues of uncertainty with their patients. Ethical principles of importance include respect for autonomy, nonmaleficence, beneficence, and justice, as well as professional duties including truth-telling, respect for privacy, maintenance of competency/proficiency, accountability, and other normative standards of appropriate behavior learned in the surgical context [3]. An ethics education can ideally prepare surgical residents to approach complex cases by teaching residents to clarify their values, principles, contexts, and hone their negotiating skills as they learn to effectively listen and communicate [16, 17].

S. Ganai, MD, PhD, FACS (✉)
Department of Surgery, Southern Illinois University School of Medicine,
315 W. Carpenter Street, Springfield, IL 62794-9638, USA
e-mail: sganai@siumed.edu

K.M. Devon, MD, MSc, FRCSC
Department of Surgery, Faculty of Medicine, University of Toronto, Toronto, ON, Canada

Joint Center for Bioethics, Dalla Lana School of Public Health, University of Toronto, Toronto, ON, Canada

Women's College Hospital, Toronto, ON, Canada

University Health Network, Toronto, ON, Canada

T.S. Köhler, B. Schwartz (eds.), *Surgeons as Educators*,
https://doi.org/10.1007/978-3-319-64728-9_21

Deficiencies have been noted in the formal education of surgical residents in processes of moral reasoning [6, 9, 12]. While 98% of surgical program directors agreed that an ethics education could improve one's ability to handle ethically challenging situations, 47% reported that limited faculty with ethics expertise was an impediment to this process [12]. While an excellent case-based curriculum is currently available through an American College of Surgeons (ACS) textbook [21], with a new edition forthcoming, textbooks alone may be considered time-consuming and onerous for busy surgical residents who need to prioritize their learning objectives. In particular, if their ethics curriculum is informally structured, there may be deficiencies in their ability to effectively address the spectrum of real-world scenarios they will see in practice. Skills including learning effective communication and negotiation may be better facilitated in a small group setting or from a video than from a textbook.

The reported prevalence of the six ethical issues discussed in the ACS text is encountered at least once per rotation by surgical residents and when surveyed ranges from 75% for competition of interests to 100% for end-of-life issues [25]. During their junior years, surgical residents are exposed to dilemmas in truth-telling, confidentiality, professional obligations, surrogate decision-making, and end-of-life care several times per rotation and deal with conflicts of interest several times per year [6]. While these issues are seen in practice by surgeons, barriers to formally teaching ethics have included (1) a preoccupation with scientific and technical aspects of medicine, (2) time constraints, (3) a lack of support by faculty in planning ethics sessions, and (4) a tendency of residents to view ethics as peripheral to their learning agenda [9].

The Impact

Ethical dilemmas are ubiquitous in surgery. They impact the surgeon-patient relationship and interactions between physicians, patients, nurses, and other healthcare providers. They influence society at large when distributive justice considerations are made, including policy changes secondary to advocacy as exemplified by passage of the 2013 HIV Organ Policy Equity (HOPE) Act, a surgeon-led initiative that has expanded transplantation allocation between HIV-infected donors and recipients [4, 10]. Justice considerations related to structures, processes, and outcomes of healthcare delivery are commonplace, including addressing disparities in access due to socioeconomic and geographic disparities (using deontological, duty-based frameworks) and allocation of resources for trauma and combat triage (using utilitarian, outcome-based frameworks). The potential impact of improper handling of ethics in practice also includes communication breakdowns leading to distrust and possible malpractice liability and inappropriately increased costs due to mishandled end-of-life decision-making.

The impact of a lack of teachers (surgeons and non-surgeons educated in ethics or interested in teaching it) has direct effects on learners by creating a void in the process of education that may need to be filled later in their careers. Conversely, teaching ethics becomes an opportunity to address "difficult to teach" Accreditation Council for Graduate Medical Education (ACGME) core competencies including professionalism, communication skills, and systems-based practice, allowing residency programs to fulfill ongoing milestone-based assessments that are required according to the Next Accreditation System [22]. While surgical ethics is still a developing field, there are numerous exciting prospects for scholarship and discourse related to its role as an applied philosophy exploring ever-expanding technical advances and their impact on clinicians and patients.

Prior Inquiry

A small body of literature serves as the basis for guidance in the development of future ethics curricula. Most of the empiric studies on surgical ethics education have been summarized in a systematic review [13], which synthesized overarching educational goals related to (1) cultivating virtuous physicians and (2) teaching skills for the recognition and management of ethical dilemmas that develop in the ordinary course of patient care. While cultivating virtuous physicians is challenging to measure, an Aristotelian virtue-ethics-based framework has been suggested as an ideal way to discuss, evaluate, and remediate the six ACGME core competencies through exploration of associated virtues and vices [18]. Recently, interviews and focus groups have shown that ethics issues are naturally dealt with in the "hidden curriculum" of surgical training, yet when they are presented formally, they gain significance and become identifiable to the learner for discussion [15]. Further integration of ethics into objective standardized clinical exams (OSCEs) for assessment and evaluation was found to add greatly to the educational process for learners [13, 15].

From the perspective of both program directors and learners, surveys suggest that the ideal method for ethics education is by case-based learning, which can be reasonably implemented in traditional surgical teaching conferences [9, 12]. Expert opinion suggests that ethics curricula can be designed with a focus on different learner levels [17], as well as by covering different topics using a modular approach, as done in the ACS textbook [21]. An interventional study on teaching informed consent to surgical residents that used pre- and posttest evaluations demonstrated that psychomotor processes of ethics can be taught using mixed methods and result in an improvement in a resident's level of confidence over time [2].

While many of the aforementioned studies demonstrate enthusiasm for designing and implementing curricula, there are few studies in which there is rigorous evaluation of the process of teaching ethics other than pre- and posttest surveys. Brewster and colleagues utilized standardized patients to simulate three aspects of a complex case: informed consent for resection of a retroperitoneal sarcoma, an inanimate team-based simulation of their handling of an intraoperative catastrophe during caval dissection, and a videotaped review of the resident disclosing the adverse outcome to the patient's (simulated) wife [5]. Residents found this to be a valuable learning experience, with particular value gained from debriefing their emotions and performance. Another study showed that implementation of elements of the

ACS-sponsored textbook on surgical ethics [21] in the form of four faculty-facilitated seminars improved the confidence of residents [25].

An assessment of a formal bioethics curriculum across 67 residency programs within an academic center demonstrated that (1) bioethics teaching was considered valuable by teachers and trainees, (2) there appeared to be mismatch between educational agendas of the staff and ethical issues faced by residents, and (3) staff and students indicated that they felt that ethics teaching had a positive impact, but there was a lack of formal evaluation to confirm the impression [19]. The global impact of ethics education is uncertain. If the ultimate intended goal of teaching ethics is to change behavior, it is unclear whether acquisition of new ethics knowledge and skills actually accomplishes this task or improves patient-centered outcomes. There is clearly room for scholarship and discourse on the subject of surgical ethics education.

Approaches

Current formal approaches to ethics education for surgical residents include independent study (e.g., providing residents the ACS textbook), didactic lectures, small group discussions, and larger group case-based learning paradigms. Among responding programs in 2008, 76% of surgical residency programs incorporate elements of ethics education into either their core curriculum or grand rounds, with only 2% using standardized patients or simulated scenarios [11].

Ethics education also occurs in a variable fashion throughout residency training and is often dependent on random encounters and patient interactions. The learning may rely on modeling the behavior of other faculty or more senior residents, which creates risk of promoting unprofessional conduct via the hidden curriculum [20]. Ethics education occasionally occurs in simulation sessions and is sometimes evaluated as a component of assessments of competency, such as informally during the American Board of Surgery Certifying Examination, where oral exam questions occasionally focus on ethics issues such as informed consent and the disclosure of risk associated with a surgical procedure. Also infrequently, specific cases may be discussed with a focus on a real or theoretical ethical dilemma during required surgical morbidity and mortality conferences. While these can be engaging to learners, these discussions are often time limited and without defined objectives or forms of assessment of knowledge transfer. Such opportunities require intentionality and the initiative of an attending or resident to bring up the discussion points and frame the ethical considerations. While there may be an expectation of competency in surgical ethics at the completion of training, the lack of a structured educational curriculum has not guaranteed that surgical residents will be formally trained in how to approach these issues.

Integrated Clinical Ethics

Ethics curricula that integrate with the clinical and other education experiences of trainees and rely less on teaching theoretical aspects of ethics have been advocated as an approach to encourage lifelong learning and teaching of bioethics [14]. Future approaches for an innovative ethics curriculum would utilize a combination of educational strategies chosen to complement specific content and learning objectives. Such approach might still center on case-based learning events, but also use additional teaching modalities that may better address specific goals and objectives. For instance, conceptual learning could be supplemented by short didactic sessions or videos provided for independent study. Examples of topics are included in Box 21.1. Modules for learning ethical principles could be integrated into clinical rotations such as breast oncology (e.g., genetic testing), transplantation (e.g., distributive justice), thoracic (e.g., innovation), and trauma (e.g., competence and surrogate decision-making), making the material more immediately relevant to the learner. Assessment may be enhanced by evaluating competencies within a virtue-ethics-based framework that emphasizes caring for the patient as a primary goal [18]. Brief oral exams for assessment and feedback can be initiated by a designated instructor within each rotation and integrated into the resident's portfolio to allow for achievement of Next Accreditation System milestones [22]. OSCEs focusing on ethics principles can also be designed to capitalize instances when learners are already in technical skills simulation sessions.

One example of this approach has been implemented during the Southern Illinois University (SIU) surgical resident readiness course designed for fourth year medical students with interest in entering a career in surgery. In their first week, students are instructed on the processes of informed consent through a didactic lecture that covers topics ranging from establishing the doctor-patient relationship to professional norms including documentation of operative notes and consent discussions. Subsequently, during their curriculum, they are asked to simulate these conversations with their partner prior to performance of procedures in a cadaveric skills lab. During a PGY2 "Residents as Teachers" curriculum, SIU residents participate in didactic lectures on teaching followed by three hands-on sessions where they provide supervised sign-out of multiple patients to a colleague and obtain and critique performance of informed consent for placement of a central line, followed by teaching a colleague on how to place a central line using a patient simulator. In these scenarios, the processes of how to communicate well with others become important areas for self-evaluation and peer-to-peer feedback. Through a change in context and perspective with the learner, we allow informed consent to transition from a low-level task "checked off" prior to operating to a necessary process element of fundamental importance for establishing the surgeon-patient relationship.

Optimally, ethics education ought to be provided at multiple time points of training so that the learner can build upon and reflect on prior knowledge and experiences and engage in a transformative learning experience. In a longitudinal fashion, teaching and assessing confidence in informed consent could be part of a multilevel simulation curriculum, allowing for assessments before a PGY1 places a central line in a patient simulator, at the PGY2 level when they use a colonoscopy simulator, or at the PGY3 level when they rehearse for Fundamentals of Laparoscopic Surgery testing.

Written narrative reflection may also help residents process the emotional aspects of dealing with conflicts and dilemmas they encounter longitudinally during residency [23]. Written self-reflections of ethical dilemmas encountered by the resident may be included in a learning portfolio, a method that has been shown to promote professional growth and development [27]. Real-time observations by faculty of residents interacting with patients may also be included in their portfolio to provide feedback on the resident's abilities to handle ethical dilemmas.

Ethics Morbidity and Mortality Conferences

Recently, the use of ethics morbidity and mortality (M&M) case discussions was integrated into five general surgery sites at the University of Toronto [24]. This consisted of 30 min per month allocated during M&M conference where the case discussed is selected because of the inherent ethical dilemma rather than a traditional complication. The scope of issues discussed was extremely wide ranging from patient requesting an inappropriate intervention to the conflict of obligations in surgical teaching. Residents present the case as they would a standard M&M, along with a literature review of a relevant ethics dilemma that arises out of the case. Prior to this intervention, learners saw ethics content as abstract and unimportant to everyday practice (Snelgrove, et al. unpublished data [24]). After the intervention, learners felt that ethics could be taught and enhanced their awareness and ability to tackle issues in real life. This occurred through the learning of a new language which allowed dialogue, debriefing, and critical reflection to occur [24]. Components of successful "Ethics M&M Rounds" included maintaining a safe learning environment; discussing relevant, real-time cases; and having good faculty moderation.

Addressing Limited Resources to Teach Ethics

While case-based learning has been identified as an important modality for teaching surgical ethics [9, 12], it is not always effectively used across residency programs. A lack of faculty support has been identified as a critical barrier in the implementation of surgical ethics educational sessions [9]. While this may simply be an issue of faculty interest, there may be additional challenges posed by instructors having a lack of formal training in ethics and related disciplines. In an effort to consolidate limited faculty resources, case-based learning may also be considered using teleconferencing or Webinar capabilities that allows sharing of moderators (ethics-trained faculty or clinicians with a strong interest in teaching ethics) among many learners. The moderators would then be prepared to ask questions to the presenter or other participating sites, as well as further case discussion and exploration of relevant ethical principles. Multiple-choice polling can be done in real time through audience response systems. After completion of a session, learning and feedback by participants can be further facilitated through web-based methods of sharing articles, surveys, and assessment tools.

While standard case-based conferences are often seen as ideal for discussions among groups for reasons of convenience, they can also serve to enhance discussions of normative and applied ethics because of their focus on the narrative aspects of clinical practice. Case-based teaching strategies can optimally provide learners with models on how to think professionally about problems, allow them to develop critical thinking skills, and enhance their ability to learn from their own experiences, whether real or simulated [8]. Case studies allow conversation of the moral principles at stake, with discussion of the stakeholders, conflicting rights and values, and clinicians' reasoning, as well as their obligations, interpersonal skills, and decision-making [26]. Case-based methods allow development of problem-solving skills in a safe environment for learners to receive feedback; understand conflicting attitudes, beliefs, and values; and allow social collaboration for analysis and discussion [7].

By teleconferencing surgical ethics case conferences across multiple institutions, we may be able to pool expertise in teaching ethics as well as capitalize on the shared and diverse experience of surgeons on a national or even international level. This would potentially create opportunities for mentorship in surgical ethics which residents may not have at their home institution. Ultimately, encouraging surgical ethics discourse will require training faculty on how to effectively teach surgical ethics. While opportunities are limited, the ACS Division of Education offers a structured fellowship in surgical ethics at the Maclean Center for Clinical Medical Ethics of the University of Chicago [1]. The University of Toronto offers a "Teaching the Teachers" retreat offering interactive workshops for their faculty and residency coordinators directed toward facilitating teaching bioethics [14]. The challenge of teaching surgical ethics will only be facilitated through prioritizing ethics within the surgical curriculum and fostering enthusiasm and interest in including ethics discourse in the daily practice of surgeons.

Summary

Although seemingly routine, the act of choosing to perform an operation is a moral decision requiring agency. While surgeons encounter ethical dilemmas frequently, they are not always well equipped to manage and discuss problems that are often unique to their discipline. Despite increasing interest in providing surgical residents a formal education in ethics, current curricula may be difficult to implement or be dependent on the presence of motivated faculty. We recommend a mixed-methods modular ethics curriculum that centers around traditional case-based learning methodology, focusing on the M&M conference. Via multi-institutional collaboration, we foresee using teleconferencing as a tool to enhance ethics education over a network of residency programs using distance learning techniques; however, even these methods will compete for learner and faculty time. Further research needs to be performed on the value and effectiveness of various modalities for teaching surgical ethics. Teaching surgical ethics should be prioritized as it appears to be of importance for maintaining professional conduct by surgeons, fostering the surgeon-patient relationship, and improving patient-centered outcomes, but further inquiry must be performed to verify this and show how to do this effectively.

Box 21.1 Topics in Surgical Ethics

- Shared decision-making and informed consent
- Disclosure of adverse events and errors
- Required reconciliation of DNR orders
- Surrogacy rules and advanced directives
- Frameworks for resource allocation
- Surgical innovation versus research
- Negotiating futility disputes
- Prognostication and communicating uncertainty
- Professional accountability and competency
- Surgery and the Jehovah's witness patient
- Conflicts of interest
- Withdrawal and withholding of support
- Brain death and transplantation ethics
- Confidentiality, privacy, and social media
- Genetic testing and prophylactic surgery
- Stress management and surgeon impairment

References

1. American College of Surgeons. ACS cosponsors fellowships in ethics and leadership. Bull Am Coll Surg. 2016;101(3):57.
2. Angelos P, Da Rosa DA, Derossis AM, Kim B. Medical ethics curriculum for surgical residents: results of a pilot project. Surgery. 1999;126:701–5.
3. Bosk CL. Forgive and remember. Chicago: University of Chicago Press; 1979.
4. Boyarsky BJ, Segev DL. From bench to bill: how a transplant nuance became 1 of only 57 laws passed in 2013. Ann Surg. 2016;263:430–3.
5. Brewster LP, Risucci DA, Joehl RJ, Littooy FN, Temeck BK, Blair PG, Sachdeva AK. Management of adverse surgical events: a structured education module for residents. Am J Surg. 2005;190:687–90.
6. Brewster LP, Hall DE, Joehl RJ. Assessing residents in surgical ethics: we do it a lot; we only know a little. J Surg Res. 2011;171:395–8.
7. Dailey MA. Developing case studies. Nurse Educ. 1992;17:8–11.
8. Dowd S, Davidhizar T. Using case studies to teach clinical problem-solving. Nurse Educ. 1999;24:42–6.
9. Downing MT, Way DP, Caniano DA. Results of a national survey on ethics education in general surgery residency programs. Am J Surg. 1997;174:364–8.
10. Durand CM, Segev D, Sugarman J. Realizing HOPE: the ethics of organ transplantation from HIV infected donors. Ann Intern Med. 2016;165(2):138–42.
11. Grossman E, Angelos P. Futility: What Cool Hand Luke Can Teach the Surgical Community. World J Surg. 2009;33:1338–40.
12. Grossman E, Posner MC, Angelos P. Ethics education in surgical residency: past, present, and future. Surgery. 2010;147:114–9.
13. Helft PR, Eckles RE, Torbeck L. Ethics education in surgical residency programs: a review of the literature. J Surg Educ. 2009;66:35–42.

14. Howard F, McKneally MF, Levin AV. Integrating bioethics into postgraduate medical education: the University of Toronto Model. Acad Med. 2010;85:1035–40.
15. Howard F, McKneally MF, Upshur RE, Levin AV. The formal and informal surgical ethics curriculum: views of resident and staff surgeons in Toronto. Am J Surg. 2012;203:258–65.
16. Keune JD, Kodner IJ. The importance of an ethics curriculum in surgical education. World J Surg. 2014;38:1581–6.
17. Kodner IJ. Ethics curricula in surgery: needs and approaches. World J Surg. 2003;27:952–6.
18. Larkin GL, McKay MP, Angelos P. Six core competencies and seven deadly sins: a virtues-based approach to the new guidelines for graduate medical education. Surgery. 2005;138:490–7.
19. Levin AV, Berry S, Kassardjian CD, Howard F, McKneally M. Ethics teaching is as important as my clinical education: a survey of participants in residency education at a single university. UTMJ. 2006;84(1):60–3.
20. Mahajan R, Aruldhas BW, Sharma M, Badyal DK, Singh T. Professionalism and ethics: a proposed curriculum for undergraduates. Int J Appl Basic Med Res. 2016;6(3):157–63.
21. McGrath MH. Ethical issues in clinical surgery. Chicago: American College of Surgeons; 2007. 84 pages.
22. Nasca TJ, Philibert I, Brigham T, Flynn TC. The next GME accreditation system – rationale and benefits. N Engl J Med. 2012;366:1051–6.
23. Pearson AS, McTigue MP, Tarpley JL. Narrative medicine in surgical education. J Surg Educ. 2008;65(2):99–100.
24. Snelgrove R, Ng S, Devon K. Ethics M&Ms: toward a recognition of ethics in everyday practice. J Grad Med Ed. 2016;8(3):462–264.
25. Thirunavukarasu P, Brewster LP, Pecora SM, Hall DE. Educational intervention is effective in improving knowledge and confidence in surgical ethics – a prospective study. Am J Surg. 2010;200:665–9.
26. Waithe ME, Duckett L, Schmitz K, Crisham P, Ryden M. Developing case situations for ethics education in nursing. J Nurs Educ. 1989;28:175–80.
27. Webb TP, Merkley TR. An evaluation of the success of a surgical resident learning portfolio. J Surg Educ. 2012;69:1–7.

Surgical Ergonomics

22

Carrie Ronstrom, Susan Hallbeck, Bethany Lowndes, and Kristin L. Chrouser

What is Ergonomics?

Definition

The term ergonomics, also described as human factors, derives from the Greek roots "ergon" and "nomos" meaning work and law, respectively. The International Ergonomics Association defines ergonomics as "the scientific discipline concerned with the understanding of interactions among humans and other elements of a

C. Ronstrom, MD (✉)
University of Minnesota Medical School, 420 Delaware Street SE, Minneapolis, MN 55455, USA
e-mail: ronst003@umn.edu

S. Hallbeck, PhD, PE, CPE
Department of Health Sciences Research, Division of Health Care Policy and Research, Mayo Clinic, Rochester, MN, USA

Robert D. and Patricia E. Kern Center for the Science of Health Care Delivery, Mayo Clinic, 200 First St SW, Rochester, MN 55905, USA

Department of Surgery, Mayo Clinic, 200 First St SW, Rochester, MN 55905, USA
e-mail: Hallbeck.susan@mayo.edu

B. Lowndes, PhD, MPH
Department of Health Sciences Research, Division of Health Care Policy and Research, Mayo Clinic, Rochester, MN, USA

Robert D. and Patricia E. Kern Center for the Science of Health Care Delivery, Mayo Clinic, 200 First St SW, Rochester, MN 55905, USA
e-mail: Lowndes.Bethany@mayo.edu

K.L. Chrouser, MD, MPH
Minneapolis VA Health Care Center, University of Minnesota, Department of Urology, 420 Delaware St SE, Minneapolis, MN 55455, USA
e-mail: Chrouser@umn.edu

T.S. Köhler, B. Schwartz (eds.), *Surgeons as Educators*,
https://doi.org/10.1007/978-3-319-64728-9_22

system, and the profession that applies theory, principles, data, and methods to design in order to optimize human well-being and overall system performance" [1]. Ergonomic principles may be applied to many aspects of the surgeon's work including operating room layout, equipment design, and surgeon posture with the goal to enhance safety, effectiveness, and quality of life and to decrease the risk of workplace injury.

Prevalence of Musculoskeletal Injuries Among Surgeons

The US Bureau of Labor Statistics publishes data annually reviewing the distribution of nonfatal occupational injuries and illnesses stratified by private sector. In 2015, the Health Care and Social Assistance sector ranked number one for total number of injuries with 5,623,000 reported that year alone [2]. To put in proper context, more injuries were reported in the Health Care and Social Assistance private sector than the combined private sectors of construction, transportation, agriculture, and mining. Despite the recognition of employment in health care as high risk for occupational injury, relatively few studies focused on injuries sustained by surgeons until the advent of minimally invasive techniques in the late 1980s [3–5].

With the introduction of laparoscopic surgery, patients enjoyed the benefits of less postoperative pain, fewer surgical site infections, and shorter hospital stays [6]. These benefits, however, came with drawbacks for surgeons [7]. Shortly after the incorporation of minimally invasive techniques in the operating room, a rise in surgeon musculoskeletal strain and injury was noted. Surveys show that 77–100% of laparoscopic surgeons experience physical symptoms or discomfort attributed to operating [8–15]. Table 22.1 further describes pain by surgical modality. Common sites of pain include the neck, shoulder, and upper and lower back [5, 7, 17, 18]. Table 22.2 demonstrates specialty-specific prevalence and location of pain.

Table 22.1 Prevalence and location of musculoskeletal pain by surgical modality

Surgical modality	Prevalence of musculoskeletal pain attributed to operating	Location of discomfort
Open surgery	75% [8]	Neck: 6% [16], 50% [17] Shoulder: 10% [16]
Laparoscopic surgery/ MIS	77–100% [8–15]	Neck: 78% [14], 56% [17], 52% [5], 42% [18], 15% [7] Back: 77% [14], 72% [18], 26% [7] Shoulder: 77% [14], 55% [5], 45% [7], 43% [18] Wrist/hand: 47% [5] Leg: 37% [18]
Robotic	41–53% [8, 19, 20]	Neck: 74% [20], 23% [17] Shoulder: 53% [20] Lower back: 42% [20] Wrist/hand: 37% [20]

Table 22.2 Prevalence and location of musculoskeletal discomfort and common injuries by surgical specialty

Surgical specialty	Prevalence of musculoskeletal discomfort attributed to operating	Location of discomfort	Reported injuries
General	80–83% [13, 21]	Neck: 83% [13] Lower back: 68% [13] Shoulder: 58% [13] Upper back: 53% [13]	40% Digital nerve injury (with laparoscopic surgery) [22]
Thoracic	77% [15]	Back: 83% [15] Neck: 82% [15] Shoulder: 76% [15]	
Colorectal	36% [23]		42% Hand/finger injury [23] 10% Neck injury [23] 9% Back injury [23]
Obstetrics-gynecology	67% [24]	Back: 77% [25], Lower back: 76% [26] Neck: 74% [25], 73% [26] Shoulder: 67% [26] Upper back: 62% [26] Wrist/hand: 70% [25], 61% [26] Eyestrain: 17% [12]	15% Vertebral disc prolapse [25]
Gynecology-oncology	61–88% [9, 27]	Neck: 59% [9] Back: 54% [9] Shoulder: 54% [9]	
Neurosurgery	80% [21]		7% Lumbar disc disease requiring surgery [28] 5% Cervical disc disease [28]
Ophthalmology	73% [29] 52% [30]	Neck: 58% [29], 33% [30] Mid-back: 30% [29] Lower back: 33% [30], 31% [29] Shoulder: 27% [29] Upper extremity: 33% [30]	26% Bulging or herniated discs [29] 8% Spinal injury [29]
Oral and maxillofacial	87% [31]	Back: 87% [32], 64% [31] Neck: 73% [32], 53% [31] Ankle/foot: 53% [32] Knee: 47% [32] Wrist: 37% [32] Hip/thigh: 33% [32] Hand: 30% [32] Shoulder: 21% [32] Elbow: 20% [32]	

(continued)

Table 22.2 (continued)

Surgical specialty	Prevalence of musculoskeletal discomfort attributed to operating	Location of discomfort	Reported injuries
Orthopedics	67% [21]	Lower back: 50% [33] Neck: 39% [33] Shoulder: 32% [33] Upper back: 24% [33]	27% Chronic lower back pain [34] 17% Wrist or forearm tendinitis [34] 15% Lateral elbow epicondylitis [34] 14% Plantar fasciitis [34] 13% Carpal tunnel syndrome [34] 13% Shoulder tendinitis [34] 9% Knee osteoarthritis [34]
Otolaryngology	62–84% [21, 35–37]	Neck: 82% [38], 60% [35] Back: 57% [35] Lower back: 56% [38] Upper back: 40% [38] Shoulders: 40% [38] Wrist/hand: 19% [35]	
Pediatrics	45–67% [39–41]	Lower back: 44% [41] Upper extremity: 34% [41] Shoulder: 23% [41] Neck: 24% [41]	15% Lateral elbow epicondylitis [41] 13% Shoulder tendinitis/ impingement [41] 10% Cervical radiculopathy [41] 10% Carpal tunnel syndrome [41]
Plastics	82–94% [21, 42]		Cervical disc herniation [43] 15% Carpal tunnel syndrome [42] 14% Epicondylitis [42]
Urology	86% [44]	Wrist/hand: 67% [45], 63% [46], 42% [44] Neck: 59% [44], 58% [46] Back: 57% [44], 53% [46], 33% [45] Shoulder: 51% [44], 34% [46] Arm: 26% [44] Leg: 22% [46] Eyestrain: 22% [45]	43% Chronic back or neck pain [17] 49% Chronic pain [44] 30% Arthritic or neuromuscular symptoms [47] 18% Paresthesias, most commonly in the thumb and/or middle finger 18% Finger numbness during laparoscopy [16]
Vascular	83% [48]		

Despite the wide prevalence of surgeon discomfort and injury illustrated by numerous anonymous surveys, few surgeons report the injuries to their institution [9, 21, 49]. Even in nonsurgical literature, musculoskeletal disorders are highly underreported and are hard to link directly to work-related activities [50]. In a survey performed by the Tennessee Chapter of the American College of Surgeons in 2014, 40% of respondents noted that they experienced a work-related injury. Of those injured, only 50% received medical care and even fewer (19%)

reported the pain to their institution [49]. With these percentages in mind, the high rate of injuries reported by the US Bureau of Labor Statistics, data collected solely from institutional reporting, may be a gross underestimation of reality.

It is largely unknown why surgeons do not report their injuries. One study suggests that 30% of surgeons do not know how to report an occupational injury [29] and many may not see a need to report. Another possibility is that surgeons believe an injury could impact his or her training or professional reputation. Alternatively, while maintaining focus on patient care, surgeons may overlook their own well-being, accepting pain as just another part of the job [13]. Regardless of the reason, the low rate of reporting occupational injuries among surgeons is concerning as it may represent a culture of silence. Culture change may be required to prevent further repercussions to both provider and patient.

Consequences of Surgeon Musculoskeletal Pain

Surgeon musculoskeletal pain has theoretical downstream consequences, including poor outcomes, lost revenue, and surgeon burnout. The impact of surgeon discomfort on patient outcomes has not yet been fully described. A surgeon distracted by pain is unlikely to operate with maximum precision and focus. Over 50% of surgeons with musculoskeletal pain report that pain negatively affects their performance in the operating room [39, 40, 51]. It has also been found that surgeon's symptoms may influence their choice of operative approach, some opting to perform open surgeries over laparoscopy [8, 17].

Of those surgeons who report discomfort, approximately 25% have taken time off work [34, 51–53] with even more surgeons opting to decrease their operative caseload [9, 26, 51]. When an injury results in leave from work, an average of 7.3 days is lost [49]. One week of lost work for a general surgeon results in the loss of approximately $36,000 in hospital revenue, extrapolated from data published by Merritt Hawkins in 2016 [54]. This is in addition to the surgeon's own loss in personal income. Further, some surgeons consider early retirement and are concerned that pain will shorten their surgical careers [38, 48, 53, 55, 56]. This may have greater societal repercussions than lost revenue in an era already anticipating a shortage of surgeons. With a projected shortfall of between 25,200 and 33,200 surgeons by 2025, increasing numbers of early retirements could further exacerbate this situation and lead to patients without access to surgical care [57].

For surgery residents, injury may have direct consequences on their training. Training programs abide by rules put in place by the Accreditation Council for Graduate Medical Education (ACGME) in regard to total weeks of training. Residents are allowed 1 month of absence per year for illness, vacation, and other reasons. Absence longer than 1 month may result in an extension of resident training time [58]. In a study of work-related injuries sustained during obstetrics and gynecology training, Yoong et al. found that out of 97 residents, 28 (29%) had suffered injuries at work. Eight respondents required time off from residency, and one had to prolong training by 3 months [59].

Surgeon burnout is another potential ramification of workplace injury. Overall surgeon burnout is reported to be around 40% [60, 61]. A relationship between pain and burnout has been established in nurses [62] and may also be present in surgeons. Self-reported burnout has been found to positively correlate to increased pain, with burned-out vascular surgeons reporting more pain both during and after operating [48].

Risk Factors for Surgeon Injury

Identification of risk factors predisposing surgeons to occupational injury is the first step toward an ergonomic solution. Many risk factors correlate with the surgical modality and equipment used. Non-modifiable risk factors such as gender, hand size, and height are important to understand as they may be addressed with proper ergonomic adjustment. Additionally, both lack of surgical experience and poor ergonomic training are risk factors for injury. The latter can fortunately be mitigated with ergonomic education during residency.

Surgical Modality

Open Surgery

Overall, open surgery is considered more ergonomic than laparoscopic surgery because it allows direct visualization, greater range of motion, less confined postures, and ease of movement [63, 64]. For this reason, the ergonomics of open surgery have not been as well researched as minimally invasive surgery (MIS) [8, 63, 65]. There are, however, unique ergonomic challenges during open procedures. Specifically, surgeons spend up to 54% of the time with their head bent forward (see surgeon on the right in Fig. 22.1) and 27% of the time spent with their

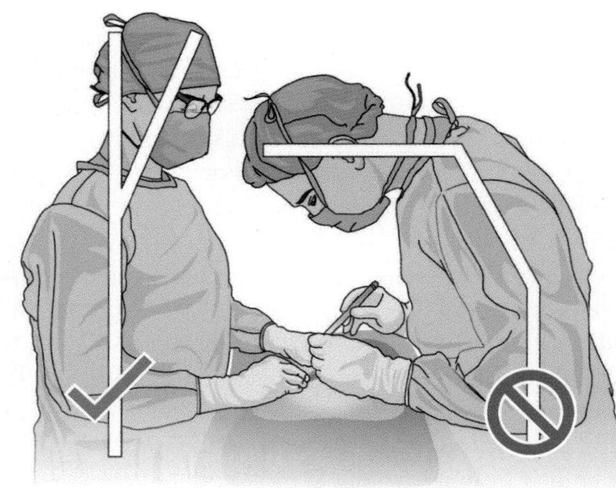

Fig. 22.1 The surgeon on the left is standing with correct posture with her head at a slight inclination of approximately 20°. The surgeon on the right has incorrect posture with his back and head extremely flexed

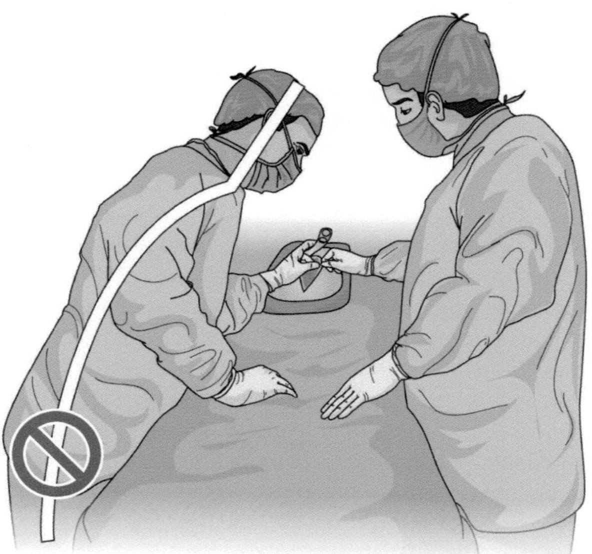

Fig. 22.2 An example of a common but incorrect body posture with the back twisted and laterally flexed

back twisted and laterally flexed (Fig. 22.2) [66]. The asymmetric loading of the spine that occurs in these postures leads to an increased risk of vertebral disc herniation [67, 68]. Further, the traditional belief that open surgery is more ergonomic than laparoscopic is now being challenged as electromyography studies of the upper extremities show increased activity during open cases as compared to laparoscopic cases [65].

Laparoscopic Surgery

Laparoscopic surgeons often assume an upright, straight-back stance with fewer trunk movements and less weight shifting than surgeons performing open surgery [63, 69]. Long periods in such static postures lead to prolonged isometric muscle contraction which decreases muscle perfusion and can increase muscle fatigue and pain [70–72]. Given the use of monitors for visualization, minimally invasive surgeons, including endoscopists, have increased eye strain and mental stress due to loss of depth perception with a two-dimensional image [73, 74]. Increased mental stress has been directly related to worsening neck strain [75]. Additionally, poor monitor placement can greatly influence neck posture and lead to neck and shoulder strain [76, 77]. Repetitive motions such as looking back and forth from the monitor to the surgical site increase the risk of overuse injuries [78]. Laparoscopic instruments pose significant challenges as they decrease tactile feedback, magnify natural hand tremor, and require four to six times more force to complete the same task as in open surgery [5, 66, 79]. The physical demands of MIS, specialized equipment, and mental intensity in the operating room are only a few factors that may contribute to muscular strain and injury [80].

Robotic-Assisted Surgery

Robotic-assisted surgery is widely considered to be more ergonomic than laparoscopic; however, challenges remain [8, 81, 82]. Approximately half of surgeons experience physical discomfort due to robotic surgery [8, 19, 20]. Symptoms include neck stiffness, as well as finger and eye fatigue [27, 83]. Eye fatigue improved with the introduction of enhanced high-definition visualization with the da Vinci Si™ [83]. The robotic console will adjust to appropriate heights for surgeons between 64 and 73 inches. However, surgeons shorter than 64 inches will need to extend their necks or raise the height of the chair to use the eyepiece. Raising the chair makes it more difficult to reach the pedals without applying extensive pressure on the popliteal area or requiring foot rests that interfere with pedal operation. Surgeons taller than 73 inches will assume a flexed neck position while using the eyepieces [84]. Professions utilizing similar seated positions, such as microscopists, have an increased risk of chronic kyphosis due to years spent bending over the scope [85]. As robotic surgery becomes more prevalent, ergonomic shortfalls and the accompanying physical repercussions for robotic surgeons may manifest in the future.

Gender and Anthropometry

Studies suggest female surgeons have greater than a twofold risk for physical discomfort associated with laparoscopy when compared to their male counterparts [9, 26]. This may be because women are more likely to have small hand size and short stature [86, 87]. Surgeons with a glove size less than 6.5 report more difficulty with using laparoscopic instruments than those with a larger glove size [88]. Female surgeons are more likely to describe laparoscopic instruments as too big and are over three times more likely than men to receive treatment for hand injuries [89]. A more ergonomic design for laparoscopic instruments should consider varying hand sizes and strengths. Women are also more likely than men to experience shoulder and neck pain [90]. Short stature has been correlated with shoulder and neck pain during laparoscopy due to excessive shoulder abduction to accommodate for the length of the instruments [89, 91]. In general, females are more likely to seek medical treatment for their injuries [92]. Therefore, higher rates of physical discomfort and injury could also be due to increased reporting.

Surgical Inexperience

Surgery residents may also have unique risk factors for occupational injury. Hemal and colleagues reported that those with less than 2 years of experience have significantly higher rate of finger numbness and eye strain than their more senior colleagues, despite having an equivalent laparoscopic workload. The researchers hypothesize that inexperience or anxiety may contribute to ergonomic errors such as higher grip force of instruments or incorrect body posture [16, 46]. This is consistent with a study by Uhrich et al., which showed that residents experienced significantly greater discomfort than attending surgeons as well as increased muscle load of several muscle groups while performing the same tasks as staff surgeons [7, 46, 72]. In other professions, workers with less experience have higher prevalence of musculoskeletal problems due to poorer job skills and insufficient practice [93, 94].

In addition, assisting during laparoscopic surgery, a common resident role, comes with unique disadvantages. Specifically, assistants have been found to disproportionately bear 70–80% of their body weight on one leg during laparoscopic surgery while retracting or holding the camera, leading to postural instability and asymmetric muscle activation [95, 96]. Therefore, since residents have less experience and are often required to perform physically demanding tasks such as retracting, they could be at an increased risk of musculoskeletal pain and occupational injury.

The fact that less-experienced surgeons report more complaints justifies an enhanced focus on ergonomics during surgical residency. Junior surgeons are less familiar with operative procedures and may intrinsically experience higher mental and physical stress levels. Consequently, their main intraoperative focus will be on the surgical procedure, with less attention paid to their own physical status, surgical setup, or other ergonomic conditions. Implementing ergonomic training for surgical residents will increase their understanding of the human-system interactions in the operating room.

Lack of Ergonomic Education

One of the most important risk factors for surgeon injury appears to be lack of awareness of ergonomic principles. Up to 90% of surgeons have no prior training in ergonomics [14, 35], and a lack of ergonomic training has been directly linked to occupational injury in surgeons [10, 14, 83, 97]. Without an understanding of ergonomic factors to prevent strain, surgeons are at a greater risk for injury. Surgeons as educators may alleviate this risk by implementing and educating residents in ergonomic principles that can be easily applied to the surgeon's work within and outside the operating room. Learning ideal ergonomic practices could improve physical health and well-being for surgeons as well as support career longevity.

Prevention of Injury in the Operating Room

Using knowledge of human-system interactions to one's advantage in the operating room has been shown to reduce musculoskeletal strain and injuries and increase performance [91, 98, 99]. Surgeons as educators are provided many opportunities to implement ergonomic practices in the operating room such as awareness of body position, posture, and how the body interacts with equipment in the room. The surgeon may also include a warm-up prior to the first case, take scheduled breaks during surgery, and add variety to operative days. The following are high-yield ergonomic interventions that may be used to prevent injuries and enhance performance.

Surgeon Posture

The importance of posture cannot be overstated, yet it is often overlooked. While operating, surgeons are often found in awkward positions that create musculoskeletal strain. Even proper body alignment, if static and held with tension, may decrease circulation and lead to muscle fatigue [70–72]. In addition, poor body positioning can impair technical performance [100]. Ideal posture maintains neutral joint positions with the least possible amount of strain. The Alexander technique is an educational process to avoid muscular and mental tension through correct postural alignment [101]. A study evaluating the impact of surgeon education in Alexander technique showed an improvement in tremor, discomfort, and fatigue [102]. In addition to the Alexander technique, there are other ways to encourage proper posture such as focusing on awareness of body positioning and limiting muscle tension.

Proper Standing Posture

Operating while standing is ideal for cases that require large movements or significant force. Ideal standing posture is with the head directly over the shoulders and with the chin slightly tucked so that the neck is in a flexion of 15–25° (see surgeon on left in Fig. 22.1) [103–105]. The shoulders are directly over the pelvis and the feet are hip-width apart. The knees are soft and not locked. During laparoscopic surgery, the shoulders should be in approximately 20° of abduction and 40° of internal rotation [106]. The elbows should be flexed 90–120°, and the wrists should not exceed greater than 15° of deviation or flexion in any direction (Fig. 22.5) [106, 107]. To vary position, the surgeon may place a foot on a step stool while being mindful of maintaining pelvic girdle alignment so that weight is equally distributed between both feet [108]. Additionally, an anti-fatigue mat may improve comfort especially during long cases [109, 110]. The mat acts as a cushion between the feet and hard-surfaced floor. Anti-fatigue mats are used in many industries where workers must stand for long periods [111] and are marketed for use in the operating room.

Correct Seated Body Alignment

Sitting while operating is ideal for cases with a small surgical window such as vaginal surgery and microsurgery. Sitting is especially advantageous as it allows the body to be supported by several surfaces such as the floor, seat, backrest, and occasionally armrests. For this reason, stools and chairs with backrests are more comfortable than those without [24]. When seated, the feet should rest flat on the ground with the knees flexed at an angle of 90° or greater [84]. If a foot pedal is required, it should be placed directly in front of the working foot. Sitting may be alternated with periods of standing as prolonged sitting is associated with low back pain [112].

Seated posture during robotic surgery is slightly different than open surgery as the surgeon leans forward while working at the console. Prior to beginning a case, the chair and console height should be adjusted to a comfortable viewing position. The console is optimized for surgeons between 64 and 73 inches tall. The feet should rest on the floor behind the pedals with the knees at a 90° or greater angle, while the forehead rests gently on the headpiece. The forearms relax onto the armrests with the arms near the body and the elbows at a 90° angle [82, 84]. Prolonged work with outstretched and unsupported arms loads the muscles of the trunk and shoulder. This strain may be decreased 25% by using armrests [84, 113]. For this reason, surgeons should frequently clutch so that the forearms are supported in a neutral position.

Postural Resets

It is difficult to maintain good posture, especially if it is not a habit. It may be necessary to employ a postural reset, a moment to check in with your posture and readjust as necessary [108]. The postural reset could be implemented during intraoperative breaks or at any natural transitions during the procedure. As a surgeon educator, direct feedback may be given in the operating room or in training facilities regarding the resident's posture in the same way that one would comment on proper surgical technique. For some, it may be necessary to provide visual feedback by videotaping the surgeon or resident and reviewing the video for correct body alignment.

Operating Room Setup

One important step to preventing injury while operating is proper setup of the operating room. In 2012, Miller et al. reported that surgeons who agree with the statement, "The equipment and overall layout of my operating room is designed for and encourages surgeon comfort," are less likely to experience neck, shoulder, and arm pain or stiffness [10]. It takes only a few moments before cases, and at natural transitions during cases, to properly adjust operating room equipment. Yet the benefits may be significant.

Proper Monitor Placement

Incorrect monitor placement is one of the factors most likely to cause discomfort in the operating room [11, 114] and is associated with neck and upper back discomfort as well as eye strain [72, 74, 115]. Many problems arise when monitors are placed on top of a high instrument tower. Ceiling-suspended monitors and those on easily adjustable arms are ideal as they allow for versatile positioning [116, 117]. Optimal monitor placement is dependent on the location, height, and distance of the monitor in relation to the surgeon so that the surgeon's neck, back, and eye musculatures maintain neutral positions.

In regard to location, the monitors should be placed directly in front of each surgeon and assistant so that there is a straight line between the surgeon and assistant's body orientation, target organ, and monitor [91, 98, 118]. This is shown in Fig. 22.3 and is described as the straight-line principle. To accomplish this, there should always be at least two monitors in the operating room [107]. This positioning helps to avoid repetitive or prolonged spine rotation which leads to asymmetric contraction of the spinal musculature and may increase the risk for vertebral disc prolapse [67, 68]. Often, perfect positioning of the monitor directly in front of the surgeon is not possible due to the location of the first assistant or intervening equipment. In these cases, the surgeon may need to change his or her body orientation to avoid rotation of the spine [91].

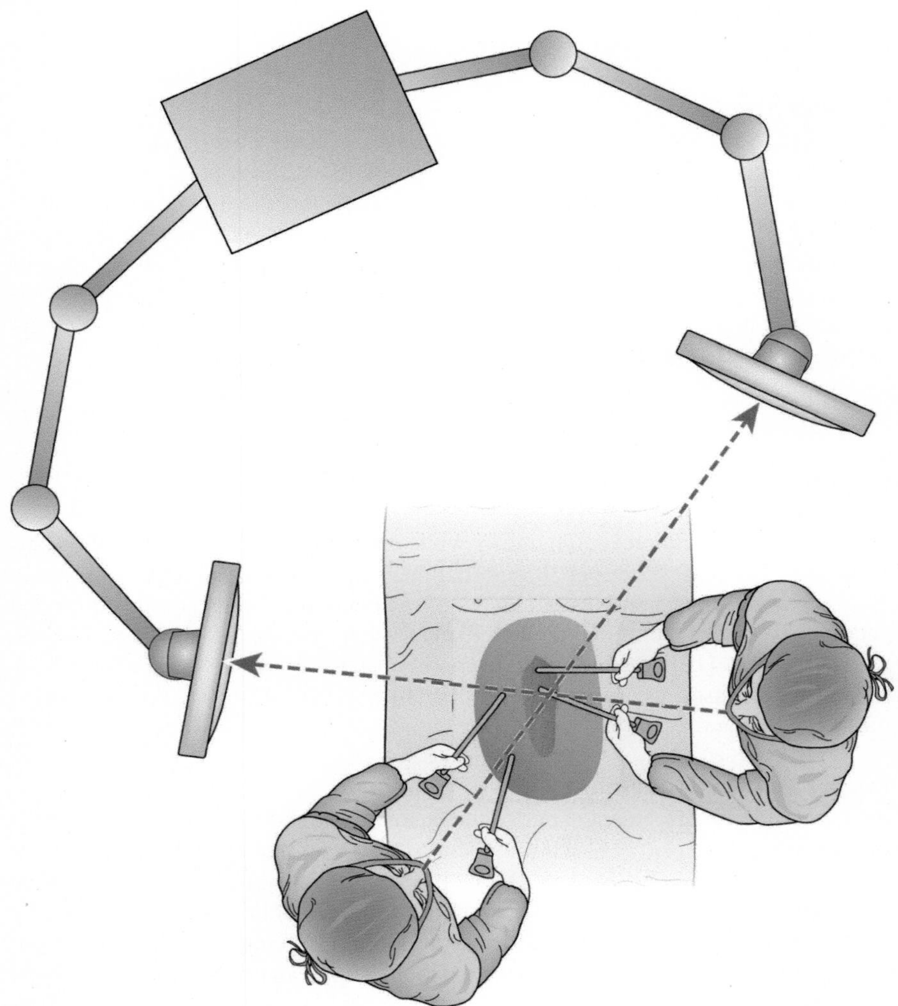

Fig. 22.3 Proper monitor placement in the operating room is shown with a straight line between the surgeon and assistant's body orientation, target organ, and monitor

Proper monitor height is guided by the gaze-down technique, which is placing the center of the screen approximately 10–20° below eye level [119]. This positioning mimics the neutral orientation of the human eye in its orbit, which is at an inclination of 15°, and prevents neck extension [120]. *An easy way to approximate proper monitor height is to place the top of the screen at eye level* as seen in the top image of Fig. 22.4 and in Fig. 22.5. In this position, electromyography registers the lowest

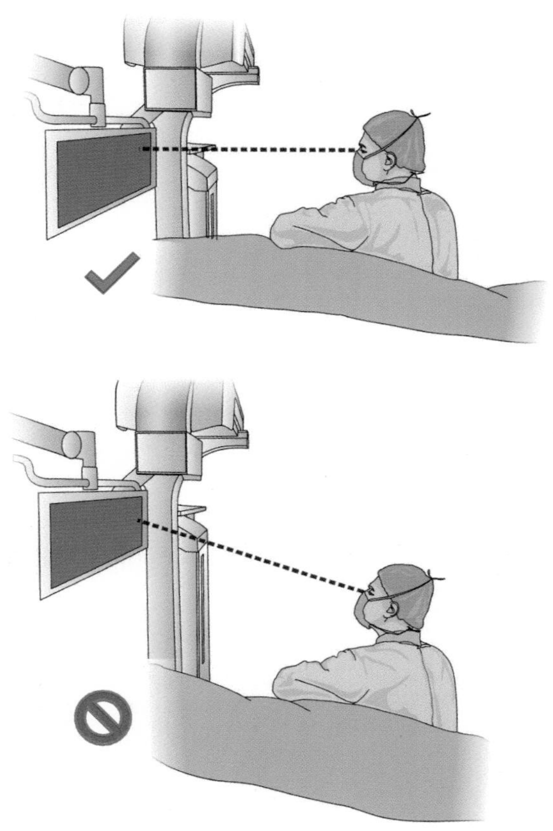

Fig. 22.4 Correct monitor height is shown in the top image. The top of the monitor is placed at eye level and approximately 3 feet away from the surgeon. Incorrect monitor height, with the monitor above eye level, is shown in the bottom image

cervical muscle activity indicating muscle ease [103–105]. The gaze-down technique not only improves neck and eye discomfort, it may improve performance as several simulation studies have shown shorter task times and fewer errors [46, 98, 121–123].

The optimal monitor distance for a standard 19-inch monitor is 2.5–4 feet from the surgeon's eye which allows for the extraocular and ciliary musculature to be in its most relaxed state [124]. However, this distance is dependent on monitor diameter and resolution. Large, high-definition screens may need to be placed slightly further away [114, 115]. During close-up visual activity, the eyes converge and the lenses accommodate which leads to strain on the eye musculature if close-up activity is prolonged [120, 125–127]. Conversely, visual acuity decreases with increasing distance which may result in forward projection of the head to compensate for

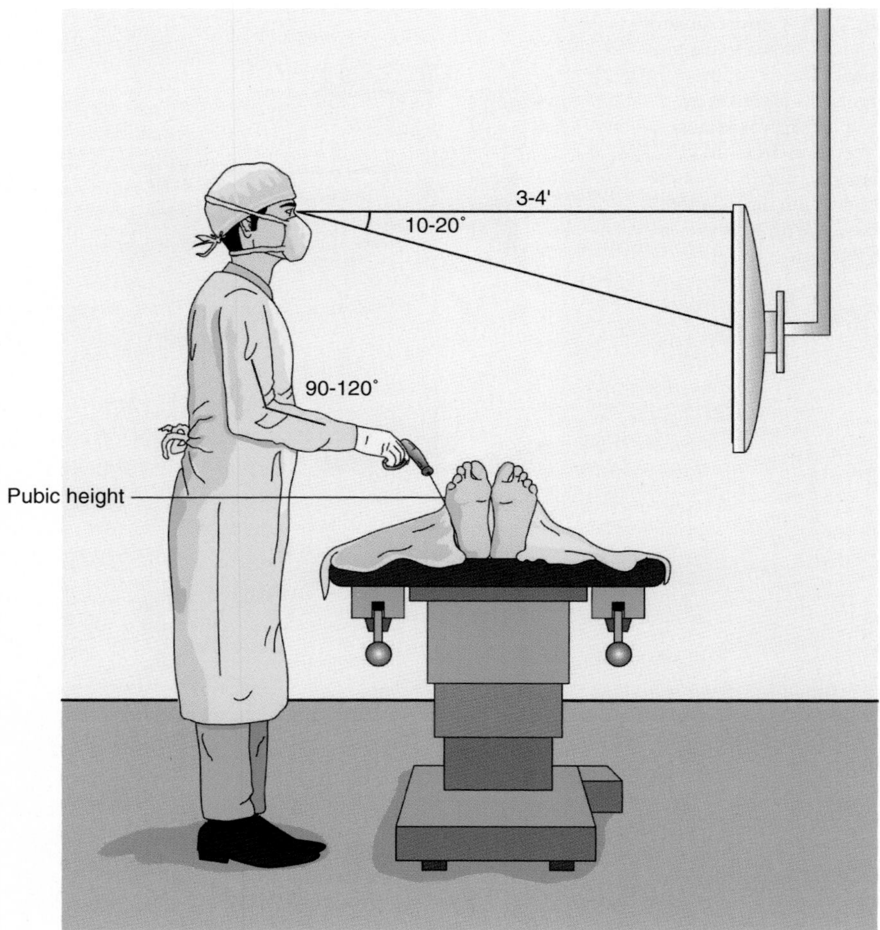

Fig. 22.5 Proper laparoscopic surgery posture is shown with the operating surface at pubic height and the elbows in 90–120° of flexion. The foot pedal is directly in front of the working foot. The monitor is 3–4 feet from the surgeon with the top of the screen at eye level so that the center of the screen is 10–20° below eye level

loss of detail. *A simple approximation for proper monitor distance is 3 feet from the surgeon with minor adjustments made based on the monitor specifications and surgeon comfort.* If the monitor must be placed closer to the surgeon, it should be lowered and tilted upward [114, 115].

Correct Table Height Adjustment

Open Surgery

Improper table height can lead to wrist, hand, shoulder, neck, and back pain [9, 14, 71, 91]. Appropriate adjustment of the operating table height reduces the risk of

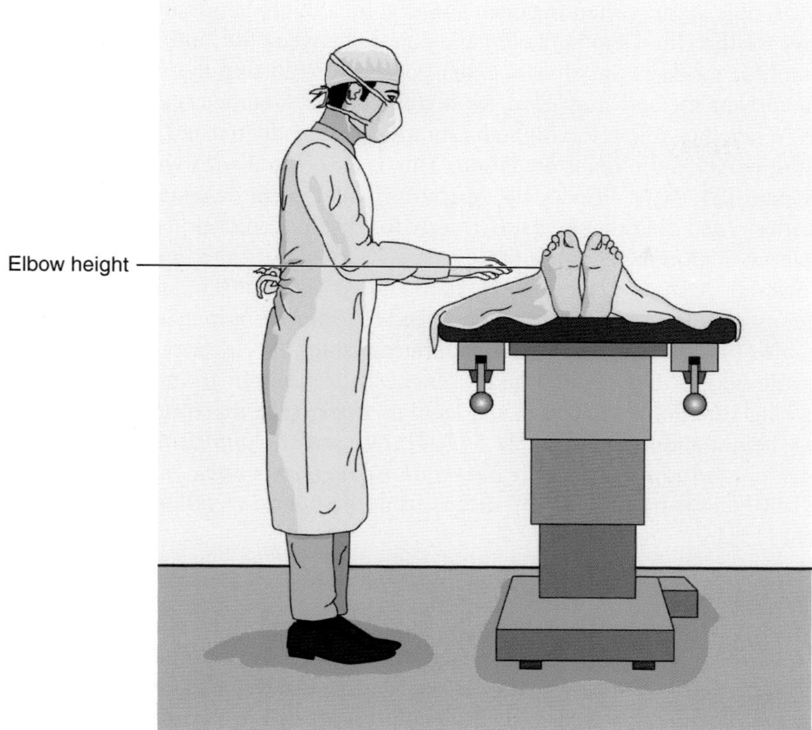

Fig. 22.6 Proper operating table height for open surgery is shown with the operating surface at the level of the elbow

developing musculoskeletal pain by 83% [128]. For manual work, a working height about 5 cm below the elbow is recommended with an acceptable range of 10 cm below (for heavy work) to 5 cm above elbow height (for precision work) [129]. *During open procedures, most surgeons adjust the table, so the patient is at elbow height* (Fig. 22.6). There are variations in table height based on procedure. For example, during spine surgery requiring loupes, a working surface which is at the midpoint between the umbilicus and sternum is optimal for reducing musculoskeletal fatigue [97]. With multiple surgeons, the table height should be adjusted to the height of the tallest person on the operating team as the other team members may use step stools to accommodate. Ideally, however, step stools should be avoided as they limit the surgeon's movement and make foot pedals more difficult to use given the step's small platform area [130].

Laparoscopic Surgery

Given the long length of laparoscopic instruments and elevation of the operating surface with pneumoperitoneum, the operating table needs to be lower for laparoscopic surgery than for open surgery. Ideal table height during laparoscopy allows for the elbows to be flexed at an angle between 90° and 120° [130]. When the table is too low, the elbows extend past 120° limiting the freedom of instrument movement and may lead to uncomfortable, compensatory flexion of the back. When the table is too high, the shoulders are abducted and internally rotated, and the wrists are in ulnar deviation. This is associated with wrist, shoulder, and neck pain [71, 107]. Previously, operating tables were designed solely for open procedures and did not lower sufficiently for laparoscopic surgery [107]. To allow for elbow flexion to be in the proper range during MIS, the operating table must be lowered. A study performed in 2006 showed that 70% of minimally invasive surgeons desired that the table be equipped to lower more than what was currently possible [14]. In response, modern operating tables have been redesigned to allow for table heights between 23 and 43 inches. Ideal height from the ground to the operating surface, described as the level of trocar skin insertion, is 70%–80% of elbow height and seen in Fig. 22.5 [107]. *This may be approximated by positioning the operating surface at the height of the surgeon's pubic bone* (Fig. 22.5) [5, 107, 130] and is roughly 25–30 inches from the floor depending on the surgeon's height [131].

Hand-Assisted Laparoscopic Surgery

Hand-assisted laparoscopic surgery (HALS) involves simultaneous aspects of open and laparoscopic surgery; however, the ideal table height is more consistent with that of open surgery. During simulations, Manasnayakorn et al. found that the optimum table height for HALS is the height at which the laparoscopic instrument handle is 2 inches above the elbow level. Although this height is not ideal for laparoscopic surgery, during HALS, this height results in fewer errors, faster task time, and decreased muscle workload on electromyography [132].

Appropriate Foot Pedal Placement

Foot pedals are used by 87% of laparoscopic surgeons [14]. Over half of surgeons who use foot pedals find them uncomfortable and annoying [14, 133]. Van veelen et al. found that one third of surgeons allow the surgical nurse to position the foot pedal. Often, the foot pedal is under the operating table or sterile sheet and unable to be directly visualized [133]. This results in 75% occasionally hitting the wrong switch and 91% occasionally losing contact with the foot pedal. In addition, 100% believe the foot pedal limits their freedom of movement resulting in a static posture [133]. Often, the surgeon maintains dorsiflexion of the foot over the pedal to avoid losing contact. This results in distribution of the body weight to the standing leg and the heel of the working foot for prolonged periods of time. These ergonomic concerns with the foot pedal are exaggerated when the surgeon must use a step stool as the small space further limits the ability to shift body weight, leading to a static position [77]. Ergonomic principles to improve ease of use and discomfort with the foot pedal include placing the pedal directly in front of the main foot and in line with the target instruments, ideally before the operation begins, thus limiting prolonged dorsiflexion of the foot and dorsiflexion past 25° [133].

Ergonomic Challenges and Benefits of Visualization Adjuncts

Various forms of retraction are used during surgery to assist with exposure and visualization. Handheld retractors, especially during long open cases, are associated with musculoskeletal discomfort of the hands, arms, shoulders, neck, and back [78] as well as the development of peripheral neuropathies [134, 135]. Self-retaining retractors are available for a wide variety of open and laparoscopic cases and alleviate the need for handheld retraction [136]. Given that the flexor muscles of the hand fatigue after only 60 s of maximal isometric contraction [137], self-retaining retractors are also more stable than handheld retractors [138]. Whenever possible, opt for self-retaining retractors over handheld.

Loupes and microscopes are used to magnify fine detail and support proper upright neck posture with the downward inclination of the lenses. However, there is significant concern that loupes and microscopes are associated with career-limiting neck pain [55]. Sivak-Callcott and colleagues showed that over half of the oculoplastic surgeons surveyed agreed that loupes can lead to spinal disorders and are concerned about long-term effects that result from prolonged use of loupes [29]. This risk partially results from the weight of the loupes. The higher the magnification of the loupes, the heavier they are. For this reason, surgical residents may find that 2.5× magnification is adequate as well as more comfortable than higher magnifications [139]. The loupe frames must also be lightweight and properly fitted so that the frame does not slip down the nose or apply too much postauricular pressure. In addition, for proper neck posture, the angle of declination of the loupes should be approximately 30° from the horizontal plane at the level of your eyes to lessen eye and neck strain. Loupes must also be properly adjusted to the correct depth of convergence so that the working distance, or distance from the lenses to the surgical field, supports an ideal posture [139].

In regard to microscopes, 83% of otolaryngologists report experiencing symptoms during microsurgery with the most common locations being the neck, upper back, and shoulders [38]. A common etiology of pain is the static posture of the neck and upper body while operating under a microscope. Arm supports can decrease upper back and shoulder tension [84, 113]. In addition, using a microscope with an articulated eyepiece allows for improved neck posture and the ability to more easily change position while operating to reduce neck strain [38]. Ocular extenders can be added to the assistant's side to prevent neck overextension during non-midline procedures.

Adequate light is necessary in the operating room for proper visualization of the surgical field. Headlamps improve visualization by providing coaxial illumination in line with the eyes which limits shadows. Unfortunately, they also add weight to the head and increase the risk of neck and upper back pain [29]. In addition, fiber-optic headlights limit freedom of movement since they are plugged into a light box. It is important to ensure that, when using loupes and headlamps simultaneously, both are properly adjusted to the same line of sight, and neither are used longer than necessary [139].

Adequate visualization sometimes requires intraoperative imaging using fluoroscopy. In order to limit radiation exposure, protective aprons are worn.

Unfortunately, these aprons weigh an average of 10 pounds and lead to increased muscle strain of the trunk, most notably the trapezius and pectoral muscles [140, 141]. Back pain is reported in over half of interventional cardiologists and vascular surgeons who routinely use lead aprons [48, 142]. It is important to have an appropriately fitted radioprotective apron, not only for comfort of fit but also to avoid the extra weight from an apron that is too large. Ideal lead aprons are two pieces because the weight on the lower section is distributed on the pelvis rather than entirely on the shoulders [143].

Surgical Warm-Up

Warm-up exercises are a standard activity for professional sports players, musicians, and singers. Physical warm-up decreases injury in other professions by increasing flexibility, circulation, and muscle temperature [144, 145]. Many surgeons perform "mental warm-up" exercises by reviewing imaging and discussing the surgical approach prior to cases. However, physical warm-up exercises have not been widely adopted by surgeons. Although surgical skill warm-up has not yet been proven to decrease the risk of musculoskeletal discomfort in surgeons, many other important benefits have been noted. In 2012, Lee et al. studied the effect of a 20-min warm-up 1 h prior to laparoscopic renal surgery as compared to no warm-up. The warm-up involved completing an electrocautery skill task on a simulator and 15 min of laparoscopic suturing and knot tying in a pelvic box trainer. Following the warm-up, video analysis of operative technique showed an improvement in hand movement smoothness, tool movement smoothness, and posture stability. Pupillary eye tracking showed an increase in attention, and mental workload was significantly decreased as analyzed by electroencephalogram [146]. Chen et al. performed a similar study and found that a brief (<15 min) warm-up on a low-fidelity laparoscopic trainer immediately prior to laparoscopic surgery improved the intraoperative performance of the resident irrespective of resident level of training or case complexity [147]. Similar results have been shown using a robotic simulator for warm-up prior to robotic-assisted surgery [99, 148–150].

Intraoperative Breaks

Many high-risk professions have mandated breaks, including airplane pilots, nuclear power plant employees, and air-traffic control workers to mitigate fatigue, improve employee health, and enhance safety [151–153]. Studies of intraoperative breaks during MIS and open surgery have varied in break timing and duration and range from 20s breaks every 20min to 5min breaks every 40 min [56, 154, 155]. More frequent short breaks are superior to fewer long breaks in reducing muscular fatigue [112]. Intraoperative breaks have been shown to decrease salivary cortisol, suggesting that breaks decrease stress [56]. They also have been shown to almost entirely prevent the effects of musculoskeletal discomfort, specifically decreased strength and precision of movement [154]. Significant improvement in upper extremity discomfort is due to less time spent in static positions. Eye fatigue scores improve by 50% when incorporating intraoperative breaks into laparoscopic surgery [155]. Short, regular breaks do not significantly prolong the operation duration [56, 155].

Recent studies advocate for stretching during 90 s of intraoperative breaks every 20–40 min during laparoscopic and open surgery [56, 156]. Stretching increases circulation and eases muscle fatigue [157]. Park et al. studied intraoperative stretches performed while maintaining sterility. Stretches included neck flexion and extension, backward shoulder rolls with chest stretch, upper back and hand stretch, low back flexion and extension with gluteus maximus squeeze, and forefoot and heel lifts for lower extremity and ankle stretches. They found significant improvement in neck, shoulder, hand, and lower back pain when compared to control. Surgeons reported perceived improvements in physical performance and mental focus, and 87% of the surgeons enrolled in the study planned to continue intraoperative stretching breaks even after the study concluded [56]. Anecdotally, we have used this technique during long microsurgery cases, noting decreased pain and stiffness, not only in surgeons and assistants but also in circulating nurses who spend long periods of time at the computer.

A potential drawback of this intervention is that breaks create interruptions. This can decrease compliance by surgeons who do not want to pause the procedure [154]. However, during a typical procedure without planned intraoperative breaks, workflow is interrupted on average 4 min per hour due to personnel- or equipment-related events [158]. During a study of intraoperative breaks by Dorion and colleagues, it was subjectively noted that nursing staff will frequently use the timed breaks to take care of many of these other potential disruptions [154].

Prevention of Injury Outside of the Operating Room

Although the operating room is where the majority of ergonomic interventions are implemented, there are factors outside the operating room which can contribute to musculoskeletal pain. These factors may be addressed using proper office ergonomics and by maintaining good health through routine exercise and stretching.

Proper Office Ergonomics

Whether it be reviewing charts and films or writing patient notes, a surgeon spends significant time in front of a computer. The ergonomic considerations for computer monitor use share similarities with MIS monitors. However, computer viewing tends to be more near-vision reading work. For this reason, the center of the computer screen should be lowered even more than the MIS monitor as the downward gaze increases the ability of the eye to accommodate and converge by 25–30%. Ideal positioning of the computer screen is with the center 20–50° below the eye

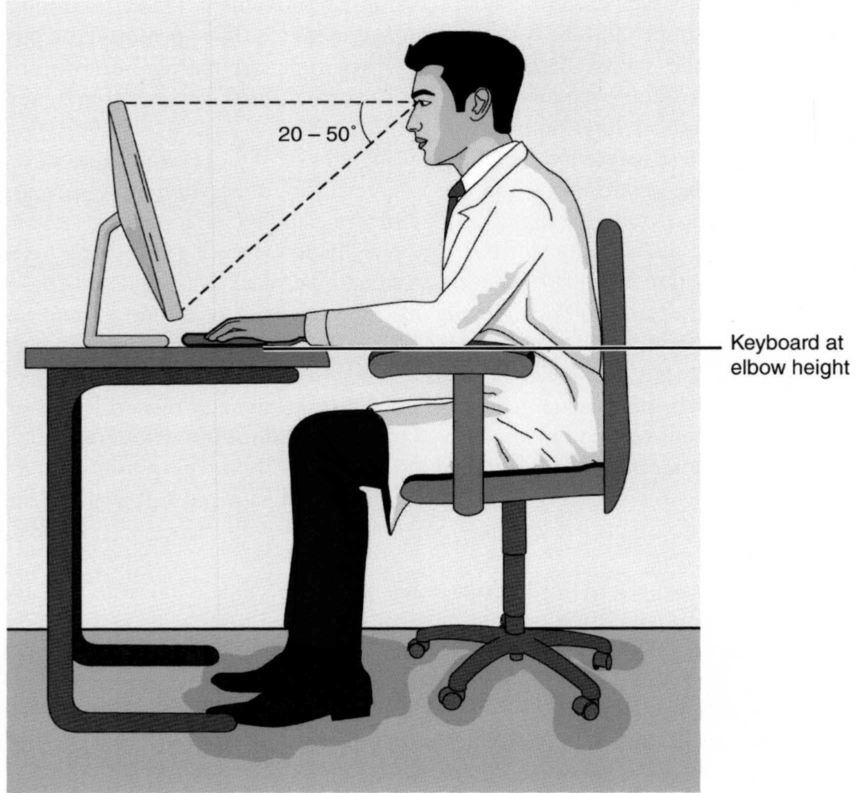

Fig. 22.7 The center of the computer screen is 20–50° below the eye level and the monitor tilted so that the upper part of the screen is further back than the lower. The keyboard is at elbow height and at least 5 inches from the edge of the desk

level [125, 127] and with the monitor tilted so that the upper part of the screen is further back than the lower (Fig. 22.7) [72, 78].

In regard to chairs, there are many ergonomically designed office chairs available. Overall, a chair with lumbar support and adjustable height and inclination is recommended. The seat should be padded with the front edges curved so that there is minimal pressure on the popliteal area [159]. Ideally, seated work is alternated with standing work [112]. This can be implemented using a standing desk or a desk with an adjustable height.

Surgeons may also experience discomfort with using the keyboard and mouse. Typing and clicking have been associated with multiple musculoskeletal disorders including carpal tunnel syndrome [160]. Carpal tunnel pressure increases with typing when the wrists are in flexion and with mouse use when the wrists are extended [161–163]. For those surgeons experiencing discomfort with these activities, ergonomic intervention has been shown to provide 89% improvement in symptoms. Ergonomic intervention includes maintaining a light touch and neutral wrist position. The keyboard should be placed at a distance of at least 5 inches from the edge of the desk. The chair height should be adjusted so that the keyboard is at elbow height and the shoulders relaxed to avoid upper extremity strain [160]. Dictation and use of voice recognition software are other options that can decrease the amount of typing required.

Regular Exercise

Exercise is important to reduce the risk of occupational injury. A study by Sivak-Callcott et al. suggests that surgeons who exercise an average of 5 h per week are less likely to experience pain or spinal disorders that result in the need to modify operating practice, when compared to surgeons who exercise less [29]. Core-strengthening exercises can prevent pain with standing while operating. Tse and colleagues found that those who received trunk muscle training for 6 weeks experienced significantly less discomfort and fewer errors during laparoscopic simulation than those who did not train [164]. Strength training is often accompanied by transient muscular soreness especially when beginning a new program; however, the long-term benefits of strength training appear to outweigh the initial increase in discomfort. A 10-week training program consisting of 20 min of trapezius-focused exercises 3 days a week was shown to significantly reduce neck discomfort in women with chronic neck pain [165]. General fitness training, such as bicycling, swimming, and performing other aerobic exercises, has been shown to increase the pain threshold transiently for about 2 h in non-exercised muscles and has also been shown to result in a reduction of the use of medications for back pain [165, 166].

Stretching is important to improve flexibility and range of motion and increase circulation to improve or prevent musculoskeletal injuries [144, 157]. Stretching exercises should be performed following a brief (<10 min) cardio warm-up three times a week. Static stretches should be maintained for 20–30 s with three repetitions to promote elongation of the muscle and other soft tissues. Dynamic stretching involves repeated movements which gradually increase in movement size and range of motion. Dynamic stretching and static stretching with a warm-up reduce muscular injuries [157].

Ergonomics for the Surgeon Educator

A lack of adherence to ergonomic principles in the operating room increases the risk of musculoskeletal discomfort [10, 14, 83, 97]. This may be especially true for residents who, while focusing on the operative procedure, pay less attention to ergonomic conditions including their own posture. If an occupational injury occurs, surgical training may be prolonged, directly affecting a resident's career as well as the residency program [59]. Evidence suggests that trainee and surgeon performance improves when optimizing posture [102], monitor position [46, 98, 121–123], and table height [97, 132]. Surgical warm-up [99, 146–150] and intraoperative breaks [56, 154, 155] have similar benefits.

Ergonomic education may be as simple as providing in-person feedback in the operating room. Franasiak and colleagues found that, following in-person ergonomic training in robotic surgery, 88% changed their practice and 74% noted reduced muscular strain. All these surgeons found in-person education helpful and felt formal ergonomic training should be required for robotics [20]. In-person ergonomic education should encompass walking the resident through proper operating room setup. This includes placing the top of the monitor at eye level and directly in front of the surgeons [91, 119, 122, 123], placing the foot pedal directly in front of the working foot [133], and adjusting the operating surface to pubic height for laparoscopic cases [130, 131] and to elbow height for open cases while taking into account the height of the resident [129]. Staff surgeons may also implement intraoperative breaks allowing all members of the surgical team to reap the benefits.

Given that the ACMGE requires all surgery programs to have access to a simulation lab, ergonomic training may take place in a simulated setting [58]. Xiao et al. found that a series of exercises simulating various table and monitor heights and ideal ergonomic setup helped surgeons understand human factors in the operating room [99]. Residents may practice operating with correct posture in the simulation lab without concern for distraction from the operative case. We have found that a short course of didactic instruction, self-assessment of postures from their own surgical videos, and simulation lab practice are effective in raising awareness of ergonomics among both residents and attending surgeons. This is best followed up with in-person intraoperative coaching to help with implementation. Residents can also use simulators to warm-up prior beginning the operative day. Ergonomists are available at some institutions and can work directly with staff surgeons and residents, especially in the office environment.

Finally, attending surgeons have the opportunity to help change some negative aspects of surgical culture. Surgical culture not only tends to deny the presence and negative impact of musculoskeletal discomfort but is also resistant to changes in surgical practice. Surgeon educators play a key role in demonstrating to residents how competent leaders facilitate changes in practice, set up ergonomically friendly operating rooms, demonstrate proper instrument use, maintain correct postures, and incorporate breaks and warm-ups into their routines. Understanding the impact of ergonomics on intraoperative performance will lead to innovative research and intervention strategies for prevention of musculoskeletal injury to improve the performance and well-being of the next generation of surgeons.

Acknowledgments This material is the result of work supported with resources and use of facilities at the Minneapolis VA Health Care System.

Disclaimer The contents of this publication do not represent the views of the US Department of Veterans Affairs or the US government.

References

1. Definition and Domains of Ergonomics. In: What is ergonomics? International Ergonomics Association. 2017. http://www.iea.cc/whats/. Accessed 4/11/2017.
2. Bureau of Labor Statistics. In: Occupational employment statistics. U.S Department of Labor. 2015. www.bls.gov/oes/. Accessed 4 Nov 2017.
3. Goodman GR. Electrosurgery burns and the urologist. J Urol. 1976;116(2):218–20.
4. Neuberger J, Vergani D, Mieli-Vergani G, Davis M, Williams R. Hepatic damage after exposure to halothane in medical personnel. Br J Anaesth. 1981;53(11):1173–7.
5. Berguer R, Forkey DL, Smith WD. Ergonomic problems associated with laparoscopic surgery. Surg Endosc. 1999;13(5):466–8.
6. Buia A, Stockhausen F, Hanisch E. Laparoscopic surgery: a qualified systematic review. World J Methodol. 2015;5(4):238–54. https://doi.org/10.5662/wjm.v5.i4.238.
7. Sari V, Nieboer TE, Vierhout ME, Stegeman DF, Kluivers KB. The operation room as a hostile environment for surgeons: physical complaints during and after laparoscopy. Minim Invasive Ther Allied Technol. 2010;19(2):105–9. https://doi.org/10.3109/13645701003643972.
8. Plerhoples TA, Hernandez-Boussard T, Wren SM. The aching surgeon: a survey of physical discomfort and symptoms following open, laparoscopic, and robotic surgery. J Robot Surg. 2012;6(1):65–72. https://doi.org/10.1007/s11701-011-0330-3.
9. Franasiak J, Ko EM, Kidd J, Secord AA, Bell M, Boggess JF, et al. Physical strain and urgent need for ergonomic training among gynecologic oncologists who perform minimally invasive surgery. Gynecol Oncol. 2012;126(3):437–42. https://doi.org/10.1016/j.ygyno.2012.05.016.
10. Miller K, Benden M, Pickens A, Shipp E, Zheng Q. Ergonomics principles associated with laparoscopic surgeon injury/illness. Hum Factors. 2012;54(6):1087–92. https://doi.org/10.1177/0018720812451046.
11. Park A, Lee G, Seagull FJ, Meenaghan N, Dexter D. Patients benefit while surgeons suffer: an impending epidemic. J Am Coll Surg. 2010;210(3):306–13. https://doi.org/10.1016/j.jamcollsurg.2009.10.017.
12. Stomberg MW, Tronstad SE, Hedberg K, Bengtsson J, Jonsson P, Johansen L, et al. Work-related musculoskeletal disorders when performing laparoscopic surgery. Surg Laparosc Endosc Percutan Tech. 2010;20(1):49–53. https://doi.org/10.1097/SLE.0b013e3181cded54.
13. Szeto GP, Ho P, Ting AC, Poon JT, Cheng SW, Tsang RC. Work-related musculoskeletal symptoms in surgeons. J Occup Rehabil. 2009;19(2):175–84. https://doi.org/10.1007/s10926-009-9176-1.
14. Wauben LS, van Veelen MA, Gossot D, Goossens RH. Application of ergonomic guidelines during minimally invasive surgery: a questionnaire survey of 284 surgeons. Surg Endosc. 2006;20(8):1268–74. https://doi.org/10.1007/s00464-005-0647-y.
15. Welcker K, Kesieme EB, Internullo E, Kranenburg van Koppen LJ. Ergonomics in thoracoscopic surgery: results of a survey among thoracic surgeons. Interact Cardiovasc Thorac Surg. 2012;15(2):197–200. https://doi.org/10.1093/icvts/ivs173.
16. Hemal AK, Srinivas M, Charles AR. Ergonomic problems associated with laparoscopy. J Endourol. 2001;15(5):499–503. https://doi.org/10.1089/089277901750299294.
17. Bagrodia A, Raman JD. Ergonomics considerations of radical prostatectomy: physician perspective of open, laparoscopic, and robot-assisted techniques. J Endourol. 2009;23(4):627–33. https://doi.org/10.1089/end.2008.0556.
18. Quinn D, Moohan J. The trainees' pain with laparoscopic surgery: what do trainees really know about theatre set-up and how this impacts their health. Gynecol Surg. 2015;12(1):71–6.
19. Giberti C, Gallo F, Francini L, Signori A, Testa M. Musculoskeletal disorders among robotic surgeons: a questionnaire analysis. Arch Ital Urol Androl. 2014;86(2):95–8. https://doi.org/10.4081/aiua.2014.2.95.
20. Franasiak J, Craven R, Mosaly P, Gehrig PA. Feasibility and acceptance of a robotic surgery ergonomic training program. JSLS. 2014;18(4). https://doi.org/10.4293/JSLS.2014.00166.

21. Soueid A, Oudit D, Thiagarajah S, Laitung G. The pain of surgery: pain experienced by surgeons while operating. Int J Surg. 2010;8(2):118–20. https://doi.org/10.1016/j.ijsu.2009.11.008.
22. Lawther RE, Kirk GR, Regan MC. Laparoscopic procedures are associated with a significant risk of digital nerve injury for general surgeons. Ann R Coll Surg Engl. 2002;84(6):443.
23. Liberman AS, Shrier I, Gordon PH. Injuries sustained by colorectal surgeons performing colonoscopy. Surg Endosc. 2005;19(12):1606–9. https://doi.org/10.1007/s00464-005-0219-1.
24. Singh R, Carranza Leon DA, Morrow MM, Vos-Draper TL, Mc Gree ME, Weaver AL, et al. Effect of chair types on work-related musculoskeletal discomfort during vaginal surgery. Am J Obstet Gynecol. 2016;215(5):648 e1–9. https://doi.org/10.1016/j.ajog.2016.06.016.
25. Cass GK, Vyas S, Akande V. Prolonged laparoscopic surgery is associated with an increased risk of vertebral disc prolapse. J Obstet Gynaecol. 2014;34(1):74–8. https://doi.org/10.3109/01443615.2013.831048.
26. Adams SR, Hacker MR, McKinney JL, Elkadry EA, Rosenblatt PL. Musculoskeletal pain in gynecologic surgeons. J Minim Invasive Gynecol. 2013;20(5):656–60. https://doi.org/10.1016/j.jmig.2013.04.013.
27. McDonald ME, Ramirez PT, Munsell MF, Greer M, Burke WM, Naumann WT, et al. Physician pain and discomfort during minimally invasive gynecologic cancer surgery. Gynecol Oncol. 2014;134(2):243–7. https://doi.org/10.1016/j.ygyno.2014.05.019.
28. Auerbach JD, Weidner ZD, Milby AH, Diab M, Lonner BS. Musculoskeletal disorders among spine surgeons: results of a survey of the Scoliosis Research Society membership. Spine (Phila Pa 1976). 2011;36(26):E1715–21. https://doi.org/10.1097/BRS.0b013e31821cd140.
29. Sivak-Callcott JA, Diaz SR, Ducatman AM, Rosen CL, Nimbarte AD, Sedgeman JA. A survey study of occupational pain and injury in ophthalmic plastic surgeons. Ophthal Plast Reconstr Surg. 2011;27(1):28–32. https://doi.org/10.1097/IOP.0b013e3181e99cc8.
30. Dhimitri KC, McGwin G Jr, McNeal SF, Lee P, Morse PA, Patterson M, et al. Symptoms of musculoskeletal disorders in ophthalmologists. Am J Ophthalmol. 2005;139(1):179–81. https://doi.org/10.1016/j.ajo.2004.06.091.
31. Kazancioglu HO, Bereket MC, Ezirganli S, Ozsevik S, Sener I. Musculoskeletal complaints among oral and maxillofacial surgeons and dentists: a questionnaire study. Acta Odontol Scand. 2013;71(3–4):469–74. https://doi.org/10.3109/00016357.2012.696688.
32. Shaik AR, Rao SB, Husain A, D'sa J. Work-related musculoskeletal disorders among dental surgeons: a pilot study. Contemp Clin Dent. 2011;2(4):308–12. https://doi.org/10.4103/0976-237X.91794.
33. Mirbod SM, Yoshida H, Miyamoto K, Miyashita K, Inaba R, Iwata H. Subjective complaints in orthopedists and general surgeons. Int Arch Occup Environ Health. 1995;67(3):179–86.
34. AlQahtani SM, Alzahrani MM, Harvey EJ. Prevalence of musculoskeletal disorders among orthopedic trauma surgeons: an OTA survey. Can J Surg. 2016;59(1):42–7.
35. Cavanagh J, Brake M, Kearns D, Hong P. Work environment discomfort and injury: an ergonomic survey study of the American Society of Pediatric Otolaryngology members. Am J Otolaryngol. 2012;33(4):441–6. https://doi.org/10.1016/j.amjoto.2011.10.022.
36. Babar-Craig H, Banfield G, Knight J. Prevalence of back and neck pain amongst ENT consultants: national survey. J Laryngol Otol. 2003;117(12):979–82. https://doi.org/10.1258/002221503322683885.
37. Rimmer J, Amin M, Fokkens WJ, Lund VJ. Endoscopic sinus surgery and musculoskeletal symptoms. Rhinology. 2016;54(2):105–10. https://doi.org/10.4193/Rhin15.217.
38. Wong A, Baker N, Smith L, Rosen CA. Prevalence and risk factors for musculoskeletal problems associated with microlaryngeal surgery: a national survey. Laryngoscope. 2014;124(8):1854–61. https://doi.org/10.1002/lary.24367.
39. Esposito C, Najmaldin A, Schier F, Yamataka A, Ferro M, Riccipetitoni G, et al. Work-related upper limb musculoskeletal disorders in pediatric minimally invasive surgery: a multicentric survey comparing laparoscopic and sils ergonomy. Pediatr Surg Int. 2014;30(4):395–9. https://doi.org/10.1007/s00383-013-3437-y.
40. Filisetti C, Cho A, Riccipetitoni G, Saxena AK. Analysis of hand size and ergonomics of instruments in pediatric minimally invasive surgery. Surg Laparosc Endosc Percutan Tech. 2015;25(5):e159–62. https://doi.org/10.1097/SLE.0000000000000125.

41. Alzahrani MM, Alqahtani SM, Tanzer M, Hamdy RC. Musculoskeletal disorders among orthopedic pediatric surgeons: an overlooked entity. J Child Orthop. 2016;10(5):461–6. https://doi.org/10.1007/s11832-016-0767-z.
42. Capone AC, Parikh PM, Gatti ME, Davidson BJ, Davison SP. Occupational injury in plastic surgeons. Plast Reconstr Surg. 2010;125(5):1555–61. https://doi.org/10.1097/PRS.0b013e3181d62a94.
43. Tzeng YS, Chen SG, Chen TM. Herniation of the cervical disk in plastic surgeons. Ann Plast Surg. 2012;69(6):672–4. https://doi.org/10.1097/SAP.0b013e3182742743.
44. Tjiam IM, Goossens RH, Schout BM, Koldewijn EL, Hendrikx AJ, Muijtjens AM, et al. Ergonomics in endourology and laparoscopy: an overview of musculoskeletal problems in urology. J Endourol. 2014;28(5):605–11. https://doi.org/10.1089/end.2013.0654.
45. Wolf JS Jr, Marcovich R, Gill IS, Sung GT, Kavoussi LR, Clayman RV, et al. Survey of neuromuscular injuries to the patient and surgeon during urologic laparoscopic surgery. Urology. 2000;55(6):831–6.
46. Liang B, Qi L, Yang J, Cao Z, Zu X, Liu L, et al. Ergonomic status of laparoscopic urologic surgery: survey results from 241 urologic surgeons in china. PLoS One. 2013;8(7):e70423. https://doi.org/10.1371/journal.pone.0070423.
47. Gofrit ON, Mikahail AA, Zorn KC, Zagaja GP, Steinberg GD, Shalhav AL. Surgeons' perceptions and injuries during and after urologic laparoscopic surgery. Urology. 2008;71(3):404–7. https://doi.org/10.1016/j.urology.2007.07.077.
48. Davila V, Stone W, Hallbeck M, Money S. Physical discomfort in vascular surgeons. Society of clinical vascular surgeons 45th annual symposium, 18–22 Mar.
49. Davis WT, Fletcher SA, Guillamondegui OD. Musculoskeletal occupational injury among surgeons: effects for patients, providers, and institutions. J Surg Res. 2014;189(2):207–212.e6. https://doi.org/10.1016/j.jss.2014.03.013.
50. Gerr F. Surveillance of work-related musculoskeletal disorders. Occup Environ Med. 2008;65(5):298–9. https://doi.org/10.1136/oem.2007.037515.
51. Davis WT, Sathiyakumar V, Jahangir AA, Obremskey WT, Sethi MK. Occupational injury among orthopaedic surgeons. J Bone Joint Surg Am. 2013;95(15):e107. https://doi.org/10.2106/JBJS.L.01427.
52. Janki S, Mulder EE, JN IJ, Tran TC. Ergonomics in the operating room. Surg Endosc. 2016. https://doi.org/10.1007/s00464-016-5247-5.
53. Vijendren A, Yung M, Sanchez J. The ill surgeon: a review of common work-related health problems amongst UK surgeons. Langenbeck's Arch Surg. 2014;399(8):967–79. https://doi.org/10.1007/s00423-014-1233-3.
54. Company MHAH. 2016 Physician inpatient/outpatient revenue survey. https://www.merritthawkins.com/uploadedFiles/MerrittHawkins/Surveys/Merritt_Hawkins-2016_RevSurvey.pdf. 2017.
55. Howarth A, Hallbeck S, Mahabir R, Lemaine V, Evans G, Noland S. Work-related physical discomfort in ASRM members: a survey. New York: American Society of Reconstructive Microsurgery; 2017.
56. Park AE, Zahiri HR, Hallbeck MS, Augenstein V, Sutton E, Yu D, et al. Intraoperative Micro Breaks with targeted stretching enhance surgeon physical function and mental focus: a multicenter cohort study. Ann Surg. 2016. https://doi.org/10.1097/SLA.0000000000001665.
57. The Complexities of Physician Supply and Demand: Projections from 2014 to 2025 [database on the Internet]. IHS Inc. Accessed.
58. ACGME program requirements for graduate medical education in general surgery. Accreditation Council for Graduate Medical Education. 2016.
59. Yoong W, Sanchez-Crespo J, Rob J, Parikh M, Melendez J, Pillai R, et al. Sticks and stones may break my bones: work-related orthopaedic injuries sustained during obstetrics and gynaecology training. J Obstet Gynaecol. 2008;28(5):478–81. https://doi.org/10.1080/01443610802091396.
60. Balch CM, Freischlag JA, Shanafelt TD. Stress and burnout among surgeons: understanding and managing the syndrome and avoiding the adverse consequences. Arch Surg. 2009;144(4):371–6. https://doi.org/10.1001/archsurg.2008.575.
61. Shanafelt TD, Balch CM, Bechamps GJ, Russell T, Dyrbye L, Satele D, et al. Burnout and career satisfaction among American surgeons. Ann Surg. 2009;250(3):463–71. https://doi.org/10.1097/SLA.0b013e3181ac4dfd.

62. Armon G, Melamed S, Shirom A, Shapira I. Elevated burnout predicts the onset of musculoskeletal pain among apparently healthy employees. J Occup Health Psychol. 2010;15(4):399–408. https://doi.org/10.1037/a0020726.
63. Berguer R, Rab GT, Abu-Ghaida H, Alarcon A, Chung J. A comparison of surgeons' posture during laparoscopic and open surgical procedures. Surg Endosc. 1997;11(2):139–42.
64. Berguer R, Smith WD, Chung YH. Performing laparoscopic surgery is significantly more stressful for the surgeon than open surgery. Surg Endosc. 2001;15(10):1204–7. https://doi.org/10.1007/s004640080030.
65. Wang R, Liang Z, Zihni AM, Ray S, Awad MM. Which causes more ergonomic stress: laparoscopic or open surgery? Surg Endosc. 2016. https://doi.org/10.1007/s00464-016-5360-5.
66. Kant IJ, de Jong LC, van Rijssen-Moll M, Borm PJ. A survey of static and dynamic work postures of operating room staff. Int Arch Occup Environ Health. 1992;63(6):423–8.
67. Kelsey JL, Githens PB, White AA 3rd, Holford TR, Walter SD, O'Connor T, et al. An epidemiologic study of lifting and twisting on the job and risk for acute prolapsed lumbar intervertebral disc. J Orthop Res. 1984;2(1):61–6. https://doi.org/10.1002/jor.1100020110.
68. Ng JK, Richardson CA, Parnianpour M, Kippers V. EMG activity of trunk muscles and torque output during isometric axial rotation exertion: a comparison between back pain patients and matched controls. J Orthop Res. 2002;20(1):112–21. https://doi.org/10.1016/S0736-0266(01)00067-5.
69. Szeto GP, Cheng SW, Poon JT, Ting AC, Tsang RC, Ho P. Surgeons' static posture and movement repetitions in open and laparoscopic surgery. J Surg Res. 2012;172(1):e19–31. https://doi.org/10.1016/j.jss.2011.08.004.
70. McGill SM, Hughson RL, Parks K. Lumbar erector spinae oxygenation during prolonged contractions: implications for prolonged work. Ergonomics. 2000;43(4):486–93. https://doi.org/10.1080/001401300184369.
71. Nguyen NT, Ho HS, Smith WD, Philipps C, Lewis C, De Vera RM, et al. An ergonomic evaluation of surgeons' axial skeletal and upper extremity movements during laparoscopic and open surgery. Am J Surg. 2001;182(6):720–4.
72. Uhrich ML, Underwood RA, Standeven JW, Soper NJ, Engsberg JR. Assessment of fatigue, monitor placement, and surgical experience during simulated laparoscopic surgery. Surg Endosc. 2002;16(4):635–9. https://doi.org/10.1007/s00464-001-8151-5.
73. Berguer R, Forkey DL, Smith WD. The effect of laparoscopic instrument working angle on surgeons' upper extremity workload. Surg Endosc. 2001;15(9):1027–9. https://doi.org/10.1007/s00464-001-0019-1.
74. Boppart SA, Deutsch TF, Rattner DW. Optical imaging technology in minimally invasive surgery. Current status and future directions. Surg Endosc. 1999;13(7):718–22.
75. Elfering A, Grebner S, Gerber H, Semmer NK. Workplace observation of work stressors, catecholamines and musculoskeletal pain among male employees. Scand J Work Environ Health. 2008;34(5):337–44.
76. Albayrak K, Meijer B. Current state of ergonomics of operating rooms of Dutch hospitals in the endoscopic era. Minim Invasive Ther Allied Technol. 2004;13(3):156–60. https://doi.org/10.1080/13645700410034093.
77. Kranenburg G. Ergonomic problems encountered during video-assisted thoracic surgery. Minim Invasive Ther Allied Technol. 2004;13(3):147–55. https://doi.org/10.1080/13645700410033661.
78. Reyes DA, Tang B, Cuschieri A. Minimal access surgery (MAS)-related surgeon morbidity syndromes. Surg Endosc. 2006;20(1):1–13. https://doi.org/10.1007/s00464-005-0315-2.
79. Ballantyne GH. The pitfalls of laparoscopic surgery: challenges for robotics and telerobotic surgery. Surg Laparosc Endosc Percutan Tech. 2002;12(1):1–5.
80. Sánchez-Margallo F, Sánchez-Margallo J. Ergonomics in laparoscopic surgery. In: Malik AM, editor. Laparoscopic surgery: InTech; 2017.
81. Yu D, Dural C, Morrow MM, Yang L, Collins JW, Hallbeck S, et al. Intraoperative workload in robotic surgery assessed by wearable motion tracking sensors and questionnaires. Surg Endosc. 2017;31(2):877–86. https://doi.org/10.1007/s00464-016-5047-y.

82. Craven R, Franasiak J, Mosaly P, Gehrig PA. Ergonomic deficits in robotic gynecologic oncology surgery: a need for intervention. J Minim Invasive Gynecol. 2013;20(5):648–55. https://doi.org/10.1016/j.jmig.2013.04.008.
83. Lee GI, Lee MR, Green I, Allaf M, Marohn MR. Surgeons' physical discomfort and symptoms during robotic surgery: a comprehensive ergonomic survey study. Surg Endosc. 2017;31(4):1697–706. https://doi.org/10.1007/s00464-016-5160-y.
84. Lux MM, Marshall M, Erturk E, Joseph JV. Ergonomic evaluation and guidelines for use of the daVinci Robot system. J Endourol. 2010;24(3):371–5. https://doi.org/10.1089/end.2009.0197.
85. Sillanpaa J, Nyberg M, Laippala P. A new table for work with a microscope, a solution to ergonomic problems. Appl Ergon. 2003;34(6):621–8. https://doi.org/10.1016/S0003-6870(03)00051-6.
86. Webb Associates Yellow Springs Ohio. Anthropology Research Project. A Handbook of anthropometric data. Anthropometric source book, vol 2. Washington Springfield: National Aeronautics and Space Administration for sale by the National Technical Information Service; 1978.
87. Webb Associates Yellow Springs Ohio. Anthropology Research Project. Anthropometry for designers. Anthropometric source book, vol 1. Washington Springfield: National Aeronautics and Space Administration for sale by the National Technical Information Service; 1978.
88. Berguer R, Hreljac A. The relationship between hand size and difficulty using surgical instruments: a survey of 726 laparoscopic surgeons. Surg Endosc. 2004;18(3):508–12. https://doi.org/10.1007/s00464-003-8824-3.
89. Sutton E, Irvin M, Zeigler C, Lee G, Park A. The ergonomics of women in surgery. Surg Endosc. 2014;28(4):1051–5. https://doi.org/10.1007/s00464-013-3281-0.
90. Voss RK, Chiang YJ, Cromwell KD, Urbauer DL, Lee JE, Cormier JN, et al. Do no harm, except to ourselves? A survey of symptoms and injuries in oncologic surgeons and pilot study of an intraoperative ergonomic intervention. J Am Coll Surg. 2017;224(1):16–25. e1. https://doi.org/10.1016/j.jamcollsurg.2016.09.013.
91. Aitchison LP, Cui CK, Arnold A, Nesbitt-Hawes E, Abbott J. The ergonomics of laparoscopic surgery: a quantitative study of the time and motion of laparoscopic surgeons in live surgical environments. Surg Endosc. 2016;30(11):5068–76. https://doi.org/10.1007/s00464-016-4855-4.
92. Strazdins L, Bammer G. Women, work and musculoskeletal health. Soc Sci Med. 2004;58(6): 997–1005.
93. Szeto GP, Lam P. Work-related musculoskeletal disorders in urban bus drivers of Hong Kong. J Occup Rehabil. 2007;17(2):181–98. https://doi.org/10.1007/s10926-007-9070-7.
94. Anderson R. The back pain of bus drivers. Prevalence in an urban area of California. Spine (Phila Pa 1976). 1992;17(12):1481–8.
95. Lee G, Lee T, Dexter D, Godinez C, Meenaghan N, Catania R, et al. Ergonomic risk associated with assisting in minimally invasive surgery. Surg Endosc. 2009;23(1):182–8. https://doi.org/10.1007/s00464-008-0141-4.
96. Zihni AM, Cavallo JA, Ray S, Ohu I, Cho S, Awad MM. Ergonomic analysis of primary and assistant surgical roles. J Surg Res. 2016;203(2):301–5. https://doi.org/10.1016/j.jss.2016.03.058.
97. Park JY, Kim KH, Kuh SU, Chin DK, Kim KS, Cho YE. Spine surgeon's kinematics during discectomy according to operating table height and the methods to visualize the surgical field. Eur Spine J. 2012;21(12):2704–12. https://doi.org/10.1007/s00586-012-2425-6.
98. Matern U, Faist M, Kehl K, Giebmeyer C, Buess G. Monitor position in laparoscopic surgery. Surg Endosc. 2005;19(3):436–40. https://doi.org/10.1007/s00464-004-9030-7.
99. Xiao DJ, Jakimowicz JJ, Albayrak A, Goossens RH. Ergonomic factors on task performance in laparoscopic surgery training. Appl Ergon. 2012;43(3):548–53. https://doi.org/10.1016/j.apergo.2011.08.010.
100. Bhatnager V, Drury CG, Schiro SG. Posture, postural discomfort, and performance. Hum Factors. 1985;27(2):189–99. https://doi.org/10.1177/001872088502700206.
101. Ernst E, Canter PH. The Alexander technique: a systematic review of controlled clinical trials. Forsch Komplementarmed Klass Naturheilkd. 2003;10(6):325–9. doi:75886

102. Reddy PP, Reddy TP, Roig-Francoli J, Cone L, Sivan B, DeFoor WR, et al. The impact of the alexander technique on improving posture and surgical ergonomics during minimally invasive surgery: pilot study. J Urol. 2011;186(4 Suppl):1658–62. https://doi.org/10.1016/j.juro.2011.04.013.
103. Bauer W, Wittig T. Influence of screen and copy holder positions on head posture, muscle activity and user judgement. Appl Ergon. 1998;29(3):185–92.
104. Seghers J, Jochem A, Spaepen A. Posture, muscle activity and muscle fatigue in prolonged VDT work at different screen height settings. Ergonomics. 2003;46(7):714–30. https://doi.org/10.1080/0014013031000090107.
105. Turville KL, Psihogios JP, Ulmer TR, Mirka GA. The effects of video display terminal height on the operator: a comparison of the 15 degree and 40 degree recommendations. Appl Ergon. 1998;29(4):239–46.
106. Matern U, Waller P. Instruments for minimally invasive surgery: principles of ergonomic handles. Surg Endosc. 1999;13(2):174–82.
107. van Veelen MA, Kazemier G, Koopman J, Goossens RH, Meijer DW. Assessment of the ergonomically optimal operating surface height for laparoscopic surgery. J Laparoendosc Adv Surg Tech A. 2002;12(1):47–52. https://doi.org/10.1089/109264202753486920.
108. Rosenblatt PL, McKinney J, Adams SR. Ergonomics in the operating room: protecting the surgeon. J Minim Invasive Gynecol. 2013;20(6):744. https://doi.org/10.1016/j.jmig.2013.07.006.
109. Graversen JA, Korets R, Mues AC, Katsumi HK, Badani KK, Landman J, et al. Prospective randomized evaluation of gel mat foot pads in the endoscopic suite. J Endourol. 2011;25(11):1793–6. https://doi.org/10.1089/end.2011.0155.
110. Cook J, Branch TP, Baranowski TJ, Hutton WC. The effect of surgical floor mats in prolonged standing: an EMG study of the lumbar paraspinal and anterior tibialis muscles. J Biomed Eng. 1993;15(3):247–50.
111. Aghazadeh J, Ghaderi M, Azghani MR, Khalkhali HR, Allahyari T, Mohebbi I. Anti-fatigue mats, low back pain, and electromyography: An interventional study. Int J Occup Med Environ Health. 2015;28(2):347–56. 10.13075/ijomeh.1896.00311.
112. Dul J, Weerdmeester BA. Ergonomics for beginners : a quick reference guide. 2nd ed. London/New York: Taylor & Francis; 2003.
113. Jafri M, Brown S, Arnold G, Abboud R, Wang W. Kinematical analysis of the trunk, upper limbs and fingers during minimal access surgery when using an armrest. Ergonomics. 2015;58(11):1868–77. https://doi.org/10.1080/00140139.2015.1039603.
114. van Det MJ, Meijerink WJ, Hoff C, Totte ER, Pierie JP. Optimal ergonomics for laparoscopic surgery in minimally invasive surgery suites: a review and guidelines. Surg Endosc. 2009;23(6):1279–85. https://doi.org/10.1007/s00464-008-0148-x.
115. El Shallaly G, Cuschieri A. Optimum view distance for laparoscopic surgery. Surg Endosc. 2006;20(12):1879–82. https://doi.org/10.1007/s00464-005-0162-1.
116. Kelts GI, McMains KC, Chen PG, Weitzel EK. Monitor height ergonomics: a comparison of operating room video display terminals. Allergy Rhinol (Providence). 2015;6(1):28–32. https://doi.org/10.2500/ar.2015.6.0119.
117. van Det MJ, Meijerink WJ, Hoff C, van Veelen MA, Pierie JP. Ergonomic assessment of neck posture in the minimally invasive surgery suite during laparoscopic cholecystectomy. Surg Endosc. 2008;22(11):2421–7. https://doi.org/10.1007/s00464-008-0042-6.
118. Erfanian K, Luks FI, Kurkchubasche AG, Wesselhoeft CW Jr, Tracy TF Jr. In-line image projection accelerates task performance in laparoscopic appendectomy. J Pediatr Surg. 2003;38(7):1059–62.
119. Zehetner J, Kaltenbacher A, Wayand W, Shamiyeh A. Screen height as an ergonomic factor in laparoscopic surgery. Surg Endosc. 2006;20(1):139–41. https://doi.org/10.1007/s00464-005-0251-1.
120. Jaschinski-Kruza W. Eyestrain in VDU users: viewing distance and the resting position of ocular muscles. Hum Factors. 1991;33(1):69–83. https://doi.org/10.1177/001872089103300106.
121. Omar AM, Wade NJ, Brown SI, Cuschieri A. Assessing the benefits of "gaze-down" display location in complex tasks. Surg Endosc. 2005;19(1):105–8. https://doi.org/10.1007/s00464-004-8141-5.

122. Hanna GB, Shimi SM, Cuschieri A. Task performance in endoscopic surgery is influenced by location of the image display. Ann Surg. 1998;227(4):481–4.
123. Haveran LA, Novitsky YW, Czerniach DR, Kaban GK, Taylor M, Gallagher-Dorval K, et al. Optimizing laparoscopic task efficiency: the role of camera and monitor positions. Surg Endosc. 2007;21(6):980–4. https://doi.org/10.1007/s00464-007-9360-3.
124. Kroemer KH, Hill SG. Preferred line of sight angle. Ergonomics. 1986;29(9):1129–34. https://doi.org/10.1080/00140138608967228.
125. Hill SG, Kroemer KH. Preferred declination of the line of sight. Hum Factors. 1986;28(2):127–34. https://doi.org/10.1177/001872088602800201.
126. Sommerich CM, Joines SM, Psihogios JP. Effects of computer monitor viewing angle and related factors on strain, performance, and preference outcomes. Hum Factors. 2001;43(1):39–55. https://doi.org/10.1518/001872001775992480.
127. Ripple PH. Variation of accommodation in vertical directions of gaze. Am J Ophthalmol. 1952;35(11):1630–4.
128. Rodigari A, Bejor M, Carlisi E, Lisi C, Tinelli C, Toffola ED. Identification of risk factors for fatigue and pain when performing surgical interventions. G Ital Med Lav Ergon. 2012;34(4):432–7.
129. Ayoub MM. Work place design and posture. Hum Factors. 1973;15(3):265–8. https://doi.org/10.1177/001872087301500309.
130. Matern U, Waller P, Giebmeyer C, Ruckauer KD, Farthmann EH. Ergonomics: requirements for adjusting the height of laparoscopic operating tables. JSLS. 2001;5(1):7–12.
131. Berquer R, Smith WD, Davis S. An ergonomic study of the optimum operating table height for laparoscopic surgery. Surg Endosc. 2002;16(3):416–21. https://doi.org/10.1007/s00464-001-8190-y.
132. Manasnayakorn S, Cuschieri A, Hanna GB. Ergonomic assessment of optimum operating table height for hand-assisted laparoscopic surgery. Surg Endosc. 2009;23(4):783–9. https://doi.org/10.1007/s00464-008-0068-9.
133. van Veelen MA, Snijders CJ, van Leeuwen E, Goossens RH, Kazemier G. Improvement of foot pedals used during surgery based on new ergonomic guidelines. Surg Endosc. 2003;17(7):1086–91. https://doi.org/10.1007/s00464-002-9185-z.
134. Gordon DJ, Wilkinson P. Prolonged use of a surgical retractor causing neuropathy in an assistant. J R Coll Surg Edinb. 1991;36(2):132.
135. Sackier JM, Berci G. A laparoscopic hazard for the surgeon. Br J Surg. 1992;79(7):713.
136. Steele PR, Curran JF, Mountain RE. Current and future practices in surgical retraction. Surgeon. 2013;11(6):330–7. https://doi.org/10.1016/j.surge.2013.06.004.
137. Blackwell JR, Kornatz KW, Heath EM. Effect of grip span on maximal grip force and fatigue of flexor digitorum superficialis. Appl Ergon. 1999;30(5):401–5.
138. Putzer D, Klug S, Haselbacher M, Mayr E, Nogler M. Retracting soft tissue in minimally invasive hip arthroplasty using a robotic arm: a comparison between a semiactive retractor holder and human assistants in a cadaver study. Surg Innov. 2015;22(5):500–7. https://doi.org/10.1177/1553350615586110.
139. Chang BJ. Ergonomic benefits of surgical telescope systems: selection guidelines. J Calif Dent Assoc. 2002;30(2):161–9.
140. Alexandre D, Prieto M, Beaumont F, Taiar R, Polidori G. Wearing lead aprons in surgical operating rooms: ergonomic injuries evidenced by infrared thermography. J Surg Res. 2017;209:227–33. https://doi.org/10.1016/j.jss.2016.10.019.
141. van Veelen MA, Nederlof EA, Goossens RH, Schot CJ, Jakimowicz JJ. Ergonomic problems encountered by the medical team related to products used for minimally invasive surgery. Surg Endosc. 2003;17(7):1077–81. https://doi.org/10.1007/s00464-002-9105-2.
142. Moore B, van Sonnenberg E, Casola G, Novelline RA. The relationship between back pain and lead apron use in radiologists. AJR Am J Roentgenol. 1992;158(1):191–3. https://doi.org/10.2214/ajr.158.1.1530763.
143. Pelz DM. Low back pain, lead aprons, and the angiographer. AJNR Am J Neuroradiol. 2000;21(7):1364.

144. Small K, Mc Naughton L, Matthews M. A systematic review into the efficacy of static stretching as part of a warm-up for the prevention of exercise-related injury. Res Sports Med. 2008;16(3):213–31. https://doi.org/10.1080/15438620802310784.
145. Neiva HP, Marques MC, Barbosa TM, Izquierdo M, Marinho DA. Warm-up and performance in competitive swimming. Sports Med. 2014;44(3):319–30. https://doi.org/10.1007/s40279-013-0117-y.
146. Lee JY, Mucksavage P, Kerbl DC, Osann KE, Winfield HN, Kahol K, et al. Laparoscopic warm-up exercises improve performance of senior-level trainees during laparoscopic renal surgery. J Endourol. 2012;26(5):545–50. https://doi.org/10.1089/end.2011.0418.
147. Chen CC, Green IC, Colbert-Getz JM, Steele K, Chou B, Lawson SM, et al. Warm-up on a simulator improves residents' performance in laparoscopic surgery: a randomized trial. Int Urogynecol J. 2013;24(10):1615–22. https://doi.org/10.1007/s00192-013-2066-2.
148. Abdalla G, Moran-Atkin E, Chen G, Schweitzer MA, Magnuson TH, Steele KE. The effect of warm-up on surgical performance: a systematic review. Surg Endosc. 2015;29(6):1259–69. https://doi.org/10.1007/s00464-014-3811-4.
149. Lendvay TS, Brand TC, White L, Kowalewski T, Jonnadula S, Mercer LD, et al. Virtual reality robotic surgery warm-up improves task performance in a dry laboratory environment: a prospective randomized controlled study. J Am Coll Surg. 2013;216(6):1181–92. https://doi.org/10.1016/j.jamcollsurg.2013.02.012.
150. Moran-Atkin E, Abdalla G, Chen G, Magnuson TH, Lidor AO, Schweitzer MA, et al. Preoperative warm-up the key to improved resident technique: a randomized study. Surg Endosc. 2015;29(5):1057–63. https://doi.org/10.1007/s00464-014-3778-1.
151. Varela-Mato V, Yates T, Stensel DJ, Biddle SJ, Clemes SA. Time spent sitting during and outside working hours in bus drivers: a pilot study. Prev Med Rep. 2016;3:36–9. https://doi.org/10.1016/j.pmedr.2015.11.011.
152. Caldwell JA, Mallis MM, Caldwell JL, Paul MA, Miller JC, Neri DF, et al. Fatigue countermeasures in aviation. Aviat Space Environ Med. 2009;80(1):29–59.
153. Fatigue Management for Nuclear Power Plant Personnel. US Nuclear Regulator Commission Regulator Guide 2009;March(5.73).
154. Dorion D, Darveau S. Do micropauses prevent surgeon's fatigue and loss of accuracy associated with prolonged surgery? An experimental prospective study. Ann Surg. 2013;257(2):256–9. https://doi.org/10.1097/SLA.0b013e31825efe87.
155. Engelmann C, Schneider M, Kirschbaum C, Grote G, Dingemann J, Schoof S, et al. Effects of intraoperative breaks on mental and somatic operator fatigue: a randomized clinical trial. Surg Endosc. 2011;25(4):1245–50. https://doi.org/10.1007/s00464-010-1350-1.
156. Hallbeck MS, Lowndes BR, Bingener J, Abdelrahman AM, Yu D, Bartley A, et al. The impact of intraoperative microbreaks with exercises on surgeons: a multi-center cohort study. Appl Ergon. 2017;60:334–41. https://doi.org/10.1016/j.apergo.2016.12.006.
157. Micheo W, Baerga L, Miranda G. Basic principles regarding strength, flexibility, and stability exercises. PM R. 2012;4(11):805–11. https://doi.org/10.1016/j.pmrj.2012.09.583.
158. Zheng B, Martinec DV, Cassera MA, Swanstrom LL. A quantitative study of disruption in the operating room during laparoscopic antireflux surgery. Surg Endosc. 2008;22(10):2171–7. https://doi.org/10.1007/s00464-008-0017-7.
159. Woo EH, White P, Lai CW. Ergonomics standards and guidelines for computer workstation design and the impact on users' health – a review. Ergonomics. 2016;59(3):464–75. https://doi.org/10.1080/00140139.2015.1076528.
160. Bleecker ML, Celio MA, Barnes SK. A medical-ergonomic program for symptomatic keyboard/mouse users. J Occup Environ Med. 2011;53(5):562–8. https://doi.org/10.1097/JOM.0b013e31821719af.
161. Rempel DM, Keir PJ, Bach JM. Effect of wrist posture on carpal tunnel pressure while typing. J Orthop Res. 2008;26(9):1269–73. https://doi.org/10.1002/jor.20599.
162. Keir PJ, Bach JM, Hudes M, Rempel DM. Guidelines for wrist posture based on carpal tunnel pressure thresholds. Hum Factors. 2007;49(1):88–99. https://doi.org/10.1518/001872007779598127.

163. Feuerstein M, Armstrong T, Hickey P, Lincoln A. Computer keyboard force and upper extremity symptoms. J Occup Environ Med. 1997;39(12):1144–53.
164. Tse MA, Masters RS, McManus AM, Lo CY, Patil NG. Trunk muscle training, posture fatigue, and performance in laparoscopic surgery. J Endourol. 2008;22(5):1053–8. https://doi.org/10.1089/end.2007.0409.
165. Andersen LL, Kjaer M, Sogaard K, Hansen L, Kryger AI, Sjogaard G. Effect of two contrasting types of physical exercise on chronic neck muscle pain. Arthritis Rheum. 2008;59(1):84–91. https://doi.org/10.1002/art.23256.
166. Sculco AD, Paup DC, Fernhall B, Sculco MJ. Effects of aerobic exercise on low back pain patients in treatment. Spine J. 2001;1(2):95–101.

Evaluation and Management Documentation, Billing, and Coding

23

Tobias S. Köhler

Why You Should Care and Why I Care You Care

You have perfected your left-handed knot tying, finally mastered the anatomy of the inguinal canal, and are ready to start your new surgical career and then comes your first day of surgery clinic. You do a great job of staying on time, being professional, and having a solid set of patient encounters. At the end of the day, your nurse hands you a stack of billing tickets to fill out (and by the way, your first 20 notes will be audited by the practice manager). Are you prepared? Hint – charging all of your patients level E3 (established level 3) is not the right answer.

E & M codes are billed in the office, hospital, skilled nursing facility, home care, inpatient, observation, emergency, and outpatient settings. Codes run levels 1–5. For established codes, one can bill E1, E2, E3, E4, and E5. Similarly for new and consult patients, one can bill N1–N5 and C1–C5. There are higher levels of billing for visits that take an inordinate amount of time which we won't get into. Tables 23.1 and 23.2 display the difference in relative value units (RVUs) for the different levels. RVUs are a standardized way of attributing value to medical labor and how you get paid. Study the tables and memorize the relative increases in value of the different strata. Also listed here are the time requirements for timed billing (more on that later).

When I went through orientation for my first job as a surgical attending, I officially spent more time learning how to properly manage toxic waste than how to document and bill properly (I'm a urologist, not a nuclear power plant worker). After a series of billing audits and several heated discussions, I vowed to learn billing better than my "auditor." I also planned to get hold of that secret book with all the answers to the tough billing nuances (still searching by the way). I read a billing

T.S. Köhler, MD, MPH, FACS
Urology, Mayo Clinic, Rochester, MN, USA
e-mail: Kohler.tobias@mayo.edu

T.S. Köhler, B. Schwartz (eds.), *Surgeons as Educators*,
https://doi.org/10.1007/978-3-319-64728-9_23

Table 23.1 Relative value of established visit and timing thresholds

Established visits data			
	RVU	% increase	Time (min)
E1	0.18		5
E2	0.48	166	10
E3	0.97	102	15
E4	1.5	54	25
E5	2.I	40	40

Table 23.2 Relative value of new and consult visits and timing thresholds

New and consult data				
	RVU	% increase	% change N→C	Time (min)
Nl	0.48			10
N2	0.93	94		20
N3	1.42	53		30
N4	2.43	71		45
N5	3.17	30		60
Cl	0.64		33	15
C2	1.34	109	44	30
C3	1.88	40	32	40
C4	3.02	61	24	60
C5	3.77	25	19	80

book over a weekend (it only took a few hours) and felt eminently more prepared. My interest blossomed, and I attended a few billing courses. All of sudden, boom, I became the go-to guy for billing in surgery at my institution. For 8 years I gave yearly lectures for many of our divisions in surgery, and I am still learning.

Why is some random urologist *passionate* about a topic other than the strength of your urinary stream? In a word: anger, annoyance, and pride. Fine, three words. *Anger* (and thanks) stems from all the chart audits stating I overbilled (still arguing about those) but never told me I under-billed had I just done this or that. This fueled me to learn the coding and billing system. *Annoyance* that when I talked to some of the brass about what I perceived as a clear deficiency ("improvement opportunity") in rampant under-billing and how I was willing to help, the crickets became deafening. Thanks to those who have encouraged and propelled my cause forward (you know who you are). *Pride* in that I want you and your new practice to do well. In retrospect, I can honestly say that learning E & M documentation and billing improves the following:

- Patient care
- Medicolegal concerns
- Resident and medical student learning
- Research opportunities

- Clinical efficiency
- Information back to referring providers
- Performance and reputation compared to peers
- Salary
- Free time
- Environment (yup as in save the dolphins)

Integrating E & M Coding into Surgical Training

Multiple studies across various subspecialties have reported resident uncertainty in clinical billing [1–2]. Furthermore, educational programs for system-based practice are not routine among US training programs [3–4]. One study showed 82% of residents felt inadequately trained and 85% labeled themselves “novices” at coding clinical encounters [5]. When queried, 70% of general surgery program directors believed their own residents were inadequately trained in business principles [6]. This is true despite the fact that 87% of program directors agreed that residents should be trained in practice management. The good news is that instillation of programs to teach coding and billing has shown great success in improving billing where average E & M codes increased by about one tier in both established new patient visits [7]. The key is active educator involvement and someone to take the initiative to get quality programs implemented. The occasional guest or outside lecturer on E & M coding seems wholly inadequate as the concepts are abstract and quickly forgotten unless reinforced in the clinic itself. A strong surgical educator will review and correct resident documentation and make a point to review this skill set in a semiannual review. Surgical mentors should get into the habit of asking what and why residents would bill encounters as a standard part of every clinic presentation.

Ethical Billing (Bake Me a Cake with a File in It Please)

I have less than zero interest in undergoing a government audit, having a patient complaint about excess charges, or going to prison. Fraud is “a deliberate act intended to obtain improper payment.” Abuse is “a repeated act that may not be deliberate but results in improper payments.” Innocent errors will not result in criminal or civil penalties. However, penalties will be imposed if the offense is committed with actual knowledge of the falsity of the claim, reckless disregard, or deliberate *ignorance* of the falsity of the claim. Physicians and their staff have a duty to make sure that claims are filed accurately.

Medicare estimates that primary care providers routinely under-bill by 45%. Considering that E & M coding is the sole revenue source for these providers, this is astonishing to me. Medicare also states that *both* overbilling and *under-billing* constitute fraud.

Under-billing: A great way to be inefficient and go to jail?

Although I am unaware of an actual case of someone going to prison for under-billing, here's my opinion on how it could work:

Clinic A

Urologist Frank – Dr. Frank is an all-around good guy, sees patients, and bills appropriately for his new patient visit and its inclusive preoperative counseling. Any time he books a laser surgery of the prostate; he appropriately bills new patient level 4 maybe even level 5 if the surgery is complex (i.e., higher rate of complications – that folks are foreshadowing). Frank charges the patient and insurance appropriately to the level earned.

Clinic B

Urologist Beans – Dr. Beans is not that ethical. He hangs his shingle and invites patients and sees them for free regardless of appropriate counseling. No charge but books a surgery. Do not pass go, do not collect $200 – that my friends is a monopoly. Inappropriately under-billing to increase surgical volume (ultimately where the higher payment comes from) seems to be an instance where the Feds may get interested.

If you don't want the Feds to get interested (9/10 MDs agree this is a good thing), remember the story of Dr. Frank and Beans.

Overbilling: Excellent Strategies to Earn Prison Time

Here it is, the fear of quality alone time that ultimately prevents people from billing appropriately. Plain and simple, it is *ignorance* of what the billing rules actually are that is the problem. If you know the rules cold, you won't worry about prison (instead you can focus on plane crashes, spiders, and public speaking) and will bill with confidence. Later on in this chapter, I will attempt to distill down the tomes of rules to a few key concepts. For now, I'd like to list some great ways to get behind bars quickly and list the most common mistakes I have encountered:

1. Billing for patient visits when you are actually on the golf course (or in bed asleep). Unless you have some fancy telemedicine apparatus in your golf cart or a futuristic state-of-the-art foam pillow, this is definitely a no-no. It goes without saying you shouldn't bill for clinic patients or operations in which you weren't actually available (I guess I said it). Same thing with attesting notes written by others (NPs, residents, etc.). The phrase "I have seen and examined the patient and agree with the above findings" does actually mean you saw the patient. Remember, residents are paid by the government for their efforts. If you bill for a procedure or consult in which you are not present, that constitutes double billing. Imagine a scenario where you bill for an unattended procedure in the ER that ultimately has a complication (probably more likely since you weren't there), and the case goes to trial, and you are called as a witness. Not only will the plaintiff likely win but you will be on the hook for fraud as well – not a good

day!!! Now for those who want to get technical, there is something called subject to billing which is beyond the scope of the brief chapter.

2. Billing on time when there isn't that much time in a day. If you are billing on time alone (which can be done with minimal documentation – minstrels are rejoicing), it is pretty easy to add up the numbers – 6 hours of "face-to-face" timed billed in a 4-hours morning clinic will probably raise some suspicion (minstrels unemployed).
3. Billing for consults when there is no documentation to support a consult request. Consult notes differ from new patient visits in only three key ways:
   1. It says at the request of Dr. X, I was asked to see this patient for problem Y.
   2. It says report to Dr. X at the bottom (and correspondence occurred).
   3. Most important there is a retrievable consult request form in the medical record somewhere. It cannot say transfer of care; it has to say consult from Dr. X. This component is most often missed.

Billing tip – Develop a system with your office staff that ensures this document from the consulting provider is available and retrievable at the time of the appointment. Some clinics go so far as to not seeing the patient if this consult form is not completed. When completed, it guarantees an average 30% increase in revenue per encounter (see Table 23.2*).*

4. Billing both procedure and E & M code in the same visit (use of a 25 modifier). Remember that any procedure you perform has some inherent counseling built into it (that's why it pays so much more). If performing a cystoscopy for blood in the urine, a urologist cannot charge both a procedure and a visit by explaining the normal landmarks during the exam. However, if bladder cancer is found and this leads to a new discussion, it is appropriate to use a modifier and charge for both. I make a point to let the patient get dressed from their procedure (patients never remember anything you tell them if they don't have pants on), perhaps have the bladder cancer discussion in a different room, and start a whole separate note detailing that portion of the visit.
5. Billing at a high level because you wrote a lot and the patient was very "stressful." Here again, ignorance bears its ugly head – a 5-page note is only billable on its weakest section. Time and time again, I've seen overbilling from deficiencies in the history portion of the review of systems (ROS). Residents excel at missing a complete ROS.
6. Billing established patients at high levels when medical decision-making required is low. This is *super* important. As you read on, you will later on be delighted (dare I say tickled pink) to discover that established visits require only two-thirds of the basic components of billing. A great way to commit fraud is to take a level 5 history, do a level 5 physical exam, make a level 2 decision (like prescribe gargles), and bill level 5 – more on this later.

After all is said and done, if you bill appropriately based on your medical decision-making, specifically risk within decision-making, you will never go wrong. If you make a level 5 risk decision, bill level 5 – you simply need to ensure your history and physical exam meet level 5 criteria as well.

Billing Excuses: Ignorance Abounds and the Dog Ate My Billing Ticket?
Here is the list of the most common reasons I have heard people justify their poor billing:

1. "My attendings told me to bill all level 2s and 3s" – Seriously? I guess the people at the print shop had a penchant for symmetrical ink use on the billing sheet, so they decided to include level 4 and level 5 as bonus options? I hear this so often I could vomit. It vexes me. I am very vexed. Not only are the "attendings" ignorant to billing rules they also pass on bad habits to learners. Arguably, physicians are some of the brightest and most industrious humans we have, yet they can't be bothered to learn this stuff? My vexation is your gain (whispers of billing superhero doesn't it). Read on.
2. "People who bill at high levels are just trying to game the system." In the immortal words of either Ice T or Gandhi – "Don't hate the playa." The billing system (to my amazement) is actually quite logical and fair. If one bills based on risk within medical decision-making, you are charging appropriately – not too much or too little. In addition, you can be rest assured that any flaw, omission, or tardiness your billing contains will happily be unpaid by payers.
3. "I don't want to overcharge the patient" – I would argue that there are better avenues to provide charity care. Additionally, a patient will often have the same co-pay for clinic visits regardless of level billed. Finally, the true cost of health care stems from the proverbial $32 box of tissues and the paradoxical effect of improved primary care increasing prevalence of chronic nonfatal disease and nursing home costs (shout out to my med economics prof).
4. If I charge level 3 instead of 4, my attending does not have to come into the room to see the patient. I wish I could somehow produce a tritonic fog horn sound singing "la-zy" for you right now.
5. I'm too lazy to learn how to document properly – refreshingly honest, but once again nauseating. Improper documentation is bad care and leads to medical errors. Once I understood the billing system, my notes became… wait for it…. Wait for it … hold … Hold… NOW … SHORTER. I stopped babbling with useless diatribe (in hopes of meeting billing criteria). Show of hands for who reads the 22-point med list and 18-point problem list from a consultant? Anyone? Bueller? Anyone? Here's a concept; list only those things that are necessary to the patient's problem and your plan. That's what the billing system encourages and wants you to do (you'll see this later on in the history section). My notes are so short now; I have saved over a million trees and dolphins (see, you can save the environment), and my notes are gloriously beautiful and readable.

Take a moment to think about your current billing skills. Are you the master who should have written this chapter, or are you a neophyte? Where does your billing stack up compared to your peers? What are your average RVUs per encounter? These questions led me to audit our entire surgery department and man were there disparities. Crazy disparities (I won't even mention that one of our most lucrative divisions charged zero consults over an entire year – their biller was under the misconception that consults no longer existed – true for Medicare patients not true for most other payers – WOOPS!!!!). If you are an outlier from the group on billing, you can be rest assured that CMS who sees the same aggregate data will look closer. A great place to start your journey toward billing excellence is having your office administrator run the numbers and give you a breakdown of your personal billing and how you compare to your peers.

Billing Mechanics

I hope I have convinced you that E & M coding is very important. Surgeons often underestimate the importance of E & M billing since they think they earn all of their revenue in the operating theater. After examining an entire surgical department, I discovered E & M RVUs made up between 20% and 45% of total RVUs (and this is with poor billing). Remember that there is rarely a dispute to an E3 charge, whereas complex surgical charges are often questioned and require appeals, etc. The good news is that billing is totally learnable.

All E & M notes rest on the foundation of the three billing pillars (Fig. 23.1): history, physical exam, and medical decision-making. A new patient visit (or consult visit) requires all three components. An established patient visit requires only two of the three!!! Thus, a follow-up established visit can be devoid of a history or physical exam (you pick which one) entirely. This is because there will always be medical decision-making. In 9 years of giving talks on billing and asking the audience what the fundamental difference is between an established and new patient, only one has answered correctly.

Before I launch into billing mechanics, I want to mention that the minimums I mention are for billing purposes only.

Minimum Billing Requirements ≠ Best Patient Care Documentation
I always will document more than the billing requirements when I feel it reveals important medical information and leads to better patient care. But I do not list anything more than necessary if it doesn't add to the note. Have you seen the notes that EHRs produce these days?

Pillar 1: History (Fig. 23.2)
The term history often conjures an image of the six-page H and P one performed on their first internal medicine rotation. This type of note and notes for billing efficiently couldn't be more different.

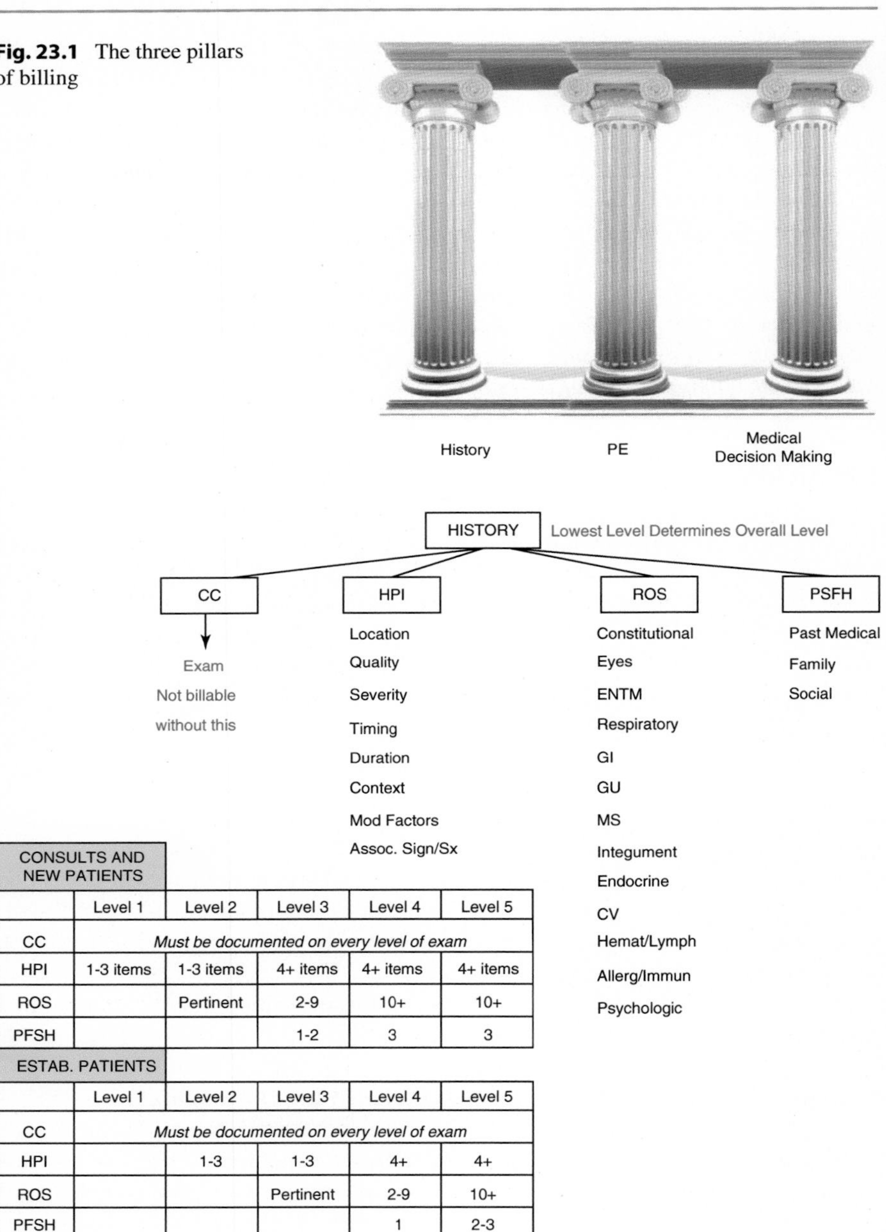

Fig. 23.1 The three pillars of billing

CONSULTS AND NEW PATIENTS					
	Level 1	Level 2	Level 3	Level 4	Level 5
CC	*Must be documented on every level of exam*				
HPI	1-3 items	1-3 items	4+ items	4+ items	4+ items
ROS		Pertinent	2-9	10+	10+
PFSH			1-2	3	3

ESTAB. PATIENTS					
	Level 1	Level 2	Level 3	Level 4	Level 5
CC	*Must be documented on every level of exam*				
HPI		1-3	1-3	4+	4+
ROS			Pertinent	2-9	10+
PFSH				1	2-3

Fig. 23.2 History billing rules

Pillar 1a: All Notes Require a Chief Complaint

Pillar 1b: HPI (History of Present Illness)

Most HPIs are rarely inadequate for billing. To bill maximally (or level 5), one has to have at least four bullets under the HPI. The bullets to choose from include location, quality, severity, timing, duration, context, modifying factors, and associated signs and symptoms. Keep in mind that location is sometimes a freebie; for example, erectile dysfunction is typically located in the penis, but this does not need to be explicitly stated. Thus HPIs can be relatively brief from a billing standpoint. However, you may want to include more bullets if it improves patient care.

Pillar 1c: ROS (Review of Systems)

The most common error performed by MDs is an insufficient ROS. A weak ROS instantly drops a level 5 visit to level 2 or 3!!! This is because the lowest billable section of the history is what determines what one can charge. For example, the billing level from a history with a CC, a seven-item HPI, and a complete past medical family and social history (PMFShx) but a poor ROS takes the history section down to level 1 or 2. When submitting the final bill, one can only charge the lowest charge section from history, PE, and MDM – no matter how good a physical exam you performed or how complex your decision was, the note is doomed to level 1 or 2.

At level 5, ROS requires ten systems with one bullet each. Again for patient care you may wish to include more bullets in specific sections. The ROS list to choose from includes constitutional, eyes, ENTM, respiratory, GI, GU, musculoskeletal, integument, endocrine, CV, heme/lymph, allergy/immunity, neurologic, and psychologic. Do not make the mistake of stating ROS per HPI or "all systems negative." This is inadequate. It is easiest (and most bulletproof) to simply list ten systems with one bullet each. Alternatively, you can "update" someone else's complete ROS if you document who wrote it and when and if this note is retrievable in the electronic medical record. This seems like more work to me than just listing ten systems. Another alternative particularly in clinic is using a scanned form that the patient fills out – this again needs to be retrievable from the record and requires your signature and date verifying you indeed reviewed it. In this case, the ROS can look like ROS reviewed from the scanned patient clinic form, pertinent positive include x, y, and z.

You may have noticed that this section came before the PMFShx. This is on purpose; it is way more important. A good doctor thinks about how each body system relates to the chief complaint.

Pillar 1d: PMFShx (Past Medical, Family, and Social History)

The highest level note for billing requires only one bullet each from these three sections. Thus, this section can be very brief. No need to list 40 medications, 17 medical problems, etc. unless you think they are relevant to the CC or to optimize patient care.

Take another look at Fig. 23.2, and you can easily see how this works. As an example, an E3 history section requires a CC, one HPI bullet, and one pertinent ROS bullet. Peruse the N3/C3 requirement: CC, four HPI bullets, two ROS bullets, and one of the three PMFShx bullets. Finally check out the C4/N4

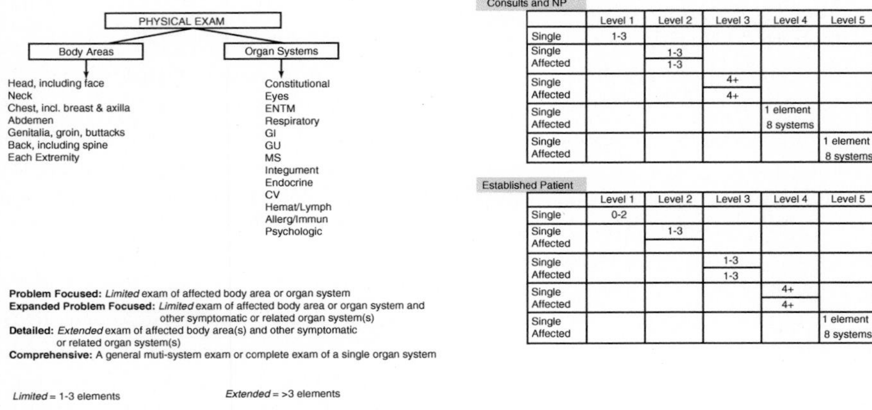

Fig. 23.3 Physical exam billing rules

requirements (the same as C5/N5): CC, four HPI bullets, ten ROS, and three (one each) of PMFShx. Some providers choose not to remember the table and instead use the last sentence in all of their notes to ensure they meet all history billing requirements.

Pillar 2: PE (Physical Exam) (Fig. 23.3)

Physical exam requirements for a level 5 visit are very straightforward. Recall that there are two systems: 1995 and 1997. Surgeons for the most part are better served utilizing the 1995 system. If you prefer to do more work, feel free to look up the 1997 system on your own (a 1997 level 5 PE exam requires more than double the bullets of the 1995 system of eight bullets). The organ systems to choose from in the 1995 system include constitutional, eyes, ENTM, respiratory, GI, GU, musculoskeletal, integument, endocrine, CV, heme/lymph, allergy/immunologic, neurologic, and psychologic. Pick eight of these symptoms and describe one physical finding. Of course, a more detailed physical exam is often required for optimum patient care. To optimize billing, a very reasonable approach is to do an eight-system exam on all patients.

Summary of Pillars 1 and 2 (and a Fibonacci Sequence… Not Really)

C5 Note = CC + 4 HPI + 10 ROS + 1 PMhx +1 + PFhx + 1 PShx + 8 PE = {5 = C, 4, 10, 1, 1, 1, 8}

Pillar 3: MDM (Medical Decision-Making) (Fig. 23.4)

MDM is the most complex part of billing. Good thing you have already mastered the two other pillars. The level billable from MDM is derived from the second highest-scored section available. The three categories are DDR, diagnoses, data,

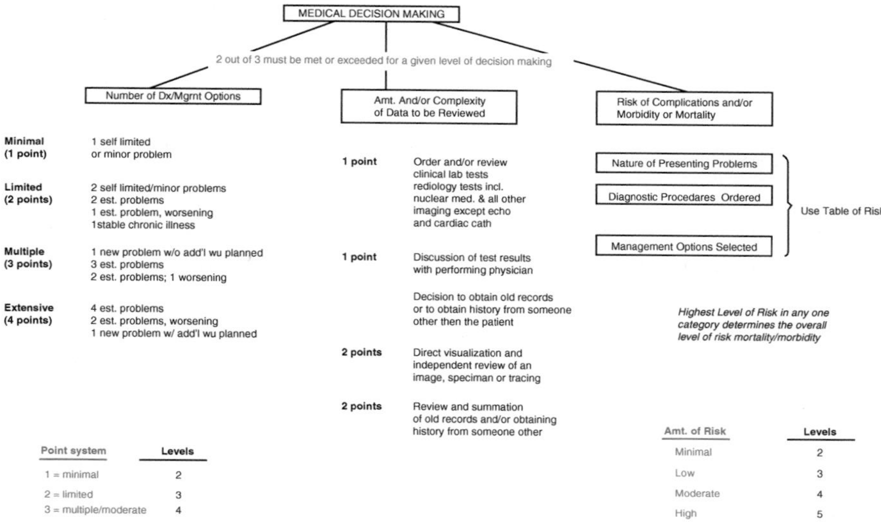

Fig. 23.4 Medical decision-making rules

and risk (not to be confused with Deutsche Democratic Republic). Assuming pillars 1 and 2 meet level 5 criteria then:

Diagnoses level 5, data level 3, risk level 5 – Bill level 5
Diagnoses level 5, data level 4, risk level 3 – Bill level 4
Diagnoses level 5, data level 3, risk level 3 – Bill level 3

Pillar 3a: Diagnoses (And/or Management Options)

The more diagnoses you address and mark as being considered allows for higher billing. A level 2 visit is a "minimal" diagnosis: a self-limited or minor problem or one established problem. A level 3 visit is a "limited" diagnosis – this can fall into four different scenarios: two self-limited minor problems, two established problems, one established problem worsening, or one stable chronic illness. A level 4 visit is a "multiple" diagnosis – this can fall into three different scenarios: one new problem with no additional work-up planned, three established problems, or two established problems one of which is worsening. Finally, a level 5 visit is an extensive diagnosis – this also has three possibilities: four established problems, two established problems both worsening, and a new problem with further work-up planned. Dizzying I know but really, you only have to remember two things here:

1. If the patient presents with a new problem that you have to work up or do something about (order a lab or X-ray, etc.), you get level 5 instantly – not too tough.
2. Add one billing level to the number of established problems you are treating. If a patient has many problems (remember you have to address these not just arbitrarily list them), it is again very simple to get to the highest level.

This is why many clinics will limit the number of diagnoses you can list on your charge tickets for billing purposes to 4.

Pillar 3b: Data (Both Amount and Complexity Considered)

For surgeons, it is often tough to get to a high-level visit based on data. Different activities are assigned "points." A level 5 visit requires four points, a level 4 visit three points, a level 3 visit two points, and a level 2 visit one point. The activities that earn points are a bit deceptive. There are five ways to earn one point: ordering or reviewing a lab (but you still only get one point even if you do both and review a gazillion different labs), ordering and/or reviewing radiology report (again only one point even if you review several reports and order several new ones), ordering and reviewing "other" tests (EEG, EKG, PFT, echo, cardiac catheterization, noninvasive vascular studies), doing a discussion of test results with performing physician, and making decision to obtain old records or obtaining history from someone other than patient. There are two ways to earn two points: personally review a film, specimen, or tracing (again only two points if you look at six different films and specimens and tracings), and review and summate old records or obtain history from someone other than the patient.

The thing to remember here is if you personally review a film, specimen, or tracing, it is possible to get to a level 5 visit.

Pillar 3c: Risk (This Is the LeBron James (King) of Billing)

Risk is the trump element and should be the basis for your billing when in doubt. Table 23.3 lists minimal-, low-, moderate-, and high-level risks which designate level 2, 3, 4, and 5 visits, respectively. Note the table is split into three columns of presenting problem(s), diagnostic procedure(s) ordered, and management options selected. If you can obtain one bullet in high risk for any column, you can bill level 5. Thus, it is worth reviewing the table and seeing where things you commonly do fall in the table.

Noteworthy level 2 categorizations include gargles – you should definitely make an effort to recommend gargles soon. More seriously, noteworthy level 3 categorizations include recommending over-the-counter drugs or treating two or more self-limited problems or one stable chronic illness. *Wait, What?* I said diagnoses (pillar 3a) were determined by number of problems?!? Indeed there is overlap between 3a and 3c, and this definitely adds to the confusion.

Noteworthy level 4 visit includes prescription drug management or opting for minor surgery with risk factors or opting for major surgery without risk factors. This sentence should prompt two questions.

Q1 What is the difference between minor and major surgery?

A1 Global period (a procedure with a 90-day global period is considered major); < 90 day global is minor. A vasectomy has a 90-day global which means you get paid only once for all the work you do in relation to the vasectomy for 3 months.

Table 23.3 Risk

Table of risk			
Level of risk	Presenting problem(s)	Diagnostic procedure(s) ordered	Management options selected
Minimal	One self-limited or minor problem, e.g., cold, insect bite, tinea corporis	Laboratory tests requiring venipuncture Chest x-rays EKG/EEG Urinalysis Ultrasound, e.g., echocardiography KOH prep	Rest Gargles Elastic bandages Superficial dressings
Low	Two or more self-limited or minor problems One stable chronic illness, e.g., well-controlled hypertension, non-insulin-dependent diabetes, cataract. BPH Acute uncomplicated illness or injury, e.g., cystitis, allergic rhinitis, simple sprain	Physiologic tests not under stress, e.g., pulmonary function tests Non-cardiovascular imaging studies with contrast, e.g., barium enema Superficial needle biopsies Clinical laboratory tests requiring arterial puncture Skin biopsies	Over-the-counter drugs Minor surgery with no identified risk factors Physical therapy Occupational therapy IV fluids without additives
Moderate	One or more chronic illnesses with mild exacerbation, progression, or side effects of treatment Two or more stable chronic illnesses Undiagnosed new problem with uncertain prognosis, e.g., lump in breast Acute illness with systemic symptoms, e.g., pyelonephritis, pneumonitis, colitis Acute complicated injury, e.g., head injury with brief loss of consciousness	Physiologic tests under stress, e.g., cardiac stress test, fetal contraction stress test Diagnostic endoscopies with no identified risk factors Deep needle or incisional biopsy Cardiovascular imaging studies with contrast and no identified risk factors, e.g., arteriogram, cardiac catheterization Obtain fluid from body cavity, e.g., lumbar puncture, thoracentesis, culdocentesis	Minor surgery with identified risk factors Elective major surgery (open, percutaneous or endoscopic) with no identified risk factors Prescription drug management Therapeutic nuclear medicine IV fluids with additives Closed treatment of fracture or dislocation without manipulation

(continued)

Table 23.3 (continued)

Table of risk			
Level of risk	Presenting problem(s)	Diagnostic procedure(s) ordered	Management options selected
High	One or more chronic illnesses with severe exacerbation. progression, or side effects of treatment Acute or chronic illnesses or injuries that pose a threat to life or bodily function, e.g., multiple trauma, acute MI, pulmonary embolus, severe respiratory distress, progressive severe rheumatoid arthritis, psychiatric illness with potential threat to self or others, peritonitis, acute renal failure An abrupt change in neurologic status, e.g., seizure, TIA, weakness, sensory loss	Cardiovascular imaging studies with contrast with identified risk factors Cardiac electrophysiological tests Diagnostic endoscopies with identified risk factors Discography	Elective major surgery (open, percutaneous, or endoscopic) with identified risk factors Emergency major surgery (open, percutaneous, or endoscopic) Parenteral controlled substances Drug therapy requiring intensive monitoring for toxicity Decision not to resuscitate or to de-escalate care because of poor prognosis

Considering it is primarily an office procedure, it seems counterintuitive, that is, a major procedure, but I didn't make the rules.

Q2 What is a surgical risk factor?

A2 Any patient condition that increases the surgical risk of complication (i.e., obesity, diabetes, blood thinners, etc.). The majority of patients have a risk factor. It is important to explicitly state in your note what these risks are. Something like, we discussed the risks and benefits of major penile implant surgery and specifically described his infection rate increased from <1 up to 3% based on his diabetes diagnosis.

Noteworthy level 5 categorizations include elective major surgery with risk factors, giving parenteral controlled substance (narcotics, etc.) or acute or chronic illness or injury that poses a threat to life or body function (MI, acute renal failure, etc.).

After studying the risk table for a short time, you will memorize the most common things you do in your practice and automatically know how to bill. You will quickly learn that anytime you write a script, it should be a level 4 visit (because of course you have already completed a level 4 history and physical exam portion of the note). Anytime you schedule surgery, it should be a level 4 or 5 visit. Take a moment to review the difference in RVUs between levels 3, 4, and 5 visits.

Billing on Time

It is the last appointment of the day, and you are tired. The patient encounter starts off pleasant enough, but then the patient reaches into a book bag and proceeds to pull out three pages of meticulously handwritten questions. You covertly text your spouse you will be late for dinner. You spend a total of 45 min with the patient and answer myriad questions. You quickly realize you didn't actually take any history and don't know what to document. All is not lost; this is the perfect patient to bill on time. With the last of your strength, you log in to your computer and type:

I spent a total of 45 min of face-to-face time with the patient discussing his myriad questions on the risks and benefits of penile implant surgery with > 50% in direct patient counseling.

Boom, you can bill E5 since this was not a new patient, and you consulted Table 23.1. The above sentence is all you need, nothing else whatsoever.

You should bill on time when counseling or coordination of care dominated (>50%) the MD/patient encounter. In this case, time can be considered the key or controlling factor to qualify for particular level of service. The total length of time *as well as the counseling or activities to coordinate care* should be documented. Remember that office or other outpatient activities need to be *your face-to-face time* (not the resident or your PA or the med student). Hospital or nursing facility is floor time and DOES NOT need to be face-to-face when billing on time. Review the time thresholds again (Tables 23.1 and 23.2), and realize that timed billing sets itself up very well for E4 and E5 visits. The time requirements for new appointments are pretty steep. There is controversy over time increments (see next section on ambiguity); some groups state that a unit of time is attained when the midpoint has passed. When codes are sequential, some state you should pick that which is closer. Others state you need to spend all of the threshold times face-to-face with the patient.

Billing tip – If you look at films or patient records in the midst of your clinic day, make a concerted effort to do it with the patient present. A simple explanation like "With your permission, before we begin our appointment, I would like to review your records and films to make sure I totally understand your history." This accomplishes two things: it lets the patient actually see how much time you are spending on their case (as well as see their own films – they love that), and it sets the stage to bill on maximized face-to-face time.

Putting It All Together and Knowing Your Auditors

So now you know how to bill each individual section. How do you determine the bill to submit? Quite simple really, you may only bill the lowest of the three pillars. Thus, if you bill a level 5 visit for a new patient, history, PE, and MDM, all need to reach level 5. If your history section only qualifies for level 3 and your PE and MDM are level 5, you may only bill level 3. Another important point is to think about who is potentially reviewing your notes. It is not physicians, so they will not understand any unmentioned nuances. I always picture some kid out of high school in a Metallica T-shirt with a red pen and an abacus. Thus, I make the notes as clear as and easy to follow as possible. I make a concerted effort to make obvious summary statements like 54-year-olds with erectile dysfunction scheduled for penile implant, a major procedure with risk factors given his diabetes and use of Plavix.

Do your best to restate the key words and phrases found in the risk table in your headings and assessment and plan (major surgery, parenteral controlled substances, prescription drug management). Also label each separate section, and make the subsections clear; don't make the auditor dig out your ten ROS from the body of the HPI.

A Word on Defense: Overrated

I have personally undergone several medical school compliance billing and coding audits now – if you read carefully, you'll know that is why I am writing this text. Of all my audits, not once have I been told you should have billed a higher level here. Further, not once have I heard, you know your medical decision-making was very high level, yet your documentation met only level 3 – had you only done this in the history, you could have billed level 4. I've tried to change this part of the audit system. Thus far, audits have only told me I have done things wrong, further perpetuating the cycle of fearful billing and undercharging. There is a reason for this; compliance has a competing goal – protecting you and the university from costly, extensive government audits and fines. This is why institutions self-audit and default to more conservative policies. They want a paper trail of self-policing to show to CMS how they have found, corrected, and educated providers about their errors. However, the auditor salary has to get paid somehow. In the end, appropriate level billing benefits everyone.

Ambiguity in Coding and Billing: It is Out There

One of the underlying reasons for defensive billing from the compliance department's perspective is the fact that there is ambiguity in the billing system. There are several phrases and/or descriptions in the official Medicare guidelines which leave one scratching their head. Here are some examples that I struggle with:

1. New problem with further work-up – We all know what a new patient is, but what does further work-up mean? If one orders a lab or X-ray for a problem, this seems pretty straightforward. But what if a patient comes in for an elective procedure like a vasectomy – is the future appointment for the vasectomy a work-up? My personal opinion is yes, but I'm not really sure.
2. "Prescription drug management" qualifies as a level 4 risk maneuver according to the risk table. Assuming all other parts of the note are up to snuff, does a yearly renewal of medications count as drug management? A new script, dosing change, and recommendation on how it should be taken to alter side effect profile

meet criteria in my book. However, I personally do not think medication renewal qualifies as drug management, but others do.

3. The level 4 physical exam in the 95 system. Level 3 exam is easy with one bullet (i.e., NAD, vital signs as below or normal affect – yeah I know it is ridiculously little). Level 5–8 organ systems – one bullet each. But the rule makers couldn't be clear for level 4 – it is listed as two total systems, one system detailed. I interpret this as one system with one bullet and another system with four bullets (e.g., general – NAD, vitals as below, GU penis circ'd (1), urethra normotopic without discharge (2), testes bilaterally present without masses (3), and cord structures present without varicocele (4)). To me, this seems very straightforward, but to our compliance and billing section, it is not.

Let me elaborate (I know you don't have a choice). There are two systems – one created in 1995 and the other in 1997. My understanding is the 1997 system was created to help specialists (like psychiatry) be able to charge for a level 5 exam without a stethoscope by being superduper thorough on certain systems (for psychiatrist – psych and neuro systems related… please, tell me about your mother). Medicare states you can use one or the other in a note but should not combine elements of the two in the same patient's note. I personally toggle between 95 and 97 in clinic for whatever is easiest for that particular patient encounter. However, my previous compliance people taught me only the 97 system?!? You really should be asking why at this point. The answer they give is that there is less ambiguity. Now take a guess which of the two systems is much more labor intensive and hard to remember. Yup, it is 97.

4. Billing on time – The thresholds for billing on time for an E3 and E4 visits are 15 and 25 min, respectively. So if you spend 21-min face-to-face with the patient (> 50% in direct patient counseling), should you bill E3 or E4? This is up for debate; I've had some experts tell me you should bill E4 (have to eclipse halfway point), but others vehemently disagree (need to hit the entire 25 min).

I still am unaware of a resource where specific billing questions like these can be answered. Institutions tend to set their own policies for various reasons. When I previously asked our billing people, that person will ask their supervisor. The supervisor has the same information you do (not some magical book with the specific answers). Try calling CMS people, and they will refer you to the document that creates ambiguity in the first place. So, ultimately for matters of dispute, it's up to interpretation of vague phrasing. This is why you can argue with the people who audit your notes, as long as there is some logic and justification why you picked what you did. Remember to fall back on medical risk as the trump card for what to decide, and you'll be fine. In billing courses I've attended, expert billers in the same room often come up with different answers on how they would bill the same encounter documentation.

Important point on ambiguity – I sometimes struggle with how to bill between levels and if unsure will err on the side of caution and bill the lower level. This is a conscientious decision not a blind one based on ignorance. I personally feel the fear of audit and punishment is greatly exaggerated and irrational. Ethical providers with logical justification for their billing will be just fine. The government would much rather focus on people double billing, billing without being present, billing without proper documentation, or billing by gaming the system (e.g., by doing elaborate histories and physical exams when medical decision-making and risk are low).

Conclusion

Congrats on reading to the end. Most people start reading about billing and have the same reaction I have to embryology lectures – gloriously refreshing somnolence. Despite its soporific qualities, my knowledge of billing has greatly benefited my surgical career in many ways. I will elaborate since you may still be on the fence.

My patient care is improved because my notes are more concise and contain only the information necessary for excellent patient care and the billing requirement minimums. Medicolegally, I do not have concerns about over- or under-billing since I know the rules extremely well. I have been able to teach many resident and medical students (and staff) the billing basics. Many of them have run with the little bit of knowledge I gave them and created their own billing templates and cheat sheets. Research opportunities abound in all of your patient encounters. You can easily incorporate validated questionnaires that cover all of the elements required for the HPI. My notes are cleaner, and thus the information and communication with referring MDs have improved. Compared to my peers who primarily bill E3 appointments for follow-ups (0.97 RVU), I am on average 50% more efficient by appropriately billing E4 (1.5 RVUs). This obviously increases my take-home pay and leaves me with more free time to spend with my family. Finally, my daughters and I roughly estimate that I have saved 7 ½ acres of rain forest over my lifetime because my notes are shorter.

Self-Check Quiz

1. List the three core elements of all E & M notes? Which is the trump element?
2. Name the three components to medical decision-making? What is the trump MDM component?
3. Besides having seen the patient within a practice for 3 years, what is the fundamental documentation difference between established and new patient visits?
4. True or false: The middle-level billing of the three categories is used to determine MDM billing.
5. True or false: For history billing, the middle-level billing of the three categories is used to determine history component billing.
6. For overall billing, the middle-level billing of the three pillars determines the submitted billing charge.

7. True or false: A vasectomy which has a 90-day global period is considered a major procedure.
8. Assuming adequate documentation, what determines picking a level 4 or 5 visit when making a decision for surgery?
9. In regard to billing on time, which is correct?
   (a) Time spent reviewing a patients' chart and films outside the clinic room is counted.
   (b) Time spent discussing the case with a colleague for an inpatient is counted.
   (c) The time threshold for a level 3 consult is the same as a level 3 new patient.
   (d) When billing on time, only one of the three core billing elements is required.
   (e) For a clinic visit, 50% of the total time must be face-to-face.
10. The difference between new patient and consult documentation is:
   (a) History documentation requirement by coding level.
   (b) Medical decision-making documentation requirement by coding level.
   (c) An increase in 16% revenue (RVUs) for C3 versus N3.
   (d) Other than a reference to the consulting MD for a specific diagnosis and proof of consult request and correspondence, there is no documentation difference.
   (e) This question is irrelevant since the majority of payers no longer honor consults.

Key:

1. History, physical exam, medical decision-making (trump core element)
2. Diagnoses, data, and risk (trump element)
3. Only two of the three pillars required for established patients, three of the three required for new patients
4. True
5. False
6. False
7. True
8. Surgical risk factors that increase chance for complication (e.g., obesity)
9. B
10. D

References

1. Adiga K, Buss M, Beasley BW. Perceived, actual, and desired knowledge regarding Medicare billing and reimbursement. A national needs assessment survey of internal medicine residents. J Gen Intern Med. 2006;21(5):466–70.
2. Howell J, Chisholm C, Clark A, Spillane L. Emergency medicine resident documentation: results of the 1999 American board of emergency medicine in-training examination survey. Acad Emerg Med. 2000;7(10):1135–8.

3. Jones K, Lebron RA, Mangram A, Dunn E. Practice management education during surgical residency. Am J Surg. 2008;196(6):878–81. [discussion 81–2].
4. As-Sanie S, Zolnoun D, Wechter ME, Lamvu G, Tu F, Steege J. Teaching residents coding and documentation: effectiveness of a problem-oriented approach. Am J Obstet Gynecol. 2005;193(5):1790–3.
5. Fakhry SM, Robinson L, Hendershot K, Reines HD. Surgical residents' knowledge of documentation and coding for professional services: an opportunity for a focused educational offering. Am J Surg. 2007;194(2):263–7.
6. Lusco VC, Martinez SA, Polk HC Jr. Program directors in surgery agree that residents should be formally trained in business and practice management. Am J Surg. 2005;189(1):11–3.
7. Ghaderi KF, Schmidt ST, Drolet BC. Coding and billing in surgical education. A Systems-Based Practice Education Program. 2017;74(2):199–202. https://doi.org/10.1016/j.jsurg.2016.08.011. Epub 2016 Sep 16.

Resources

Department of Health and Human Services: Evaluation and Management Services, August 2016 https://www.cms.gov/Outreach-and-Education/Medicare-Learning-Network-MLN/MLNProducts/Downloads/eval-mgmt-serv-guide-ICN006764.pdf

Simulation in Surgery

24

Wesley Baas, Matthew Davis, and Bradley F. Schwartz

Introduction

Medical training has always relied upon the patient serving as the instruments of medical education. Halsted's apprenticeship model was centered around the mantra: "See one, do one, teach one" [1]. Under this model, trainees practice their craft on patients and are required to learn quickly, often through their mistakes. Although this objective was intended to function with proper oversight and controls, this method of learning has long been the subject of debate about the safety and ethicality of training on patients [2]. As such, finding ways to bypass or accelerate the early learning curve has become paramount. One way physicians are amending their training while keeping patient safety paramount is through simulation. This is a relatively new and emerging field with the aim to allow trainees to practice techniques and procedures in a controlled environment that does not jeopardize patient health [3].

Urology is a specialty that has been pushing the boundaries of new technologies since the early 1900s. Simulation is particularly enticing in urology, because with new technology and techniques comes significant learning curves. Even urologists who have been in practice for many years are finding that they have to learn new procedures outside of their traditional training. This is especially challenging to attending physicians, as they are responsible for helping teach residents procedures that they are also relatively inexperienced with.

W. Baas, MD • M. Davis, MD • B.F. Schwartz, DO, FACS (✉)
Department of Surgery, Urology, Southern Illinois University
School of Medicine, Springfield, IL, USA
e-mail: bschwartz@siumed.edu

T.S. Köhler, B. Schwartz (eds.), *Surgeons as Educators*,
https://doi.org/10.1007/978-3-319-64728-9_24

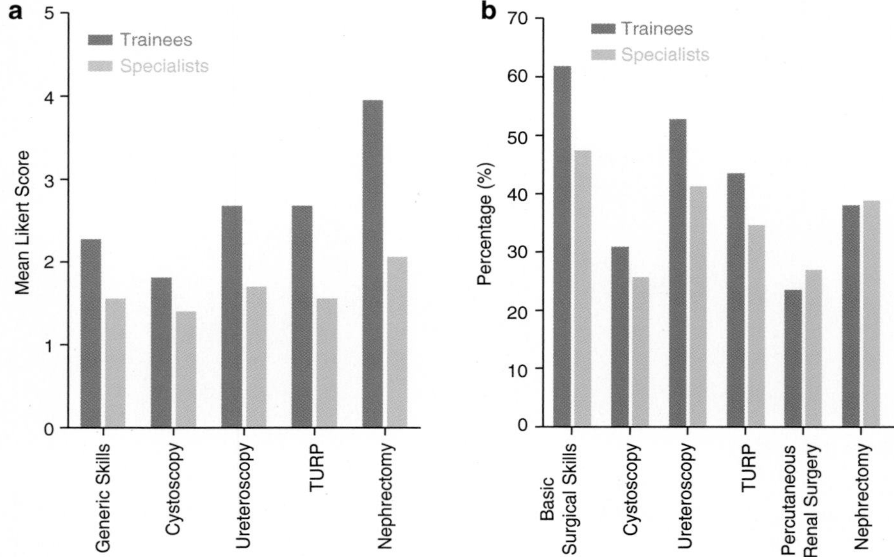

Fig. 24.1 Results of survey of 263 urological trainees and specialists comparing perception of need for additional training and whether or not simulation had been used for training [173]. (**a**) Is additional training required to develop technical skills? Likert scale: (1 = strongly disagree – 5 = strongly agree) Key: *TURP* transurethral resection of the prostate. (**b**) Percentage of trainees and specialists who had simulation experience in technical skills training. Likert scale: (1 = strongly disagree – 5 = strongly agree) Key: *TURP* transurethral resection of the prostate

The Accreditation Council for Graduate Medical Education (ACGME), the governing body of American medical residencies, is tasked with assuring that residents are properly trained before independent practice. In their most recent release of requirements for urology residencies, the ACGME states that residencies are responsible for "developing the skills, knowledge, and attitudes leading to proficiency in all the domains of clinical competency requires the resident physician to assume personal responsibility for the care of individual patients." The way in which residencies need to reach this goal is never explicitly stated. Despite no requirements from the ACGME at the time of this writing, residencies are increasingly using simulation and skills laboratories to help residents master a number of surgical skills (Fig. 24.1). In the following chapter, the currently available simulation options in urology will be discussed including open surgery, laparoscopy, robotics, and endoscopy.

Open Surgery

Despite more minimally invasive surgical approaches at the urologists disposal today, open surgery remains the backbone of urological surgery. Because of the growing number of surgeries being done in a minimally invasive manner, trainees have had less exposure to open surgery. Therefore, simulation in open surgery is one way of gaining open experience without putting patients at risk. Currently available simulators for open surgery are comprised of bench models, cadavers, and animal models.

Human cadavers likely represent the best option for open surgery simulation, but cadavers are expensive and often not readily available. In a large study comprised of 81 urology residents and 27 urology faculty members, Ahmed et al. recently put forth a simulation program in which participants performed a number of procedures on fresh-frozen cadavers [4]. These procedures included circumcision, vasectomy, orchiopexy, hydrocele repair, radical orchiectomy, open cystotomy, management of bladder perforation, transureteroureterostomy, Boari flap, psoas hitch, open surgical packing of the pelvis, and nephrectomy [4, 5]. Questionnaires of the participants indicated that the cadaveric simulations had face validity (mean score 3/5) and all procedures scored ≥3 out of 5 in terms of usefulness for learning anatomy and improving surgical skills (content validity). Interestingly, participants rated human cadaveric simulation to be the best form of training, followed by live animal simulation, animal tissue models, bench models, and virtual reality.

Because cadaver simulations are simply "surgeries" performed the same way as they would be in living patients, these will not be discussed individually. Described below are the few currently validated non-cadaveric models of open surgery.

Bladder

Suprapubic Tube Placement

Suprapubic tube (SPT) placement is a rather common procedure performed by urologists, but trainees often have to "learn on their feet" as this is a procedure often done alone and sporadically in an emergent setting. Because of this, trainees often have difficulty acquiring the skill and confidence to perform the procedure and many times elect to attempt difficult urethral catheter placement, which may put a patient at increased harm. To bolster the skills necessary for SPT placement, there are currently three validated bench models that can be used by trainees for procedural simulation.

The first SPT model called the "UroEmerge™ Suprapubic Catheter Model" was described by Shergill et al. in 2008 [6]. The authors created the model by injecting a 3 liter bag of irrigation fluid with 10 cc of povidone-iodine, giving the fluid a urine color, and tying the bag with two tourniquets to simulate a full bladder (Fig. 24.2). This "bladder" was then placed within a plastic trainer housing and covered with a commercially available abdominal open and closure pad which simulates abdominal skin, subcutaneous fat, and rectus sheath (Limbs & Things, UK) (Fig. 24.3).

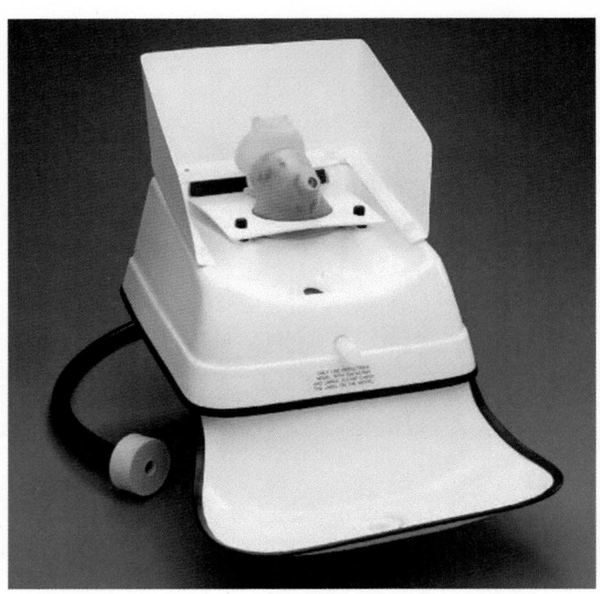

Fig. 24.2 Bristol TURP simulator [110]

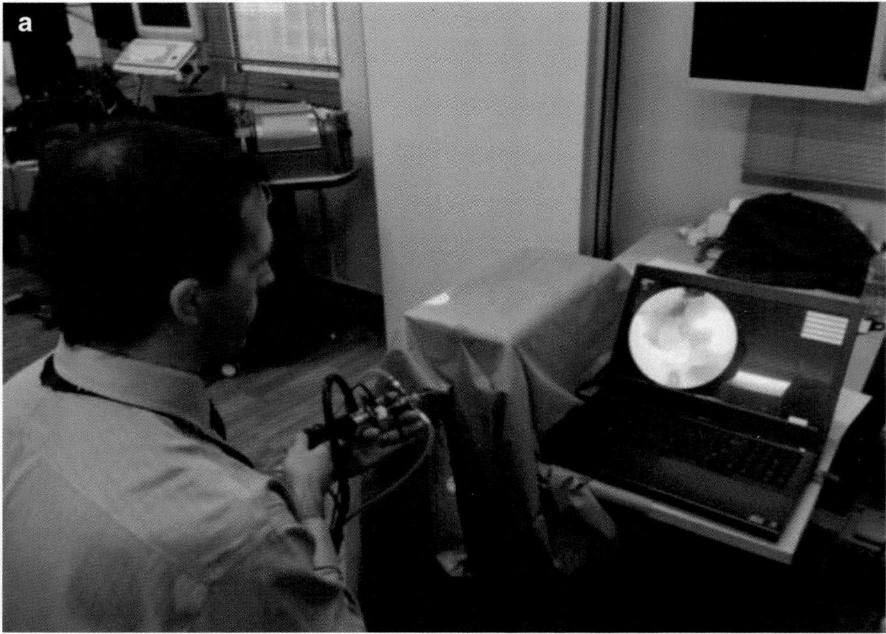

Fig. 24.3 (**a**) The UroSim simulator with resectoscope and display in use, (**b**) view of simulated prostatic anatomy, (**c**) mid-procedure view notable for circular fibers seen at bladder neck [128]

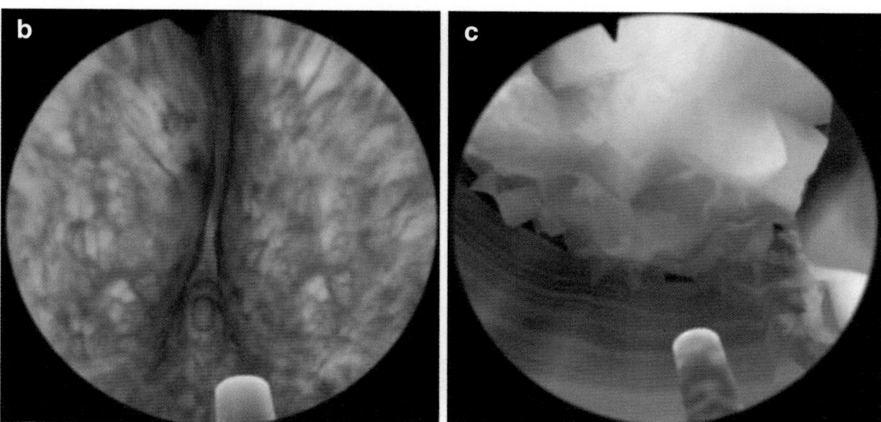

Fig. 24.3 (continued)

Shergill et al. had 36 participants use the model for SPT insertion and scored their ability using a 0–5 visual analog scale. The authors found that before training, the participants had an average score of 3.14 for ability to do SPT placement, which increased to 4.48 after the course. This suggests that this model may be a viable and easy method to help junior residents learn this procedure.

A second model was published by Hossack et al. in 2013, which, again, is relatively simple in nature [7]. The model is made by filling a standard party balloon with tap water and affixing it with tape. The authors recommended "Mefix" tape (Molnlycke Health Care, Sweden) because it kept adherence to the balloon even when wet, prevented the balloon from popping, and provided realistic resistance to trocar placement. The balloon was then placed within a plastic container with a hole cut in the lid. On top of the balloon, a standard household sponge was placed (representing perivesical fat), on top of which a three-layer square of Transpore (3 M) tape was placed (rectus sheath), and finally covered with another sponge (abdominal wall fat). In their study with 30 surgical resident participants, the authors found that 96% felt the model accurately represented a bladder and 84% felt much more confident in performing SPT insertion [7].

Singal et al. described the most recently published model in 2015 [8]. The model was created by first making a bony pelvis from urethane foam and stabilized with resin glue. Plastic parts simulating the anterior superior iliac spine and pubic symphysis were embedded within the foam to provide palpable bony landmarks. The bladder was constructed from silicone rubber with attached IV tubing and Luer Lock syringe for instillation of fluid. This was then filled and placed within the bony pelvis and covered with multiple skin and fat layers (made of silicone rubber and gel wax). The model was studied with 25 rural general surgeons under the supervision of urologists. The surgeons scored the model well in terms of value as a training or testing model (4.1/5) and overall realism (3.9/5) [8].

Vas Deferens

Vasovasostomy

Vasovasostomy (VV), or vasectomy reversal, is an option for men who have undergone sterilization vasectomy but wish to regain their fertility. Vasovasostomy is a very technically demanding procedure because the structures are small and suturing is usually performed under a microscope. Sutures are often quite small (9-0, 10-0, and/or 11-0).

In the only validated study of VV simulation, Grober et al. randomly assigned junior surgery residents to learn VV via a high-fidelity model (live rat vas deferens), a low-fidelity model (silicone tubing), or didactic training alone (control group) [9]. After training in their given randomization group, participants returned 4 months later for retention testing on the two models. The authors found that those who were randomized to either bench model performed significantly better than the didactic control group as evidenced by higher retention test checklist scores (25.5 vs 18.6, $p < 0.001$), higher global rating scores (27.0 vs 16.4, $p < 0.001$), and patency rates (69% vs 20%, $p = 0.05$) [9]. The authors did not distinguish scoring between the low- and high-fidelity model trained groups.

Laparoscopy

Laparoscopy is a growing field of urology, as urologists continue to push the boundaries of what is possible within the realm of laparoscopic surgery. Laparoscopic surgery was first introduced in the 1970s by gynecologists attempting laparoscopy for oophorectomies and myomectomies, but it did not become mainstream until expansion into general surgery with two of the most commonly performed surgeries today—laparoscopic cholecystectomy and appendectomy [10]. Since the early 1990s, minimally invasive surgery (MIS) has grown tremendously in the field of urology, with an increasing number of indications for MIS. Although, with its advances, laparoscopy has a steep learning curve that requires unique skills which do not translate well from skills learned in other modalities, such as open surgery [11]. When performing laparoscopy, one is required to navigate a three-dimensional space on a two-dimensional monitor using unique instruments that often have limited degrees of freedom of movement [12]. For urology residents training in laparoscopy, the ACGME has placed the current requirement upon graduation to be 50 cases, although it is unknown if this is enough to be truly proficient at laparoscopy. Fortunately, there have been a number of laparoscopy-specific simulators created to help bypass the steep learning curve seen with laparoscopic surgery.

Basic Laparoscopic Skills

General Training

A number of unique skills are required to be proficient in laparoscopic surgery. One example is the requirement of good hand-eye coordination to achieve accurate movements while watching a monitor that is producing a two-dimensional image of a three-dimensional space. Given the amplification of small movements by the length of the instruments, manual dexterity is also very important. At the same time, there is the fulcrum effect of the body causing movements of the hands to mirror that of the instrument. These are just a few of the basic skills that must be mastered to be proficient in laparoscopy. Because of this, several simple bench models have been created that aim to help trainees master the basic skills of laparoscopy. In addition to acquiring skills, there is also evidence to suggest that practicing on a simulator prior to real surgery improves surgical performance [13].

The field of bench trainers (also termed "box trainers" or "video trainers") for laparoscopy is vast. There are many variations of trainers, with the basic premise of having a box through which instruments can be passed to perform a variety of tasks while using a camera to project the images onto a monitor. In their 2014 Cochrane review on the topic of laparoscopic surgical box trainers (limited to those with no prior laparoscopic experience), Nagendran et al. found an astounding 770 publications requiring screening, of which 32 were ultimately included on the topic [14].

Within the confines of a standard box trainer, a number of tasks can be performed depending on the desired skill to be practiced. The Fundamentals of Laparoscopic Surgery (FLS) simulator is one such box trainer that is considered by many to be the "gold standard" for the development of laparoscopic skills [15]. Based on the McGill Inanimate System for Training and Evaluation of Laparoscopic Skills (MISTELS), the FLS consists of five tasks: peg transfer, pattern cutting, ligating loop, extracorporeal suturing, and intracorporeal suturing. The complete program also has an online didactic portion. The FLS has been extensively studied, with all five tasks being validated, and proficiency on FLS has been shown to improve operative performance [16–19]. In fact, in 2009, FLS was added by the American Board of Surgery as a requirement before being able to sit for board examinations in general surgery [20].

Munz et al. have put forth a number of suggested tasks to be performed on box trainers that can easily be done at any institution [21]. To practice instrument navigation, Munz et al. had trainees conduct preset calculations on a calculator inside the box by using a pair of graspers. Coordination was practiced by placing a 30 cm piece of twine marked at 1 cm intervals with blue lines inside the box. Users then "walked" their way down the twine by only grasping at the lines. To practice grasping, a simple setup of two dishes can be placed inside the box, and objects can be transferred back and forth between dishes (chickpeas or small bolts are common objects to grasp). Cutting can be accomplished with a number of setups including grasping twine as above and cutting every centimeter on a marked line or cutting out along the lines of a circle drawn on a piece of cloth or examination glove. An added element of difficulty can be added to any of these tasks by timing the exercises and working on improving efficiency to improve times to accomplish tasks.

As evidenced above, box trainers allow many tasks to be practiced. An added benefit is that they're relatively simple to create. As such, there has recently been a publication on making a "homemade" lap simulator [22]. Using only a translucent storage box, an LED light source, and a webcam hooked to a monitor, Aslam et al. created a relatively simple and cost-effective box trainer. In their study of 34 trainees, 96.9% found the homemade box trainer to be satisfactory, and there was no significant difference in the completion of a variety of tasks on the homemade box trainer versus a commercially available model.

Box model training appears to improve technical skills of trainees, particularly in those with no prior laparoscopic experience. This was demonstrated in a recent Cochrane review [14]. The authors found in their meta-analysis that when comparing box model training to no training, those who used box trainers took significantly less time to complete tasks (0.54 standard deviations (SD) lower), they made less errors (0.69 SD lower), they had better accuracy scores (0.67 SD higher), and they had overall higher composite scores (0.49 SD higher). The authors also noted that there appears to be no significant difference when comparing the skills obtained on any one box trainer versus another [14].

Training of basic laparoscopic skills is not limited to box trainers. With the ever-increasing advances in technology, virtual reality has become an increasing popular option for skill acquisition and surgical simulation. Of all the VR simulators, MIST-VR (Minimally Invasive Surgical Trainer, Virtual Reality; Virtual Medical Presence, UK) is likely the most studied. First described in 1997, the MIST-VR is a computer-based system that consists of a frame holding two laparoscopic instruments whose movements are tracked and translated into virtual reality movements displayed on a standard monitor [23]. A foot pedal is also present to control simulated diathermy. MIST-VR allows users to work through a series of surgical tasks of increasing complexity, with an emphasis on developing the unique skills stated above that are necessary to perform laparoscopic surgery proficiently. Based on its numerous validations from several studies, MIST-VR has been integrated into many training programs around the globe [24]. Many of these studies have shown MIST-VR to demonstrate both construct and face validity [25–31].

A slight modification to the MIST-VR is EndoTower (Verefi Technologies, Inc., Elizabethtown, PA). EndoTower is additional software that can be downloaded onto the MIST-VR computer system and also requires a slightly different handpiece. A specific focus of the EndoTower is the use of the angled laparoscopic camera, which has been known to create problems with novices because of its off-axis viewing. EndoTower creates a virtual tower that serves as an obstacle course for users to navigate and find hidden objects [29]. In a study by Ganai et al., training on the EndoTower was found to significantly improve the performance of third-year medical students on a porcine navigational assessment with better object visualization and scope orientation scores than controls ($p < 0.05$) [32].

Released in 2002, the LS500 (Xitact, Switzerland) was a groundbreaking virtual reality simulator that combined haptics with high-fidelity simulation software. A focus of the LS500 was on laparoscopic cholecystectomy, and it has been validated in a number of studies [33–35]. It was from the LS500 platform that LAP Mentor™ (Simbionix, Cleveland, OH) was launched in 2003. Now on its third edition, the LAP Mentor is a validated VR laparoscopic simulator that has expanded from a number of laparoscopic-specific tasks to include modules on a number of operations [36]. The LAP Mentor helps develop many basic laparoscopic skills, such as translocation of objects, camera manipulation, clip applying, clipping and grasping, cutting, and a variety of two handed maneuvers. Several skills necessary for suturing can also be learned on LAP Mentor, including needle loading, knot tying, interrupted suturing, continuous suturing, and more advanced techniques such as the "backhand" technique and anastomosis suturing. Because FLS is considered the "gold standard" for laparoscopic training, Simbionix set to mirror FLS with the introduction of the "essential tasks module." Included in this module are peg transfer, pattern cutting, and placement of ligating loop, as are seen in the FLS program. In a study by Pitzul et al., the LAP Mentor "essential tasks module" demonstrated moderate concurrent validity with FLS, suggesting construct validity [15].

While both box trainers and VR simulators have their own merits, it is natural to question if one modality is better than the other. Gurusamy et al. did a meta-analysis of all studies that directly compared VR training versus box trainers and found two studies that attempted to answer this question [37]. The first study found operative time was significantly shorter for the VR group compared to the box-trainer group, but there were no reported numerical values ($p < 0.004$). In the second study, the VR group was found to have a 36% improvement in terms of operative performance versus 17% for the box trainer group ($p < 0.05$) [38]. Given the low power in these studies, as well as the few number of studies that compare between the two simulation modalities, the question of superiority of training continues to go unanswered. This question also becomes more complex when considering cost-effectiveness. This will ultimately require further studies.

Adrenal and Kidney

Clayman and coworkers performed the first laparoscopic nephrectomy in 1990. Since then, laparoscopy has found its way to nearly every indication for renal surgery. In contrast to open surgery, laparoscopic renal surgery has been found to decrease hospital stays and postoperative pain and improve cosmesis without sacrificing surgical outcomes [39–42]. One could argue that the majority of renal procedures done today, including radical nephrectomy, partial nephrectomy, and pyeloplasty, should be performed with laparoscopy or robotics.

Radical/Partial Nephrectomy

There are many current simulation options specific to radical and partial nephrectomy, many of which have been validated in a number of studies. The simplest is a bench model out of the University of Western Ontario. Using a commercially available polyvinyl alcohol (PVA) powder (Air Products and Chemicals, Inc., Allentown,

PA), researchers were able to create a PVA liquid that could be poured into a custom mold and freeze-thawed into a renal model. Once the model was made, tumors could be suspended within the mold using a custom tumor mold [43]. The model was initially created for practice in renal ablative therapy, but now the model has now been expanded to use for partial nephrectomy. A unique feature of this model is its echogenic properties when scanned with an ultrasound probe, allowing trainees to use ultrasound to define tumor borders before simulating laparoscopic partial nephrectomy (LPN). Fernandez et al. studied the model's utility in LPN by having the model placed within a standard laparoscopic box trainer and having five MIS fellows do ten LPNs each. In the study, participants successfully identified 98% of tumors in a mean time of 1.12 min using a 7.5 MHz laparoscopic ultrasound probe. The researchers also found that positive surgical margins increased in the first three cases of each fellow, but steeply declined until none of the fellows had positive margins on their ninth and tenth cases. This model was recommended by four of the five fellows for training in LPN [44]. Abdelshehid et al. further expanded this model when they created an entire case scenario surrounding LPN. They created a simulated operating room (OR) environment with other team members including anesthesia, circulators, surgical assistants, pathologist, and scrub technician. Nine urologists underwent a simulated LPN, using the PVA kidney model with a 3 cm exophytic tumor placed within a standard box trainer and the SimMan 3G mannequin simulator. The authors found that the simulation-based team training was not only beneficial for its surgical simulation but also because it allowed multiple team members to practice and prepare for a complex surgery with an emphasis on improved communication [45].

Using a bench model for laparoscopic radical nephrectomy (LRN), Lee et al. created a scenario in which urology residents were told to do a LRN, but the case was complicated by a renal hilar vessel injury [46]. To create the scenario, the authors placed a commercially available rubberized kidney part-task trainer (the Chamberlain Group, Great Barrington, MA) inside a standard box trainer. Standard silicone IV tubing and a half-inch Penrose drain were passed into the hilar region of the model to simulate the renal artery and renal vein, respectively. Irrigation fluid dyed red to resemble blood was then hooked up to both sides of the IV tubing and Penrose drain. The fluid was placed under pressure to allow for brisk bleeding. The model was then draped to hide all irrigation tubing. Residents were unaware there would be any vessel injuries, which were two 1 cm lacerations made to the superior portion of the renal vein (Penrose drain). When users began ligation of the renal artery (IV tubing), the water irrigation system hooked to the Penrose was initiated, creating "venous bleeding." The residents then had to deal with the injury in any way necessary. Endpoints of the study were complete hemostasis or a 2 L blood loss. All eight of the residents (PGY-2 to PGY-5) were able to complete the exercise before the 2 L blood loss endpoint. Senior residents (PGY 4–5) were found to perform significantly better than junior residents (PGY 2–3) in terms of task-specific checklist scoring (75.0 vs 57.9, $p = 0.004$), global rating scale (4.00 vs 1.75, $p = 0.002$), and "blood loss" (462 vs 1075 mL, $p = 0.022$), suggesting construct validity.

Animal models also represent a viable and frequently used modality for surgical simulation. Often, animal models are used in proof of concept studies to demonstrate new surgical techniques and instruments. Some of the more popular laparoscopic simulation models are porcine models as the pig abdominal cavity is of similar size and has comparable anatomy to humans. In addition to porcine models, rabbit models are also sometimes used for laparoscopic nephrectomy simulation. Molinas et al. studied ten gynecologists and ten medical students in a rather large study of 200 laparoscopic nephrectomies on live rabbits [47]. Participants were evaluated during laparoscopic nephrectomy using standard laparoscopic instruments on live rabbits. Each participant performed a total of 20 nephrectomies, and the study found that both the gynecologists and students improved performance when comparing his or her first nephrectomy to the last. Overall time to perform the surgery decreased for students from 44 min to 11 min and from 29 min to 11 min in the gynecologists, with the gynecologists having significantly shorter operation times for the first nephrectomy ($p < 0.0001$) but not significantly different for the last. The students also had more episodes of heavy or mortal bleeding than the gynecologists ($p = 0.0003$), but both groups significantly improved in this category until no bleeding episodes were seen in either group after the 15th nephrectomy for each participant.

There are several virtual reality simulators for laparoscopic nephrectomy, with the Procedicus MIST™ (Mentice AB, Sweden) nephrectomy VR simulator remaining the most thoroughly evaluated [5]. The Procedicus MIST™ is a VR simulator launched in December 2007, which simulates both retroperitoneal and transperitoneal LRN. The simulator uses a standard computer, three foot pedals, haptic devices with instrumentation, and two monitors—of which one is touch screen [12]. Because of Xitact™ Instrument Haptic Port devices, the simulator allows the user to "feel" tissues, adding realism. Using a number of metrics to evaluate user performance, the LRN simulation is divided into three separate tasks. The first task is dissection and transection of the ureter, beginning with the user in the retroperitoneum after balloon dissection, at which point they must identify the gonadal vessel and ureter, dissect the ureter from its adventitia, and divide it. The second task is dissection of the hilar fat to identify the renal vessels, which then must be further dissected and divided. Adding reality to this VR model, the perihilar fat and renal vessels are capable of bleeding. The final task is complete dissection of the kidney. The Procedicus MIST™ was first validated by Brewin et al. in a study of eight experts, ten urology residents, and ten students. Face validity was demonstrated with the experts rating all components of the simulator ≥3 on a 1–5 Likert scale of realism, with particular emphasis on realistic graphics (mean 3.9) and instrument movements (mean 3.8). The simulator also demonstrated construct validity, with it being able to differentiate the experts, trainees, and novices by assessing hemorrhage (experts 236 mL, trainees 377 mL, and novices 1110 mL; $p < 0.01$), errors (181 vs 294 vs 419, $p < 0.01$), task time (1310 vs 1459 vs 2240 s, $p < 0.01$), and instrument travel (24.5 vs 28.4 vs 37.0 m, $p < 0.01$). However, Wijn et al. contrasted the study performed by Brewin et al., finding that the Procedicus MIST™ did not distinguish between intermediate (<10 LRN performed)

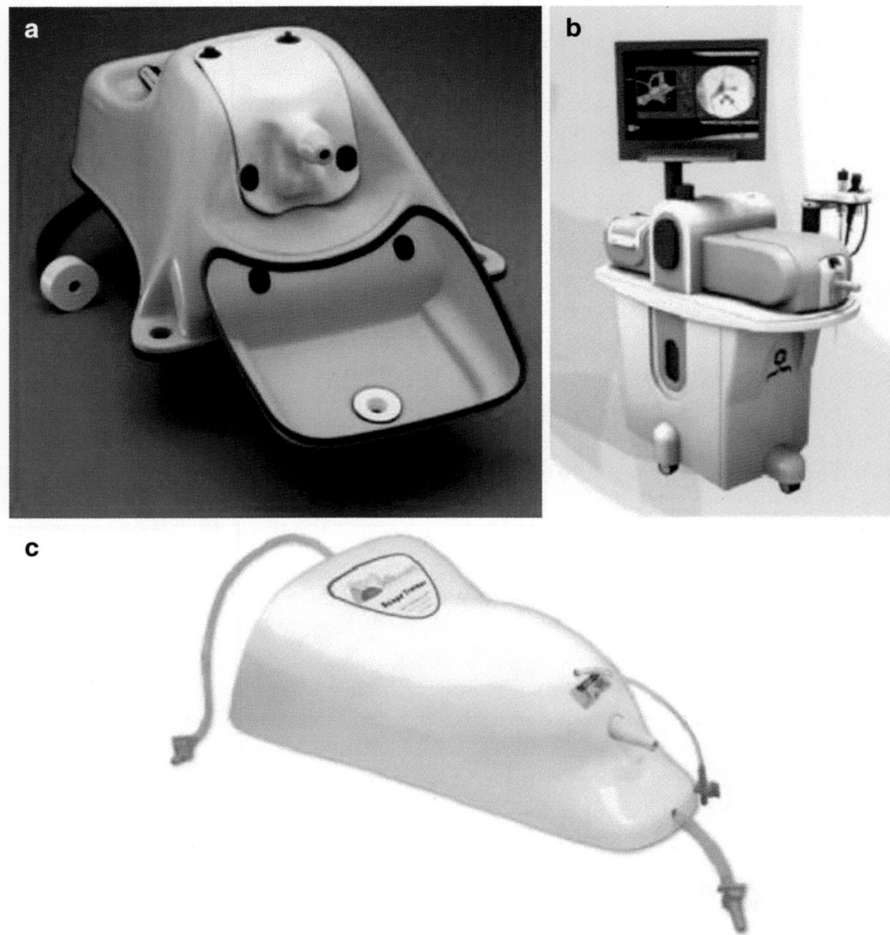

Fig. 24.4 Currently available commercial ureteroscopy simulators, (**a**) Uro-Scopic Trainer, (**b**) URO Mentor, (**c**) Scope Trainer [137]

and experts (≥10 LRN) and, therefore, was "not suitable for implementation in a urologic training program" in its present form [48].

Recently created, there are now patient-specific simulations that allow surgeons to rehearse before surgery. Makiyama et al. first developed this technology, in a study in which they successfully generated a VR simulator with specific patient anatomy (Fig. 24.4) [49]. The simulator uses dynamic CT images (1 mm slice early phase CT on 64 detector spiral CT) of the patient of interest, and a complex model data generator then extracts anatomic information and enters it into the simulator. The simulator allows for both transperitoneal and retroperitoneal approaches, and the kidney moves according to positioning (supine vs lateral). The simulator allows the surgeon to place the trocars and camera anywhere on the body, allowing generous autonomy on deciding one's surgical approach. Once trocar placement has been decided, users can use a number of instruments including forceps, Maryland dissectors, scissors, hook device, clips, laparoscopic stapling devices, and entrapment bags. A foot pedal allows for the use of simulated electrocautery, and a scope handled by an assistant can be changed between 0°, 30°, and 45° lens. The simulator also includes haptics, giving tactile feedback. Realistic bleeding is also included with the simulator, with the degree of bleeding depending upon the injury and type of vessel involved. Surgeons have the option of achieving hemostasis with gauze, forceps, or clips. In a follow-up study by Makiyama et al., face and content validity of the simulator was demonstrated in 13 preoperative simulations (7 nephrectomies, 4 partial nephrectomies, and 2 pyeloplasties) carried out by three surgeons [50]. On a 1–5-point Likert scale, the surgeons rated anatomical integrity to be 3.4 ± 1.1 (face validity), utility of the simulations to be 4.2 ± 1.1 (content validity), and confidence during subsequent surgery to be 4.1 ± 1.1.

Pyeloplasty

There are five procedures currently identified by the American Urological Association's (AUA) Laparoscopic, Robotic, and New Surgical Technology (LRNST) Committee for which simulation would be beneficial [51]. One of those procedures is laparoscopic pyeloplasty (LPP). LPP is done most often for ureteropelvic junction (UPJ) obstruction. This is a technically challenging procedure when done laparoscopically because it requires excision of the UPJ obstruction, spatulation of the renal pelvis and proximal ureter, and suturing of the anastomosis—all which must be accomplished intracorporeally. Without surprise, the learning curve for laparoscopic pyeloplasty can be steep for beginners [52].

Currently, the simulation options available for laparoscopic pyeloplasty include bench and animal models. The Simulation PeriOperative Resource for Training and Learning (SimPORTAL) from the University of Minnesota is responsible for the creation of a number of surgical simulation models. One model is a high-fidelity physical renal pelvis/ureter tissue analog bench model that allows for simulation of laparoscopic pyeloplasty. Using organosilicate-based materials, Poniatowski et al. created the pyeloplasty simulation model by 3D printing a patient-specific mold [51]. The renal pelvis is approximately 6 cm in the superior-inferior direction and 3 cm in the anterior-posterior direction, with an attached 18 cm ureter with 0.8 cm diameter. The UPJ obstruction has an outer diameter of 0.5 cm with an inner diameter of 0.2 cm. The model can then be placed in a standard laparoscopic box trainer, and the procedure can be performed. Additionally, the creators of this model integrated lines going down the length of the model that can only be seen under UV light. These lines allow for Black Light Assessment of Surgical Technique (BLAST™) to be done after the exercise, specifically looking for alignment of the UV-sensitive lines, indicating proper alignment of the UPJ anastomosis. Poniatowski et al. demonstrated face, content, and construct validity of the pyeloplasty model in a study of 31 attending clinical urologists. Face validity was demonstrated with a questionnaire given to participants after using the

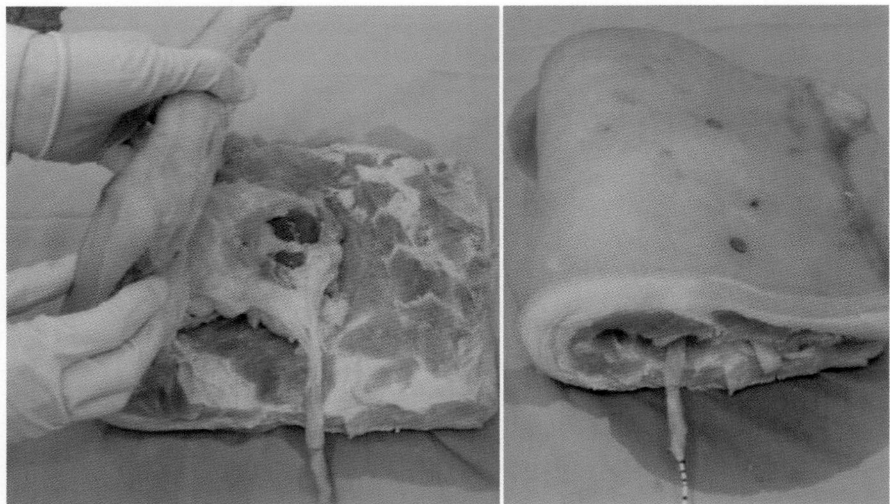

Fig. 24.5 Ex vivo porcine kidney wrapped in full-thickness skin flap [165]

model with participants giving the model an average score of 4.17 on a 5-point Likert scale for anatomical accuracy of the renal pelvis, ureter, and UPJ obstruction. Scores of 4.42 and 4.33 were given for the model reproducing skills for the anastomotic suturing and reproducing the skills of spatulation, respectively (content validity). Construct validity was shown as those who had experience in performing a LPP in the previous 5 years performed better than those who had not in terms of increased patency ($p < 0.05$), decreased twisting ($p < 0.05$), and decreased leakage ($p < 0.10$) [51].

A simpler model is the "latex glove" laparoscopic pyeloplasty model set forth by Raza et al. [53]. The authors used a standard latex glove with a knot tied at the base of one of the fingers to create a model in which the knot represents a strictured UPJ and the palm represents the dilated renal pelvis (Fig. 24.5). The model was placed within a standard laparoscopic box trainer, and a laparoscopic dismembered pyeloplasty was then performed. In their small study of five participants ranging from an experienced surgeon (>20 laparoscopic pyeloplasties) to an inexperienced medical student, Raza et al. touted construct validity for this model. The more experienced participants were found to perform the procedure in significantly less time (47 vs 160 min, $p = 0.043$) and with better suturing [53]. Further studies into the applicability of this model into urological training are yet to be seen.

Yang et al. have set forth a benchtop model for the simulation of a retroperitoneal laparoscopic dismembered pyeloplasty [54]. The model consists of a kidney made of commercially available plastic clay (such as Play-Doh®) with the middle part of the model being imbedded with a metal clip, allowing for the attachment of a carp swim bladder, to simulate a dilated renal pelvis. A separate 10 cm portion of porcine ureter is used as the model ureter, with it already being connected, as if the UPJ obstruction had already been excised. The model is then placed within a box consisting of five hinged boards, which can be adjusted to mimic the limited working space of the retroperitoneum. As would be done with a standard box trainer, the box is then used with standard laparoscopic equipment. The authors found in a cohort of five surgeons that operative time significantly reduced after using the trainer (41.84 vs 25.04 min, $p < 0.01$) and the surgeons rated themselves better on a general self-efficacy score (22.20 vs 27.60, $p < 0.01$). The authors also compared complication rates of the surgeons in real patient cases before and after simulation. Analyzing 15 patients prior to simulation for an average of 6.6 months follow-up, one patient experienced a restenosis and another patient experienced a prolonged urine leak. They then compared this to a group of 15 additional patients, followed at an average of 7.4 months after model simulation, and found there were no reported complications [54]. However, it is unclear if this study was powered to be able to detect significant differences in complications.

Animal models are also available to simulate LPP training. Ramachandran et al. were the first to describe the unique anatomy of the chicken esophagus to simulate LPP by using the chicken crop and esophagus to simulate the renal pelvis and ureter, respectively [55]. The crop of the chicken is a dilated segment of esophagus proximal to the stomach that primarily functions in food storage. Ramachandran et al. exposed the crop and esophagus of a dead chicken and then cleaned and filled the crop/esophagus with water to simulate a dilated renal pelvis. An 8F feeding tube was then passed down the esophagus into the crop, and the esophagus was ligated with a silk suture. The model was then placed into a standard box trainer, and a dismembered LPP was performed. Three urology residents initially studied this model in their final year of study, with each resident doing four LPPs over the period of a month. The study found that at the first attempt, only one of the three residents could complete the task because of technical difficulties experienced during laparoscopic suturing. However, after the fourth attempt, all the subjects could complete a good quality LPP in a mean time of 67.7 min, with each attempt taking less time and with better anastomosis suturing scores [55]. Jiang et al. then went on to demonstrate construct validity for this model in a separate study of 15 participants divided into three groups based off of experience. Participants were studied on the time to completion, as well as with a quality score on a scale of 1–10 assessed by a blinded evaluator (exact tissue sutured, equality of bite sizes, equal stitch intervals, lack of tissue tear, and water-tight anastomosis). The study found that the model was able to distinguish level of experience both by time to perform the task (33.80 min for experts vs 55.20 min for limited experience group vs 92.60 min in no experience group; $p < 0.001$) and in regard to a quality score (9.0 vs 7.2 vs 4.0; $p < 0.001$) [56].

There is one model currently described that uses live animals for LPP. Fu et al. were able to perform 60 LPPs (each side done three times) on ten anesthetized Guangxi Bama minipigs (20–30 kgs) using their own specialized proposed method [57]. Ten hours before surgery, the pigs fasted and underwent bowel preparation and then were placed under anesthesia and placed supine on an operating table. After getting access in a standard laparoscopic fashion, the renal hilum was exposed, and the ureter was divided close to the hilum and spatulated. Next, a piece of small bowel adjacent to the renal hilum was selected as a surrogate for an enlarged renal pelvis. The lower portion of the small intestine was then cut open, and after an antegrade stent was placed down the ureter, the "pyelotomy" was sutured to the previously spatulated ureter. Fu et al. studied this model with five trainees in an advanced laparoscopic urology fellowship, with each subject completing 12 LPPs over a 10-day period. The authors found that operative time significantly reduced after the trainees had performed 12 LPPs (135 vs 62 min, $p < 0.001$), and all subjects commented that the simulation was helpful and improved their laparoscopic skills [57].

Prostate

Urethrovesical Anastomosis

Since its introduction in 1997, the laparoscopic radical prostatectomy has largely been abandoned in favor of using robotic-assisted laparoscopy [58]. This is attributable to the extreme difficulty of intracorporeal suturing and knot tying deep within the pelvis, particularly the urethrovesical anastomosis (UVA), when performing with straight laparoscopy. Thus, there have been models created to help simulate and improve the skills needed to perform this task.

There are currently three described bench models for simulation of the UVA, two of which include animal tissues. The first is a relatively simple model introduced by Nadu et al. [59]. The authors used pieces of chicken skin available at local supermarkets to fashion a urethra and bladder that could be sewn together in a laparoscopic box trainer. This was accomplished by fashioning the chicken skin into a 4 cm tubular structure (urethra) over a 16F urethral catheter. The bladder is created by folding over a piece of chicken skin and cutting a 1 cm orifice in the folded edge. The model is then secured into a standard box trainer, and a UVA can be simulated at that time. Nadu et al. found in their initial study that two advanced laparoscopy urology fellows substantially reduced the time required to perform the anastomosis, from 75 min initially to 20 min after performing 20 UVAs on the model [59]. These results were confirmed in a subsequent study by Yang et al., suggesting this simple model may at least help improve operative time in performing the UVA in a laparoscopic radical prostatectomy [60].

A second bench model, described by Sabbagh et al., introduced a low-fidelity model for perfecting the UVA. This very simple model consists of a piece of latex tubing through which a Foley catheter can be passed and sutured to another piece of latex in the form of the bladder neck while placed in a standard laparoscopic box trainer. In their initial study, Sabbagh et al. randomly divided 28 senior surgery residents, fellows, and staff surgeons into two groups. The first group was the intervention group which practiced UVA on their low-fidelity model. Meanwhile, the second group practiced basic laparoscopic skills such as knot tying on a foam pad. The groups were later evaluated by a blinded grader on their ability to do five interrupted intracorporeal sutures on both the low-fidelity model and the foam pad. The study found that the intervention group scored significantly higher on a task-specific checklist (10.9 vs 8.1, $p = 0.017$) and global rating score (29.6 vs 22.8, $p = 0.005$) and in significantly less time (27.6 vs 38.3 min, $p = 0.004$) compared to the control group [61]. The authors subsequently published a prospective, single-blind, randomized study of their model in which the same cohort of 28 participants was again divided into the same intervention and control groups, but this time, the participants were evaluated on their ability to do a UVA on an anesthetized pig. Again, the group that trained on the low-fidelity model did significantly better than the control group in terms of checklist score, global rating score, and end product rating, demonstrating that skills acquired in a low-fidelity trainer can be translated to more "real-life" situations [62].

The third bench model is a combination bench-and-animal model simulating UVA, which has been proposed by Laguna et al. [63]. The authors used dead, plucked chickens that were at least 2.5 kilograms for their simulation. Using two subcostal incisions extended to the thighs, the authors removed all thoracoabdominal organs except for the esophagus and the stomach. An 18F catheter was placed through the esophagus, and the chicken was then placed within a Pelvic Trainer through which a standard laparoscopic camera and instruments could be used. Once in the box trainer, the specimen was transected completely at the gastroesophageal junction. In their study of the model, five urologists of varying experience (ranging from never having done a laparoscopic radical prostatectomy to >250 performed) were instructed to sew the UVA with two different suturing methods (six interrupted sutures vs running single-knot suture). The study found that suturing time and operator experience were linearly related ($r = -0.724$, $p < 0.001$) and that the most inexperienced surgeon significantly reduced the time required to complete the anastomosis with interrupted sutures (320.5 vs 146.7 s per stitch, $p = 0.001$) [63].

Female Urology

Sacrocolpopexy

Commonly performed by urologists with a focus in female urology, sacrocolpopexy is considered by many to be the "gold standard" procedure to repair vaginal prolapse. Sacrocolpopexy can be performed open, laparoscopically, or robotically, but as with many other surgeries, there is an increasing trend to perform this procedure more often in a minimally invasive fashion. However, with minimally invasive surgery comes with the added difficulty of laparoscopic suturing. Therefore, a model for laparoscopic sacrocolpopexy was created. Tunitsky-Bitton et al. created a simple bench model for laparoscopic sacrocolpopexy in which a RUMI Advanced Uterine Manipulation System (Cooper Surgical, Inc., Trumbull, CT) with attached sacrocolpopexy tip was covered with swimsuit material and placed within a standard FLS box trainer [64]. The authors studied this model with 5 experts (female pelvic medicine and reconstructive surgeons experienced with laparoscopic sacrocolpopexy) and 15 trainee participants (fourth-year gynecology residents and fellows). Participants used the model to perform the most difficult step of the laparoscopic sacrocolpopexy procedure—posterior mesh attachment. The authors found that the model demonstrated construct validity with experts performing significantly better than the trainee group in total score and every domain of the GOALS scale (33 vs 20.5, $p = 0.002$). Face and content validity was also suggested as 75% (all experts) "agreed" or "strongly agreed" that the model was realistic and useful for training laparoscopic sacrocolpopexy [64].

Robotic-Assisted Surgery

Robotic surgery, utilized by the urologic specialty more than any other, is an additional surgical tool that represents the next step up from laparoscopy. With it come a number of advantages over traditional laparoscopy, including improved ergonomics, instruments with "wrists," higher camera magnification, three-dimensional vision, and improved depth perception [65, 66]. Since it was first introduced, the number of robotic surgeries done around the world has grown exponentially. In 2014, Intuitive Surgical, makers of the da Vinci Surgical System (the only robotic surgical device in use today), reported 570,000 robotic cases had been performed [67]. However, with its incorporation, there is concern that many surgeons have been inadequately trained prior to doing robotic cases [67]. Even within residency programs, which are specifically designed to train residents, many residents feel inadequately prepared to perform minimally invasive surgery at graduation [68, 69].

Similar to the creation of the Fundamentals of Laparoscopic Skills curriculum, there has been the creation of the Fundamentals of Robotic Surgery (FRS), representing a push toward standardization of training in robotic surgery. They have formed a curriculum based around the development of basic robotic skills through simulation exercises that can be applied to a number of specialties. As the result of a conglomeration of 14 international surgical societies, FRS is the first consensus robotic curriculum [20]. Robotic simulation is similar to other surgical simulation modalities, consisting of physical models, animal models, and virtual reality.

Basic Robotic Skills

A cornerstone of the FRS program is the acquisition of basic robotic skills. These skills are absolutely essential to become a safe and proficient surgeon. For simulation purposes, the development of psychomotor skills is paramount, since it has been shown to have a steep learning curve. The FRS program has 10 tasks which teach 16 psychomotor skills. These tasks are FLS peg transfer, FLS suturing and knot tying, FLS pattern cutting, running suture, dome with four towers for ambidexterity, vessel dissection and clipping, fourth-arm retraction and cutting, energy and mechanical cutting, docking task, and trocar insertion task [20]. For simplicity, these tasks are all performed on a single device, the "FRS dome" (Fig. 24.6).

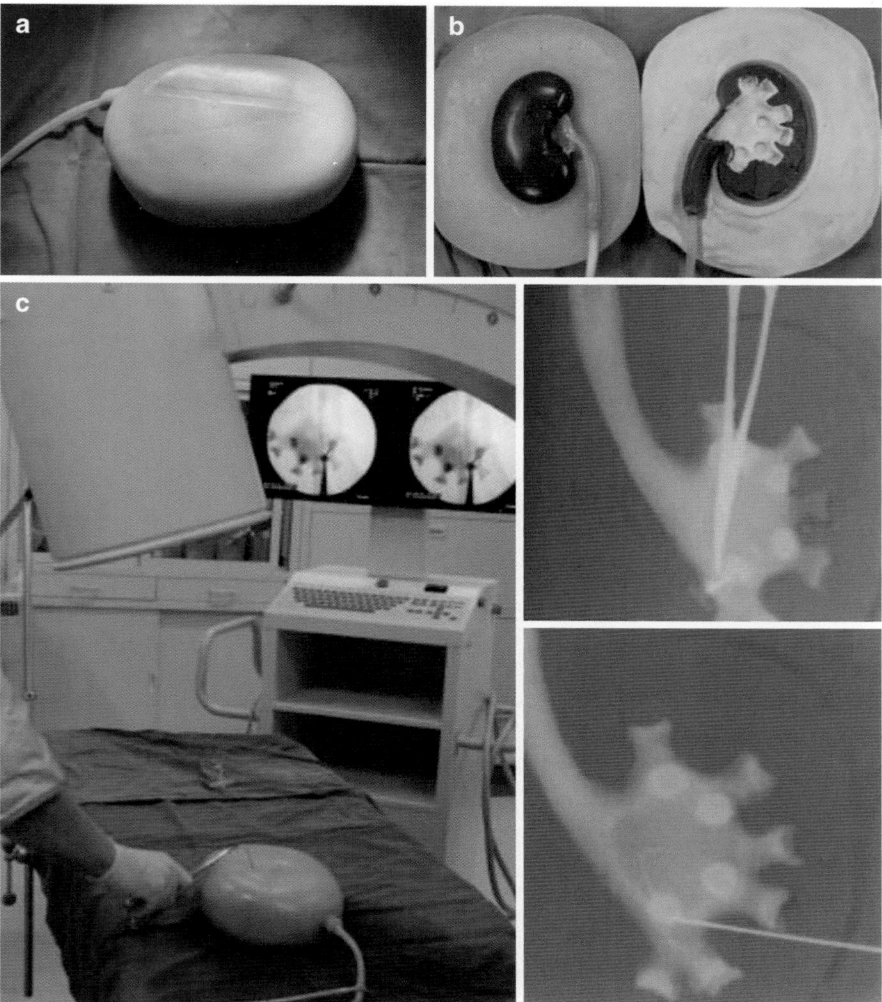

Fig. 24.6 Validated PCNL model compatible with both fluoroscopy and ultrasound [167]. (**a**) Practice of fluoroscopy guided PRA; (**b**) Puncture, C-arm at 20°; (**c**) Guidewire placement, C-arm upright

In addition to physical models, there have also been virtual reality simulations used in FRS to develop robotic skills. Robotic VR training has been dominated by three validated platforms: Robotic Surgical Simulator (Simulated Surgical Systems, Williamsville, NY), dV-Trainer (Mimic Technologies, Seattle, WA), and the da Vinci Skills Simulator (Intuitive Surgical, Sunnyvale, CA) [70]. The Robotic

Surgical Simulator (Robotic Surgical Simulator) and dV-Trainer are both standalone devices with hand controls and foot pedals designed to imitate the da Vinci robot, whereas the da Vinci Skills Simulator (dVSS) is a "backpack" to a standard da Vinci surgeon's console where the trainee uses the console with a training interface [71]. All three simulators work on basic robotic skills including grasping, suturing, and psychomotor exercises such as peg transfer and letter-board tasks. Several studies are available that show validated face, content, and construct validity of all three simulators [71–77]. Hung et al. presented an interesting study in which the three platforms were cross-correlated by using structured inanimate exercises (bench models), the three VR simulators, and an in vivo robotic skills assessment on a porcine model [70]. The authors were able to confirm construct validity of each of the training tools and demonstrated that virtual reality performance was strongly correlated with in vivo tissue performance.

Adrenal/Kidney

There is currently very little that is published in the literature regarding simulation surgery on kidneys or adrenals for robotic surgery. This is hardly surprising, as robotic surgery has not been around as long laparoscopic surgery. There will likely be a movement to produce more kidney-specific robotic surgery simulations, as just like in laparoscopy a steep learning curve is present to master nephron-sparing robotic surgery. Mottrie et al. published that the learning curve of robotic partial nephrectomy for an experienced robotic surgeon is estimated to be approximately 30 cases to achieve a warm ischemia time of less than 20 min and improved complication rates [78].

Partial Nephrectomy

The first kidney-specific robotic simulation currently described comes from Hung et al. at the University of Southern California from 2012. They describe an ex vivo porcine kidney model with an embedded 1.5 inch Styrofoam ball, simulating a renal tumor [79]. The model was created by using a 1 inch melon scooper to score the renal capsule, with a 15-blade scalpel then used to create the defect, with care taken to avoid involvement of the collecting system. Once the defect was created, the commercially available Styrofoam ball was simply affixed within the defect with super glue (Fig. 24.7). The authors estimated that the model costs approximately 15 USD and took an average of 7 min to create. They studied this model in a group of 46 participants divided into experts, intermediates, and novices based upon level of robotic experience. The participants used a robot with Prograsp forceps and curved scissors (cautery and fourth robotic arm where not given) to excise the tumor (Styrofoam ball) with a clear margin of renal parenchyma (Fig. 24.8). The authors boasted excellent results with this cohort of participants, with experts giving the model a "very realistic" rating (face validity) and "extremely helpful" for training of residents and fellows (construct validity). The model was also able to distinguish between levels of experience with experts performing significantly better than intermediates and novices in overall score, time, depth perception, bimanual dexterity,

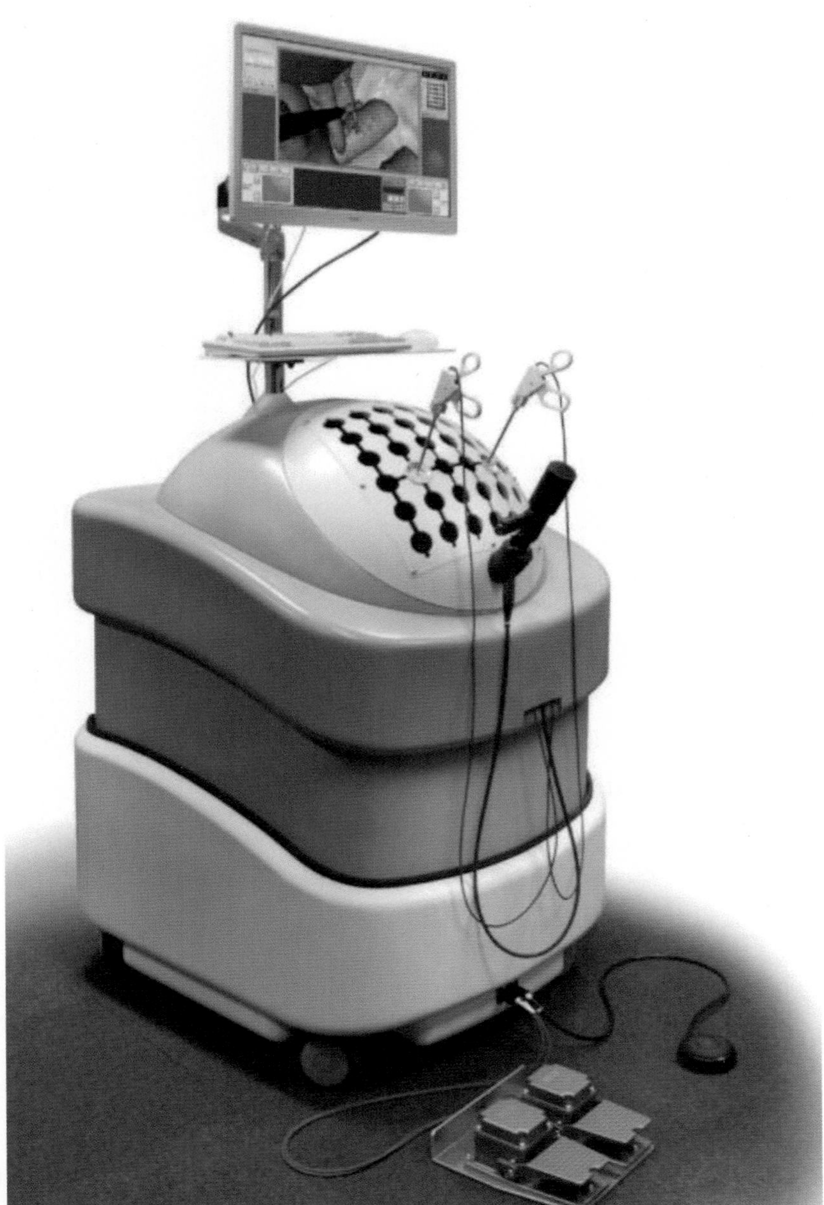

Fig. 24.7 Patient-specific VR simulator [50]

efficiency, tissue handling, and instrument and camera awareness [79]. However, the reality of blood loss and hemorrhage is not available with this model and poses a weakness to its use—especially for a model examining a procedure like partial nephrectomy.

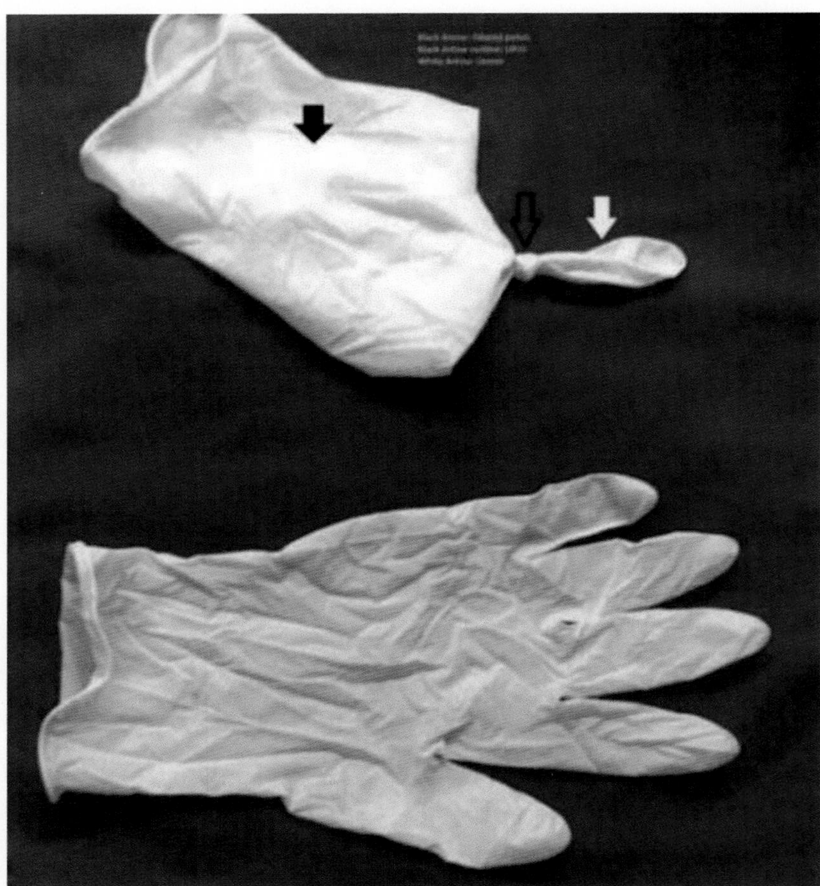

Fig. 24.8 "Latex glove" laparoscopic pyeloplasty model [53]

Coming from the same group, a recently published simulation platform created for robotic partial nephrectomy was made that utilizes both augmented reality and virtual reality [80]. The authors created this simulation platform from the existing dV-Trainer platform. The first component of the simulator is augmented reality (AR) in which actual surgical footage is overlaid with virtual instruments which the user can manipulate. During this time, there is also narration from the operating surgeon, allowing for cognitive and technical tips to be learned by the user. The goal of the augmented reality portion of the simulation is to learn key aspects of the procedure via a number of interactive exercises. The simulation is divided into five modules each representing a key aspect of the procedure (colon mobilization, kocherization of the duodenum, hilar dissection, kidney mobilization, and tumor resection and repair). In the final module, there is an imbedded virtual reality exercise in which the user performs renorrhaphy on a modification of a previously validated suture sponge exercise from the Mimic Simulation library. In their study of this new simulator, Hung et al. again divided 42 participants into expert, intermediate, and novice

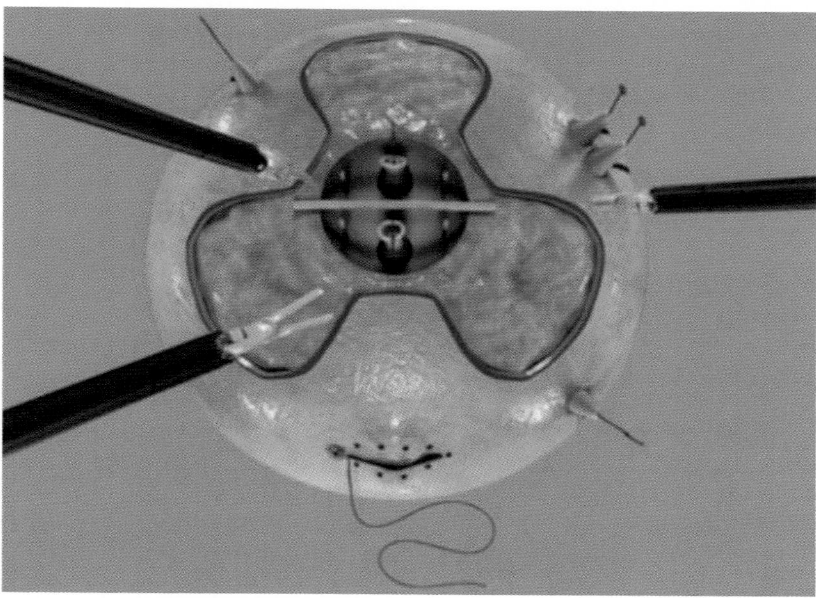

Fig. 24.9 Fundamentals of Robotic Surgery Dome for acquisition of basic robotic skills [20]

categories based upon robotic surgery experience. The authors found that the experts gave the simulation a median score of 8/10 in terms of realism (face validity). Experts also rated the platform highly in terms of its ability to teach relevant anatomy (9/10) and operative steps (8.5/10), suggesting content validity. Construct validity was suggested with experts performing significantly better than both novices and intermediates in a number of categories. Interestingly, the authors had the participants perform an in vivo porcine partial nephrectomy and found performance on the simulator correlated strongly with performance in the porcine partial nephrectomy ($r = 0.8$, $p < 0.0001$), demonstrating concurrent validity [80].

Bladder/Ureter

As with kidney simulation, there is currently little availability in the way of bladder- and ureter-specific robotic simulators. This may be a consequence of the relatively recent move toward doing more bladder/ureter procedures in a robotic fashion. Hung et al. have published a relatively simple cystotomy repair simulation in which a 2.5 cm incision is made on the anterior surface of a porcine bladder and a watertight closure is made using a robot [71].

Ureteral reimplantation represents a growing field in minimally invasive surgery, as minimally invasive techniques have been shown to have similar functional outcomes similar to those of open procedures [81, 82]. Despite its increased prevalence, ureteral reimplantation remains a relatively infrequently done procedure that may be lacking in traditional urologic training, particularly those done in a minimally invasive nature. As such, simulation-based training has been developed for this procedure. There is currently one validated ureteral reimplantation model described in the literature. This model consists of a plastic box which has a simulated bladder and ureter held in place by alligator clips (Fig. 24.9). The bladder and ureters are made of a commercially available hydrogel material (LifeLike BioTissue, Canada). The simulated bladder was created with a 12 × 15 cm rectangular piece of the hydrogel. The simulated ureter was created with hydrogel as well with a 0.5 mm wall thickness, 6 mm in diameter, and 15 cm in length. A 1 cm incision was made in the "bladder," and a 6F ureteral stent was passed through the ureter, and the anastomosis was then performed using a standard robot. Tunitsky et al. studied this model with 21 participants divided into "procedure experts" (>10 robotically assisted ureteral reimplant procedures performed), "robot experts" (fellowship-trained gynecologic surgeons with experience in a number of robot procedures), and "trainees" (fourth-year urology residents as well as urology and urogynecology fellows) [83]. After completing the simulation, all of the experts "agreed" or "strongly agreed" that the model was realistic and useful (face validity). Using a Global Operative Assessment of Laparoscopic Skills (GOALS) scale, the authors demonstrated construct validity by showing that procedure experts score significantly higher than both robotic experts and trainees ($p = 0.02$ and $p = 0.004$, respectively), and robotic experts performed significantly better than the trainees ($p = 0.05$). The authors have suggested that the model can be reused about ten times with an approximate cost of $22 (excluding stent and suture cost).

Prostate

Robot-Assisted Laparoscopic Radical Prostatectomy

The radical prostatectomy represents one surgery that has seen significant changes since the introduction of robot-assisted surgery. Because of the robot's ability for vision magnification and the use of small, long instruments which work well deep within the pelvis, there has been a dramatic shift in prostatectomies being done primarily open to now most being done with robotic assistance (RALRP) [84]. There have been multiple studies which have shown a rather steep learning curve for RALRP, with some suggesting that 250 cases may be necessary to gain proficiency at RALRP [85]. Increased experience with RALRP has been shown to result in fewer anastomotic strictures and a lower rate of cancer recurrence [86, 87]. As such, simulation training for RALRP has been developed to supplement the often inadequate RALRP exposure experienced during residency.

Alemozaffar et al. first described a unique simulation for RALRP in which a female porcine genitourinary tract tissue is fashioned into a male pelvic genitourinary model which can be used to simulate RALRP [88]. The authors started by making a plaster replica of the male pelvis with a fitted rubber pad to simulate the urogenital diaphragm. They then harvested the vagina, bladder, and ureters from a female pig. Through a number of steps, the porcine vagina was fashioned into a rectum and prostatic pedicle with the introitus becoming the prostate gland. The fallopian tubes were used to create seminal vesicles and the dorsal venous complex (DVC). Ureters were used to represent the neurovascular bundles running along the prostate. The recreated porcine anatomy is then placed into the pelvis model, which can then be used for simulation with a standard robot. The authors then had ten novices and ten experts perform the following steps of RALRP on the model: ligation of the DVC, division of the bladder neck, seminal vesicle dissection, ligation of the prostatic pedicle with sparing of the nerves, apical prostatic dissection with division of the urethra, bladder neck reconstruction, and UVA. The model demonstrated face validity with experts giving it a 3.7/5 score of realism, with a particularly impressive 4.5/5 for the UVA portion of the simulator. Experts also supported content validity with a score of 4.7/5 regarding the usefulness of the model for training of RALRP. Construct validity was demonstrated as experts performed the procedure significantly faster (60.8 vs 121.4 min, $p < 0.001$) and with significantly higher OSATS performance scores (4.6/5 vs 2.6/5, $p < 0.001$) [88].

While not a specific RALRP, Volpe et al. recently validated a curriculum specific for RALRP called the European Association of Urology Robotic Training Curriculum (ERUS curriculum) [89]. The ERUS curriculum was developed by a panel of experts in robotic surgery and consisted of 12 weeks of training divided into three stages: e-learning; an intensive week of simulation-based laboratory training including virtual reality, cadaveric, and animal simulations; and 3 weeks of supervised modular training in RALRP until they ultimately carried out a full RALRP. Despite being a small study of only ten urology fellows, the authors demonstrated that the training program resulted in significant improvement of the fellows' performance during RALRP, with 80% being deemed by their mentors as safe and effective to perform a RALRP independently after the training program [89].

Urethrovesical Anastomosis

As was discussed previously in the laparoscopy section, the urethrovesical anastomosis (UVA) is one of the most integral steps in a prostatectomy with a steep learning curve requiring surgeons to master intracorporeal suturing and anastomosis deep within the pelvis. As more and more prostatectomies are done robotically, there is a need for simulation for the robotic radical prostatectomy. By gaining proficiency in performing the UVA, one could go a long way toward becoming proficient at robot-assisted laparoscopic radical prostatectomy (RARP).

One such simulator is the virtual reality-based "Tube 3" module designed by Kang et al. [90]. The Tube 3 is a module specifically made for simulation of the UVA on previously discussed Mimic dV-Trainer (MIMIC Technologies, Seattle, WA). On the Tube 3 modules, users can perform a virtual reality UVA using a number of techniques, and scoring metrics are automatically tracked by the Mimic Technology. Kang et al. validated the Tube 3 module by dividing 20 urology attendings and residents into expert and novice categories and having them perform a UVA with a single-knot technique previously described by Van Velthoven et al. [90, 91]. The authors demonstrated face and content validity in which the ten experts answered questionnaires about the Tube 3 module. All of the experts "agreed" or "totally agreed" that the technical skills required to complete Tube 3 were compared to those that performed a UVA during radical prostatectomy. Eighty percent of the experts deemed it to be useful for training others to do UVAs and that it would be helpful in measuring proficiency at performing UVAs. Construct validity was also demonstrated with Tube 3's ability to distinguish the expert from the novice group. The experts performed significantly better than the novices in a number of categories including total task time, total score, economy of motion, and number of instrument collisions ($p < 0.05$). In a separate study, Kim et al. found the Tube 3 module to have concurrent and predictive validity by having 11 urology residents and fellows train on the Tube 3 module and then perform a robotic double bowel layer closure (concurrent validation) and a robotic UVA, both on commercially available models [92]. The authors demonstrated that participants who trained with the Tube 3 module were significantly faster to perform the above tasks than those who did not train on Tube 3.

A second described UVA simulator comes from the University of New York at Buffalo, which developed a haptic-enabled augmented reality-based training module for UVA. The system referred to as "HoST," hands-on surgical training, augments a real surgery with virtual reality components in which users are given audio and visual didactics of a given procedure (in this case, UVA) and then perform the steps themselves in the previously described Robotic Surgical Simulator. In a multi-institutional randomized controlled trial by Chowriappa et al., the HoST was found to improve technical skills for performing a UVA with little cognitive demand. Fifty-two urology residents and fellows (all with less than 25 h on a robotic console) were randomized to either the HoST training group or to control. All participants became familiar with the robot via fundamental skills of robotic surgery (FSRS) training on a RoSS console. The HoST training group then completed four, 20 min HoST modules, while the control group watched videos of UVA surgery for an equal amount of time. The groups were then scored on their ability to perform UVA on an inanimate model using a da Vinci robot. Face and content validity was suggested as 70% or more of the participants deemed the simulator to be realistic and would be helpful in learning to do UVA. The HoST group performed significantly better than the control group in terms of needle driving, needle positioning, suture placement, and on overall Global Evaluative Assessment of Robotic Skills (GEARS) score ($p < 0.05$) [93]. Participants also performed a NASA Task Load Index assessment, and the HoST group was found to have less temporal demand and effort and less mental fatigue than the control group ($p < 0.05$).

Endoscopy

Endoscopy has come a long way since Antonin Desormeaux excised a urethral papilloma using an endoscope with lighting from a kerosene lamp in the 1850s [94]. Endoscopy is perhaps now the most routine procedure performed by urologists, so a strong foundation of endoscopic skills is essential. Urologists have many tools at hand to perform endoscopy, most commonly using cystoscopes and ureteroscopes, which are made both rigid and flexible and in a number of sizes. Endoscopy is used for a number of procedures both diagnostic and therapeutic in nature; as such, a number of simulators for endoscopic procedures have been developed and will be discussed below.

Bladder/Urethra

Cystourethroscopy

Cystourethroscopy, occurring both in the operating room and in the office, represents one of the most commonly performed procedures by urologists. A rigid or flexible cystoscope is typically used to thoroughly examine the bladder and urethra in both males and females. There are currently several options for simulation of cystourethroscopy, including both bench models and virtual reality (VR) simulators. The URO-Mentor™ (Simbionix Corp, Cleveland, OH, USA) can be used for both flexible and rigid cystoscopy as well as ureteroscopy. The URO-Mentor uses a novel, sophisticated visual engine that is able to offer high-fidelity simulation with a number of features, including two- and three-dimensional rendering, collision detection, texture mapping, x-ray rendering, and special effects such as blood, smoke, and stone fragments [95]. In a study by Schout et al., the URO-Mentor system was used in training of flexible cystoscopy by both novice and expert endoscopists. The study demonstrated good construct validity and found that simulation with the URO-Mentor system resulted in large improvements in novice performance in terms of time, trauma caused, areas inspected, and global rating scale score [96]. In another study from the same group, study participants who received training on the URO-Mentor virtual reality system performed significantly better doing cystourethroscopy on real patients than those who did not receive VR training [97].

Despite the proven benefits that high-fidelity trainers and simulators provide, they come with significant cost, as new simulators often cost tens of thousands of dollars. It has been questioned if low-fidelity models could allow for the same learning experience for novices. Matsumoto et al. demonstrated that a low-fidelity model consisting of a Penrose drain representing the urethra, an inverted Styrofoam cup representing the bladder, and drinking straws inserted into the cup as ureters was just as effective for skill improvement in a group of 40 medical students when compared to a $3,700 high-fidelity model [98]. The same authors also presented a low-fidelity model of Styrofoam tubing, representing the urethra, leading into a bell pepper, representing the bladder, with 18 gauge Angiocaths puncturing the bell pepper, representing the ureters. This model has an advantage of a very low cost and the use of similar equipment used in the operating room, as trainees are able to practice cystoscopy and cannulation of ureters with various types of wires.

The use of cadavers in medical education is invaluable; however, there is scant literature available on using human cadavers in cystourethroscopy simulation. In one study from Bowling et al., they used fresh-frozen cadavers to assess cystoscopy skills in 29 OB/GYN residents. Various clinical scenarios were created, such as vaginal mesh eroding into the urethra. The residents were divided into a control group versus a study group who received training via a didactic session with bench models. The authors found that residents who underwent didactic training had significant decreases in scope assembly time and increases in task-specific checklists (92.9% vs 52.5%, $p < 0.001$) and global rating scores (87.8% vs 57.6%, $p < 0.001$) versus that of the controls [99]. Despite these benefits, cadavers are very expensive, cannot be used repeatedly, and can be difficult to obtain in various parts of the world.

Transurethral Resection of Bladder Tumor (TURBT)

Bladder cancer is one of the most common cancers in the world, with incidence increasing yearly. As such, transurethral resection of bladder tumor (TURBT) is one of the more common procedures performed by urologists [100]. There is a steep learning curve with inexperienced endoscopists performing TURBT. New learners are liable to inadequate inspection of the bladder, incomplete tumor resection, inadvertent bladder perforation, and/or increased bleeding. Additionally, patient outcomes have proven to be tied to experience, as inexperience with TURBT has been found to be a predictor of higher readmission rates and higher recurrence rates after TURBT for Ta and T1 tumors [101]. Therefore, TURBT represents a profitable target for simulation.

Currently there is one major TURBT simulator described in the literature, the Uro-Trainer® (Karl Storz GmbH, Tuttlingen, Germany) [102]. The Uro-Trainer is a VR simulator with both visual perception and haptic feedback, enabling users to resect papillary bladder tumors as well as carcinoma in situ (CIS) [102, 103]. The Uro-Trainer is commercially available and features a customary resectoscope, two flat screens, multiple instrumentations with varied resection loops, as well as laser instruments [103]. First presented by Reich et al., the Uro-Trainer was proven as a valuable teaching tool for both medical students and urology residents [104]. In a subsequent study, Kruck et al. demonstrated increased area of inspection (36.8–54.3%, $p < 0.05$) and improvements in resection rates (26.5% to 52.0%, $p < 0.05$) among novice endoscopists [103]. The Uro-Trainer was also used in this study to teach new techniques to experienced urologists. They found that experienced urologists gained significant improvement in both bladder inspection (52.2% vs 62.7%, $p = 0.003$) and resection rates (43.8% vs 57.1%, $p = 0.002$) with integrated photodynamic diagnostics (a type of fluorescence cystoscopy) versus standard white-light cystoscopy [103].

A second TURBT simulator was recently validated in the medical literature, the Simbla TURBT simulator (SAMED GmbH, Dresden, Germany). It is a high-fidelity simulator that has a resectable bladder with anatomical structures and embedded tumors within [105]. The Simbla model provides a realistic feel and scenario to trainees by allowing the use of standard OR instruments with connected monopolar or bipolar diathermy. It can also be connected to irrigation for continuous flow throughout the system. In an interesting study by de Vries et al., they identified 21 procedural steps and 17 pitfalls associated with TURBT. The Simbla simulator was found to cover 13 steps and 8 pitfalls. This simulator was found to have face, content, and construct validity [105]. Obviously, the major advantage of the Simbla model over its VR counterparts is its ability to use real instruments and irrigation.

Intravesical Botulinum Toxin Injection (Botox)

The use of intra-detrusor injection of Botox® (botulinum toxin) for overactive bladder was approved in 2011 by the FDA. This provided yet another new procedure to be learned by urologists. This procedure is done cystoscopically under local or general anesthesia with the goal to deliver an even distribution of botulinum toxin into the detrusor muscle, usually via 20–30, 1 cc injections [106]. There is currently only one VR trainer in the literature, which was developed at the University of Minnesota. Their system provides virtual bladder models of multiple sizes and bladder wall thickness, which allows learning of variable injection patterns with optimum penetration depth and dose control [106]. However, this simulator is currently not commercially available and is yet to be formally verified. Nonetheless, it presents a potential source of simulation for an increasingly more performed procedure.

Prostate

Transurethral Resection of the Prostate (TURP)

Transurethral resection of the prostate (TURP) is the classic, gold-standard procedure for the treatment of medically refractory lower urinary tract symptoms secondary to benign prostatic hyperplasia (BPH). However, as pointed out by Wignall et al., the learning curve to properly perform TURP is steep for several reasons. Users must work in a small three-dimensional space represented on a two-dimensional monitor, which requires substantial visual-spatial coordination [107]. This procedure is made more difficult as it is very common to experience intraoperative visual impairment from tissue and blood. Furthermore, serious adverse events can occur from this procedure, including urinary incontinence, erectile dysfunction, profuse bleeding, hyponatremia, and injury to a number of key structures including the urethra, ureter, or rectum [107]. Once a popular procedure is performed during residency, there has been a halving in the number of TURPs done by graduating urology residents over the last 15–20 years [107, 108]. Therefore, there is a demand for TURP simulators to help augment the learning of this procedure.

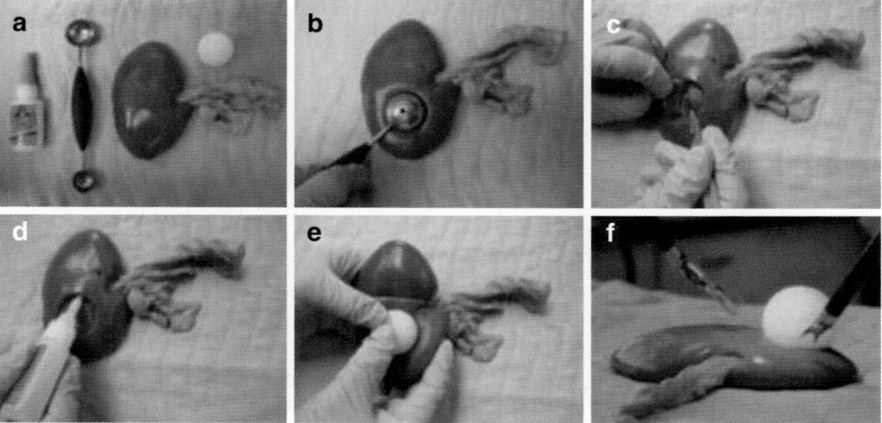

Fig. 24.10 Partial nephrectomy model proposed by Hung et al., (**a**) equipment used in model, (**b**) melon scooper used to score renal capsule, (**c**) a 15-blade scalpel is used to create a defect, (**d**) superglue applied to defect, (**e**) foam ball affixed to model, (**f**) excision of foam tumor [79]

TURP simulators can be broadly divided into high-fidelity virtual reality models versus non-virtual reality physical models—each with their own advantages and disadvantages. Physical simulators rely upon standard TURP equipment used on prostatic tissue surrogates, such as chicken breast, vegetable matter, or pig liver. Trainees at the authors' home institution use a standard TURP resectoscope with associated electrocautery capabilities in an OR-like environment with irrigation fluid and a standard endoscopy tower to resect portions of porcine liver. This model is particularly useful for more inexperienced trainees who can gain experience with assembling and using equipment likely identical to that used in the OR. The main disadvantage of this physical surrogate models is the lack of bleeding and other intraoperative complicating issues when resecting the tissue [109].

Another physical model, the Bristol TURP Trainer (Limbs & Things, UK), is a disposable bench model containing a synthetic prostate within a latex bladder on a plastic base [110] (Fig. 24.10). Trainees use a resectoscope with attached monopolar or bipolar diathermy to resect the prostate model, which is complete with irrigation fluid, realistic anatomy including ureteral orifices and verumontanum, and is made of a synthetic material that can be cut with the resectoscope diathermy loop. This is one of few physical models that has demonstrated face, content, and construct validity [111]. Advantages of this model are the lifelike anatomy, as well as the technical aspects it provides such as using actual resectoscopes, managing fluids, and handling resected prostatic chips. However, similar to other physical models, the Bristol TURP Trainer does not allow for bleeding or other potential complications of the procedure.

The first VR TURP trainer was developed in 1990 by Lardennois et al. Since its introduction, the use of virtual reality for TURP simulation has grown significantly [107, 112]. Many of the earlier models were limited in utility due to their lack of haptics, inaccurate deformation of tissues, and lack of bleeding [107]. Hemostasis was recognized as a critical learning point by Oppenheimer et al. in successful TURP training, so they developed simulated bleeding through the creation of a bleeding movie texture map library [113]. This subsequently initiated the creation of the University of Washington VR TURP trainer (UWTURP), in partnership with Gyrus/ACMI (Reading, Berkshire, United Kingdom), which has become the most extensively validated TURP trainer to date [111, 114]. Created in 2000, the UWTURP comprises a physical model of the penis and pelvis with digital recreations of urothelium and resection bed being based off of digital footage from actual TURP procedures. The simulator has the advantage of being able to track both motion and force data, allowing for objective measures of operative errors, blood loss, grams resected, irrigant volume, and amount of electrocautery use. Numerous studies have validated the model; thus, the UWTURP can successfully distinguish experts from novices. In a study by Sweet et al., no TURP experts had an operative error on a 5 min resection task, whereas novices resected the sphincter 50% of the time and 16% had to stop the operation because of blood loss making vision impossible [114]. Simulated practice with this heavily validated model is invaluable, as novices will learn from their mistakes in a simulated setting rather than harming patients during the early learning curve.

The PelvicVision TURP simulator is another VR TURP simulator that has shown construct validity in two small studies. This model consists of a modified resectoscope attached to a robotic arm, foot pedals, and a standard desktop computer [115]. The simulator gives haptic feedback as well as real-time tracking of variables such as resectoscope movements, blood loss, resection volumes, flow of irrigation, and operative errors, such as bladder perforation, resection of sphincter, and perforation of prostatic capsule. Källström et al. proved construct and content validity in a small study with this model that involved students. These students were able to demonstrate a positive learning curve and improving self-assessments in which they found the procedure to be easier with an increasing numbers of simulations [115].

Photoselective Vaporization of the Prostate (PVP)

Introduced in 1998, the GreenLight™ (American Medical Systems, Inc. Minnetonka, MN) laser photoselective vaporization of the prostate (PVP) has proven to be an effective treatment of bladder outlet obstruction secondary to BPH with significantly less morbidity than traditional TURPs [116–118]. GreenLight PVP uses a potassium-titanyl-phosphate (KTP) laser, of which it has a wavelength that is selectively absorbed by hemoglobin. Thus, tissue containing hemoglobin is preferentially vaporized with near instantaneous hemostasis [119]. AMS created a model, the GreenLight Simulator (GL-SIM), due to the popularity of GreenLight PVP. This simulator has shown both face and content validity [120]. The GL-SIM consists of a camera, scope, laser fiber, and foot pedal which are all pre-attached to a module. A standard laptop is used to run its VR software and display the video output. The system comes pre-loaded with five task-training modules, including anatomy identification, sweep speed, tissue-fiber distance, power settings, and bleeding coagulation. It also is pre-loaded with six full operative cases consisting of increasingly larger and more challenging prostates. Herlemann et al. have shown the GL-SIM to have face, construct, and content validity. Face and content validity was later confirmed by Aydin et al. [121]. They showed in their study that construct validity was demonstrated in two of the five training modules, as well as in operative time, errors made, and instrument cost [120]. Interestingly, Herlemann et al. found improved simulation outcomes in those that were able to play a musical instrument [121].

Holmium Laser Enucleation of the Prostate (HoLEP)

Similarly to PVP, Holmium Laser Enucleation of the Prostate (HoLEP) embodies an emerging alternative to the standard TURP. HoLEP uses a holmium:yttrium-aluminum-garnet (Ho:YAG) laser to enucleate entire lobes of the prostate via emission of pulsed 2140 nm energy [122]. There are some urologists stating that HoLEP has become the new "gold standard" for surgical management of BPH based on its efficacy and low morbidity [123]. However, due to its significantly different technique when compared to TURP, HoLEP has a very steep learning curve—much longer than that of a standard TURP [124]. This unfortunately is a major disadvantage of HoLEP and a reason that many in the urological community have not adopted

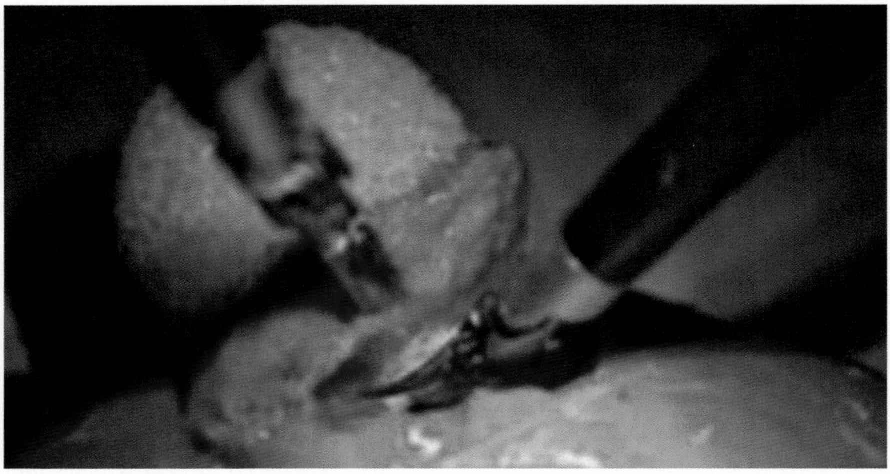

Fig. 24.11 Robotic-assisted partial nephrectomy foam ball excision operative view [79]

the technique [125]. Consequently, a bench-top model has been created to address this steep learning curve.

Developed by Kinoshita et al. and referred to as the Kansai Medical University HoLEP bench model [126], it contains a prostatic hyperplasia model that can be installed into a box simulator along with standard cystoscopic equipment and holmium lasers used to enucleate the model. Additionally, trainees are responsible for real-time fluid management to complete the procedure. The Kansai Medical University HoLEP bench model demonstrated face and content validity in a study of 36 participants by Aydin et al. [127].

There is a virtual reality simulator, the UroSim HoLEP simulator (VitraMed, Zurich, Switzerland), that has been developed and uses a cystoscope module connected to a computer system to simulate the procedure (Fig. 24.11). The simulator is equipped with haptic feedback and six different operative cases with varying anatomical variations and degrees of prostatic hyperplasia. In a study of 53 participants, Kuronen-Stewart et al. divided participants into three groups—novices, intermediate, and experts. The investigators were able to demonstrated face, content, and construct validity with significant differences in the enucleation efficiency, measured as grams enucleated per hour, between each group and a realism score of 5.6 out of 10 among experts [128].

Transrectal Ultrasound (TRUS) Prostate Biopsy

The TRUS-guided prostate biopsy currently is the gold standard to histologically diagnose prostate cancer. However, this relatively simple procedure is not without risk, with 0.69% of men requiring hospitalization to treat complications and reported mortality rates of 1.3% at 120 days [129, 130]. As such, there is a demand to develop simulators that could help bypass the early learning curve of the procedure and help avoid errors made in human patients. This is especially important given the more recent technology of targeted therapies for prostate cancer and the necessity for more accurate sampling of the prostate to avoid areas of untreated cancer.

It was at the University of Western Ontario where Chalasani et al. developed the first prostate biopsy simulator [131]. Simulator images come from a TRUS image bank that was created by collecting 3D TRUS images from 50 patients at the time of live biopsy. These images were incorporated into a mock pelvis which allowed for multiple simulated biopsies to be done with either a standard endfire or sidefire TRUS probe. Consisting of a rectangular box made using polyoxymethylene plastic, the mock pelvis is complete with dense elastic foam imbedded within to simulate the rectal wall as well as a tight elastic port of entry representative of the anus. The box can be manipulated such that simulated biopsies can be performed in either the left lateral decubitus or lithotomy positions. An embedded magnetic sensor tracks movement of the probe, and biopsies are fired with a foot pedal. Chalasani et al. demonstrated face, content, and construct validity in a small study involving 26 physicians; however, they did not reach statistical significance—likely because of the small sample size.

Recently, second prostate biopsy simulator has been created by Fiard et al. [132]. The simulator (unnamed, Grenoble University Hospital, Grenoble, France) is a laptop computer attached to a Phantom Omni haptic device and a stylus representing the ultrasound probe. Moving the stylus allows the user to explore the virtual prostate. Prostate images were obtained from human biopsy procedures. The software is also equipped with an evaluation system that evaluates users on their ability to accurately sample 12 sectors of the prostate. Fiard et al. demonstrated face and content validity in their small study 21 participants, consisting of 7 experts and 14 novices. The median rating of realism was remarkable, being rated 9/10 by novices and 8.2/10 by experts. However, construct validity did not reach statistical significance due to the small sample size, despite a 12% difference in scoring between novices and experts.

Kidney/Ureter

Ureteroscopy

Ureteroscopy (URS) incorporates an extensive range of multiple instruments used for a number of purposes. Some of the indications for URS include the management of upper tract urolithiasis, ureteral strictures, ureteropelvic junction (UPJ) obstruction, ureterocele incision/excision, upper tract biopsies, and ablation/excision of upper tract tumors. URS is accomplished with the use of either a semirigid or flexible ureteroscopes, of which there are many choices depending upon the manufacturer and the indication. With the ever-increasing incidence of urolithiasis in the United States, the incorporation of URS in the urologists' repertoire has also increased, especially since URS is a first-line treatment in stones <2 cm [133, 134].

There is not an established outcome currently for expertise of URS, but several studies on the learning curve for URS have used varying endpoints to estimate

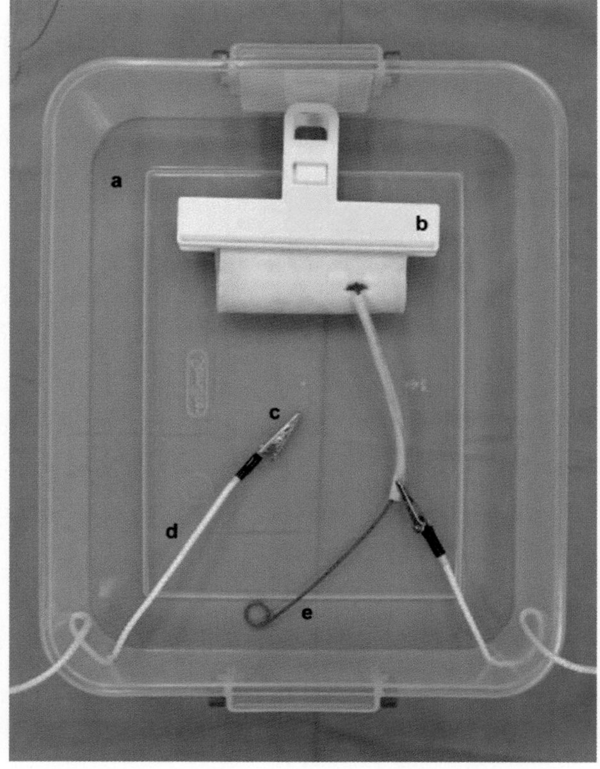

Fig. 24.12 Robotic-assisted ureteral reimplantation model [83]. (*a*) Storage container 15 × 11 × 3 inches (approximately US $5); large bag clip (approximately US $3) attached with Velcro adhesive tape (approximately US $4), (*b*) alligator clips × 2 (approximately US $3) (*c*) twine (approximately US $5), (*d*) ureteral 6-F JJ stent, (*e*). **The cost does not include ureteral stent and suture

competence. Operating room time, total fluoroscopy time, stone-free rates, complication rates, instrument damage, and cost have all been used as surrogate outcomes in the measurement of a URS learning curve [135]. As such, there is a documentable improvement in the complication and success rates of URS with surgeon experience [135]. Making sure residents are well trained upon graduation from residency, the ACGME has placed a minimum number of 60 URS cases for graduating residents. However, they also note "the minimum requirement for procedures does not supplant the requirement that, upon a resident's completion of the program, the program director must verify that he or she has demonstrated sufficient competence to enter practice without direct supervision" (http://www.acgme.org/portals/0/pfassets/programresources/480-urology-case-log-info_.pdf). Consequently, teaching programs and their trainees are starting to become objectively measured. The Objective Structured Assessment of Technical Skills (OSATS), based on a 14-point curriculum, has been designed to assess the necessary cognitive and psychomotor skills of trainees, and it has indeed shown to correlate ureteroscopic performance with experience [136].

As discussed previously, there has been a push to augment training programs with simulators to potentially bypass the early error-prone learning curve of procedures. URS is a particular procedure that has seen significant innovations in simulation options over the last decade. Currently available URS simulators are broadly categorized into virtual reality, bench, animal, and human models (Fig. 24.12).

Regarding bench URS models, there are three main validated simulator models currently available. The first is the URO-Scopic™ trainer from Limbs & Things (Bristol, United Kingdom). The URO-Scopic™ trainer is a high-fidelity physical model that incorporates the training of standard semirigid and flexible ureteroscopes. The model includes a male pelvis with a urethra, bladder, bilateral ureters, and collecting systems [137]. Three studies have analyzed the URO-Scopic™ trainer. In the first study, Matsumoto et al. demonstrated construct validity of the model in a study of 17 urology residents, showing improved performance as evidenced by OSATS, pass rating, and time of procedure [138]. Mishra et al. further studied URO-Scopic™ by comparing URO-Scopic™ versus a VR simulator (URO Mentor™, discussed later). Lastly, in a study of 21 urologists with no experience in URS, the trainees gave URO-Scopic™ a realism score of 6.74/10, and users were found to improve their performance of URS via a global rating score system with each attempt at URS [139].

The second available URS bench model is the Scope Trainer (Mediskills Ltd., United Kingdom). The model is high fidelity, comprised of a distensible bladder and a single collecting system. The Scope Trainer has many helpful features, including a transparent dome that allows visualization of instruments within the model. Other features include reproduction of lumbar lordosis to enhance realism, a collecting system containing stones and papillary tumors, and a "percutaneous" access tract for antegrade passage of a scope. Two studies are currently available that evaluate the Scope Trainer, both performed by Brehmer and colleagues. In their first study, 14 urologists were observed and scored using a task-specific checklist when performing rigid URS on both patients and the Scope Trainer model. Impressive to note is that all study participants claimed the model was similar to surgery and that participants scored identically between human and model cases [140]. Predictably, the study participants who had underwent an endourology fellowship scored significantly higher than their counterparts on both human and model surgery (18.2 vs 16.8, $p = 0.0084$). In their second study, 26 urology residents used the Scope Trainer for semirigid URS. Participants on first use of the model recorded baseline scores, then they trained on the model under supervision, and then finally a post-training procedure was done. Baseline and post-training procedures were scored on a task-specific checklist and a global score (maximum = 19). Residents were found to significantly improve their skills from an average baseline score of 7.7 to a post-training score of 17.2 [141]. Notably, the Scope Trainer showed promise as a tool for improving URS manual dexterity skills. Construct validity was also demonstrated in this study, with experienced residents scoring an average total score of 17.6 versus an average score of 7.7 by inexperienced residents.

The third validated bench URS model is the "adult ureteroscopy trainer" (Ideal Anatomic Modeling, Holt, Michigan). White et al. used CT images of the upper tract of a patient who had difficulty spontaneously passing renal calculi to make their model via rapid prototyping, which involves the creation of thin, virtual, horizontal cross sections from animation modeling software to transform those virtual cross sections into a physical model. With this technology, they were able to essentially "clone" that patient's collecting system into a durable silicon mold. In their initial study of 46 participants, ranging from urology attendings to medical students, results were rather impressive. One hundred percent of participants rated the model as realistic, 98% thought it would serve as a good training format, and 96% recommended it for urology training [142]. Construct validity was verified with expert and novice endoscopists removing a lower pole calculus and being scored by a global rating scale and ureteral checklist, modified for absence of bladder and urethra. Expert endoscopists scored significantly better than their novice counterparts (33.1 vs 15.0, $p < 0.0001$) and performed the task in less time (141.2 vs 447.2 s, $p = 0.01$). The authors touted that the model cost $485, a bargain in comparison to other models—which can range from $3700 to $60,000! However, one notable limitation of this model is the lack of bladder and urethra, which eliminates the technically heavy steps of guidewire manipulation and cannulation of the ureteral orifice.

Recently a flexible URS model called the K-Box® (Porgès-Coloplast, France) was created and published [143]. The K-Box® consists of four independent boxes made of polyurethane and has a number of features not been seen in previous models. Each box allows a number of trays that can be swapped in and out, allowing for multiple configurations to challenge the user. The model uses a standard ureteroscope along with wires and baskets, and to assist users, the model's lid can be removed, and the scope's location can be seen, acting as a surrogate for fluoroscopy. The model allows users to practice tasks such as advancing guidewires, placing ureteral sheaths, and basketing stones. Trainees also have the capability to use water in the model, allowing the use of laser to fragment stones. The K-Box® seems to be a viable and potentially very useful model, but it still needs further studying in order to establish validity.

In contrast to physical bench models, VR model simulators use computer-based systems to simulate particular procedures. Preminger et al. showed the feasibility of a VR URS simulator in 1995, and since that time, the field of VR URS simulators has seen significant advances, particularly with the concurrent advances in technologies [144]. The most studied VR ureteroscopy simulator is the URO Mentor (Simbionix, Israel), which was briefly mentioned previously. The URO Mentor consists of a male pelvic mannequin incorporated with a Windows-based computer interface. The simulator allows users to practice with both flexible and semirigid ureteroscopes, which are passed through the interface device into the mannequin. Once inside the mannequin, the system converts movements that tracked multiple sensors into realistic images on the monitor. Additionally, the simulator also allows for realistic 2D fluoroscopic imaging during simulations. An array of virtual working instruments is available to users when using URO Mentor, including guidewires, baskets, forceps, stents, dilators, and a number of lithotripsy probes [95].

Michel et al. first described the URO Mentor in 2002, and since that time, there have been a number of validation studies performed [95, 137]. Their initial study aspired to demonstrate face validity, stating that both trainees and endourological instructors felt the URO Mentor displayed a high degree of realism, but their study was flawed in that they never disclosed how many participants were in the study nor how it was done [95]. However, there have been several other studies that have demonstrated construct validity for the URO Mentor simulator. Watterson et al. and Wilhelm et al. did similar studies in 2002, both of which verified construct validity. In their studies, they used 20 and 21 medical students, respectively, and randomized them to teaching on the URO Mentor system versus control groups. Both found that the trained participants did significantly better than the control groups (Watterson: global rating score 23.6 vs 14.7, $p < 0.001$; Wilhelm: 21.3 vs 16.1, $p < 0.001$) [145, 146].

Jacomides et al. studied the completion time of training modules on the URO Mentor for 16 medical students and 16 urology residents. They discovered that the students significantly decreased their completion times of the module after training on the URO Mentor for 5 h. However, they found no significant difference in the completion times among the residents. Notably, they found the medical students were able to complete the task in similar times to first-year residents, who had a median 14 clinical URS procedures after training [147]. This is significant in that medical students may be able to bypass the early learning curve and catch up to residents in terms of operating times by using the VR simulator. Matsumoto et al. further exhibited construct validity by assessing 16 urology residents using several parameters in the task of basketing a distal ureteral stone on the URO Mentor. Their study found that senior residents scored significantly better than junior residents in terms of global rating scores, examiner checklist assessment, pass/fail rating, time to complete task, and incidence of scope trauma [148]. In a study of 89 participants that consisted of both urologists and urology residents, Dolmans et al. found that URO Mentor scored a mean global realism score of 3.14 on a 1–5 Likert scale for URS. Eighty-two percent of participants rated it ≥3.5 on a scale of 1–5 in terms of usefulness as an educational tool. In this study, the overall rating for the URO Mentor on a 10-point scale (1 = poor, 10 = excellent) was 7.3 [149].

Criterion validity for URO Mentor has also been evaluated in multiple studies. The importance of criterion validity is that it helps answer the question if a simulator can effectively translate to improve clinical performance. Ogan et al. studied 16 medical students and 16 urology residents for criterion validity on the URO Mentor. Participants underwent a baseline evaluation on the URO Mentor, and the medical students underwent an additional 5 h of supervised training on the simulator. After the medical students received training, all participants then underwent a second evaluation on the URO Mentor in addition to a similar task on a fresh-frozen cadaver. The study found that the medical students significantly improved performance from their baseline assessment to their second simulated task, but they still underperformed against the residents in the cadaveric URS in multiple subjective and objective measurements. In terms of criterion validity, the student performance on the post-training simulation strongly correlated with performance on the cadaver in areas of time =, global rating score anatomy, and overall scores. Unfortunately, these correlations did not hold for urology residents. This suggests that the URO Mentor is helpful in predicting the performance of inexperienced endoscopists, but likely does not predict performance improvement for those with more experience [150]. Knoll et al. studied 20 urologists of varying experience in their performance in treating a lower calyceal stone. Cases performed ranged from 21 to 153. The authors found that those that had performed less than 40 URS cases scored significantly worse than those who had greater than 80 cases, thus exhibiting construct validity. Criterion validity was also proposed by comparing five inexperienced urology residents versus five inexperienced urology residents trained on the URO Mentor. When compared, they found that the simulator-trained group performed significantly better on their first four URS cases on humans, as assessed by operative times between the groups [151].

The use of live animals for surgical training is controversial. Therefore, ex vivo animal models are advocated by a number of authors. By using organs obtained from pigs already being slaughtered for food, legal and ethical issues have been essentially erased [152]. Looking for a more realistic feel than plastic models at the time, Strohmaier and Giese were some of the first authors to describe the use of an ex vivo porcine model [153]. They used an en bloc resection of all retroperitoneal organs (kidneys with ureters, bladder, urethra, aorta, vena cava, intestine, rectum, and anus) from freshly slaughtered adult pigs, with subsequent isolation of the urinary tract. The authors describe that 7.5–9 F ureteroscopes could successfully be navigated through the porcine GU system, giving more realistic and accurate tissue feeling than physical models. Subsequent authors have since described using similar porcine ex vivo setups [109, 154, 155].

Soria et al. did a validation study that was divided into three levels. During the second level of their study, an ex vivo porcine renoureteral unit was used for training of laser lithotripsy on a mid-ureteral stone. Their model demonstrated face validity in the study of 40 participants with a global realism score of 4.25 ± 0.13 on a 5-point Likert scale [156]. Unfortunately, further validation and data regarding educational value for ex vivo models are currently still lacking.

Percutaneous Access/Litholopaxy

Since being first described by Fernström and Johansson in 1976, percutaneous nephrolithotomy (PCNL) has signified a viable and increasingly popular way to manage complex renal calculi [157]. Due to further advances in technique since its inception, PCNL has essentially eliminated the use of open surgery in the removal of renal calculi [158]. However, PCNL is still a risky procedure with a high incidence of overall complications at 83% [159]. The most common complications include hemorrhage requiring transfusion, with overall mean incidence ranging 11.2–17.5%. Colonic or pleural injuries are highly associated with the access portion of the procedure. PCNL is also known for its steep learning curve. Current literature suggests that 36–45 cases are needed to become competent and 105–115 cases are needed to achieve proficiency for PCNL [160, 161]. Additionally, as few as 11% of urologists are able to obtain percutaneous access without the help of an interventional radiologist, which suggests that many trainees are uncomfortable or untrained in achieving percutaneous renal access [162]. As such, simulation in PCNL has become increasingly popular.

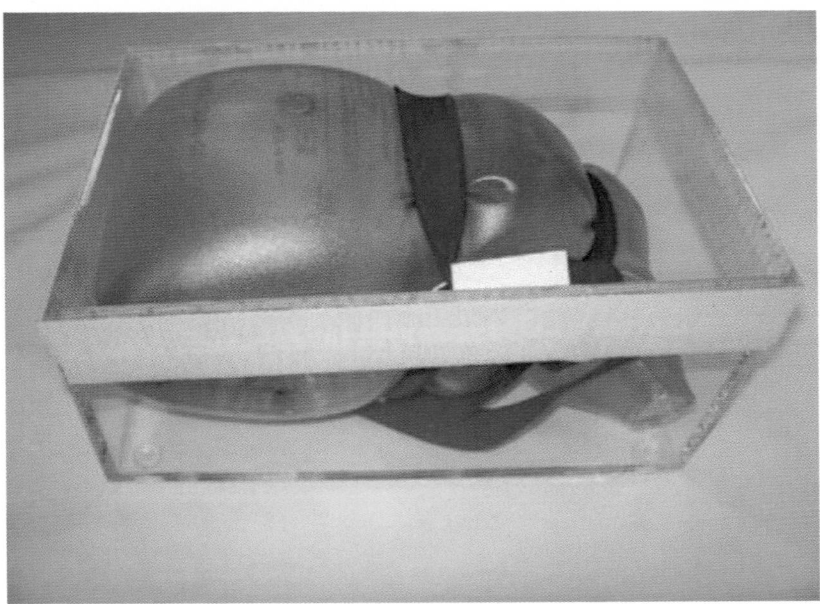

Fig. 24.13 UroEmerge™ Suprapubic Catheter Model with plastic trainer housing the simulated full bladder [6]

Four bench models of PCNL are currently described in the literature—three of them utilize ex vivo porcine renoureteral units. The initial model was described by Hammond et al. in which the authors placed pebbles within a porcine kidney/ureter, which was then placed inside a chicken carcass [163]. Urology residents were then taught needle access, guidewire placement, tract dilation, retrograde and antegrade pyelograms, renal access sheath insertion, and rigid and flexible nephroscopy with the assistance of fluoroscopy. This model has never been validated, but through anonymous surveys, it is suggested that trainees are satisfied with the model, allowing them to become more comfortable with the technique and equipment of renal access.

A second bench model, developed by Strohmaier and Giese, also used ex vivo porcine kidneys and ureters but in a considerably different way [164]. Calculi are placed into the cadaveric porcine renoureteral units via opening the collecting system and then secured by a watertight closure with a running suture. Then, ureters can be cannulated with catheters through which saline is instilled to mimic hydronephrosis. The model is then placed upon a rectangular silicone mold, and the entire setup is covered with liquid silicone, which takes approximately 3 h to solidify and lasts about 1 week. Trainees can then perform the usual steps to perform nephrolithotomy via ultrasound or fluoroscopic guidance into the collecting system. Other procedures and techniques that can be performed with this model include endopyelotomy, incision of calyceal neck stenosis, antegrade stent placement, and inserting percutaneous drainage catheters.

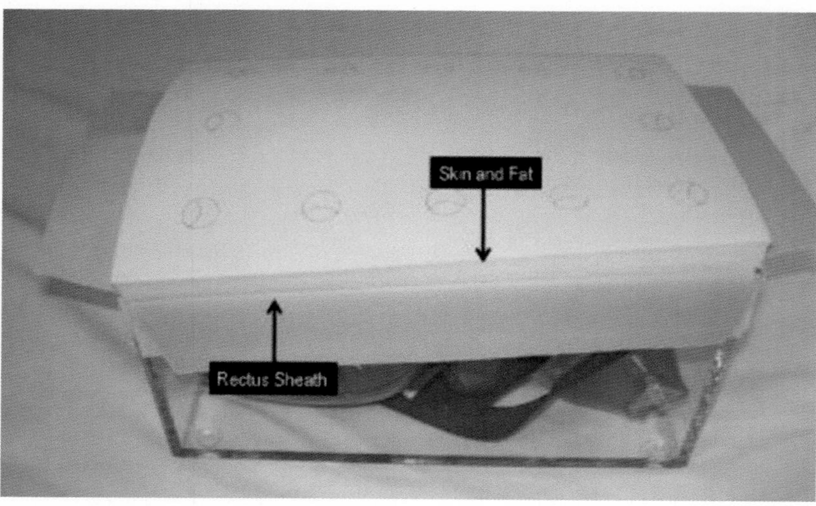

Fig. 24.14 UroEmerge™ Suprapubic Catheter Model contains an abdominal pad that simulates skin and rectus sheath [6]

A unique ex vivo porcine model was created by Zhang et al. in 2008 by wrapping a porcine kidney in a full-thickness skin flap complete with fascia and muscle (Fig. 24.13) [165]. Trainees using this model found it to be quite useful; however, the authors note that the 12th rib is an important anatomical landmark for percutaneous renal access. Therefore, they modified their model to incorporate a portion of porcine thoracic or abdominal wall that contained at least two ribs [166]. One hundred twenty-six urologists tried the modified model, and 90.5% rated the model as "helpful" or "very helpful" for simulation of PCNL.

Currently, there is a single validated PCNL bench model as described by Zhang et al. [167]. The model is 36 × 32 × 12 cm and composed of three components made of mixed silicon materials (Fig. 24.14). Consisting of a kidney with a dilated collecting system with an attached ureteral stump, the model is encased within simulated perirenal tissue of approximately 4 cm thickness. The goal of this model was to simulate the texture of the human body as much as possible. Similar to previous bench models, trainees can practice both fluoroscopy and ultrasound techniques on this model to obtain renal access. A significant advantage of this model was that multiple trainees could repeatedly use it as it is tolerant to multiple sticks for needle access; however, the cost-effectiveness of this model versus ex vivo animal models has never been studied. In their study, Zhang et al. demonstrated face, content, and construct validity for the model. Nine experts—considered experts as they've logged over 60 cases—and thirty novices were enrolled in the study and performed fluoroscopy-guided percutaneous renal access on the model. The experts rated the model an overall appraisal of 4 out of 5 points on a 1–5-point Likert scale, a score of 5 for utility as a training tool, and a score of 4 as an assessment tool, thus giving the model both face and content validity. Significant differences were found between experts and novices, with experts taking less total time (183.11 vs 278.00 s, $p < 0.001$), shorter fluoroscopy time (109.22 vs 183 s, $p < 0.001$), and fewer attempts (1.28 vs 2.35,$p < 0.001$), thus exhibiting construct validity. After two 1 h skills sessions on the models, novices significantly improved their total time (278.00 vs 189.93 s, $p < 0.001$), fluoroscopy time (183.13 vs 121.97, $p < 0.001$), and number of attempts (2.35 vs 1.43, $p < 0.001$). After extensive training, it was found that there was no significant difference in performance of the novices versus the experts in the aforementioned categories.

Similar to other procedures, a virtual reality simulator has been developed and validated for percutaneous renal access. The PERC Mentor™ (Simbionix, Israel) is one such simulator, which has a number of fascinating features. The PERC Mentor™ uses a torso mannequin linked to a computer-based simulation system. The mannequin can be added onto the previously discussed URO Mentor system and is considered a high-fidelity flank model, designed to provide haptics of skin, muscle, connective tissue, and ribs similar to real human tissue. A virtual C-arm and mock angiographic instruments are included with the simulator, allowing users to make percutaneous access under simulated fluoroscopic guidance that is controlled by a foot pedal. A metal needle containing a spatial sensor is placed through the simulated torso into a digitally projected renal collecting system. Contrast medium can be delivered through a ureteral catheter, and placement can be confirmed in real time with aspiration of "urine" from the collecting system. Unique to this model is its simulation on the displacement of organs with respirations, something that has not been feasible with bench models. A number of tasks and case scenarios are available, with difficulty ranging on a scale of 1–10. Endpoints are measured during tasks and case scenarios, including operative time, number of puncture attempts, fluoroscopy time, rib collisions, collecting system perforations, and vascular injuries [168].

Knudsen et al. initially validated the PERC Mentor™, where 63 novices, including medical students and inexperienced residents, used the PERC Mentor™ to learn percutaneous renal access [169]. Participants initially underwent baseline testing on the simulator, the goal of which was to gain percutaneous access into the kidney and pass a wire into the collecting system. Then the users were randomly divided into two groups. The first group underwent two 30-minute training sessions on the simulator, while the second group received no training. They then attempted to gain percutaneous renal access again but in a different case scenario, for which they were assessed using a global rating scale by the study evaluators as well as measured parameters collected by the simulator. The study showed that the two groups were insignificantly different at baseline, but after training, the intervention group significantly improved their performance on 11 of the 14 measured outcomes, but the untrained group made no improvements. Furthermore, the trained group performed significantly better than the untrained group on the posttest in all but two parameters—the number of rib collisions and the amount of contrast used on antegrade nephrostogram. Face validity was demonstrated because the high-fidelity flank model, fluoroscopy foot pedal, and realistic needle allowed all participants to effectively gain percutaneous renal access. The authors also asserted that content validity was demonstrated because the simulator was developed with the input of a number of experts in the field, who helped create the varied case scenarios, anatomy, and imaging data. The PERC Mentor™ also demonstrated construct validity by correlating the subjective global rating score with objective measures such as Spearman rank correlations, which helps to establish convergent validity. This was further validated by a follow-up study from Park et al., in which nine experts, comprising five urologists and four interventional radiologists, were compared against 63 novice medical students and residents on a case scenario using the PERC Mentor™ [170]. Construct validity was demonstrated due to the experts significantly outperforming the novices, as measured by the global rating score (24/25 vs 12/25). Experts rated the PERC Mentor™ very highly on five of six domains (mean 8.1 on 10-point scale), thus giving the model substantial face and content validity.

Achieving better performance in the operating room is the ultimate goal of any simulator. Termed predictive validity, Margulis et al. performed a follow-up study to the initial PERC Mentor™ validation study to see if users trained on the PERC Mentor™ performed better in the OR [171]. The authors used the same 63 novices from the initial study, for which they evaluated the trained and untrained groups in their ability to gain percutaneous renal access in anesthetized pigs. The study found that the trained group performed significantly better than their control counterparts in terms of number of punctures (1.9 vs 2.7, $p = 0.005$), number of infundibular punctures (0.3 vs 1.1, $p = 0.002$), and number of collecting system perforations (0.4 vs 0.8, $p = 0.003$) and scored higher on the global rating score (3.8 vs 2.7, $p < 0.001$). A crossover study was then performed in which the control group underwent training on the PERC Mentor™. This group was subsequently found to perform at a level with no statistical difference of the initially trained group. Although surgery on an anesthetized pig may not translate to operating on humans, the study still provides promising evidence that the simulator improves performance without putting humans in undue danger.

Recently described, an unvalidated hybrid simulator called the SimPORTAL (University of Minnesota) is an additional VR PCNL model. The SimPORTAL is a fluoro-less "C-arm" trainer that was paired with a transparent silicon flank bench model during its initial study [172]. This model unit consists of two webcams mounted onto a small C-arm that is produced with a 3D printer. The C-arm can be tilted (−30°/+30°) and rainbowed (−15°/+15°). The cameras are attached to a MacBook Pro™, and via a special video processing technique, the camera images are fused, overlaid, and processed to achieve a simulated x-ray image which can be seen on a screen by the user. In their initial trial study with 14 participants, Veneziano et al. found that 92.8% of participants found it to be of at least equal value to currently the PERC Mentor™ and as such warrants further validation studies [172].

Conclusion

Surgical simulation is an emerging field aimed at providing learners with an environment to sharpen skills in a setting that does not put patients in harm's way. In the field of urology, the majority of procedures performed by a urologist have some sort of simulation with simulators being developed and validated for open, endoscopic, laparoscopic, and robotic procedures. Future advancements will aim toward increasing realism and applicability to real-life scenarios.

References

1. Preece R. The current role of simulation in urological training. Cen Eur J Urol. 2015;68:207–11.
2. Scott DJ, Dunnington GL. The new ACS/APDS skills curriculum: moving the learning curve out of the operating room. J Gastrointest Surg : Off J Soc Surg Aliment Tract. 2008;12:213–21.
3. Aggarwal R, Darzi A. Technical-skills training in the 21st century. N Engl J Med. 2006;355:2695–6.
4. Ahmed K, Aydin A, Dasgupta P, Khan MS, McCabe JE. A novel cadaveric simulation program in urology. J Surg Educ. 2015;72:556–65.
5. Aydin A, Shafi AM, Khan MS, Dasgupta P, Ahmed K. Current status of simulation and training models in urological surgery: a systematic review. J Urol. 2016;196(2):312–20.
6. Shergill IS, Shaikh T, Arya M, Junaid I. A training model for suprapubic catheter insertion: the UroEmerge suprapubic catheter model. Urology. 2008;72:196–7.
7. Hossack T, Chris BB, Beer J, Thompson G. A cost-effective, easily reproducible, suprapubic catheter insertion simulation training model. Urology. 2013;82:955–8.
8. Singal A, Halverson A, Rooney DM, Davis LM, Kielb SJ. A validated low-cost training model for suprapubic catheter insertion. Urology. 2015;85:23–6.
9. Grober ED, Hamstra SJ, Wanzel KR, et al. Laboratory based training in urological microsurgery with bench model simulators: a randomized controlled trial evaluating the durability of technical skill. J Urol. 2004;172:378–81.
10. Blum CA, Adams DB. Who did the first laparoscopic cholecystectomy? J Minim Access Surg. 2011;7:165–8.
11. Figert PL, Park AE, Witzke DB, Schwartz RW. Transfer of training in acquiring laparoscopic skills. J Am Coll Surg. 2001;193:533–7.
12. Brewin J, Nedas T, Challacombe B, Elhage O, Keisu J, Dasgupta P. Face, content and construct validation of the first virtual reality laparoscopic nephrectomy simulator. BJU Int. 2010;106:850–4.
13. da Cruz JA, Dos Reis ST, Cunha Frati RM, et al. Does warm-up training in a virtual reality simulator improve surgical performance? A prospective randomized analysis. J Surg Educ. 2016;73(6):974–8.
14. Nagendran M, Toon CD, Davidson BR, Gurusamy KS. Laparoscopic surgical box model training for surgical trainees with no prior laparoscopic experience. Cochrane Database Syst Rev. 2014;(1):CD010479.
15. Pitzul KB, Grantcharov TP, Okrainec A. Validation of three virtual reality fundamentals of laparoscopic surgery (FLS) modules. Stud Health Technol Inform. 2012;173:349–55.
16. Derossis AM, Fried GM, Abrahamowicz M, Sigman HH, Barkun JS, Meakins JL. Development of a model for training and evaluation of laparoscopic skills. Am J Surg. 1998;175:482–7.
17. Fried GM, Feldman LS, Vassiliou MC, et al. Proving the value of simulation in laparoscopic surgery. Ann Surg. 2004;240:518–25; discussion 25–8
18. Keyser EJ, Derossis AM, Antoniuk M, Sigman HH, Fried GM. A simplified simulator for the training and evaluation of laparoscopic skills. Surg Endosc. 2000;14:149–53.
19. Sroka G, Feldman LS, Vassiliou MC, Kaneva PA, Fayez R, Fried GM. Fundamentals of laparoscopic surgery simulator training to proficiency improves laparoscopic performance in the operating room-a randomized controlled trial. Am J Surg. 2010;199:115–20.
20. Smith R, Patel V, Satava R. Fundamentals of robotic surgery: a course of basic robotic surgery skills based upon a 14-society consensus template of outcomes measures and curriculum development. Int J Med Robot + Comput Assist Surg : MRCAS. 2014;10:379–84.

21. Munz Y, Kumar BD, Moorthy K, Bann S, Darzi A. Laparoscopic virtual reality and box trainers: is one superior to the other? Surg Endosc. 2004;18:485–94.
22. Aslam A, Nason GJ, Giri SK. Homemade laparoscopic surgical simulator: a cost-effective solution to the challenge of acquiring laparoscopic skills? Ir J Med Sci. 2016;185:791–6.
23. Wilson MS, Middlebrook A, Sutton C, Stone R, McCloy RF. MIST VR: a virtual reality trainer for laparoscopic surgery assesses performance. Ann R Coll Surg Engl. 1997;79:403–4.
24. Debes AJ, Aggarwal R, Balasundaram I, Jacobsen MB. A tale of two trainers: virtual reality versus a video trainer for acquisition of basic laparoscopic skills. Am J Surg. 2010;199:840–5.
25. Chaudhry A, Sutton C, Wood J, Stone R, McCloy R. Learning rate for laparoscopic surgical skills on MIST VR, a virtual reality simulator: quality of human-computer interface. Ann R Coll Surg Engl. 1999;81:281–6.
26. Gallagher AG, Lederman AB, McGlade K, Satava RM, Smith CD. Discriminative validity of the minimally invasive surgical trainer in virtual reality (MIST-VR) using criteria levels based on expert performance. Surg Endosc. 2004;18:660–5.
27. Gallagher AG, Richie K, McClure N, McGuigan J. Objective psychomotor skills assessment of experienced, junior, and novice laparoscopists with virtual reality. World J Surg. 2001;25:1478–83.
28. Gallagher AG, Satava RM. Virtual reality as a metric for the assessment of laparoscopic psychomotor skills. Learning curves and reliability measures. Surg Endosc. 2002;16:1746–52.
29. Maithel S, Sierra R, Korndorffer J, et al. Construct and face validity of MIST-VR, Endotower, and CELTS: are we ready for skills assessment using simulators? Surg Endosc. 2006;20:104–12.
30. McNatt SS, Smith CD. A computer-based laparoscopic skills assessment device differentiates experienced from novice laparoscopic surgeons. Surg Endosc. 2001;15:1085–9.
31. Taffinder N, Sutton C, Fishwick RJ, McManus IC, Darzi A. Validation of virtual reality to teach and assess psychomotor skills in laparoscopic surgery: results from randomised controlled studies using the MIST VR laparoscopic simulator. Stud Health Technol Inform. 1998;50:124–30.
32. Ganai S, Donroe JA, St Louis MR, Lewis GM, Seymour NE. Virtual-reality training improves angled telescope skills in novice laparoscopists. Am J Surg. 2007;193:260–5.
33. Schijven M, Jakimowicz J. Face-, expert, and referent validity of the Xitact LS500 laparoscopy simulator. Surg Endosc. 2002;16:1764–70.
34. Schijven M, Jakimowicz J. Construct validity: experts and novices performing on the Xitact LS500 laparoscopy simulator. Surg Endosc. 2003;17:803–10.
35. Schijven MP, Jakimowicz JJ. Introducing the Xitact LS500 laparoscopy simulator: toward a revolution in surgical education. Surg Technol Int. 2003;11:32–6.
36. Ayodeji ID, Schijven M, Jakimowicz J, Greve JW. Face validation of the Simbionix LAP mentor virtual reality training module and its applicability in the surgical curriculum. Surg Endosc. 2007;21:1641–9.
37. Gurusamy KS, Aggarwal R, Palanivelu L, Davidson BR. Virtual reality training for surgical trainees in laparoscopic surgery. Cochrane Database Syst Rev. 2009;(1):CD006575.
38. Hamilton EC, Scott DJ, Fleming JB, et al. Comparison of video trainer and virtual reality training systems on acquisition of laparoscopic skills. Surg Endosc. 2002;16:406–11.
39. Dunn MD, Portis AJ, Shalhav AL, et al. Laparoscopic versus open radical nephrectomy: a 9-year experience. J Urol. 2000;164:1153–9.
40. Gill IS, Kavoussi LR, Lane BR, et al. Comparison of 1,800 laparoscopic and open partial nephrectomies for single renal tumors. J Urol. 2007;178:41–6.
41. Kerbl K, Clayman RV, McDougall EM, Kavoussi LR. Laparoscopic nephrectomy: the Washington University experience. Br J Urol. 1994;73:231–6.
42. Tan HJ, Wolf JS Jr, Ye Z, Wei JT, Miller DC. Population-level comparative effectiveness of laparoscopic versus open radical nephrectomy for patients with kidney cancer. Cancer. 2011;117:4184–93.
43. Fernandez A, Chen E, Moore J, et al. Preliminary assessment of a renal tumor materials model. J Endourol. 2011;25:1371–5.

44. Fernandez A, Chen E, Moore J, et al. A phantom model as a teaching modality for laparoscopic partial nephrectomy. J Endourol. 2012;26:1–5.
45. Abdelshehid CS, Quach S, Nelson C, et al. High-fidelity simulation-based team training in urology: evaluation of technical and nontechnical skills of urology residents during laparoscopic partial nephrectomy. J Surg Educ. 2013;70:588–95.
46. Lee JY, Mucksavage P, McDougall EM. Simulating laparoscopic renal hilar vessel injuries: preliminary evaluation of a novel surgical training model for residents. J Endourol. 2012;26:393–7.
47. Molinas CR, Binda MM, Mailova K, Koninckx PR. The rabbit nephrectomy model for training in laparoscopic surgery. Hum Reprod. 2004;19:185–90.
48. Wijn RP, Persoon MC, Schout BM, Martens EJ, Scherpbier AJ, Hendrikx AJ. Virtual reality laparoscopic nephrectomy simulator is lacking in construct validity. J Endourol. 2010;24:117–22.
49. Makiyama K, Nagasaka M, Inuiya T, Takanami K, Ogata M, Kubota Y. Development of a patient-specific simulator for laparoscopic renal surgery. Int J Urol : Off J Jpn Urol Assoc. 2012;19:829–35.
50. Makiyama K, Yamanaka H, Ueno D, et al. Validation of a patient-specific simulator for laparoscopic renal surgery. Int J Urol : Off J Jpn Urol Assoc. 2015;22:572–6.
51. Poniatowski LH, Wolf JS Jr, Nakada SY, Reihsen TE, Sainfort F, Sweet RM. Validity and acceptability of a high-fidelity physical simulation model for training of laparoscopic pyeloplasty. J Endourol. 2014;28:393–8.
52. Jarrett TW, Chan DY, Charambura TC, Fugita O, Kavoussi LR. Laparoscopic pyeloplasty: the first 100 cases. J Urol. 2002;167:1253–6.
53. Raza SJ, Soomroo KQ, Ather MH. "Latex glove" laparoscopic pyeloplasty model: a novel method for simulated training. Urol J. 2011;8:283–6.
54. Yang B, Zhang ZS, Xiao L, Wang LH, Xu CL, Sun YH. A novel training model for retroperitoneal laparoscopic dismembered pyeloplasty. J Endourol. 2010;24:1345–9.
55. Ramachandran A, Kurien A, Patil P, et al. A novel training model for laparoscopic pyeloplasty using chicken crop. J Endourol. 2008;22:725–8.
56. Jiang C, Liu M, Chen J, et al. Construct validity of the chicken crop model in the simulation of laparoscopic pyeloplasty. J Endourol. 2013;27:1032–6.
57. Fu B, Zhang X, Lang B, et al. New model for training in laparoscopic dismembered ureteropyeloplasty. J Endourol. 2007;21:1381–5.
58. Schuessler WW, Schulam PG, Clayman RV, Kavoussi LR. Laparoscopic radical prostatectomy: initial short-term experience. Urology. 1997;50:854–7.
59. Nadu A, Olsson LE, Abbou CC. Simple model for training in the laparoscopic vesicourethral running anastomosis. J Endourol. 2003;17:481–4.
60. Yang RM, Bellman GC. Laparoscopic urethrovesical anastomosis: a model to assess surgical competency. J Endourol. 2006;20:679–82.
61. Sabbagh R, Chatterjee S, Chawla A, Kapoor A, Matsumoto ED. Task-specific bench model training versus basic laparoscopic skills training for laparoscopic radical prostatectomy: a randomized controlled study. Can Urol Assoc J. 2009;3:22–30.
62. Sabbagh R, Chatterjee S, Chawla A, Hoogenes J, Kapoor A, Matsumoto ED. Transfer of laparoscopic radical prostatectomy skills from bench model to animal model: a prospective, single-blind, randomized, controlled study. J Urol. 2012;187:1861–6.
63. Laguna MP, Arce-Alcazar A, Mochtar CA, Van Velthoven R, Peltier A, de la Rosette JJ. Construct validity of the chicken model in the simulation of laparoscopic radical prostatectomy suture. J Endourol. 2006;20:69–73.
64. Tunitsky-Bitton E, King CR, Ridgeway B, et al. Development and validation of a laparoscopic sacrocolpopexy simulation model for surgical training. J Minim Invasive Gynecol. 2014;21:612–8.
65. Guru KA, Kuvshinoff BW, Pavlov-Shapiro S, et al. Impact of robotics and laparoscopy on surgical skills: a comparative study. J Am Coll Surg. 2007;204:96–101.

66. Zihni AM, Ohu I, Cavallo JA, Ousley J, Cho S, Awad MM. FLS tasks can be used as an ergonomic discriminator between laparoscopic and robotic surgery. Surg Endosc. 2014;28:2459–65.
67. Moglia A, Ferrari V, Morelli L, Ferrari M, Mosca F, Cuschieri A. A systematic review of virtual reality simulators for robot-assisted surgery. Eur Urol. 2016;69:1065–80.
68. Duchene DA, Moinzadeh A, Gill IS, Clayman RV, Winfield HN. Survey of residency training in laparoscopic and robotic surgery. J Urol. 2006;176:2158–66; discussion 67
69. Preston MA, Blew BD, Breau RH, Beiko D, Oake SJ, Watterson JD. Survey of senior resident training in urologic laparoscopy, robotics and endourology surgery in Canada. Can Urol Assoc J. 2010;4:42–6.
70. Hung AJ, Jayaratna IS, Teruya K, Desai MM, Gill IS, Goh AC. Comparative assessment of three standardized robotic surgery training methods. BJU Int. 2013;112:864–71.
71. Hung AJ, Patil MB, Zehnder P, et al. Concurrent and predictive validation of a novel robotic surgery simulator: a prospective, randomized study. J Urol. 2012;187:630–7.
72. Hung AJ, Zehnder P, Patil MB, et al. Face, content and construct validity of a novel robotic surgery simulator. J Urol. 2011;186:1019–24.
73. Kenney PA, Wszolek MF, Gould JJ, Libertino JA, Moinzadeh A. Face, content, and construct validity of dV-trainer, a novel virtual reality simulator for robotic surgery. Urology. 2009;73:1288–92.
74. Korets R, Mues AC, Graversen JA, et al. Validating the use of the Mimic dV-trainer for robotic surgery skill acquisition among urology residents. Urology. 2011;78:1326–30.
75. Seixas-Mikelus SA, Kesavadas T, Srimathveeravalli G, Chandrasekhar R, Wilding GE, Guru KA. Face validation of a novel robotic surgical simulator. Urology. 2010;76:357–60.
76. Seixas-Mikelus SA, Stegemann AP, Kesavadas T, et al. Content validation of a novel robotic surgical simulator. BJU Int. 2011;107:1130–5.
77. Sethi AS, Peine WJ, Mohammadi Y, Sundaram CP. Validation of a novel virtual reality robotic simulator. J Endourol. 2009;23:503–8.
78. Mottrie A, De Naeyer G, Schatteman P, Carpentier P, Sangalli M, Ficarra V. Impact of the learning curve on perioperative outcomes in patients who underwent robotic partial nephrectomy for parenchymal renal tumours. Eur Urol. 2010;58:127–32.
79. Hung AJ, Ng CK, Patil MB, et al. Validation of a novel robotic-assisted partial nephrectomy surgical training model. BJU Int. 2012;110:870–4.
80. Hung AJ, Shah SH, Dalag L, Shin D, Gill IS. Development and validation of a novel robotic procedure specific simulation platform: partial nephrectomy. J Urol. 2015;194:520–6.
81. Kozinn SI, Canes D, Sorcini A, Moinzadeh A. Robotic versus open distal ureteral reconstruction and reimplantation for benign stricture disease. J Endourol. 2012;26:147–51.
82. Rassweiler JJ, Gozen AS, Erdogru T, Sugiono M, Teber D. Ureteral reimplantation for management of ureteral strictures: a retrospective comparison of laparoscopic and open techniques. Eur Urol. 2007;51:512–22; discussion 22-3
83. Tunitsky E, Murphy A, Barber MD, Simmons M, Jelovsek JE. Development and validation of a ureteral anastomosis simulation model for surgical training. Female Pelvic Med Reconstr Surg. 2013;19:346–51.
84. Stitzenberg KB, Wong YN, Nielsen ME, Egleston BL, Uzzo RG. Trends in radical prostatectomy: centralization, robotics, and access to urologic cancer care. Cancer. 2012;118:54–62.
85. Freire MP, Choi WW, Lei Y, Carvas F, Hu JC. Overcoming the learning curve for robotic-assisted laparoscopic radical prostatectomy. Urol Clin North Am. 2010;37:37–47, Table of Contents
86. Hu JC, Wang Q, Pashos CL, Lipsitz SR, Keating NL. Utilization and outcomes of minimally invasive radical prostatectomy. J Clin Oncol : Off J Am Soc Clin Oncol. 2008;26:2278–84.
87. Vickers AJ, Bianco FJ, Serio AM, et al. The surgical learning curve for prostate cancer control after radical prostatectomy. J Natl Cancer Inst. 2007;99:1171–7.
88. Alemozaffar M, Narayanan R, Percy AA, et al. Validation of a novel, tissue-based simulator for robot-assisted radical prostatectomy. J Endourol. 2014;28:995–1000.

89. Volpe A, Ahmed K, Dasgupta P, et al. Pilot validation study of the European Association of Urology robotic training curriculum. Eur Urol. 2015;68:292–9.
90. Kang SG, Cho S, Kang SH, et al. The Tube 3 module designed for practicing vesicourethral anastomosis in a virtual reality robotic simulator: determination of face, content, and construct validity. Urology. 2014;84:345–50.
91. Van Velthoven RF, Ahlering TE, Peltier A, Skarecky DW, Clayman RV. Technique for laparoscopic running urethrovesical anastomosis: the single knot method. Urology. 2003;61:699–702.
92. Kim JY, Kim SB, Pyun JH, et al. Concurrent and predictive validation of robotic simulator Tube 3 module. Korean J Urol. 2015;56:756–61.
93. Chowriappa A, Raza SJ, Fazili A, et al. Augmented-reality-based skills training for robot-assisted urethrovesical anastomosis: a multi-institutional randomised controlled trial. BJU Int. 2015;115:336–45.
94. Shah J. Endoscopy through the ages. BJU Int. 2002;89:645–52.
95. Michel MS, Knoll T, Kohrmann KU, Alken P. The URO Mentor: development and evaluation of a new computer-based interactive training system for virtual life-like simulation of diagnostic and therapeutic endourological procedures. BJU Int. 2002;89:174–7.
96. Schout BM, Muijtjens AM, Hendrikx AJ, et al. Acquisition of flexible cystoscopy skills on a virtual reality simulator by experts and novices. BJU Int. 2010;105:234–9.
97. Schout BM, Ananias HJ, Bemelmans BL, et al. Transfer of cysto-urethroscopy skills from a virtual-reality simulator to the operating room: a randomized controlled trial. BJU Int. 2010;106:226–31; discussion 31.
98. Matsumoto ED, Hamstra SJ, Radomski SB, Cusimano MD. The effect of bench model fidelity on endourological skills: a randomized controlled study. J Urol. 2002;167:1243–7.
99. Bowling CB, Greer WJ, Bryant SA, et al. Testing and validation of a low-cost cystoscopy teaching model: a randomized controlled trial. Obstet Gynecol. 2010;116:85–91.
100. Siegel R, Naishadham D, Jemal A. Cancer statistics, 2013. CA Cancer J Clin. 2013;63:11–30.
101. Jancke G, Rosell J, Jahnson S. Impact of surgical experience on recurrence and progression after transurethral resection of bladder tumour in non-muscle-invasive bladder cancer. Scand J Urol. 2014;48:276–83.
102. Schout BM, Bemelmans BL, Martens EJ, Scherpbier AJ, Hendrikx AJ. How useful and realistic is the uro trainer for training transurethral prostate and bladder tumor resection procedures? J Urol. 2009;181:1297–303; discussion 303.
103. Kruck S, Bedke J, Hennenlotter J, et al. Virtual bladder tumor transurethral resection: an objective evaluation tool to overcome learning curves with and without photodynamic diagnostics. Urol Int. 2011;87:138–42.
104. Reich O, Noll M, Gratzke C, et al. High-level virtual reality simulator for endourologic procedures of lower urinary tract. Urology. 2006;67:1144–8.
105. de Vries AH, van Genugten HG, Hendrikx AJ, et al. The Simbla TURBT simulator in urological residency training: from needs analysis to validation. J Endourol. 2016;30(5):580–7.
106. Shen Y, Vasandani P, Iyer J, et al. Virtual trainer for intra-detrusor injection of botulinum toxin to treat urinary incontinence. Stud Health Technol Inform. 2012;173:457–62.
107. Wignall GR, Denstedt JD, Preminger GM, et al. Surgical simulation: a urological perspective. J Urol. 2008;179:1690–9.
108. Sweet R, Porter J, Oppenheimer P, Hendrickson D, Gupta A, Weghorst S. Simulation of bleeding in endoscopic procedures using virtual reality. J Endourol. 2002;16:451–5.
109. Hammond L, Ketchum J, Schwartz BF. Accreditation council on graduate medical education technical skills competency compliance: urologic surgical skills. J Am Coll Surg. 2005;201:454–7.
110. Brewin J, Ahmed K, Khan MS, Jaye P, Dasgupta P. Face, content, and construct validation of the Bristol TURP trainer. J Surg Educ. 2014;71:500–5.
111. Viswaroop SB, Gopalakrishnan G, Kandasami SV. Role of transurethral resection of the prostate simulators for training in transurethral surgery. Curr Opin Urol. 2015;25:153–7.

112. Lardennois B, Clement T, Ziade A, Brandt B. Computer stimulation of endoscopic resection of the prostate. Ann Urol. 1990;24:519–23.
113. Oppenheimer P, Gupta A, Weghorst S, Sweet R, Porter J. The representation of blood flow in endourologic surgical simulations. Stud Health Technol Inform. 2001;81:365–71.
114. Sweet RM. Review of trainers for transurethral resection of the prostate skills. J Endourol. 2007;21:280–4.
115. Kallstrom R, Hjertberg H, Svanvik J. Construct validity of a full procedure, virtual reality, real-time, simulation model for training in transurethral resection of the prostate. J Endourol. 2010;24:109–15.
116. Bachmann A, Muir GH, Collins EJ, et al. 180-W XPS GreenLight laser therapy for benign prostate hyperplasia: early safety, efficacy, and perioperative outcome after 201 procedures. Eur Urol. 2012;61:600–7.
117. Liberale F, Muir GH, Walsh K, Krishnamoorthy R. GreenLight laser prostatectomy: a safe and effective treatment for bladder outlet obstruction by prostate cancer. BJU Int. 2011;107:772–6.
118. Malek RS, Barrett DM, Kuntzman RS. High-power potassium-titanyl-phosphate (KTP/532) laser vaporization prostatectomy: 24 hours later. Urology. 1998;51:254–6.
119. Malek RS, Kuntzman RS, Barrett DM. Photoselective potassium-titanyl-phosphate laser vaporization of the benign obstructive prostate: observations on long-term outcomes. J Urol. 2005;174:1344–8.
120. Aydin A, Muir GH, Graziano ME, Khan MS, Dasgupta P, Ahmed K. Validation of the GreenLight Simulator and development of a training curriculum for photoselective vaporisation of the prostate. BJU Int. 2015;115:994–1003.
121. Herlemann A, Strittmatter F, Buchner A, et al. Virtual reality systems in urologic surgery: an evaluation of the GreenLight simulator. Eur Urol. 2013;64:687–8.
122. Kuntz RM. Current role of lasers in the treatment of benign prostatic hyperplasia (BPH). Eur Urol. 2006;49:961–9.
123. van Rij S, Gilling PJ. In 2013, holmium laser enucleation of the prostate (HoLEP) may be the new 'gold standard'. Curr Urol Rep. 2012;13:427–32.
124. El-Hakim A, Elhilali MM. Holmium laser enucleation of the prostate can be taught: the first learning experience. BJU Int. 2002;90:863–9.
125. Shah HN, Mahajan AP, Sodha HS, Hegde S, Mohile PD, Bansal MB. Prospective evaluation of the learning curve for holmium laser enucleation of the prostate. J Urol. 2007;177:1468–74.
126. Khan R, Aydin A, Khan MS, Dasgupta P, Ahmed K. Simulation-based training for prostate surgery. BJU Int. 2015;116:665–74.
127. Aydin A, Ahmed K, Brewin J, Khan MS, Dasgupta P, Aho T. Face and content validation of the prostatic hyperplasia model and holmium laser surgery simulator. J Surg Educ. 2014;71:339–44.
128. Kuronen-Stewart C, Ahmed K, Aydin A, et al. Holmium laser enucleation of the prostate: simulation-based training curriculum and validation. Urology. 2015;86:639–46.
129. Gallina A, Suardi N, Montorsi F, et al. Mortality at 120 days after prostatic biopsy: a population-based study of 22,175 men. Int J Cancer. 2008;123:647–52.
130. Kakehi Y, Naito S. Complication rates of ultrasound-guided prostate biopsy: a nation-wide survey in Japan. Int J Urol : Off J Jpn Urol Assoc. 2008;15:319–21.
131. Chalasani V, Cool DW, Sherebrin S, Fenster A, Chin J, Izawa JI. Development and validation of a virtual reality transrectal ultrasound guided prostatic biopsy simulator. Can Urol Assoc J. 2011;5:19–26.
132. Fiard G, Selmi SY, Promayon E, Vadcard L, Descotes JL, Troccaz J. Initial validation of a virtual-reality learning environment for prostate biopsies: realism matters! J Endourol. 2014;28:453–8.
133. Dauw CA, Simeon L, Alruwaily AF, et al. Contemporary practice patterns of flexible ureteroscopy for treating renal stones: results of a worldwide survey. J Endourol. 2015;29: 1221–30.

134. Ghani KR, Sammon JD, Karakiewicz PI, et al. Trends in surgery for upper urinary tract calculi in the USA using the Nationwide Inpatient Sample: 1999–2009. BJU Int. 2013;112: 224–30.
135. Skolarikos A, Gravas S, Laguna MP, Traxer O, Preminger GM, de la Rosette J. Training in ureteroscopy: a critical appraisal of the literature. BJU Int. 2011;108:798–805; discussion
136. Kishore TA, Pedro RN, Monga M, Sweet RM. Assessment of validity of an OSATS for cystoscopic and ureteroscopic cognitive and psychomotor skills. J Endourol. 2008;22:2707–11.
137. Brunckhorst O, Aydin A, Abboudi H, et al. Simulation-based ureteroscopy training: a systematic review. J Surg Educ. 2015;72:135–43.
138. Matsumoto ED, Hamstra SJ, Radomski SB, Cusimano MD. A novel approach to endourological training: training at the surgical skills center. J Urol. 2001;166:1261–6.
139. Mishra S, Sharma R, Kumar A, Ganatra P, Sabnis RB, Desai MR. Comparative performance of high-fidelity training models for flexible ureteroscopy: are all models effective? Indian J Urol : IJU : J Urol Soc India. 2011;27:451–6.
140. Brehmer M, Tolley D. Validation of a bench model for endoscopic surgery in the upper urinary tract. Eur Urol. 2002;42:175–9; discussion 80.
141. Brehmer M, Swartz R. Training on bench models improves dexterity in ureteroscopy. Eur Urol. 2005;48:458–63; discussion 63
142. White MA, Dehaan AP, Stephens DD, Maes AA, Maatman TJ. Validation of a high fidelity adult ureteroscopy and renoscopy simulator. J Urol. 2010;183:673–7.
143. Villa L, Somani BK, Sener TE, et al. Comprehensive flexible ureteroscopy (FURS) simulator for training in endourology: the K-box model. Cen Eur J Urol. 2016;69:118–20.
144. Preminger GM, Babayan RK, Merril GL, Raju R, Millman A, Merril JR. Virtual reality surgical simulation in endoscopic urologic surgery. Stud Health Technol Inform. 1996;29:157–63.
145. Watterson JD, Beiko DT, Kuan JK, Denstedt JD. Randomized prospective blinded study validating acquistion of ureteroscopy skills using computer based virtual reality endourological simulator. J Urol. 2002;168:1928–32.
146. Wilhelm DM, Ogan K, Roehrborn CG, Cadeddu JA, Pearle MS. Assessment of basic endoscopic performance using a virtual reality simulator. J Am Coll Surg. 2002;195:675–81.
147. Jacomides L, Ogan K, Cadeddu JA, Pearle MS. Use of a virtual reality simulator for ureteroscopy training. J Urol. 2004;171:320–3; discussion 3.
148. Matsumoto ED, Pace KT, DAH RJ. Virtual reality ureteroscopy simulator as a valid tool for assessing endourological skills. Int J Urol : Off J Jpn Urol Assoc. 2006;13:896–901.
149. Dolmans VE, Schout BM, de Beer NA, Bemelmans BL, Scherpbier AJ, Hendrikx AJ. The virtual reality endourologic simulator is realistic and useful for educational purposes. J Endourol. 2009;23:1175–81.
150. Ogan K, Jacomides L, Shulman MJ, Roehrborn CG, Cadeddu JA, Pearle MS. Virtual ureteroscopy predicts ureteroscopic proficiency of medical students on a cadaver. J Urol. 2004;172:667–71.
151. Knoll T, Trojan L, Haecker A, Alken P, Michel MS. Validation of computer-based training in ureterorenoscopy. BJU Int. 2005;95:1276–9.
152. Watterson JD, Denstedt JD. Ureteroscopy and cystoscopy simulation in urology. J Endourol. 2007;21:263–9.
153. Strohmaier WL, Giese A. Porcine urinary tract as a training model for ureteroscopy. Urol Int. 2001;66:30–2.
154. Celia A, Zeccolini G. Ex vivo models for training in endourology: construction of the model and simulation of training procedures. Urologia. 2011;78(Suppl 18):16–20.
155. Chou DS, Abdelshehid C, Clayman RV, McDougall EM. Comparison of results of virtual-reality simulator and training model for basic ureteroscopy training. J Endourol. 2006;20:266–71.
156. Soria F, Morcillo E, Sanz JL, Budia A, Serrano A, Sanchez-Margallo FM. Description and validation of realistic and structured endourology training model. Am J.Clin Exp Urol. 2014;2:258–65.

157. Fernstrom I, Johansson B. Percutaneous pyelolithotomy. A new extraction technique. Scand J Urol Nephrol. 1976;10:257–9.
158. Kim SC, Kuo RL, Lingeman JE. Percutaneous nephrolithotomy: an update. Curr Opin Urol. 2003;13:235–41.
159. Michel MS, Trojan L, Rassweiler JJ. Complications in percutaneous nephrolithotomy. Eur Urol. 2007;51:899–906; discussion.
160. Jang WS, Choi KH, Yang SC, Han WK. The learning curve for flank percutaneous nephrolithotomy for kidney calculi: a single surgeon's experience. Korean J Urol. 2011;52: 284–8.
161. Ziaee SA, Sichani MM, Kashi AH, Samzadeh M. Evaluation of the learning curve for percutaneous nephrolithotomy. Urol J. 2010;7:226–31.
162. Bird VG, Fallon B, Winfield HN. Practice patterns in the treatment of large renal stones. J Endourol. 2003;17:355–63.
163. Hammond L, Ketchum J, Schwartz BF. A new approach to urology training: a laboratory model for percutaneous nephrolithotomy. J Urol. 2004;172:1950–2.
164. Strohmaier WL, Giese A. Ex vivo training model for percutaneous renal surgery. Urol Res. 2005;33:191–3.
165. Zhang Y, Ou TW, Jia JG, et al. Novel biologic model for percutaneous renal surgery learning and training in the laboratory. Urology. 2008;72:513–6.
166. Qiu Z, Yang Y, Zhang Y, Sun YC. Modified biological training model for percutaneous renal surgery with ultrasound and fluroscopy guidance. Chin Med J. 2011;124:1286–9.
167. Zhang Y, Yu CF, Jin SH, Li NC, Na YQ. Validation of a novel non-biological bench model for the training of percutaneous renal access. Int Braz J Urol : Off J Braz Soc Urol. 2014;40:87–92.
168. Stern J, Zeltser IS, Pearle MS. Percutaneous renal access simulators. J Endourol. 2007;21: 270–3.
169. Knudsen BE, Matsumoto ED, Chew BH, et al. A randomized, controlled, prospective study validating the acquisition of percutaneous renal collecting system access skills using a computer based hybrid virtual reality surgical simulator: phase I. J Urol. 2006;176:2173–8.
170. Park S, Matsumoto ED, Knudsen BE, et al. Face, content and construct validity testing on a virtual reality percutaneous renal access simulator. J Endourol. 2006;20:A4.
171. Margulis V, Matsumoto E, Knudsen B, et al. Percutaneous renal collecting system access: can virtual reality training shorten the learning curve? J Urol. 2005;173:315.
172. Veneziano D, Smith A, Reihsen T, Speich J, Sweet RM. The SimPORTAL fluoro-less C-arm trainer: an innovative device for percutaneous kidney access. J Endourol. 2015;29:240–5.
173. Aydin A, Ahmed K, Shafi AM, Khan MS, Dasgupta P. The role of simulation in urological training – a quantitative study of practice and opinions. Surgeon: J Royal Coll Surg Edinb Irel. 2016;14(6):301–7.

Resident Physician Burnout: Improving the Wellness of Surgical Trainees

25

Laura M. Douglass and Amanda C. North

What Is Burnout?

Burnout is a syndrome characterized by emotional exhaustion, depersonalization, and a sense of decreased personal accomplishment specific to the workplace [1]. Considered the gold standard measure of burnout and the most commonly referenced measure of burnout in the medical literature, The Maslach Burnout Inventory (MBI) is a reproducible and validated 22-item survey evaluating the three components of burnout [2]. Emotional exhaustion is the extent to which a person feels emotionally overextended (nine items). Depersonalization is the degree to which a person feels detached toward or cynical about patients (five items). Personal accomplishment is the level of pride or satisfaction with one's achievements (eight items). Each item is scored on a 7-point Likert scale. Physicians with an emotional exhaustion score of 27 or higher or depersonalization score of 10 or higher are considered to have at least one manifestation of burnout [1, 2].

Who Is Burned Out?

Physicians as a whole are burned out at higher rates than population-matched controls in the United States [3]. While attending surgeons report a 40% burnout rate in a survey of 7905 members of the American College of Surgeons [4], Pulcrano et al. found that surgical residents are particularly vulnerable and are more likely to be burned out and report poor quality of life (QOL) than attending surgeons [5]. Throughout the entire medical training process, residency training appears to have the highest risk for burnout. Dyrbye et al. found that burnout, high

L.M. Douglass • A.C. North, MD (✉)
Montefiore Medical Center, Bronx, NY, USA
e-mail: anorth@montefiore.org

T.S. Köhler, B. Schwartz (eds.), *Surgeons as Educators*,
https://doi.org/10.1007/978-3-319-64728-9_25

depersonalization, and high fatigue are most common during residency and fellowship in comparison to medical students and early career physicians with less than 5 years of practice. They also found that residents and fellows were more likely to report burnout, high emotional exhaustion, and high depersonalization than the population control sample [3].

Resident burnout rates range between 50% and 69% among all medical specialties [6, 7]. One study examined 665 surgical residents and found that 69% met the criteria for burnout on at least one subscale. Female surgical residents reported higher rates of burnout than male residents (73 vs. 65%, respectively, $p = 0.02$) [8]. While surgical residents face unique challenges including the physical demands of operating and the intellectual demands of rapidly learning both surgical procedures and medical knowledge, several studies have shown no significant difference in burnout among the different specialties [6, 7]. Martini et al. compared burnout rates among different specialties and found a range between 27% in family medicine and 75% in obstetrics-gynecology, 40% burnout in general surgery residents, and no significant variation among specialties [6].

Several studies have examined the timing and persistence of burnout among internal medicine residents. Ripp et al. surveyed internal medicine residents both at the start and end of intern year. Burnout prevalence was 36% at the start of training and increased to 81% by the end of intern year. Of the residents who started free of burnout, 75% developed burnout by the end of the year [9]. Campbell et al. studied 86 internal medicine residents through all 3 years of residency and found 78% of residents were burned out at least once. Of the 58 burned-out interns, 42 (75%) continued to be burned out through their 3 years of training [10]. These studies examined internal medicine residents, and their findings may not be generalizable to surgical residents. Nonetheless these findings are provocative and suggest that some residents start residency burned out and that once burnout occurs, it tends to persist throughout training for a certain group of trainees.

Burnout and Surgical Education

While a certain level of stress can be expected during residency, burnout is pathologic and relevant to all involved stakeholders: patients, residents, and medical educators. Residency programs and surgical educators are in the unique position to positively or negatively affect patient care and resident wellness because they provide and supervise the training of residents as they care for patients in a high stress environment.

The highly publicized and tragic death of Libby Zion at New York Hospital in 1984 drew the public's attention to resident work hours and the effects on patient care. Research since then has linked resident burnout with suboptimal care and increased self-perceived medical errors. Shanafelt et al. found 76% of surveyed residents ($n = 115$) met criteria for burnout, and burned-out residents were more likely to self-report providing suboptimal care at least monthly compared to residents without burnout (53% vs. 21%, $p = 0.004$), as well as in multivariate analysis (odds ratio 8.3 [95% CI, 2.6–26.5]) [11]. In a prospective longitudinal cohort study, West et al. found that 139 residents (39%) reported at least one major medical error during the study period [12]. Residents reporting a medical error had significantly higher rates of burnout on all three subscales of the MBI ($p < 0.001$), greater fatigue (difference, 0.54; $p = 0.006$), and significantly lower QOL (difference, 10.41; $p = 0.02$). Additionally, residents reporting an error were more likely to screen positive for depression at least once during the study period (odds ratio, 2.83; $p < 0.001$). Similarly, Prins et al. also found that residents with moderate or severe burnout self-reported more medical errors overall ($p < 0.001$) and more errors due to lack of time ($p < 0.001$) [13]. It has also been reported that residents who commit self-perceived medical errors are more likely to subsequently experience burnout ($p = 0.002$ for all three subscales of MBI), decreased QOL ($p = 0.02$), and screen positive for depression (odds ratio 3.29, 95% CI 1.90–5.64) [14], suggesting a cycle of burnout with perceived medical errors. The true incidence of medical errors performed by burned-out residents vs. non-burned residents is not known, as these studies rely on self-perceived and self-report medical error.

While much focus has been on the effects of burnout on patient care, there are real and considerable negative effects on the actual residents delivering that care. In August 2014, two resident physicians committed suicide in separate incidents in New York City. While suicide represents the extreme end of the spectrum, it demonstrates the seriousness of burnout in resident physicians. No study to date has specifically looked at the rate of resident physician suicide; however it is well known that physicians in general are at increased risk for suicide. A meta-analysis found male physicians have 40% higher risk of committing suicide and female physicians have 130% higher risk of committing suicide than the general population [15]. One study specifically looked at suicidal ideation in medical residents and found 12% of residents reported having suicidal thoughts and that suicidal ideation is more prevalent in burned-out residents (20.5% vs. 7.6%, $P < 0.001$) [16].

Associated with suicide is depression, which multiple studies have found higher risk for depression in residents with burnout [3, 7, 10, 11, 17]. Holmes et al. reported that of the residents who screened positive for depression (17% total), 96% of them also met criteria for burnout [7]. Another study found that residents meeting criteria for burnout were more likely to both self-report major depression during residency (315 vs. 11%, $p = 0.031$) and screen positive on a depression screening (51% vs. 29%, $p = 0.042$) [11]. While burnout and depression are associated with each other, their causal relationship is not well understood. In addition, resident burnout is associated with decreased QOL [5], career dissatisfaction [11], increased odds of motor vehicle accidents [18], and higher levels of stress and worry [17].

The graduate medical education (GME) community also has a large stake in resident burnout because patient care and resident wellness reflect upon the training and learning environment that residency programs provide. In response to concerns about patient care and resident well-being, the Accreditation Council for Graduate Medical Education (ACGME) introduced an 80-h workweek restriction, restricted overnight shift lengths, and mandated minimum time off between shifts in 2003. The ACGME then revised restrictions in 2011 to include a 16-h shift limit for interns. The intended goals were to promote patient safety and resident well-being while maintaining educational standards. Whether these goals have been achieved will be discussed later in this chapter. The ACGME Council of Review Committee Residents (CRCR), a group of 29 residents and fellows representing all ACGME-accredited specialties, convened to discuss current resident wellness resources, to envision the ideal learning environment to promote resident wellness and how to achieve it. They concluded a national policy on resident wellness should [19]:

- Increase awareness of stress of residency and destigmatize depression in trainees
- Develop systems to identify and treat depression in trainees in a confidential way to reduce barriers to accessing help
- Enhance mentoring by senior peers and faculty
- Promote a supportive culture
- Encourage additional study of problem to deepen understanding of the issue

Also relevant to graduate medical education is the discord between the actual and perceived magnitude of the problem by residency program directors. Holmes et al. found that 69% of residents were burned out; however an overwhelming majority of program directors (92%) estimated the burnout rate in their program to be 49% or less [7]. Only one program director accurately predicted a burnout rate of 50–74%. Seventy five percentage of program directors also reported challenges managing residents suffering from burnout or other mental health issues. The authors voiced concern that despite the difficulties assisting residents with burnout, program directors still underestimated its prevalence. They hypothesized that a major obstacle for program directors is the difficulty in identifying burned-out residents outside of the rare case in which a resident comes forward or when burnout is obviously impeding the resident's clinical work. Perhaps more important to program directors is identifying at-risk residents before they become burned out or clinical work is affected. This will be further explored later in this chapter.

Another concern for surgical program directors is the disproportionately high rate of attrition in general surgery residency, which is estimated to be between 14% and 23% [20]. Program directors expend valuable time and resources to recruit replacement residents, in addition to regular recruitment and management of current residents. While burnout has not been directly associated with surgical residency attrition, it is likely related considering the most common reasons for leaving are work hours and lifestyle [20–22].

Contributing Factors

Resident burnout is a real and prevalent problem; however we are just beginning to explore and understand the contributing factors to burnout, including risk factors and protective factors. A review in 2004 by Thomas et al. reviewed 15 heterogeneous articles on resident burnout and determined that the available data was insufficient to identify causal relationships and therefore do not support using demographic (age, gender, marital status, number of children) or personality characteristics to identify at-risk residents [23]. New studies have since come out; however the continued lack of large, prospective studies should be taken into account.

Why are residents burned out? Holmes et al. found that both residents and program directors agreed that lack of time for self-care, exercise, and/or engagement in enjoyable activities outside of work; conflicting responsibilities between work, home, and family; and feeling underappreciated are the greatest contributors to burnout [7]. Ishak et al. reviewed 51 studies and identified time demands, lack of control, work planning, work organization, inherently difficult job situations, and interpersonal relationships as possible contributing factors to burnout [24]. In an exploratory study in which questionnaires were sent to residents from 13 different specialties, Eckleberry et al. sought to determine which hypothesized stressors are associated with the presence or absence of burnout [25]. Of the 32 hypothesized burnout factors, 11 factors were significantly associated with at least two of the burnout scales on the MBI. These 11 factors include perfectionism, lack of stress-coping skills, personal bad habits (smoking, drug use), lack of control over office processes, lack of control over schedule, poor relationships with colleagues, lack of time for self-care, difficult and complicated patients, not enough time in the day, excessive paperwork, and regret over chosen career. Pessimism was associated with all three subscales of the MBI. Chaukos et al. reported that residents with burnout had significantly lower levels of mindfulness and coping skills [17]. The authors hypothesized that mindfulness may enhance the ability to find meaning in one's work through self-awareness and increased coping skills may protect against depersonalization and emotional exhaustion.

Eckleberry et al. also studied 29 hypothesized wellness factors and a wellness scale defined as lower emotional exhaustion, lower depersonalization, and higher personal accomplishment [25]. Thirteen wellness factors were associated with two or more wellness scales and include using meditation, relaxation, massage, or other alternatives; using alcohol or illicit drugs; using support group for physicians; talking about feelings; using professional counseling; feeling like one has a say in the training program; feeling like one has some control over one's schedule; having a plan for the future; having enough money; having a supportive work environment; feeling connected to and compassionate toward patients; having good coping skills; and being happy with child care. The authors concluded that burnout and wellness factors should be considered when designing burnout interventions with the goal to minimize factors that cause burnout and promote wellness factors that protect from burnout. Prins et al. found that highly engaged residents were less likely to self-report medical errors ($p < 0.01$) [13]. They proposed that engagement (a positive, fulfilling feeling related to one's work characterized by vigor, dedication, and absorption) may be a protective factor for burnout. Vigor describes high levels of energy and willingness to invest in work. Dedication is defined by feelings of enthusiasm, pride, and inspiration about one's job. Absorption means time passes quickly, and other things do not matter because one is so engrossed with work. Engagement is essentially the opposite of burnout, and the authors encourage keeping residents highly engaged in their work.

Managing Burnout

Given the high prevalence of burnout, why don't more residents actively seek assistance? In one study, 42% of residents reported inability to take time off work to seek treatment as the most common barrier to treatment, while 24% reported ambivalence, avoidance, and/or denial of the problem. More revealing is only 35% of residents agreed that they knew how to get help for a burned-out colleague, and 25% of residents also incorrectly believed burnout is a reportable condition to state medical board [7]. Related to the fear of burnout being a reportable condition, stigmatization also likely plays a role [19, 26–28] and is also seen in medical students and physicians.

The biggest challenge facing the graduate medical education community is how to prevent and mitigate resident burnout. It has been suggested that burnout starts in medical school with reported rates up to 55.9% [29–31] and may develop or continue into residency [3, 24]. Medical school may therefore be an opportune time to introduce wellness programs and burnout interventions.

Proposed interventions are often categorized into physician-focused interventions and organizational interventions. Physician- or individual-focused interventions include mindfulness training [32–35], stress management [36, 37], meditation and relaxation training [38], communication skills training [39], and exercise [40]. Examples of organizational or workplace interventions are workload modifications [41], mentoring [24], teamwork and group discussions [42–45], wellness programs [46], and duty-hour restrictions. Many of the proposed interventions may reduce burnout; however most of the studies are small and report inconclusive or conflicting data. In a literature review of 51 studies by Ishak et al., they concluded current data on interventions is insufficient to recommend any particular intervention [24]. Another systematic review and meta-analysis published in 2016 reviewed 15 randomized trials and 37 cohort studies and reported overall burnout decreased from 54% to 44% ($p < 0.0001$), but no specific intervention has shown to be superior to others [47]. The most recent review by Panagioti et al. of 19 randomized control trials and controlled before-after studies similarly concluded, "At present, the low quality of research evidence does not allow firm practical recommendations" [48]. However, they did find small significant reductions in burnout with the most significant improvements seen in organization-directed interventions compared to physician-directed interventions, confirming their hypothesis that burnout is an issue of the entire health-care organization.

Of the proposed interventions, the ACGME duty-hour restrictions during surgical residency have been studied the most. As discussed earlier in the chapter, the ACGME currently limits residents to an 80-h workweek (averaged over 4 weeks) and 16-h shift limit for interns. One of the first to report the effects of the 80-h workweek restriction, Gelfand et al. found that work hours significantly decreased (100.7 to 82.6, $P < 0.05$) but there was no significant change in surgical resident burnout parameters on the MBI [49]. Antiel et al. studied the first cohort of general surgery interns to train under the new 16-h shift limit restriction enacted in 2011. They reported 44% of interns felt the restrictions decreased resident fatigue; however 28% of interns demonstrated weekly symptoms of both emotional exhaustion and

28% reported depersonalization on the MBI, and one in seven residents considered giving up a surgical career [50]. Importantly, interns felt there were decreased coordination of care (53%), decreased ability to achieve patient care continuity (70%), and decreased operating room time (57%). A systematic review of 135 articles, of which 57 were considered moderate to high quality, concluded duty-hour restrictions did show benefits to resident wellness after the 2003 regulation limiting to an 80-h workweek but no consistent improvement after the 2011 restriction to 16-h shifts for interns [51]. They also found negative impacts on patient outcomes and resident performance on certification exams. More recently, the results of the FIRST trial were published in 2016 [52]. The FIRST trial was a national, non-inferiority trial comparing current, standard ACGME duty-hour policies to flexible policies that waived rules regarding shift length and time off between shifts. The 80-h workweek remained in place for both groups. The results showed no significant difference in overall well-being between the two groups (14.9% vs. 12.0%, $p = 0.10$). They also found no significant difference in the effect of fatigue on personal or patient safety. Everett et al. also found that despite the 80-h workweek limitation, general surgery residents continue to leave general surgery at an increased rate (0.6–0.8 residents/lost/program/year, $p = 0.0013$) [22]. Overall, a significant proportion of residents remain burned out despite duty-hour restrictions.

One must consider that wellness is more than the absence of burnout. There has been recent focus on resident wellness programs (RWP) as a method to not only reduce burnout but to improve the overall well-being and health of residents. An article by Lefebvre defined resident wellness programs as a "combination of active and passive initiatives targeting the various domains of physical, mental, social, and intellectual wellness" [53]. The author proposed the key components of an effective program are a safe place to express grievances; ongoing surveillance that may include mandatory meetings; educational lectures, workshops, and exercises; and physical, mental, social, intellectual, and community wellness initiatives and should include both active and passive strategies. The effectiveness of a RWP likely relies on the effectiveness of its individual components, although the additive effects of a comprehensive program are unknown. As an example, a residency program in Texas developed a Wellness Toolbox with the hope of shifting the focus from burnout to wellness. The toolbox includes screening for burnout and then providing ongoing education on achieving wellness. There are lectures to promote wellness, retreats, support groups, social events, and other activities aimed at promoting wellness. Objective data is lacking, but the authors report a perceived culture shift within the department with an increased willingness to openly discuss wellness and participate in wellness activities [54].

Conclusion

Resident burnout is a significant issue for patients, residents, and the medical education community. Despite increased interest in resident burnout, there is a lack of large, high-quality studies to identify risk factors and protective factors for burnout. This poses a significant challenge in identifying at-risk residents and developing preventative strategies. While there are a multitude of proposed burnout interventions, the current data is not sufficient to recommend a single intervention over another but provides a framework for future research. It appears that organizational-based interventions are most effective and likely reflect an entire culture shift that must occur to improve the wellness of residents and all physicians.

References

1. Maslach C, Jackson S, Leiter M. Maslach burnout inventory manual. 3rd ed. Palo Alto: Consulting Psychologists Press; 1996.
2. Rafferty JP. Validity of the Maslach Burnout Inventory for family practice physicians. J Clin Psychol. 1986;42(3):488–92.
3. Dyrbye LN. Burnout among U.S. medical students, residents, and early career physicians relative to the general U.S. population. Acad Med. 2014;89(3):443–51.
4. Shanafelt TD. Burnout and career satisfaction among American surgeons. Ann Surg. 2009;250(3):463–71.
5. Pulcrano M. Quality of life and burnout rates across surgical specialties: a systematic review. JAMA Surg. 2016;151(10):970–8.
6. Martini S. Burnout comparison among residents in different medical specialties. Acad Psychiatry. 2004;28(3):240–2.
7. Holmes EG. Taking care of our own: a multispecialty study of resident and program director perspectives on contributors to burnout and potential interventions. Acad Psychiatry. 2017;41(2):159–66.
8. Elmore LC. National survey of burnout among US general surgery residents. J Am Coll Surg. 2016;223(3):440–51.
9. Ripp J. The incidence and predictors of job burnout in first-year internal medicine residents: a five-institution study. Acad Med. 2011;86(10):1304–10.
10. Campbell J. Predictors of persistent burnout in internal medicine residents: a prospective cohort study. Acad Med. 2010;85(10):1630–4.
11. Shanafelt TD. Burnout and self-reported patient care in an internal medicine residency program. Ann Intern Med. 2002;136(5):358–67.
12. West CP. Association of resident fatigue and distress with perceived medical errors. JAMA. 2009;302(12):1294–300.
13. Prins JT. Burnout, engagement and resident physicians' self-reported errors. Psychol Health Med. 2009;14(6):654–66.
14. West CP. Association of perceived medical errors with resident distress and empathy: a prospective longitudinal study. JAMA. 2006;296(9):1071–8.
15. Schernhammer ES. Suicide rates among physicians: a quantitative and gender assessment (meta-analysis). Am J Psychiatry. 2004;161(12):2295–302.
16. van der Heijden F. Suicidal thoughts among medical residents with burnout. Arch Suicide Res. 2008;12(4):344–6.
17. Chaukos D. Risk and resilience factors associated with resident burnout. Acad Psychiatry. 2017;41(2):189–94.
18. West CP. Association of resident fatigue and distress with occupational blood and body fluid exposures and motor vehicle incidents. Mayo Clin Proc. 2012;87(12):1138–44.
19. Daskivich TJ. Promotion of wellness and mental health awareness among physicians in training: perspective of a national, multispecialty panel of residents and fellows. J Grad Med Educ. 2015;7(1):143–7.
20. Dodson TF. Why do residents leave general surgery? The hidden problem in today's programs. Curr Surg. 2005;62(1):128–31.
21. Leibrandt TJ. Has the 80-hour work week had an impact on voluntary attrition in general surgery residency programs? J Am Coll Surg. 2006;202(2):340–4.

22. Everett CB. General surgery resident attrition and the 80-hour workweek. Am J Surg. 2007;194(6):751–7.
23. Thomas NK. Resident burnout. JAMA. 2004;292(23):2880–9.
24. Ishak WW. Burnout during residency training: a literature review. J Grad Med Educ. 2009;1(2):236–42.
25. Eckleberry-Hunt J. An exploratory study of resident burnout and wellness. Acad Med. 2009;84(2):269–77.
26. Moutier C. When residents need health care: stigma of the patient role. Acad Psychiatry. 2009;33(6):431–41.
27. Adams EFM. What stops us from healing the healers: a survey of help-seeking behaviour, stigmatisation and depression within the medical profession. Int J Soc Psychiatry. 2010;56(4):359–70.
28. Dyrbye LN. The impact of stigma and personal experiences on the help-seeking behaviors of medical students with burnout. Acad Med. 2015;90(7):961–9.
29. Dyrbye LN. Healthy exercise habits are associated with lower risk of burnout and higher quality of life among U.S. medical students. Acad Med. 2017;92(7):1006–11.
30. Dyrbye LN. Burnout and suicidal ideation among U.S. medical students. Ann Intern Med. 2008;149(5):334–41.
31. Dyrbye LN. Relationship between burnout and professional conduct and attitudes among US medical students. JAMA. 2010;304(11):1173–80.
32. Williams D. Efficacy of burnout interventions in the medical education pipeline. Acad Psychiatry. 2015;39(1):47–54.
33. Goldhagen BE. Stress and burnout in residents: impact of mindfulness-based resilience training. Adv Med Educ Pract. 2015;6:525–32.
34. Krasner MS. Association of an educational program in mindful communication with burnout, empathy, and attitudes among primary care physicians. JAMA. 2009;302(12):1284–93.
35. Rosenzweig S. Mindfulness-based stress reduction lowers psychological distress in medical students. Teach Learn Med. 2003;15(2):88–92.
36. McCue JD. A stress management workshop improves residents' coping skills. Arch Intern Med (1960). 1991;151(11):2273–7.
37. Milstein JM. Burnout assessment in house officers: evaluation of an intervention to reduce stress. Med Teach. 2009;31(4):338–41.
38. Ospina-Kammerer V. An evaluation of the Respiratory One Method (ROM) in reducing emotional exhaustion among family physician residents. Int J Emerg Ment Health. 2003;5(1):29–32.
39. Bragard I. Efficacy of a communication and stress management training on medical residents' self-efficacy, stress to communicate and burnout: a randomized controlled study. J Health Psychol. 2010;15(7):1075–81.
40. Weight CJ. Physical activity, quality of life, and burnout among physician trainees: the effect of a team-based, incentivized exercise program. Mayo Clin Proc. 2013;88(12):1435–42.
41. Linzer M. A cluster randomized trial of interventions to improve work conditions and clinician burnout in primary care: results from the Healthy Work Place (HWP) study. J Gen Intern Med : JGIM. 2015;30(8):1105–11.
42. Ghetti C. Burnout, psychological skills, and empathy: balint training in obstetrics and gynecology residents. J Grad Med Educ. 2009;1(2):231–5.
43. West CP. Intervention to promote physician well-being, job satisfaction, and professionalism: a randomized clinical trial. JAMA Intern Med. 2014;174(4):527–33.
44. Ripp JA. A randomized controlled trial to decrease job burnout in first-year internal medicine residents using a facilitated discussion group intervention. J Grad Med Educ. 2016;8(2):256–9.
45. Bar-Sela G. "Balint group" meetings for oncology residents as a tool to improve therapeutic communication skills and reduce burnout level. J Cancer Educ. 2012;27(4):786–9.
46. Brennan J. Designing and implementing a resiliency program for family medicine residents. Int J Psychiatry Med. 2015;50(1):104–14.
47. West CP. Interventions to prevent and reduce physician burnout: a systematic review and meta-analysis. Lancet (British edition). 2016;388(10057):2272–81.

48. Panagioti M. Controlled interventions to reduce burnout in physicians: a systematic review and meta-analysis. JAMA Intern Med. 2017;177(2):195–205.
49. Gelfand DV. Effect of the 80-hour workweek on resident burnout. Arch Surg (Chicago 1960). 2004;139(9):933–8; discussion 8-40
50. Antiel RM. Effects of duty hour restrictions on core competencies, education, quality of life, and burnout among general surgery interns. JAMA Surg. 2013;148(5):448–55.
51. Ahmed N. A systematic review of the effects of resident duty hour restrictions in surgery: impact on resident wellness, training, and patient outcomes. Ann Surg. 2014;259(6):1041–53.
52. Bilimoria KY. National cluster-randomized trial of duty-hour flexibility in surgical training. N Engl J Med. 2016;374(8):713–27.
53. Lefebvre DC. Perspective: resident physician wellness: a new hope. Acad Med. 2012;87(5):598–602.
54. Eckleberry-Hunt JJ. Changing the conversation from burnout to wellness: physician well-being in residency training programs. J Grad Med Educ. 2009;1(2):225–30.

Preparations Beyond Residency

26

Nikhil K. Gupta, Sumeet Batra, and Tobias S. Köhler

Introduction

Surgical Education often focuses on the how to of surgical maneuvers and the acquisition of textbook knowledge. Indeed much of this textbook's previous chapters have dealt with many of these important subjects. This chapter, however, will focus on preparing the surgical trainee for their first year out of training when pushed out of the nest into the real world. First, the trainee must pick and obtain their first job. Topics considered are building a dossier, selecting potential jobs, mastering interview techniques, and negotiating a contract. Next, the chapter will detail licensing and privileging. To follow, strategies to build a successful surgical career will be discussed. Finally, the chapter will cover basics of financial planning, including housing, disability, and cash flow. Several book recommendations and resources will be provided to help address what many first year practitioners state they wish they would have known.

Starting Practice

Finding a job can be daunting for residents. This is often the first time many of them are venturing out into the unregulated Wild West, beyond the relative structure of school applications and the residency match. The rules are sparse and the norms are unclear. Following a path can clarify much of the mud that is starting practice.

N.K. Gupta, MD
Rutgers-Robert Wood Johnson Medical School, New Brunswick, NJ, USA

S. Batra, MD, MPH
Cook Children's Healthcare System, Fort Worth, TX, USA

T.S. Köhler, MD, MPH, FACS (✉)
Urology, Mayo Clinic, Rochester, MN, USA
e-mail: kohler.tobias@mayo.edu

T.S. Köhler, B. Schwartz (eds.), *Surgeons as Educators*,
https://doi.org/10.1007/978-3-319-64728-9_26

Choosing the correct first job can set you up for life and allow you to become the superstar (academic, family, earning) you aspire to be. Choosing poorly will leave you and your family miserable, even more so if you compound a bad choice with golden handcuffs from buying too much house (a very common error).

Choose Wisely: Determining the Best First Job for You

The number of practice options available to graduating fellows and residents has expanded tremendously in recent years. Choosing a practice setting that fits the graduate's needs is an incredibly important decision, as over 50% of recent graduates switch practice settings within 5 years. The best job is your perfect mix of location, job satisfaction, lifestyle, spousal (and family) happiness, and remuneration – not necessarily in this order of ranking.

1. Location, location, location

Job location brings with it several unique variables. Proximity to family, friends, and the resources they provide are a very strong consideration. Built-in babysitting from your in-laws to allow you a night out, not having to board a plane over the holidays, and established proximal emergency contacts are paramount to many. According to the NIA and Social Security Administration sponsored Health and Retirement Study (HRS: a longitudinal panel study that surveys a representative sample of approximately 20,000 people in America), the average adult American lives within 18 miles of their mother.

Location also determines weather. According to software engineer Kelly Norton, when criteria of pleasant days where mean temp is 55–75 and range is 45–85° Fahrenheit, cities in California were victorious (LA 183 and San Diego 182 days per year), and cities in Montana were clearly suboptimal (McAllister 14 and Clancy 15 days per year). Cost of living is quite different based on location too. If groceries and housing cost three times and your job only pays two times, things may not be as clear-cut on the best location. Public transportation, traffic, and proximity to airports are very important to some. Quality of life components of location also entail city crime rate, air quality, quality of schools, nightlife, quality restaurants, and access to your favorite hobbies (hiking, biking). Also remember to consider employment and volunteer opportunities for your spouse.

2. Job Satisfaction

Regardless of work-life balance, most doctors end up spending more time at work than at home. Given the realities of modern-day practice, doctors usually have to take some of their work home as well, whether to finish charts or other responsibilities. Thus, gaining satisfaction from the job is extremely important and a huge factor when choosing your first practice.

When shifting among all the opportunities that are out there, look for things that may indicate a satisfying work environment. Before starting the job search, you should consider what practice types you would thrive in. There are many different options, summarized in a section below. New graduates should consider how they would like to practice, whether they would like to operate more or remain mostly in the clinic, whether they would prefer to specialize versus remaining generalized, or whether they would like to focus more on academic pursuits with a less clinical practice. They should consider how the call schedule, how busy each call is, and the overall clinical and academic workload would affect their desired work-life balance and time spent with family. Adequate nursing and ancillary services can alleviate much of the operational burden that goes along with a clinical practice. Collegiality among colleagues helps foster a positive work environment. A strong leader who can effectively advocate for the practice and who shows an interest in your advancement and often acts as a mentor can greatly improve your professional life. Ultimately, a satisfying job is one where you practice how you want to practice, enjoy your colleagues, the administrative and operational burden is not too high, and, most importantly, you have opportunities for advancement. This is your first job and will likely not be your only job. You want to set yourself up for your next move in however many years.

3. Lifestyle and Spousal Happiness

While you may have the greatest job in the world, if your life outside of work is nonexistent or your spouse is miserable, then you will be miserable. Quality of life outside of work allows you to recharge. Constantly thinking about work is unhealthy and fosters resentment. The brain requires a variety of activity to stimulate satisfaction and creativity. Maintain hobbies, such as hiking or playing an instrument. Experience the culture in whatever town or city you live in. Meet new people, and stimulate other parts of your brain that do not deal with how to alleviate a patient complaint. On the TV show *House*, Dr. House often comes to his most brilliant deductions when he is doing something other than caring for his patient. While Dr. House is a fictional character who encounters ridiculous medical mysteries, distracting your brain improves your overall happiness and makes you a better doctor as well.

Obviously, spousal happiness should play an important role in where you start practicing. However, sometimes, an area or a spouse's job just is not what it seemed at the outset. A spouse who feels like a fish out of water or whose job or profession becomes seriously compromised because of the area where you live will put on a brave face, but the situation will put strain on you and your family. Relationships are hard enough to maintain when both parties are happy. Spousal dissatisfaction should be acknowledged, and you should work to remedy it together, even if it requires moving to a different part of the country, closer to family and friends, or where your spouse has greater professional opportunities.

4. Remuneration

Surgeons are usually at the top of the list when it comes to American occupations. This is easy to forget as we tend to compare our salaries to our more senior peers. It is important to remember the 99% of the population that earns less than you to keep things in perspective. On the other hand, you should fight for every single salary dollar and get paid what you deserve. Recall that as a surgeon, you provide essential services that may not be available without you. If this allows a hospital to become a level 1 trauma center, the hospital gain is easily offset by your gargantuan salary. Surgeons need to make an honest assessment of the value they bring. Don't forget about the ancillaries your practice creates: imaging, pathology, and referral to high-profit treatments like radiation and some chemotherapy.

Physician compensation varies a bit based on the state. In general, physicians earn more when there is more demand and a smaller supply of physicians. For this reason, physicians in the South, Upper Midwest, or the Mountain West often earn more than their counterparts on the coasts. Similarly, physicians in large urban areas tend to earn less than their counterparts in rural areas. The more specialized the physician, the greater these pay disparities may be. Other things to consider are the costs of living, licensure, malpractice, and other regulatory burdens, which may vary significantly by state. Many of these costs tend to be lower in more rural/conservative states due to legislative actions such as tort reform.

Remuneration goes beyond just salary. Recall that benefits like life insurance, disability insurance, malpractice insurance, retirement contribution match and total allowed amount, and number of vacation days are also critical. Another form of remuneration is recognition within your work and in academia. Some will happily take a little less salary for fair and consistent methods to be recognized for your clinical, teaching, and research achievements. Indeed the latter set you up for future opportunities.

Ultimately, the best location to practice is a place that best ties family, personal, and professional interests together, whether it be in a large coastal metropolis or a small Midwestern town. Figure 26.1 summarizes key points to remember when

1. Location, location, location – Proximity to friends and family, climate, quality of life, and recreational activity all contribute to finding the right place to practice.
2. Job satisfaction – The right job will allow you to flourish professionally by providing advancement opportunities, giving you the right clinical/operative balance, minimal administrative and operational burden, collegial colleagues, and a thoughtful and supportive chairman/senior partner.
3. Lifestyle – Maintaining an active lifestyle outside of work keeps you satisfied, refreshed, and makes you a better doctor
4. Spousal happiness – Maybe the most important aspect of this list, if your spouse is happy then you will be happy
5. Money, money, money, money! Money! – Being compensated for what you are worth is important, but remuneration is more than just salary. Salary should be taken in context with cost of living, benefits, vacation time, and institutional and community recognition for your work.

Fig. 26.1 Finding the right job

selecting your first job. It is important to note that your perfect job may not be available in the year you graduate. However, a mentor of mine once told me to always keep my stick on the ice (he was a Canadian plastic surgeon). This means that you always need to be prepared for when opportunities in life (the puck) come your way. Having a strong sense of what your dream opportunity truly is combined with continued hard (and smart) work in your current position eventually pays off.

Practice Type

Traditionally, solo practice was the most common route for recent graduates, though only a small fraction of recent graduates still pursue this option. This practice setting allows for the greatest autonomy when making both medical and business decisions. It also allows the physician to develop a closer relationship with his patients. However, as the name implies, a solo practitioner has to bear all the risk of developing and running the practice. Start-up costs of creating or buying an existing practice are high, as are the time demands placed on the physician. Hours are generally longer and more unpredictable, and the solo practitioner has to develop coverage options for evening and weekend hours and vacation time. As the healthcare system continues to become more integrated and complex, so will running a solo practice.

Group practices are a much more common option for recent graduates, as they offer a preestablished patient base, income, and schedule stability and the mentorship of senior physicians. Group practices may be comprised only of physicians from one specialty or multispecialty integrated groups. These groups may operate independently and serve multiple hospitals/health systems or work exclusively with a local hospital or health system. Most group practices offer a track to partnership after a few years of practice but offer less autonomy and decision- making opportunities to younger members. Single-specialty practices tend to offer a higher salary than multispecialty group practices, whereas multispecialty practices offer easier care coordination and continuity of care among physicians of various specialties.

Depending on the state, a physician may also be employed directly by a hospital or health system (including the VA system). This often offers even greater financial stability and an improved lifestyle over group practices, as well as more robust benefits and retirement options. Many hospitals are able to provide some student loan assistance or qualify for federal loan forgiveness options (see section on debt). However, long-term earning potential and autonomy may be limited compared to solo or group practice.

Other options for employment include corporate medicine or public health roles, which are usually limited to primary care specialties. These settings often require a higher focus on administrative work than on clinical care, and significant lifestyle and income stability, at the cost of lower compensation.

Physicians in all of these employment models above may choose to be involved in academics. This commitment may vary from limited teaching or precepting of medical students/residents to full-time clinical or basic science research. Physicians who are focused on academia tend to work either as employees of a university hospital/health system or an affiliated group practice. These positions often provide financial and lifestyle flexibility but offer lower starting salaries than private practice. The opportunity to teach students and residents can be considered an attraction to academia or a burden, depending on the individual's interest in teaching. Academia also allows for, and indeed expects, clinical or basic science research, with access to resources such as grant funding, laboratory space, and statisticians as well as hungry residents and medical students eager to pad their CVs. For a successful academic physician who is able to climb the ranks within a department, the financial and professional rewards may be quite substantial.

Job Search Mechanics

In the past, jobs were often found through word of mouth, especially via professional connections developed during residency and fellowship. However, it is becoming easier to find a job online due to a variety of job boards and recruiters specializing in physicians.

While physician jobs may be found on mainstream job sites such as indeed.com, many of the positions will be found on job boards for various specialty societies. Practicematch.com and practicelink.com are large job boards specifically for physician jobs of various specialties. Doximity, which functions as a LinkedIn for physicians, also frequently has job listings as well as salary surveys and other useful tools for networking.

There are a number of third-party physician staffing and recruiting companies which can be found with a simple Web search. Providing your CV to these companies is a good way to hear about a number of opportunities quickly. Recruiters must be dealt with carefully, however, as the practice will have to pay the recruitment firm a finder's fee which will likely depress the new hire's initial salary.

Applicants interested in a specific practice or institution may look at the institution's career page or try cold calling human resources or department heads to see if there is any interest in hiring a new physician.

Applicants interested in working for the Department of Veterans Affairs or military should use usajobs.gov to find the latest available positions. Oftentimes, jobs at county hospitals or public health departments are found on that entity career page or by calling human resources.

Building a Dossier

During the job application process, the first way many practices and departments meet the applicant is through the *curriculum vitae* or CV. As a thorough accounting of the applicant's productivity and important accomplishments, the practice gets a sense of what is important to the applicant and where his or her interests lie. Building an efficient, thorough, and impactful CV makes a favorable impression on the practice and makes the applicant that much more desirable.

Keeping an up-to-date CV throughout residency is extremely important. Often residents scramble to update their CVs for job applications for the first time since they entered residency. This practice creates lapses in memory, and often many important accomplishments and publications are left off of the CV. One way a mentor can push residents to keep their CVs updated is to demand to see an updated CV at least once per year. Putting their progress down on paper not only keeps their CVs updated, but it also forces them to consider the progress they have made during the year and to consider what they want to achieve in the next.

Each updated CV should not consist of just blindly adding to a list. Each time the CV is updated, residents should reflect and consider what is important to them. If teaching is important, they should show this by highlighting teaching accomplishments in prominent positions. If academic endeavors are important, then research accomplishments and publications should be highlighted. If they find their CV is lacking in whatever their interest is, the residents can then focus on improving that aspect of their portfolio.

The Interview

While this section summarizes the interview process and gives tips to improve interviewing skills, the ability to interview well is invaluable and too large a topic for one chapter. Much of the information below is adapted from *Knock 'em Dead* by Martin Yate. Mr. Yate's book provides a thorough examination of how to prepare and how to interview well and even has scripts for certain difficult situations. Though the book is not geared specifically toward doctors, the lessons are universal and easily applied to our field.

After initially screening applicants via CV, practices schedule what they consider the most important part of the process: the interview. In fact, practices expect to have multiple conversations with qualified applicants throughout the process. For simplicity, this process is structured in three interviews, with each interview accomplishing different goals and moving the process along. Applicants may have fewer than three conversations or many, many more than three conversations, but each set of interactions generally moves along the same timeline that is described below.

When interviewing for a job, residents come from an environment where they have been told that they are not good enough and how much they need to improve for 5+ years. For their entire residencies, they strive to become better under the guidance of teachers and mentors whom the residents often feel they cannot match. Also, the last time residents interviewed for positions, they were medical students interviewing with accomplished surgeons, creating a striking and intimidating power dynamic. Thus, it is quite striking for residents on job interviews when they are treated as colleagues, with equal and often superior skills to the partners of the practice. Residents must realize they are commodities, freshly trained on the most advanced technologies and attuned to the most up-to-date understanding of pathology and treatment of disease. These are skills that practices can utilize and market to grow themselves and to increase revenue. The interview is as much about the applicant screening the practice as the practice screening the applicant. Applicants should understand the power they have during the interview.

The first interview consists of a 30,000-foot overview. The practice wants to get to the applicant personally, beyond the CV. This interview is often done over the phone as a "get to know you" conversation. The practice wants to know who the applicants are, what their goals are, and how they see themselves growing both professionally and personally and what skills the applicants would add to the practice. The practice can then evaluate whether the applicant would fit whatever need the practice is trying to fill. At the same time, this is the first time the applicant can evaluate the practice. The applicant can evaluate whether the practice seems to have a stable footing in the community, whether it is committed to growing in a similar direction as the applicant's own aspirations, and whether the practice's needs fit with what the applicant provides. This is a preliminary conversation from a macro viewpoint, so applicants should feel free to take this interview even if there is a low level of interest.

The second interview is always done in person. This interview demonstrates intent from both parties and allows the practice and the applicant to get to know each other on a more personal level, often with spouses as well. The practice wants to know if the applicant fits into the culture of the practice. The applicant should also take the opportunity to speak to as many members of the practice as possible in order to get an idea of whether the practice is a good place for him or her to grow.

At a minimum, the applicant should speak to the chairman/senior partner, the younger faculty/partners, the business manager, and the person vacating the position the applicant is filling. Applicants can learn firsthand about the leadership of the practice, how the members of the practice treat each other, opportunities for advancement, and how the practice thinks it can fully utilize the applicant's skills. If possible, applicants should have at least short conversations with support staff of the practice, including secretaries, MAs, and nurses. A happy and loyal support staff is a sign of a strong practice. High turnover is a warning sign. Applicants should also try to reach out to potential colleagues in other departments or specialties in the area to discuss possible clinical or research collaboration. This will begin the groundwork for fruitful collaborations and potentially a referral base and also give a sense of the practice's reputation in its community.

The third interview consolidates expectations and can be done in person or over the phone. The practice and the applicant discuss specifics of what they can offer to each other and often begin negotiations. Each party tries to set expectations, and as long as they are close enough, a term sheet will then result as the first salvo in the negotiation process. It is important that the applicant be honest and not lead on a practice in this, but the applicant should be ready to walk away if the practice cannot provide a suitable situation.

Applicants should be well prepared for the interview process with clear goals in mind. They should also be wary of signs of instability in a practice such as high faculty/partner/associate turnover rate, financial instability, disproportionately few women or minorities in key positions, or barriers to speaking with key staff during the interview process. Not every interview ends in a job offer. If applicants can confidently and succinctly convey their visions for their professional growth, then the applicants can consider the interview process a success.

Contract Negotiation

"In business as in life, you don't get what you deserve, you get what you negotiate" – Chester Karrass.

Negotiating contracts is often daunting for residents. Thus far they have been given a residency contract and told to sign without any discussion. Graduating residents feel pressure to simultaneously ensure they get their payday, to not leave anything on the table, and to set the foundations for a fruitful career. It is difficult to wield leverage without practice, especially when dealing with a practice that has extensive experience hiring doctors and negotiating contracts. Residents must remember that EVERYTHING is negotiable and that EVERYTHING should be in the contract. If something is not in the contract, it cannot be counted on despite verbal promises. Graduating residents have more power than they think, as practices are often desperate to fill vacancies to maintain their patient base and generate revenue. The result of the negotiation is a function of how well the resident leverages his or her position.

Residents usually see a high first year salary as the ultimate goal of a negotiation. However, first year salary is the least important part of the overall financial negotiation. More important is the payment structure. Residents should understand how they get paid more than how much they get paid. The most common pay structures are either a straight salary, regardless of production, or a low base salary with production bonuses. Production bonuses are attractive as there is no theoretical ceiling on how much can be made, but residents should keep in mind that in the first 1–2 years, they will be building their practice and thus will likely not be all that productive. Many practices offer a competitive salary, sometimes with very modest production bonuses, for the first few years to allow newly graduated surgeons to find their footing. The practice will usually lose money on their new hires for the first 2 years as the production is not in line with their salary. However, practices will often look to recoup that loss once new hires become busier with more modest salary increases than the expected increases in production in years 2–3. When negotiating salary, graduating residents should consider the entire pay structure multiple years down the line so that they are compensated fairly for their work.

Advancement pathways should be clear in the contract. Expected promotion pathways should be clear for academic practices and a clear path to partnership with any necessary buy-ins laid out in the contract for private practices. Some private practices try to take advantage of new graduates, hiring associates with promises of partnership, but when it comes to time for partnership, the associate is let go and the partnership never comes. When negotiating the contract, one should also consider how the profits are shared among the partners, whether all partners share profits equally or if the partners "eat what they kill," i.e., the partners make what they produce. Different practices may prefer different methods, as sometimes older partners slow down and do not feel it fair to take a larger proportion of income than they deserve. The profit sharing should be considered in the context of the practice and what the graduating resident thinks he or she wants in the practice.

Most benefits can be negotiated up or down, depending on the generosity of the pay structure. Generally, essential benefits such as health insurance, malpractice insurance, and retirement benefits are standardized. However, benefits such as vacation time; paid time off; sick leave; parking spot; access to a secretary, nurse, or MA; and the ability to hire a nurse practitioner or physicians' assistant can be negotiated up or down. Practices will often help with continuing medical education endeavors to maintain board certification and attending national society meetings as this helps raise the profile of the practice. The best time for the resident to ask for new equipment necessary for practice is during this period, as the practice is most willing to listen during this negotiation period and would like to get the new hire started as quickly and smoothly as possible. New hires should be mindful of their position during the contract negotiation. While they have significant leverage, overextending during the initial negotiation can foster resentment among the established surgeons in the practice and lead to a toxic work environment. New hires should push for what they want but keep expectations in line with what is reasonable. They are the low men and women on the totem pole and will have to work to earn what they deserve.

When finalizing the contract, it is extremely important for the potential new hire to thoroughly read the contract and to have a lawyer go over the contract as well. A lawyer specializing in doctor's contracts is a modest expense considering how much the lawyer can save the new hire by finding unfavorable clauses or identifying areas that can be used as negotiation leverage. Often a practice offering a high first year salary includes a clause that the new hire will have to pay back whatever portion of that salary is not earned through clinical work. A lawyer can advise on a reasonable, region-specific restrictive covenant. Generally a lawyer can advise on what is reasonable, favorable, and unfavorable in a contract, giving the new hire leverage in the negotiation and protecting the new hire from unfavorable situations.

To understand how to wield leverage and negotiate effectively, Herb Cohen's book *You Can Negotiate Anything* details how to use power, time, and information to tilt the negotiation in your favor.

Licensing and Credentialing

Licensing

If the resident is certain he or she will pursue a job in a specific state, it behooves them to apply for full state licensure as soon as possible. Many jobs will favor candidates who are already licensed, and the process of obtaining a license from start to finish can take up to 6–8 months in some states, most notoriously Texas and California. Requirements vary somewhat by state, but most state medical boards will require primary source verification of the following documents:

1. Diplomas from college/medical school/intern/residency

   Residents should save an original and digital copy of all diplomas received at the end of school and training programs, as many boards will require these as proof of completion.

2. College/medical school transcripts

   Residents should also save the contact information for their undergraduate and medical school registrars, so they can procure a primary source copy of all transcripts.
3. Contact information for medical school, internship, residency – forms for good standing

   Residents should maintain the email address and phone numbers of their residency coordinators and program directors, as this information will be required to procure letters of good standing. If a graduating resident has any gaps or changes in training programs, these letters will be essential to obtaining licensure.
4. Past malpractice information

   Licensing boards will want a detailed history of any malpractice claims against the resident, as well as the outcomes of such claims. Other adverse events such as disciplinary action by a training program will have to be explained as well.

FCVS or the Federation Credentials Verification Service is a program developed by the Federation of State Medical Boards. This program allows applicants to create a permanent repository of all primary source documents needed by state licensing boards and hospital credentialing services. There is a one-time fee involved in creating the initial portfolio, as well as a smaller fee paid each time an applicant sends his or her profile to a state or institution. This can be very helpful for residents who may be applying to jobs in a number of states or who may change jobs frequently. The FSMB also provides a uniform application for state licensure that many states accept in lieu of a state-specific application, similar to a uniform application for college. A list of states which accept the uniform application is found here: http://www.fsmb.org/licensure/uniform-application/participating-boards.

After obtaining a state medical license, a license to dispense controlled substances must also be obtained from the state medical board, which often includes a nominal fee. Information for this can be found on each individual state medical board's website. Then a DEA number can be obtained to prescribe controlled substances and medications. The application can be found at https://apps.deadiversion.usdoj.gov/webforms/jsp/regapps/common/newAppLogin.jsp.

Privileges and Credentialing

The process of obtaining hospital and operative privileges and insurance credentialing can be as arduous and time-consuming as obtaining a state medical license. Hospital and insurance plan credentialing requires many of the same documents as state licensure, as well as other information necessary to bill insurance providers. The National Provider Identifier (NPI) is a 10-digit ID number assigned to all providers who bill CMS, i.e., Medicare. Many private insurers use this number as well. Residents who have not done so already should apply for this number at https://nppes.cms.hhs.gov/#/. The Council for Affordable Quality Healthcare (CAQH) is a private, nonprofit organization that helps compile data on providers for the purposes of credentialing, directory maintenance, sanctions tracking, and electronic billing.

Residents should ask their prospective practice for details on how to enroll or visit https://proview.caqh.org/Login/Index?ReturnUrl=%2fPR for more information.

In order to obtain operative privileges, residents must submit a case log detailing procedures performed during a portion of or all of residency. The ACGME case log entry should be able to run a report sufficient for this requirement. However, residents should ensure that certain annotations are made clear, such as whether a case was performed laparoscopically or robotically.

Residents will be asked to discuss their malpractice history, if any, and the outcomes of any suits against them. Residents may be asked to perform a self-query on the National Provider Data Bank to show all cases the resident was named in. The NPDB can be found at https://www.npdb.hrsa.gov/ext/selfquery/SQHome.jsp. Graduating residents may also be asked for proof of malpractice coverage during training, with evidence of tail coverage for events occurring during training.

As part of credentialing, many hospitals will require a physician to provide a history of all immunizations, including childhood vaccinations. If proof of vaccination is not submitted, titers may be drawn for proof of immunity for MMR and varicella. Other vaccinations that will be assessed include hepatitis B and influenza. If proof of vaccination for these (or even MMRV) is not provided, many institutions will opt to revaccinate. Residents may save themselves time and frustration by obtaining these records before starting their new job.

Most institutions will also perform a two-step TB test or Quantiferon Gold/T--SPOT to assess for the presence of latent TB. Residents with a history of positive TB tests can eliminate the hassle of further testing if they can provide a recent negative chest X-ray and proof of prophylactic treatment for latent TB. Residents with a history of BCG vaccination may want to request a T-SPOT or Quantiferon Gold test to reduce the likelihood of a false positive.

Building a Career

Graduating from residency is only the beginning. When starting practice, it is important for young surgeons to remain goal oriented in order to build a career. As Yogi Berra said, "If you don't know where you're going, you might not get there."

Setting Goals

Where do you see yourself in 5, 10, 15, etc., years? What do you want your obituary to say about you? What is your definition of a successful practice? Obviously there are no right answers here. Some surgeons seek to build a high volume and strive toward technical excellence – do you want to be recognized as one of the best surgeons in your field? Some surgeons spend as much of their free time as possible doing volunteer work and surgery in third world countries – is this for you? Others want to make a significant contribution to the field through research – what questions do you want to attempt to answer? How does your family fit in?

How many friends will attend your funeral? What will your students and residents say about you? How many future patient operations will you have influenced (positively or negatively) based on your teaching of surgical learners? These questions are an exercise in your values and goals. Only you can figure them out. Picking mentors you would like to emulate as both role models and sounding boards can certainly help.

Make Yourself Indispensable, Not a Headache

Ask any chairperson or leader what is the hardest part of their job, and the vast majority will say it's dealing with personnel issues: people being unprofessional, hostile, and generally disagreeable. Don't be this person! It is clear that people most often get sued based on their personality and how they react to complications and not complications themselves. The irony is that your kindergarten teacher probably taught you all of the skills you need to thrive: be nice, compromise, and treat others as they would have them treat you. Conflict will invariably happen – but how will YOU handle it? Will you throw surgical instruments, curse, and chastise? A previous mentor of mine taught me to go to the balcony in stressful situations, that is, float outside your body and look down at the situation as an objective observer. Only the best surgeons never get rattled, remain calm, and have unyielding equanimity. DO NOT send that email (it will feel good for 5 s and then perhaps haunt you for the rest of your career) – sit on it for at least 24 h. If you have a conflict, set an appointment to talk about it at least 3 days later after it happened – ruminate on it.

So you won't be a headache, how can you make yourself indispensable? Being indispensable gives you job security and leverage to negotiate. What special skills or passions do you have that you can utilize? Will you become the go to mentor to the residents, elite researcher, and volunteer work organizer? Remember that the average work employee is thanked for what they do once per year – you can clearly do better. Be kind to your employees and office staff. Give something extra over the holidays. Remember that good employees are extremely hard to find. Fight for and earn their loyalty by making sure they feel valued, heard, and appreciated. Also, recall that it can be quite lonely at the top – who tells the chair they are doing a good job? If you think you have a great leader, let them know every once in a while too. There are several excellent leadership books (not to mention an excellent chapter on leadership elsewhere in this book) out there which will give you insight into your boss and yourself too (remember you will be leading OR teams, clinic staff, etc.) *Good to Great* by Jim Collins is my favorite – will you someday become a level 5 leader?

Optimizing initial outcomes – "You never get a second chance to make a first impression" – Oscar Wilde.

You finished your long residency and bonus fellowship and are finally ready for the real world. Your first patient walks in the door; he exposes his abdomen which reveals multiple surgical scars and states he has had several complications from the last time he was operated upon – what do you do? If you are like most surgeons, you love to operate. Combine this with the initial independence and the invariable slow start-up to any practice and you may get overeager. As we start out, our pre-patient counseling tends to minimize the complications and our lack of surgical experience and push for surgery. Do not make this mistake!!! Your first 3–6 months of surgery should be chip shots. Establish your reputation as a conscientious, meticulous surgeon with excellent outcomes. If the proverbial train-wreck walks into your clinic, either refer or arrange to do the case with the most senior partner with the best reputation, and if something goes wrong when operating with him/her, it was bad luck. If something goes wrong operating by yourself, it will be perceived as your fault because you are a bad surgeon. In counseling patients, it is always better to underpromise and overdeliver. If a patient chooses not to go with you as their surgeon because you were too thorough with your description of complications, that is great – this is a patient with unrealistic expectations who might have sued. Patient selection is key when starting out – look for warning signs from patients. If an office staff tells you the patient might be a problem, listen to them. I highly recommend reading the CURSED patient by Dr. Landon Trost; it reviews the warning signs of patients that are high risk for litigation. Remember to utilize your mentors as much as possible. If you have a tough case, call and plan with your mentor ahead of time. If you get in trouble in the OR, call them, call your partner, and call another consultant in – load the boat. Medicolegally the word of two collaborating MDs that reach a shared decision is much stronger than a first year surgeon's opinion. Avoid hubris; get the help the patient needs. Finally, when first filling out your OR scheduling sheets, allot more time than you need for the case. We have a tendency to do the opposite and list the time it took to do that fastest case that day when the stars aligned. If anesthesia and the circulator are expecting a 1 ½ h case and you finish it an hour, you are perceived as a fast surgeon; however, if you list 30 min and take an hour, all of sudden you are a slow surgeon. Building a referral base takes time and requires you to change referring MD habits. Be patient. Do a good job at correspondence and be available. Giving talks introducing your practice over lunch or dinner is a good approach to get your name out there. Some surgeons choose to partner with industry as they do a better job of ensuring attendance and cover the expenses.

Becoming an expert in documentation and coding and billing also puts you one step ahead of the game when starting out. Ample literature shows the majority of residents feel unprepared for real world when it comes to coding and billing. Most residents learn coding and billing from their mentors who unfortunately often do not bill properly either. As Medicare estimates primary care physicians underbill by 45%, surgeons likely underbill even more given the common false assumption that the operating theater is the only true revenue earner. Proper documentation leads to increased revenue, more concise notes, and decreased medical legal risk. An entire chapter is dedicated to this crucial topic elsewhere in this book.

Cultivating Your Academic Reputation

If you are in academics, letter of recommendation and establishing a national reputation are key to promotion to both associate and full professors. Those interested in academics need to make a concerted effort to try to attend every local and regional meeting and submit at least one abstract in your area of expertise. The fellow attendees to these meetings will be a strong referral base. At the meetings, make an effort to get to the microphone and ask intelligent questions. Introduce yourself and your institution, and remember to remain cordial and professional. Become a reviewer for the major journals in your field and do a good job (do them on time and make an adequate effort). Eventually, you will be asked to review, present, or moderate at national meetings. Do a great job, and you will likely be asked back. Everyone in academics is busy, so if someone asks you to do something like serve on a committee or write a book chapter, think carefully about whether or not you accept the invite. It is much better to politely decline (and ask them to ask you again next time) than accept and be late or do a poor job. One cannot stress enough the importance of saying no to book chapters, committee positions, grant review, or other tasks that you can't do well in a timely fashion. Of course, skip tasks that have little to no perceived value.

Maintaining Life Balance

Burnout rates for surgeons are about 40%. Another chapter in this book discusses this important topic entirely. Remember to keep things in perspective. Reassess your values. How much income do you really need to be happy? How many of your children's recitals or birthdays are you missing? Figure out what is really bothering you at work (the pebble in your shoe), and make a plan to address it. Camaraderie at work is often the greatest aegis to burnout. Remember to maintain healthy habits for well-being – this includes diet, exercise, laughter, gratitude, forgiveness, meditation, and sleep.

Financial Planning

A major key to professional success is financial stability. Surgeons come out of residency with huge debt burdens, unable to significantly dent this debt with their modest resident salaries. At the beginning of their careers, young surgeons should "live like a resident" for 3 years. By limiting costs early on, young surgeons can work to rid themselves of debt and to start building wealth.

Housing

Finding a home is affected by many factors for the young surgeon, including proximity to the office and hospital, family factors, and access to necessities and recreational activities.

Recent graduates should rent a home for a few years before buying. Many young surgeons want to start laying foundations in the community after finding their first job by buying a home. However, it is important to resist the urge to buy for a number of practical reasons. Financially, taking on the burden of a mortgage is difficult with the student debt young surgeons have accumulated and still have to pay back. Also, unless they have saved carefully, recent graduates cannot afford a large down payment and closing costs associated with buying a home, increasing the size of the mortgage loan and the debt burden and increasing the interest rate. Renting for some time also allows the recent graduate to become more familiar with an area and understand which neighborhoods are desirable and which areas have better schools. By waiting, a young surgeon will be able to make a better educated decision. Finally, and most importantly, there is no guarantee that the young surgeon will stay at his new position. In some surgical specialties, 50% of new graduates change jobs within 3 years. Buying a home potentially locks the young surgeon into a bad situation and limits flexibility at a time when flexibility is absolutely necessary. New graduates should carefully consider their options and strongly consider renting before plunging into buying a home.

Disability

Life insurance can provide financial assurance for dependents in the event of unexpected death. Many graduating residents may want to purchase life insurance due to the fact that their salaries are about to increase substantially. It is advised that they do this as early as possible, while most are still young and healthy in order to reduce premiums. There are a number of life insurance options available, which vary in cost and benefits. The simplest option is term life insurance, which lasts for a specific length of time or term. These plans are usually cheaper and only provide a payout in case of death. Premiums are generally fixed over the course of the plan. Another option is whole life insurance, which lasts for the insured's lifetime. These plans are somewhat more expensive, but they also include a cash-value component of the plan that will accrue over time at a steady rate, often with a minimum rate of return. This value grows tax deferred and may be withdrawn at any time. Universal life insurance plans are similar, with the exception that the insured may control how much money goes toward the death benefit and how much goes toward the cash value. Variable life insurance is similar to universal life insurance, except that the insured has the option of investing the cash value of the plan into equities, similar to other retirement plan. While this is riskier, most plans have a set guaranteed amount for the death benefit, which is the minimum payout agreed upon at the time the policy is created. Most residents obtain these policies through a financial advisor who will tailor a strategy that hopefully makes sense financially.

Many organizations, including the AMA, recommend that physicians purchase disability insurance. Though statistics vary widely, it has been shown in the past that doctors are more likely than other white-collar professionals to become disabled and to file claims with their disability insurance. It is ideal for a graduating resident to get disability insurance as soon as possible, because rates are lower the younger and healthier you are. Disability insurance can be obtained from a number of places, including specialty societies, employers, and even from private insurers affiliated with a training program. There are a few things residents should know when purchasing a disability policy.

1. Benefit period and elimination period

   Residents who purchase a policy through a private insurance broker or through a specialty society may be able to negotiate the maximum benefit period and/or elimination period on their policies. The maximum benefit period is the length of time that a policyholder would be eligible for benefits, which is commonly until age 65 or age 67, at which point retirement benefits may kick in to supplant the income from a disability policy. The elimination period is the length of time a policyholder must be disabled until they are eligible to start receiving benefits, which is most commonly 90 or 180 days.
2. Own occupation

   It is highly recommended that residents choose a policy that reflects their "own occupation" and not "any occupation." Own occupation policies are not only specific to physicians but to the physician's specialty. These policies are recommended for all physicians but especially those in procedural or vision intensive specialties, who, if they became disabled, would otherwise be compensated at a level for any occupation they're qualified to perform instead of their specific specialty. Thus for surgeons, "own occupation" disability insurance would cover the loss productivity from disability that would prevent a surgeon from operating but still allow a surgeon to function as a clinical physician.
3. Partial benefit

   Partial benefit plans allow for the payment of benefits in the case of partial disability. For instance, a surgeon who is disabled from performing certain procedures but can still see patients in clinic may be eligible for partial benefits from the loss of income.
4. Mental/nervous disorder exclusion

   Many plans either provide limited or no benefits for mental health/nervous disorders. This can be negotiated at the time of contract, though plans that cover mental health may be significantly more expensive.
5. Portability

   Short- and long-term insurance plans offered by an employer are often affordable and come without the hassles of medical underwriting. However, these plans are usually non-portable, so that once a physician leaves his or her job, the insurance coverage will cease. Private plans are generally portable so that coverage is maintained no matter what the work setting.
6. Taxability

   Plans that are paid for out of posttax income, such as plans purchased through a private broker or a specialty society, will have nontaxable benefits, meaning the benefit paid is not subject to tax. Plans with premiums that are paid pretax, such as employer-subsidized plans, pay benefits that are subject to tax.

Debt

Many residents have student loans from their time as undergraduates or medical students and have already been making payments for years before graduating. However, some residents put their loans into forbearance during training due to the financial stress of managing payments while making a relatively meager resident salary. This comes with obvious costs, such as racking up interest. Fortunately, beginning around 2007, a number of new loan forgiveness plans tethered to income were developed which made paying loans much easier. These plans have various terms and conditions that may affect a graduating resident's choice of job and tax-filing status.

Income-based repayment (IBR) was the first federal loan repayment plan offered to graduates with a significant amount of debt. These borrowers must qualify for partial financial hardship (significant debt to income ratio) in order to qualify for this plan. Graduates were required to have Federal Direct Loans or Federal Family Education Loans (FFEL) or to consolidate their loans into a federal program. At the time it was introduced in 2007, borrowers were expected to pay 15% of their discretionary income after a 6-month grace period for up to 25 years. After 25 years, the remainder of the loans would be forgiven, though this amount would be taxable. This program also included a 3-year interest subsidy, where unpaid interest would be covered. This plan was later modified to allow new borrowers after July 1, 2014, to pay just 10% of their discretionary income. Interest rates on these loans were set at 6.8%. For the sake of determining discretionary income, married borrowers who file jointly with their spouses would have to count the total household income, not their individual income. These payments were capped at the standard 10-year repayment plan amount that is determined at the beginning of the repayment period. Therefore, when an individual's income rises substantially, they would not pay more per month than that initial 10-year repayment amount.

Pay As You Earn (PAYE) is a more generous program that was introduced a few years after IBR. It applied to new borrowers after October 1, 2007, who also had a loan disbursement after October 1, 2011. This program capped monthly repayment at 10% of discretionary income and provided forgiveness after 20 years of repayment, though this forgiveness was still taxable. The other details of the plan are similar to IBR.

REPAYE or revised Pay As You Earn was introduced to cover the borrowers who initially were ineligible for PAYE due to having older loans. This program continues to require payment of 10% of discretionary income, as well as taxable forgiveness after 20 years; however, there are some important differences from IBR and PAYE. There is no longer a need for partial financial hardship, but there is also no payment cap. Therefore, if a borrower's income rose substantially, 10% of their income may exceed what would have been required as the 10-year standard repayment in other plans. This plan also counts spousal income regardless of how taxes are filed, likely raising the amount that needs to be paid monthly. Forgiveness is granted after 20 years for undergraduate loans and 25 years for graduate loans.

PSLF or Public Service Loan Forgiveness is an important program that is designed to provide even further loan forgiveness for people who work for the government, 501c3-eligible, nonprofits, or certain employers with public service missions. This program would allow borrowers to have tax-free loan forgiveness after 10 years of repayment under the IBR, PAYE, and REPAYE plans, as well as other federal loan programs. Importantly for physicians, many residency programs and even post-residency employed positions qualify for this repayment plan. Physicians who are employed by nonprofit hospitals, government/academic hospitals, public health entities, the VA, and the armed forces all qualify. Unfortunately, many politicians have targeted this program for being too generous to high earners, and there are doubts whether it will exist for new borrowers after 2018. More information can be found at https://studentaid.ed.gov/sa/repay-loans/understand/plans/income-driven or at student loan blogs such as https://studentloanhero.com/featured/ultimate-student-loan-repayment-guide-for-doctors.

Many physicians are eligible for some loan forgiveness through work in a medically underserved community such as rural, inner city or Native American reservation. Other options that can be explored include military service, which applies to active-duty military and military reservists for all the major armed forces, the National Guard, and the US Public Health Service. Many of these forgiveness options stipulate an upfront commitment that varies in the number of years.

For borrowers who either do not qualify for federal loans or would like to pay their loans down more quickly, a good option may be refinancing with a private lender. This generally allows borrowers to set more favorable loan repayment terms, at a much lower interest rate than paying back the federal government. Downsides to this include forgoing the opportunity to earn loan forgiveness and taking on a much higher monthly payment upfront. This may be worth it for borrowers who will earn high salaries and work in private settings and see no need to pursue programs like PSLF.

Building Wealth

After enduring college, medical school, and residency, surgeons finish training significantly behind their peers in other occupations in investment, saving, and retirement planning. Lack of formal education and experience, relatively low income through residency, huge debt burden, and extreme time constraints prevent residents from actively managing their money or seeking advice to do so.

Tax shelters can save money for future use while decreasing taxable income and thus tax burden. The most common instruments available to residents and young surgeons are retirement accounts. 401k and 403b accounts allow money to be saved and invested pretax with tax only being paid at the time of retirement. 401k accounts are offered by corporations, while 403b accounts are offered by nonprofit organizations like hospitals and schools. A Roth IRA account is another type of retirement saving account that saves and invests post-tax income so that no tax penalty is levied upon retirement. A healthcare savings account uses pretax income to pay for health-related bills for things such as prescription drugs and co-pays. These accounts are instruments that can reduce tax burden and help save for important expenditures like healthcare and retirement.

There are different investment vehicles available, from basic stocks and bonds on through. However most residents and surgeons do not have the time or the knowledge or experience to properly invest their money. Mutual funds collect people's money and invest it along a predetermined theme, whether in certain types of companies or certain companies. These funds all have an "expense ratio," which is the maintenance cost of these funds. The lower the expense ratio, the more of the money that gets invested as opposed to being used for operational costs. Highly managed funds that conduct a lot of trading have higher expense ratios, whereas less active funds have lower expense ratios. Index funds, a type of mutual fund, tend to have the lowest expense ratio as they are designed to merely mirror a certain stock market index such as the S&P 500 in scope and performance. Generally, index funds have outperformed most actively managed mutual funds in the long term and, with very low expense ratios, have the lowest overall cost. Before investing, it is important to understand what the short- and long-term goals of that investment are and tailor the type of investment to those goals.

Money managing and investment are a huge, often nebulous topic that cannot be completely summarized here. Residents should be encouraged to seek advice, whether from sources like the book *The White Coat Investor* (the author also runs a website, whitecoatinvestor.com) or a financial advisor. A financial advisor can aid with loan management, purchasing life insurance and disability insurance, and managing investments. However, not all financial advisors act in the best interest of their clients. Many advisors are paid according to what financial instruments they sell their clients. When looking for an advisor, it is best to find a fiduciary. A fiduciary is a financial advisor who is legally and ethically bound to act in the best interest of the client. Whatever advice residents get from whatever source, they should maintain understanding and control of their money. In giving several talks on this topic, I routinely ask what have I left out. A common answer is divorce – nothing separates you from 50% of your assets faster.

Preparing residents for life after residency is difficult, as many of these "life skills" come only with experience. Residents should be encouraged to seek out resources to gain and improve these life skills. Proper mentorship and guidance can aid a resident in developing a solid foundation right from the beginning for a personally and professionally prosperous career.

Conclusions

This chapter has focused on the important aspects of residents obtaining their first job, growing their careers, and ensuring financial stability. Figure 26.2 summarizes the key take-home points of the chapter which often overlap with the most commonly mentioned things young faculty state "I wish I had have known" before I started. An effective mentor ensures their trainees do not have to learn these lessons the hard way.

1. Picking a practice – The paramount choice combining the ideal blend of location, job satisfaction, spousal satisfaction, location, and remuneration. Residents must determine what is most important to them.
2. Dossier building – A dossier is built with a specific goal in mind and with frequent updates, not all at once.
3. Interviewing Skills – An applicant has as much power in an interview as the practice that is interviewing candidates.
4. You don't get what you deserve, you get what you negotiate – New hires have significant leverage in contract negotiation and everything is negotiable.
5. Finalizing the contract – Get everything in writing and have a lawyer review it
6. Licensing, credentialing, and obtaining Privileges is an arduous process – don't procrastinate or you'll be left in the dust.
7. Establish your goals – Progressive advancement can be accomplished with forethought and strategy.
8. Make yourself indispensable, not a headache – Be reliable and competent
9. Cultivate your research and academic reputation – Networking and collaboration spread the word of your greatness.
10. You never get a second chance to make a first impression – Be nice. You never know whose help you need or who you work with next.
11. Set yourself up for success in the operating room and clinic – Know your limits, be thorough, and collaborate.
12. Just say no – Be reliable, don't bite off more than you can chew.
13. Become a master biller – It's how you get paid, and it's not as mysterious as you think it is.
14. Live like a resident for 3 years after becoming an attending – Delayed gratification: responsible budgeting helps wipe out debt and build wealth.
15. Protect yourself and your family with disability and life insurance – When you need it, it is too late to get it.
16. No one cares about your money more than you–Invest wisely by minimizing fees and obtaining a fiduciary
17. Maintain balance – Work-life balance can be balanced however you want to. Be aware of what combination makes you happiest and strive to accomplish that goal

Fig. 26.2 Take-home points for preparation beyond residency

References

1. National Institute on Aging. Growing older in america: the health and retirement study. https://www.nia.nih.gov/health/publication/growing-older-america-health-and-retirement-study.
2. Yate M. Knock 'em Dead 2017: the ultimate job search guide. 2017th ed: Adams Media; 2016.
3. Cohen H. You can negotiate anything: the world's best negotiator tells you how to get what you want: Bantam.
4. Federation Credentials Verification Service (FCVS) – https://www.fsmb.org/licensure/fcvs.

5. Federation of State Medical Boards (FSMB) uniform application for state licensure – http://www.fsmb.org/licensure/uniform-application/participating-boards.
6. Application for DEA Number – https://apps.deadiversion.usdoj.gov/webforms/sp/regapps/common/newAppLogin.jsp.
7. National Provider Identifier (NPI) – https://nppes.cms.hhs.gov/#/.
8. Council for Affordable Quality Healthcare (CAQH) – https://proview.caqh.org/.
9. National Provider Data Bank (NPDB) – https://www.npdb.hrsa.gov/ext/selfquery/SQHome.jsp.
10. Collins J. Good to great: why some companies make the leap and others don't. 1st ed: Harper Business; 2001.
11. Trost LW, Baum N, Hellstrom WJ. Managing the difficult penile prosthesis patient. J Sex Med. 2013;10:893–906.
12. Student Loans Resources – https://studentaid.ed.gov/sa/repay-loans/understand/plans/income-driven.
13. https://studentloanhero.com/featured/ultimate-student-loan-repayment-guide-for-doctors/.
14. Dahle JM. The white coat investor: a Doctor's guide to personal finance and investing. 1st ed: The white coat investor LLC; 2014. https://www.whitecoatinvestor.com.

Index

T.S. Köhler, B. Schwartz (eds.), *Surgeons as Educators*,
https://doi.org/10.1007/978-3-319-64728-9

Printed by Printforce, the Netherlands